HEALTH AND ARCHITECTURE

HEALTH AND ARCHITECTURE

THE HISTORY OF SPACES OF HEALING AND CARE IN THE PRE-MODERN ERA

Edited by
Mohammad Gharipour

BLOOMSBURY VISUAL ARTS
LONDON • NEW YORK • OXFORD • NEW DELHI • SYDNEY

BLOOMSBURY VISUAL ARTS
Bloomsbury Publishing Plc
50 Bedford Square, London, WC1B 3DP, UK
1385 Broadway, New York, NY 10018, USA
29 Earlsfort Terrace, Dublin 2, Ireland

BLOOMSBURY, BLOOMSBURY VISUAL ARTS and the Diana logo
are trademarks of Bloomsbury Publishing Plc

First published in Great Britain 2021
Paperback edition first published 2023

Selection and editorial matter copyright © Mohammad Gharipour, 2021
Individual chapters copyright © their authors, 2021

Mohammad Gharipour has asserted his right under the Copyright, Designs
and Patents Act, 1988, to be identified as Editor of this work.

For legal purposes the Acknowledgments on p. xxiii constitute
an extension of this copyright page.

Cover design by Namkwan Cho
Cover image: Anonymous, Hospital Real de Todos-os-Santos (View of Rossio). Courtesy of
Álvaro Roquette and Pedro Aguiar Branco, Antiquary. Photo by Onshot / Rui Carvalho.

All rights reserved. No part of this publication may be reproduced or transmitted in any form or by
any means, electronic or mechanical, including photocopying, recording, or any information
storage or retrieval system, without prior permission in writing from the publishers.

Bloomsbury Publishing Plc does not have any control over, or responsibility for, any third-party
websites referred to or in this book. All internet addresses given in this book were correct at the
time of going to press. The author and publisher regret any inconvenience caused if addresses
have changed or sites have ceased to exist, but can accept no responsibility for any such changes.

A catalogue record for this book is available from the British Library.

Library of Congress Cataloging-in-Publication Data
Names: Gharipour, Mohammad, editor.
Title: Health and architecture : the history of spaces of healing and care
in the pre-modern era / [edited by] Mohammad Gharipour.
Identifiers: LCCN 2020046858 (print) | LCCN 2020046859 (ebook) |
ISBN 9781350217379 (hardback) | ISBN 9781350217416 (paperback) |
ISBN 9781350217386 (pdf) | ISBN 9781350217393 (epub) | ISBN 9781350217409
Subjects: LCSH: Architecture–Health aspects. | Health facilities–Design and construction. |
Hospital buildings–Design and construction. | Architecture–Psychological aspects.
Classification: LCC RA967 .H36 2021 (print) | LCC RA967 (ebook) | DDC 725/.52–dc23
LC record available at https://lccn.loc.gov/2020046858
LC ebook record available at https://lccn.loc.gov/2020046859

ISBN:	HB:	978-1-3502-1737-9
	PB:	978-1-3502-1741-6
	ePDF:	978-1-3502-1738-6
	eBook:	978-1-3502-1739-3

Typeset by Integra Software Services Pvt. Ltd.

To find out more about our authors and books visit www.bloomsbury.com
and sign up for our newsletters.

To my brilliant wife, Nooshin;
for her encouragement, inspiration, and support

CONTENTS

List of Illustrations ... ix
Notes on Contributors ... xiv
Preface ... xviii
Acknowledgments ... xxiii

1 Places of Care and Healing: Context, Design, and Development in History
   Mohammad Gharipour ... 1

Part I Religiosity: Healthcare in Religious Context

2 The Hospital Design in History: The Dichotomy of Religious and Secular Contexts
   Guenter B. Risse ... 25

3 A Plan for the King and the Sick: Portuguese Hospital Architecture during the Age of Exploration
   Danielle Abdon ... 35

4 Healing of the Poor: The Hospital of Our Lady of Potterie in Bruges and the Miracle Book (*c.* 1520–1)
   Miyako Sugiyama ... 56

5 "The Love of Friends Made This in the Cause of Humanity": Therapeutic Environment in Quaker Asylum Design at the York Retreat
   Ann-Marie Akehurst ... 74

Part II Polity: Public Health and Politics

6 *Dar al-shifaʾ* or *Bimaristan*? Islamic Hospitals of Damascus, Sivas, and Cairo in the Twelfth and Thirteenth Centuries
   Richard Piran McClary ... 99

7 The Body of the City: Medicine and Urban Renewal in Sixtus IV's Rome
   Johanna D. Heinrichs ... 116

8 Spaces of Healing in Early Modern Portuguese Empire: Changing Public Health and Hospital Buildings on Mozambique Island
   Eugénia Rodrigues ... 138

Contents

9   From Exigency to Civic Pride: The Development of Early Australian Hospitals
Julie Willis   162

Part III Typologies: Places of Health in History

10   House of Misericórdia: Healthcare and Welfare Architecture in Sixteenth-Century Portugal
Joana Balsa de Pinho   181

11   Making the Home a Healing Space: Self-Cultivating Practices in Late Imperial China
Ying Zhang   197

12   For Care and Salvation: Leprosy Hostels in Pre-Modern Japan, *c.* 1200–1800
Susan L. Burns   209

13   Purity and Progress: The First Maternity Hospitals in the United States
Jhennifer A. Amundson   221

Part IV Architecture: Designing Spaces of Healing

14   Health as Harmony: The *Pellegrinaio* Cycle of Santa Maria della Scala in Siena
Maggie Bell   241

15   Uterus House: Incubating Obstetrics in Early Modern Bologna
Kim Sexton   260

16   Healing by Design: An Experiential Approach to Early Modern Ottoman Hospital Architecture
Nina Macaraig   279

17   Architectural Prescriptions: Johns Hopkins Medicine and the Shift from the Pre-Modern to the Modern Hospital
Stuart W. Leslie   302

Bibliography   315
Index   348

ILLUSTRATIONS

3.1	Antonio Averlino (il Filarete), *Treatise on Architecture*, Book XI, f. 82v, *c.* 1461–4	36
3.2	Alfred Guesdon, *View of Milan*, lithograph, *c.* 1850	36
3.3	Anonymous, possibly Portuguese, *Hospital Real de Todos-os-Santos (View of Rossio)*, eighteenth century, oil on canvas, 39 × 59 cm	37
3.4	Antonio Averlino (il Filarete), *Treatise on Architecture*, Book XI, f. 83v, *c.* 1461–4	40
3.5	Georg Braun and Frans Hogenberg, Detail of *Milan*, *Civitates Orbis Terrarum*, vol. 1, 1572	40
3.6	Reconstruction of hospital complex in 1755	43
3.7	António de Holanda, Detail of *Genealogical Tree of the Kings and Queens of Portugal from Alfonso Enriquez to Alfonso II*, fol. 7, in *Genealogy of the Royal Houses of Spain and Portugal* (Ms. Add. 12531), *c.* 1530–4	46
3.8	Georg Braun and Frans Hogenberg, Detail of *Lisbon*, *Civitates Orbis Terrarum*, vol. 1, 1572	46
3.9	Anonymous artist (Flemish or Spanish), Detail of *Panoramic View of Lisbon*, *c.* 1570–80	47
4.1	Miraculous statue of Our Lady of Potterie, *c.* 1270–80, white stone, 160 cm	56
4.2	Virgin and Child, *The Miracle Book of Our Lady of Potterie*, *c.* 1520–1, pen, ink, on paper, originally fol. 2r, currently fol. 5r, 21.7 × 14.2 cm	60
4.3	Virgin Potterie helped those who venerated her, *The Miracle Book of Our Lady of Potterie*, originally fol. 11v, currently fol. 14v	61
4.4	Woman cured from water sickness, originally fol. 2v, currently fol. 5r	65
4.5	The Virgin helped women who had difficulties in becoming pregnant, *The Miracle Book of Our Lady of Potterie*, originally fol. 11r, currently fol. 14r	67
4.6	Pieter Adriaens escaped from a storm in England, *The Miracle Book of Our Lady of Potterie*, originally fol. 4r, currently fol. 7r	68
5.1	Peter Atkinson the Younger, *Perspective View of the North Front of the Retreat near York*, 1812, (BIA RET 2/1/2/1) subsequently published in Samuel Tuke, *Description of the Retreat: An Institution Near York, for Insane Persons of the Society of Friends* (York, 1813)	78
5.2	W. Strickland, *View of the North East Front of the Proposed Asylum Near Philadelphia* (1814)	79
5.3	The Retreat: Ground Story Plan showing pencil revisions (BIA RET 2/1/1/1(c))	82
5.4	South front elevation for the proposed Retreat, consultation drawing (BIA RET 2/1/1/1(b))	84
5.5	Chamber Story Plan of the Retreat, consultation drawing (BIA RET 2/1/1/1(d))	85
5.6	The Retreat Directors' Minute Book showing original subscription appeal in print and handwritten addition regarding Hannah Mills (BIA RET 1/1/1/1/, fol. 1r)	89

Illustrations

6.1	Plan of the al-Nuri Hospital, Damascus	102
6.2	Decorative elements of the al-Nuri Hospital, Damascus	103
6.3	Ground plan of the 'Izz al-Din Kay Kawus I Hospital, Sivas	105
6.4	North, east, and south iwans of the 'Izz al-Din Kay Kawus I Hospital, Sivas	105
6.5	Entrance portal of the 'Izz al-Din Kay Kawus I Hospital, Sivas	106
6.6	Plan of the al-Mansur Hospital, Cairo	109
6.7	Street entrance leading to the al-Mansur Hospital, Cairo	109
6.8	The interior of the Qalawun hospital, Cairo	110
7.1	Rome, Sistine inscription from Via Florea (Campo de' Fiori), 1483	117
7.2	View of Rome from Hartmann Schedel, *Liber Chronicarum* (Nuremberg, 1493), woodcut	117
7.3	Rome, Hospital of Santo Spirito in Sassia, east end and north facade along via Borgo Santo Spirito	118
7.4	Rome, Ponte Sisto	123
7.5	Plan of the Hospital of Santo Spirito, from Pierre Saulnier, *De capite sacri ordinis Sancti Spiritus dissertatio* (Lyons, 1649)	126
7.6	Elevations of the east and north facades of the Hospital of Santo Spirito, from Pierre Saulnier, *De capite sacri ordinis Sancti Spiritus dissertatio* (Lyons, 1649)	127
7.7	View of the interior of the Corsia Sistina, from Pierre Saulnier, *De capite sacri ordinis Sancti Spiritus dissertatio* (Lyons, 1649)	129
8.1	Map of Mozambique Island that shows the stone quarter to the west and the *macuti* palm huts scattered to the east and south of the stone town. The hospital appears in an isolated location south of the town	142
8.2	A view of a street in the stone town	144
8.3	Carved entrance door	145
8.4	Present-day *macuti* houses in the southern part of Mozambique Island	146
8.5	Detail from the 1754 map of Mozambique Island showing the hospital, convent, and church of St. John (16) and further away the church of Good Health (17)	147
8.6	The Misericórdia church with a building attached to the left, where the charitable hospital for the poor was located on the ground floor	150
8.7	A pipe system on the Misericórdia terrace to conduct water to the cistern	151
8.8	An early nineteenth-century map of Mozambique Island that shows how the stone quarter extended up to the hospital buildings (N) as well as the *macuti* houses to the east	154
9.1	Prefabricated second hospital (the long range seen at the lower left), Sydney, viewed from the western side of Sydney Cove. Sydney General Hospital, Sydney, New South Wales, Australia. Architect: Samuel Wyatt, 1790; artist: George William Evans (attrib.), *c.* 1803	164
9.2	Central range of Sydney's general hospital, colloquially known as the "Rum Hospital," Macquarie Street, Sydney. Sydney General Hospital, Sydney, New South Wales, Australia; architect: unknown, 1811–16; photographer: Charles Percy Pickering, 1870	166

Illustrations

9.3	The Parramatta Convict Hospital is typical of early Australian colonial hospitals, with two identical wards per floor, surrounded by a verandah under a large hipped roof. Paramatta Convict Hospital, Parramatta, New South Wales, Australia; architect: John Watts, 1818; photographer unknown, *c.* 1870–1920	167
9.4	The Liverpool Hospital demonstrated for the first time in Australia architectural sophistication as yet unseen in a hospital. Liverpool Hospital, Liverpool, New South Wales, Australia; architect: Francis Greenway, 1822–5; photographer: unknown, *c.* 1880s	168
9.5	The use of the Regency style for the hospital aligned it with other prominent civic buildings in Hobart. Second Hobart Hospital, Hobart, Tasmania, Australia; architect: unknown, 1843; photographer: John Watt Beattie, *c.* 1880	170
9.6	Perth finally realized a permanent hospital in 1852. The design is unusual for Australian hospitals in its use of the corner towers to bookend the verandahs. The Colonial Hospital, Perth; architect: James Austin, 1852; photographer: Alfred Hawes Stone, *c.* 1868	172
9.7	The Melbourne Hospital, with its Tudor Gothic style, represented the high aspirations of the town's citizens. Melbourne Hospital, Melbourne, Victoria, Australia; architect: Samuel Jackson, 1846–8; lithographer: Stringer, Mason & Co., *c.* 1850	174
10.1	Vila do Conde House of Misericórdia	184
10.2	Old photo of Mogadouro House of Misericórdia (*c.* mid 20th century, before the demolitions)	185
10.3	Old photo of Montemor-o-Velho House of Misericórdia (*c.* 1950, before the demolitions)	185
10.4	Renaissance cloister of the hospital of Estremoz	187
10.5	Meeting room of the brothers, Montemor-o-Velho House of Misericórdia	189
10.6	Church, Tentúgal House of Misericórdia	189
10.7	Exterior facade, Proença-a-Nova House of Misericórdia	191
10.8	Church, Santarém House of Misericórdia	192
10.9	Church, Alcochete House of Misericórdia	192
11.1	A page from a mid-seventeenth-century woodblock print showing a son and his wife preparing and tasting drugs in advance for their parents and parents-in-law in the home	198
11.2	The pages showing the recipe of "Elixir for dispelling the plague and saving the suffering" in *Yifang bianlan*.	203
11.3	The page showing the recipe for "Whole chicken ointment" in *Jiye liangfang*	205
12.1	The restored Kitayama Hall	210
12.2	Facilities of care at Gokurakuji Temple: 1. leprosy hostel; 2. bathhouse; 3. hospice; 4. clinic.	215
12.3	Architectural diagrams of Kitayama Hall, *c.* 1920s.	216
13.1	Pennsylvania Hospital (R. Scot, del. & sc.)	223
13.2	City of London Lying-in Hospital: views of the front elevation and courtyard. Engraving by B. Cole	228
13.3	The Lying-in Hospital and Rotunda, Dublin, Ireland. Steel engraving by Owen after W. H. Bartlett	229

Illustrations

13.4	Melbourne Lying-In Hospital. Charles Nettleton, photog. (State Library, Victoria.)	230
13.5	Preston Retreat, Philadelphia	231
13.6	New-York Asylum for Lying-in-Women. Colored wood engraving	232
14.1	*Pellegrinaio*, full view	242
14.2	Domenico di Bartolo, *The Expansion of the Hospital*, 1443	244
14.3	Agostino di Marsilio, Gualtieri di Giovanni, and Adamo di Colino, *Solomon* in vault above *The Expansion of the Hospital*, 1439–40 (detail)	246
14.4	Agostino di Marsilio, Gualtieri di Giovanni, and Adamo di Colino, *David* in vault above *The Care and Marriage of Foundlings*, 1439–40 (detail)	248
14.5	Domencio di Bartolo, *The Care and Marriage of Foundlings*, 1441	249
14.6	Pesellino (Francesco di Stefano), *The Construction of the Temple of Jerusalem*, 1445	250
14.7	Domenico di Bartolo, *The Expansion of the Hospital*, 1443 (detail)	251
15.1	Casa Nascentori, Bologna (via Drapperie, 8), *c.* 1527–50	261
15.2	Obstetrical models made for Giovanni Antonio Galli between 1734 and 1746/50 by Anna Morandi and Giovanni Manzolini and others, as installed in the Museo di Palazzo Poggi, Bologna	263
15.3	Palazzo Poggi, Bologna, 1549–60, with alterations after it became home to the Institute of the Sciences in 1711. Above, the facade on via Zamboni; below, plan of the ground floor, rooms 12 and 13 contained the obstetrical models	264
15.4	The geography of early modern medicine in central Bologna, showing the location of key schools and hospitals. A. Antonio Galli's house-academy (Casa Nascentori); B. Santa Maria della Vita; C. Santa Maria della Morte; D. the Archiginnasio; E. Institute of Sciences (Palazzo Poggi)	267
15.5	Palazzo Marsili, Bologna (via D'Azeglio 48), 1653–81, rebuilding of an earlier palazzo on the site, sometimes attributed to Francesco Dotti. The arrow points to the remains of the observatory tower	269
15.6	The *Spellati*, 1638–49, by Antonio Levanti, skinned atlas figures in the Anatomy Theater in the Palazzo dell'Archiginnasio, Bologna	271
15.7	Casa Nascentori, Bologna, *c.* 1527–50, passage from street to courtyard, with later alterations	273
16.1	Ground plans of the Yıldırım Darüşşifası (a), Fatih Darüşşifası (b), Hospital of Bayezid II (c), Hafsa Sultan Darüşşifası (d), Haseki Sultan Darüşşifası (e), Süleymaniye Darüşşifası (f), Atik Valide Darüşşifası (g), Sultanahmed Darüşşifası (h)	280
16.2	Overall plan of the Hafsa Sultan Mosque Complex, Manisa. Necipoğlu, *The Age of Sinan*, 54	283
16.3	Entrance of the Hafsa Sultan Darüşşifası	284
16.4	Portico of the Hafsa Sultan Darüşşifası. Kılıç, *Şifahaneler*, 247	285
16.5	Overall plan of the Süleymaniye Mosque Complex, Istanbul. No. 10 indicates the *darüşşifa*. Necipoğlu, *The Age of Sinan*, 205	286

16.6	Second courtyard of the Süleymaniye Darüşşifası. Kılıç, *Şifahaneler*, 273	287
16.7	Portico of the Hospital of Bayezid II	290
16.8	"Stage" in the Hospital of Bayezid II	292
16.9	Water runnel in the Hospital of Bayezid II	295
16.10	Courtyard of the Süleymaniye's *imaret*	296
17.1	Johns Hopkins Medicine, a twenty-first-century city within a city. Note the original dome near the middle of the complex, with the School of Nursing to its right	304
17.2	John Shaw Billings's final plan for the Johns Hopkins medical campus. The pathology laboratory, the first building to be completed, is at the upper left, with the octagon ward pavilion closest to the administrative building and the isolating ward furthest away	306
17.3	The Johns Hopkins Hospital at its opening in 1889. The administration building, with the signature dome and cupola, is at the center, with the paying wards for male and female patients, topped with turrets, to either side. Front view of buildings from northeast	307
17.4	Johns Hopkins University School of Medicine, Women's Fund Memorial Building under renovation, 1915. The Hunterian Laboratory (anatomy) and the Women's Fund Building (physiology), exemplified the institute model of German medicine, with each department in its own building	309
17.5	Chief of surgery William Halsted and his "All Star" team performing an operation in their new surgical theater, 1904. Designed for aseptic surgery, Halsted's operating room had strict protocols for sterilizing instruments, garments, and all surfaces. Note the rubber gloves on the nurse and physicians	311

CONTRIBUTORS

Danielle Abdon earned her Ph.D. in Art History from Temple University. She specializes in Renaissance architecture on the Italian and Iberian Peninsulas, as well as exchanges between Europe and the New World. Her dissertation, "Poverty, Disease, and Port Cities: Global Exchanges in Hospital Architecture during the Age of Exploration," focused on fifteenth- and sixteenth-century hospitals in Italy, Iberia, and the Americas, specifically how contemporary ideas of poor relief and public and environmental health promoted architectural and infrastructural innovations in hospital buildings. In addition to receiving a Carter Manny Award Citation of Special Recognition (2019) for the writing of her dissertation, Abdon's research has been funded by the Bibliotheca Hertziana—Max Planck Institute for Art History, the Countway Library of Medicine at Harvard University, the Getty Foundation, the Huntington Library, the John Carter Brown Library, the Society of Architectural Historians, as well as Temple University.

Ann-Marie Akehurst holds a BA in English Literature and Language from the University of Lancaster. While raising her children, she gained an MA in Fine Art (University of Leeds) and a Ph.D. in History of Art (University of York) under Professors Mark Hallett and Anthony Geraghty, where her topic was "Architecture and Philanthropy: Building Hospitals in Eighteenth-Century York" (2009). She was Postdoctoral Research Associate, IPUP, University of York (2009); has held a Paul Mellon postdoctoral fellowship (2009–10); and been a Research Associate at the University of York, where she taught History of Art (2007–14). She has published on early modern architecture and national identity, sacred space, and medical buildings. She is working on a monograph on architecture, philanthropy, place, and identity, focused on early modern York. She is now an independent researcher, affiliated to the Royal Institute of British Architects.

Jhennifer A. Amundson received her Master's in Architecture from the University of Illinois in Urbana-Champaign and her Ph.D. at the University of Delaware. An architectural historian and former architect, she serves as Dean of the O'More College of Architecture and Design, Art, and Design at Belmont University in Nashville, where she has also established its new program in architecture. Her many presentations and publications on the history, theory, and technology of nineteenth- and twentieth-century architecture and the history of the profession includes *Thomas Ustick Walter: The Lectures on Architecture* (Athenaeum of Philadelphia, 2006).

Maggie Bell received her Ph.D. in the History of Art and Architecture from the University of California Santa Barbara in 2019. Her dissertation research, which was supported by grants from the Samuel H. Kress Foundation and the Kunsthistorisches Institut in Florence, centers on the fifteenth-century frescoes in the central ward of the Hospital of Santa Maria della Scala in Siena, and the relationships among architecture, healing practices, and visual representation. She is currently an Assistant Curator at the Norton Simon Museum of Art at Pasadena, where she is developing an exhibition on the role of the bodily perception of visual art in the early modern period (April 2020).

Contributors

Susan L. Burns is Professor of Japanese History and East Asian Languages and Civilizations at the University of Chicago. She works on the history of gender, medicine, and public health in early modern and modern Japan. Her recent publications includes *Kingdom of the Sick: A History of Leprosy and Japan* (University of Hawaii Press, 2019); *Gender and Law in the Japanese Imperium* (co-edited with Barbara Brooks, University of Hawaii Press, 2013), and "Reinvented Places: Tradition, Family Care, and Psychiatric Institutions in Japan," *Social History of Medicine*, 32, no. 1 (2019): 99–120. Her research has been supported by the Fulbright-Hays Fellowship, the IIE Fulbright, the Japan Foundation, the Japan Society for the Promotion of Science, and the National Endowment for the Humanities.

Mohammad Gharipour is Professor and Director of Graduate Architecture Program at the School of Architecture and Planning at Morgan State University in Baltimore, Maryland. He obtained his Master's in Architecture from the University of Tehran and his Ph.D. in architecture at the Georgia Institute of Technology. He has received many grants and awards, including Hamad Bin Khalifa Fellowship in Islamic Art (2007), the Spiro Kostof Fellowship Award from the Society of Architectural Historians (2008), National Endowment in Humanities (2015), Fulbright-Hays (2016), Foundation for Landscape Studies (2016), National Institute of Health (2017), and Fulbright (2018). He has also authored and edited eleven books, including *Persian Gardens and Pavilions: Reflections in Poetry, Arts and History* (I.B.Tauris, 2013), *Synagogues of the Islamic World* (Edinburgh University Press, 2017), and *Gardens Renaissance and the Islamic Empires* (Pennsylvania State University Press, 2017). Dr. Gharipour is the director and founding editor of the *International Journal of Islamic Architecture*.

Johanna D. Heinrichs is Assistant Professor of Architecture in the College of Design at the University of Kentucky, where she teaches courses in the history and theory of architecture. She earned her Ph.D. in the Department of Art and Archaeology at Princeton University and an M.Phil. in History of Art from the University of Cambridge. She has published essays on villa architecture and landscape in early modern Venice and its territories, both in edited volumes and in the journal *Annali di Architettura*. She is currently preparing a book manuscript on Andrea Palladio's Villa Pisani at Montagnana and villa culture in Renaissance Venice. Her research has been supported by the Gladys Krieble Delmas Foundation and the Italian Art Society.

Stuart W. Leslie is Professor of the History of Science and Technology at The Johns Hopkins University. He has published widely on the architecture of modern science, including recent studies of nuclear laboratories in India and Pakistan, aerospace modernism in southern California, and the healthcare designs of Bertrand Goldberg and Eberhard Zeidler. Among his publications are *Boss Kettering: Wizard of General Motors* (Columbia University Press, 1983) and *The Cold War and American Science: The Military-Industrial-Academic Complex at MIT and Stanford* (Columbia University Press, 1994). He is currently completing an official history of The Johns Hopkins University.

Nina Macaraig received her Ph.D. from the University of Minnesota in 2005. She is currently Visiting Associate Professor in the Department of Archaeology and History of Art, Koç University, Istanbul. She specializes in Ottoman architectural history, particularly the "lesser" monuments within its canon, such as bathhouses and soup kitchens, and sensory aspects of the built environment. Her articles include "Ottoman Royal Women's Spaces: The Acoustic Dimension," *Journal of Women's History* 26, no. 1 (2014), and "The Fragrance of the Divine: Ottoman Incense Burners and Their Context," *The Art Bulletin* 96, no. 1 (2014), which received the journal's Third Biannual Best Article Award and the Ömer Lütfi Barkan Article Prize, respectively. She is the author of *Çemberlitaş Hamamı in Istanbul: The Biographical Memoir of a Turkish Bath* (Edinburgh University Press, 2018).

Richard Piran McClary is Lecturer at York University. Before this position, he had Leverhulme Trust Early Career Fellowship at the University of Edinburgh, where he conducted research on the Qarakhanid Architecture of Central Asia and teaches Islamic art. His first monograph, *Rum Seljuq Architecture (1170–1220): The Patronage of Sultans*, was published by Edinburgh University Press in 2017, and his second monograph is an interdisciplinary study of *mina'i* ware ceramics from Iran. He has written extensively on Islamic architecture, painting, and ceramics of the wider Iranian world, and had lectured on the topic around the world.

Joana Balsa de Pinho holds a Ph.D. in History of Art at University of Lisbon (2013). Her Ph.D. dissertation on the influence of the Confraternities of the Mercy in sixteenth-century Portuguese architecture was awarded a fellowship from the Foundation for Science and Technology. She has developed professional activities in the study and rehabilitation of historical heritage, cultural promotion, educational projects, organization of exhibitions, and training in Museology; and also received several fellowships in scientific research projects, including, since 2012, from the Centre for Lusophone and European Literatures and Cultures (University of Lisbon). Since 2018, she has integrated several research projects as a member of the research team Magister—A arquitectura tardo-gótica em Portugal: protagonistas, modelos e intercâmbios artísticos (2013–16)—and as a RIC (Hospitalis—Hospital Architecture in Portugal at the dawn of Modernity: identification, characterization, and contextualization).

Guenter B. Risse is Professor Emeritus, University of California, San Francisco, and Affiliate Professor in the Department of Bioethics and Humanities, University of Washington School of Medicine, Seattle. His research interests and publications have ranged broadly, notably concerned with the history and ecology of disease, as well as medicine during the Scottish Enlightenment. More recently, the author focused on the history of emotions driving xenophobia and the stigma of disease as well as public health policies and interventions in California. He is the author of numerous articles and several books on hospital history, including *Mending Bodies, Saving Souls: A History of Hospitals* (Oxford University Press, 1999).

Eugénia Rodrigues is a Researcher at the Centre for History of the University of Lisbon (Centro de História da Universidade de Lisboa) and she teaches History of Africa and History of Empires at the School of Arts and Humanities (Faculdade de Letras) of the same university. Her research focuses on social history in early modern Mozambique and the Indian Ocean, mainly concerning territorial appropriation, intercultural representations, slavery, gender, and circulation of knowledge. Her publications include an edited volume (with Mariana Candido), *African Women's Access and Rights to Property in the Portuguese Empire*, special issue of *African Economic History*, 43 (2015), and *Portugueses e Africanos nos Rios de Sena: Os prazos da Coroa em Moçambique nos Séculos XVII e XVIII* (Lisbon, 2013).

Kim Sexton is Associate Professor of Architecture in the Fay Jones School of Architecture at the University of Arkansas where she teaches architectural history and global humanities. Having trained at Binghamton University (BA) and Yale University (Ph.D.), she studies the history of architecture in late medieval and Renaissance Italy. She has published in the *Journal of the Society of Architectural Historians* and *The Art Bulletin*, and edited the volume *Architecture and the Body, Science and Culture* (Routledge, 2017). She is completing a book manuscript on the Italian loggia and working on a second book on medieval bodies and spaces with historian Lynda Coon.

Miyako Sugiyama is an art historian specializing in early Netherlandish art. She received her Master's in Art History from Keio University (Japan) in 2012 and her Ph.D. in Art Sciences from Ghent University (Belgium) in 2017. She has received several grants, including the Flemish Government of Belgium Scholarship (2013–14), Kress Foundation Travel Grants (2016), and a scholarship offered by Japan Student Services Organization (2015–17). Her research focuses on the functions of images and relationships between art and devotional practices in the fifteenth- and early sixteenth-century Netherlands. She has been published in *The Medieval Low Countries* (2016), *Simiolus-Netherlands Quarterly for the History of Art* (2017), and *Oud Holland* (2019). Currently, she is a postdoctoral researcher at Japan Society for the Promotion of Science.

Julie Willis is Professor of Architecture and Dean of the Faculty of Architecture, Building and Planning at the University of Melbourne, Australia. She is a distinguished architectural scholar, with expertise in Australian architectural history of the nineteenth and twentieth centuries. Her current research examines the transmission and translation of architectural knowledge through professional networks. Major works include the *Encyclopedia of Australian Architecture* (Cambridge University Press 2012, with Philip Goad), the edited collection *Designing Schools: Space, Place and Pedagogy* (Routledge 2017, with Kate Darian-Smith), and *Architecture and the Modern Hospital: Nosokomeion to Hygeia* (Routledge 2019, with Philip Goad and Cameron Logan).

Ying Zhang is an Associate Professor in the Yuelu Academy at Hunan University. She received her Ph.D. from Johns Hopkins University in 2017. Her articles are published in *Late Imperial China* and *Frontiers of History in China*. She is currently completing revisions to her book manuscript, *Household Healing: Rituals, Recipes, and Virtues in Late Imperial China*, under advance contract with the University of Washington Press. This project investigates China's rich tradition of household healing practices and reinterprets these practices in relation to religion, gender roles, and morality from the seventeenth to the early twentieth century. It demonstrates the various ways in which the home served as a central site of healing technology during this period. It also sheds new light on the circulation of healing information in the context of literati sociability, philanthropic activities, and religious practices in Ming-Qing China.

PREFACE: STRUCTURE AND CONTENTS OF THIS VOLUME

Exploring the dazzling array of approaches to healthcare and healthcare architecture in the pre-modern era in different societies, as well as the consolidation of hospitals as an independent building typology, this book takes a deep look at how different political, cultural, and scientific contexts shaped hospital designs. Each chapter employs an interdisciplinary, comparative, or new methodological approach to analyze the design and function of healthcare facilities—either a single structure or specialized typologies—in a particular city or region at a given moment in time. The chapters illustrate what constituted health in different places during the pre-modern period and how healthcare architecture responded to scientific and socio-cultural contexts, or, vice versa, how that context influenced its design. Seeking a global history that acknowledges the connections across traditions, the volume demonstrates that the binary of "Western" and "Eastern" medicine is part of the eighteenth- and nineteenth-century construct that disciplined both medical treatment and the various civilizations colonized under this rubric.

Opening with an overview of healthcare facilities from ancient times to the nineteenth century, this volume consists of four parts, each embracing case studies from various regions. The first two parts explain how healthcare facilities evolved under the influence of religious and political settings. Examining the typological development of healthcare facilities, the third part includes chapters on various building types such as houses, charity hospitals, leprosy hostels, and maternity hospitals. These studies demonstrate how hospitals in the pre-modern era evolved within various cultural and social contexts and how their transformations reflected revolutions in the medical sciences. With the first three parts focusing on the typological and contextual development of places of care, the fourth part addresses how architecture, design, and art could lead to more effective care for patients. Chapters in each part are sorted chronologically in order to provide a better understanding of the evolution of places of care across geographies. These studies demonstrate how these places in the pre-modern era evolved within various cultural and social contexts and how their transformation reflected revolutions in the medical sciences.

The first part addresses the complex interplay between religious and cultural settings and the design of healthcare facilities with a series of case studies from Portugal, Belgium, and England. This part opens with a chapter by scholar of hospital history Guenter B. Risse on the development of hospitals in both religious and secular settings. He argues that important pre-modern buildings devoted to caring for sick people disclose and confirm a range of beliefs about illnesses and strategies to treat them, often influenced by both religious and secular perspectives. As anthropological studies have demonstrated, in ancient and even medieval civilizations, illness was frequently understood within a religious framework, and elaborate doctrines sought to identify supernatural agents capable of curing and protecting people from disease. On the other hand, since sickness is a uniquely personal experience, sufferers also explored non-religious empirical and scientific dimensions of health issues. In this chapter, Risse discusses the binary and somewhat complementary impact of religion and science on the healing process. For as far back as the historical evidence goes, hospitals in any form have always been inextricably bound up with cultural beliefs.

At the beginning of the fourteenth century, as a response to the dramatic increase in the poor and sick populations in Western Europe and lack of sanitation, several European cities started reforming existing systems of public health and social welfare, primarily through creating religious and charitable networks. Danielle Abdon's chapter addresses the reformation of healthcare and the appearance and dissemination of a specific architectural typology exclusive to hospitals during the peak of the Portuguese Empire, from the fifteenth to the seventeenth centuries. Characterized by a cruciform design, Portuguese hospitals promoted medical and sanitary innovations, including triage, separation of the sick and poor, isolation, and sewage disposal. Abdon explains the adoption of the cruciform plan as the main prototype for hospitals in a period when the Portuguese monarchy struggled to increase social and sanitary infrastructure. Abdon portrays a different view of Lisbon as the first global metropolis of early modern Europe and a dynamic international center in the early modern world. She argues that the Portuguese importation of an Italian plan for hospitals reflected the monarchy's ambitions of becoming an international hub, while helping to create a shift in hospital architecture from improvised to purposefully designed buildings that incorporated local needs.

The next chapter by Miyako Sugiyama examines the context behind the construction of the Hospital of Our Lady of Potterie, which was founded in the twelfth century in the city of Bruges and provided shelter for travelers and the sick. Sugiyama's analysis focuses on a miraculous statue of the Virgin and Child on the hospital grounds in order to demonstrate relationships between images and audiences in spaces of healing. Sugiyama researches the textual and visual evidence concerning this statue to reconstruct the tripartite relationship between image, audience, and space in order to understand the religious mission of pre-modern hospitals in regard to providing social welfare. In the last chapter of the first section, Ann-Marie Akehurst turns our attention to the shift in healthcare design to a humane approach that gradually foregrounded care over containment through an analysis of the Retreat Asylum, founded by the Quaker group the Religious Society of Friends near the city of York in Britain. This facility was considered a groundbreaking psychiatric institution in the eighteenth century, as its design and program represented a new and humane attitude toward the mentally ill, affording patients dignity by encouraging them to pet animals, engage in social events, and partake in what is now called Occupational Therapy. Consulting archival documents and religious writings, Akehurst analyzes various therapeutic aspects of this asylum, which represents the evolution of early modern hospitals from places of care to spaces limiting the spread of disease and facilitating cure.

The second part of this volume includes the study of medieval, early modern, and colonial cases from the Middle East, Africa, Europe, and Australia to highlight the development of healthcare facilities as an integral part of the empire-building process. In the first chapter of this section, Richard McClary argues that hospitals served as important symbols of royal charity in the Islamic world in the twelfth and thirteenth centuries, inspiring rulers to build majestic places of healing for the benefit of their subjects. McClary looks at the design of three hospitals in Damascus (Syria), Sivas (Turkey), and Cairo (Egypt) to explore the Sultanic patronage and its impact on the construction of facilities in the medieval Islamic world. The next chapter, by Johanna Heinrichs, elucidates the connection between public health concerns and urban development in Rome in the late fifteenth century. Coming to power in a Rome that had suffered a century of population loss and neglect, Pope Sixtus IV was determined to revitalize the city's infrastructure and its flagging reputation. In this chapter, Heinrichs argues that Sixtus IV's project of urban restoration should be understood not simply as papal benevolence but explicitly as medical care, given his self-ascribed role as the "bearer of health."

What makes European powers more relevant in the debate over hospital design is the role that they played in establishing and constructing new hospitals, beyond their national boundaries and in their colonies. The next chapter by Eugénia Rodrigues explores the development of military hospitals in Mozambique Island,

Preface: Structure and Contents of this volume

the capital of colonial *Portuguese* East Africa prior to 1898. By analyzing public health policies set by the administration and their impact on the configuration of the hospitals, Rodrigues explains how the Portuguese constructed military hospitals in buildings that were adapted for the purpose or were planned from scratch. She addresses the progressive transformation of the hospital established by the Portuguese Crown on Mozambique Island in the early sixteenth century, as well as the role played by the hospital run by the Santa Casa da Misericórdia during the eighteenth century. In expanding the discussion on European colonies, the last chapter in this part, by Julie Willis, reveals the use of similar colonial policies by the British and their envoys in Australia during the eighteenth and nineteenth centuries. Willis illustrates the difficulties of creating a functioning medical infrastructure during the British colonization (1788–1850) of Australia. While the early Australian hospitals were treated as shelters in which only the most basic medical care was provided, the design of colonial hospitals drew upon the typology of the military field hospital and, more often, that of military barracks.

The chapters in the third Part of this volume analyze the development of various typologies of places of care in different geographies, including Portugal, China, Japan, and the United States. This part is opened by Joana de Pinho's discussion on the formation of Misericórdias (charity hospitals) in the city of Lisbon in 1498 and their spread throughout Portugal in the sixteenth century. She explains the crucial role that Misericórdias played in the Portuguese healthcare system, both for their territorial coverage and institutional role in assisting the poor and the sick. By fulfilling their charitable proposes, namely welcoming the poor and the sick, celebrating liturgy, and burying the dead, the Misericórdias were either constructed as new buildings or housed in preexisting autonomous spaces. By studying examples of this prevalent typology, Pinho presents a lucid understanding of their architecture and design characteristics and sheds light on their authorship, patronage, and use.

In other parts of the world and far from Portugal, healing occurred in a wide range of locations and places that were not necessarily designed as hospitals or healthcare facilities. In the next chapter, Ying Zhang discusses the use of houses in providing a physical space for regulating bodily conditions for both men and women in early modern China. She examines sixteenth- and seventeenth-century vernacular documents in order to illustrate heterogeneous healing techniques that occurred in the home, the use of artifacts, and social relations in regard to these practices in a domestic setting. Zhang also addresses how the home constitutes a meaningful healing space, how the material setting of the domestic space shapes the choice of healing methods and the meanings of healthcare, and how the practice of self-treatment informs the social identity of the practitioners. In another study of healthcare facilities in East Asia, Susan L. Burns explores the spread of leprosy hostels in early modern Japan as the result of increasing public health concerns over disease. Drawing upon textual and visual sources and modern architectural site reports, Burns demonstrates how these institutions emerged and how they functioned over the course of Japan's long pre-modern period, stretching from the thirteenth to the end of the eighteenth century. These pre-modern leprosy hostels differed fundamentally from modern institutions of care and confinement, as they were not founded to control infection, nor to treat or even care for those with the disease, but to address both spiritual and physical health through facilitating the salvation of leprosy sufferers and those who offered them compassion. Burns explains the reflections of this approach in the architectural style of monastic dormitories and temple complexes that were repurposed as leprosy hostels.

The next chapter by Jhennifer Amundson explores the formation of another healthcare typology: the first maternity hospitals in the United States. While traditional home-birth survived longer in Western Europe, the institution of maternity hospitals in the United States started in the early nineteenth century. This establishment was motivated by charitable impulses, increased professional specialization, and the desire for social improvement. Due to concerns for the well-being of mother and child, giving birth at home was preferred over hospitals, which were only utilized by women who could not afford to arrange for home-births. Amundson considers two case studies, the Preston Retreat (Philadelphia, 1830s) and the New-York Asylum for Lying-In Women (New York, 1823), to demonstrate how the design of these buildings responded to medical findings in medicine and public health.

The last part of this book consists of essays that address the impact of architecture and design on the healing process, the impact of design on the patients' experience, the interaction between their environment and their recovery, and the effectiveness of hospital design. After the medieval era, many hospitals in Italy provided various types of care that included treating the sick, caring for foundling children, distributing alms, and housing pilgrims and poor travelers. Maggie Bell's chapter studies one such hospital, the Santa Maria della Scala, a sprawling complex founded in Siena in the eleventh century. Investigating eight fifteenth-century monumental frescoes from the pilgrim's hall (*pellegrinaio*) depicting the mythologized history of Santa Maria della Scala and scenes of daily activities, she clarifies how the architecture of Scala was central to the hospital's institutional identity and self-image. She also identifies the role of the frescoes within fifteenth-century discourses on architecture and medicine. Bell proposes that these frescoes present a visual argument for the relationship between architectural enterprise and individual and public health and medicine.

The next chapter by Kim Sexton provides an in-depth study of the design of the Uterus House, originally built in the 1520s by the Nascentori, a family of glassmakers, for their business and residence in Bologna. This residence, which is a typical sixteenth-century *palazzetto*, is located in the heart of Bologna's busy market area and housed a private academy. Galli, the star scientist and surgeon in charge of this private academy in the eighteenth century, commissioned Bolognese sculptors and modelers to make about two hundred obstetrical wood, clay, wax, and papier-mâché models and devices with moving parts. Sexton examines the residence's transformation into an illustrious school and laboratory where midwives of both sexes gathered for the latest in experimental- and demonstration-based lessons. She also clarifies how the design of this academy responded to specific contextual issues, which were related to the social, medical, and cultural roles of private academies in Bologna and beyond. Contemporaneous to the powerful government in Renaissance Italy, the Ottomans' patronage of charity structures and the increasing need for both public and military healthcare resulted in the mass construction of hospitals across their empire. Nina Macaraig's chapter argues how these hospitals provided spatial qualities and sensory experiences to enhance the care of a variety of patients. She uses historical source material, such as endowment deeds, to explore the effectiveness of the Ottomans' user-centered and prescriptive approach to design by exploring how these buildings appealed to the senses, promoted well-being, and assisted in the therapeutic process.

This volume concludes with Stuart Bill Leslie's chapter, which narrates the history of the Baltimore-based Johns Hopkins Hospital, one of the best-known and most highly ranked medical centers in the world. With roots in the Pennsylvania Hospital (1751), American public hospitals were administered as charitable institutions for the worthy poor, with little input from physicians. Leslie studies the transformation of the Johns Hopkins medical school into a fully modern hospital to highlight a major shift in the American attitude toward medical care. He concludes that Johns Hopkins Medicine's greatest contribution—both medical and architectural—would not be any single innovation but rather the flexibility to adapt, improve, improvise, and combine best practice from many sources and disseminate those ideas widely.

As evident, the primary concern of this volume is not to provide an encyclopedic history of hospitals in the pre-modern age, but to propose a cohesive and comprehensive set of essays on the formation and development of spaces of care in various continents. The goal is to feature the contextual, formal, and spatial complexities of these spaces through a non-dichotomous perspective. Therefore, rather than constituting itself as a reference, this volume aims to highlight interesting and exciting aspects of health and architecture, and even challenge our perceptions of hospital history through a series of studies from various fields ranging from urban planning to architecture and art.

Preface: Structure and Contents of this volume

Connectedly, the current book questions the relationship and overlaps between health, context, and architecture. While our understanding of pre-modern hospitals is limited, especially in non-Western contexts, the records are sufficient to give us an understanding of human beings' achievements and efforts to create healthy and salutogenic spaces. While contemporary hospitals seem to be highly uniform and rigidly organized, the places of care in the pre-modern era tend to be the result of local or regional efforts to heal and cure people, reflecting a more humane approach to design and architecture. While the phenomenon of the modern hospital is often regarded as a Western invention, this book highlights the contributions of various civilizations and cultures to the development of the idea of places of care and healing in any form and function.

ACKNOWLEDGMENTS

The idea for this project originated in a panel that I organized at the Society of Architectural Historians annual meeting with my friend and colleague Bill Leslie. I am thankful to him for his enormous support for this volume and for generously agreeing to write an excellent epilogue. I should express my appreciation not only to the contributors for their patience and persistence in revising their papers in the span of four years but also to the authors whose work did not make it into this volume. Also, I owe thanks to the anonymous reviewers for providing extremely helpful feedback, Henry Johnson for copy-editing the final manuscript and Meridith Murray for making the index for this volume. Like any other scholarly project, this volume comes with its weaknesses and shortcomings, but I do hope that it represents a step forward in expanding our understanding of the history of hospitals.

My wife and best friend, Nooshin, has been extremely encouraging and supportive of this project. To her, I dedicate this book, with love and gratitude.

CHAPTER 1
PLACES OF CARE AND HEALING
CONTEXT, DESIGN, AND DEVELOPMENT IN HISTORY
Mohammad Gharipour

The word "heal" is derived from an Anglo-Saxon word "haelon," which means wholeness. As this root indicates, healing involves a holistic process that requires attention to a patient's physical, biological state as well as to his or her psychological one, which entails spiritual, mental, emotional, and social needs. In various historical contexts, places of healing have provided therapy to those in physical and mental distress. For the historian, they provide a window into the notions of health, science, and medicine as conceived by various civilizations. Whether housed in monasteries in medieval Europe, appended to Chinese palaces in fifteenth-century Beijing, or designed to sooth their patients with elegant fountains and birdsong in sixteenth-century Ottoman Istanbul, healthcare spaces provide some of the most beautiful architectural expressions of therapy—and reflect the vast, and ceaselessly changing, array of attitudes toward healing that have existed across time. As the majority of research on healthcare facilities has focused on the nineteenth century onwards, healthcare design in the pre-modern era represents fertile ground for new inquiry.

As this book aims to accomplish, an interdisciplinary study of the design of places of care across culture and time would shed light on the multitudinous perceptions and approaches to healing and health that have existed in a range of historical and geographic environments. Hospitals have long reflected the cultural attitudes of their day, as well as the predominant scientific theories and political dynamics in their broader environments. There is much about this wider context that can be teased out from hospital architecture, such as considering how medical developments affect building design and hospitals' interior spaces, or how the hospital building's style might overlap and connect with other typologies, to name a few avenues of study. While the spatial practices of healthcare architecture should be viewed in the context of urbanization and urban design, it is equally important to articulate the internal and external changes of architecture that concern cultural and medical configurations.

Primarily, this book asks: what distinguishes pre-modern hospitals from their modern counterparts, and how has evolution in building design occurred historically? While the difference between pre-modern and modern hospitals is somewhat vague and, of course, dependent on geography, a number of distinctive features characterize the era of modern healthcare. These include the shift from caring for patients as a religious, charitable act to active medicalization; the revival of environmental perspectives on disease and health; the rise of public health institutions and policies; emphasis on preventive care; and greater monitoring of patients and medical staff. These transformations have not only changed the design and construction of hospitals in both rural and urban communities but have also produced a design practice that takes into account the measurable physiological and psychological effects of an environment on the people exposed to it.[1]

This introductory chapter limns the chronological development of places of care across different geographies to demonstrate the tension evolving between practitioners acting within a worldview shaped by spiritual ritual and understanding of the body and those who adopt an emerging vocabulary of scientific diagnosis and treatment. While it could not possibly substitute for a comprehensive study of hospital history—already covered more masterfully by several extant publications[2]—the purpose of this chapter is to provide a historical summary, highlight some crucial points on the design of places of healing in various forms, and prepare the reader for the contents of this volume.

Health and Architecture

Ancient Times

Our knowledge of places of care in ancient civilizations, including the Egyptians, Mesopotamians, Persians, Greeks, and Romans, is limited, although the few historical accounts and artifacts that do exist can help us understand their context, design, and evolution. Medical organizations in ancient Egypt were guided by political states. The strict hierarchical organization of medical practice could have affected the use and design of spaces dedicated to the healing of various populations. In ancient Egypt, special institutions known as "The Houses of Life" trained healers and physicians and compiled medical texts.[3] Although physicians were said to have treated the sick in their own homes, tombs were used for more intensive surgeries and difficult procedures.[4] In the tomb of Ankh-Mahor, known as The Tomb of the Physician at Saqqara, a burial ground in ancient Egypt, wall paintings represent two men undergoing a medical procedure variously explained as a massage or surgery. The Greek historian Herodotus wrote extensively of his observations of Egyptian medical practice after he visited the country around 440 BCE.[5] Nevertheless, there is not much information on how the design of these spaces would have looked in ancient Egypt.

The medical systems of the roughly contemporaneous ancient Mesopotamian cultures were not as intricate as the Egyptians' medical sciences. Their medicinal culture depended upon magic and astrology for diagnosis and used magical and ritualistic therapeutics. Mesopotamians believed in keeping a clean spirit and body in order to prevent diseases and in purifying themselves before God. Yet, the rulers in ancient Mesopotamia promulgated surprisingly progressive regulations organizing the healthcare system. Adapting existing edicts, King Hammurabi of Babylon incorporated precepts of managed care into the *Code of Hammurabi*—a huge stone stele erected approximately in 1780 BCE. The code emphasized the following:

> Rates set for general surgery, eye surgery, setting fractures, curing diseased muscles and other specific healthcare services; fees set according to a sliding scale based on ability to pay; owners to pay for healthcare for their slaves; objective outcome measurement standards to assure quality of care; outcome information management to include data collection and evaluation; consumer and patient's rights to be publicized, explained and made known to all.[6]

The laws of the *Code of Hammurabi*, especially concerning the setting of fees and malpractice, informed not only Jewish and Islamic law but also were echoed in the modern health policy of the United States. Only a few hundred years before the disappearance of the Babylonians, the Greeks started developing a society in which health was seen as a holistic process, as they believed that the healthy mind existed in a healthy body. According to the historian C. F. Kleisiaris and her colleagues:

> Three main categories were observed in the Hippocratic provision of care: health promotion, interventions on trauma care, and mental care and art therapy interventions. Health promotion included physical activity as an essential part of physical and mental health, and emphasized the importance of nutrition to improve performance in the Olympic Games. Interventions on trauma care included surgical practices developed by Hippocrates, mainly due to the frequent wars in ancient Greece. Mental care and art therapy interventions were in accordance with the first classification of mental disorders, which was proposed by Hippocrates. In this category music and drama were used as management tools in the treatment of illness and in the improvement of human behavior.[7]

The Greek tradition of healthcare originated in Asclepieion, a healing temple where the wealthy and famous orator Aelius Aristides was healed in 145 CE after dreaming that the Greek god of healing, Asclepius, had invited him to Asclepieion.[8] From the evidence, it appears that Asclepieia (healing temples) were mostly constructed in valleys at favorable wooded locations and near natural springs, or near caves outside of towns.[9] As reflected in the Hippocratic Oath, the Asclepieia based their medical practice on an inclusive approach predicated on "understanding the patient's health, independence of mind, and the need for harmony between the individual, social and natural environment."[10]

The design of the healing temple reflected the rituals performed within its walls. The sacred land or *hieron* in the Asclepieion was always marked by an enclosure, called a *temenos*, separating it from secular spaces by a wall or stones surrounding the whole complex. A roofed gate provided access and opportunities for prayer. The roofed gate must have been in proximity to water basins that allowed guests to purify themselves symbolically before stepping into a sacred area. The enclosure guarding the sacred land included a temple, an image, and an altar. A few of the enclosures were also built next to a grove, spring, or cave in the countryside.[11]

In the Greek temples of healing, elected officials were to monitor the temple's funds and administration, as well as other peripheral buildings. People visited these temples for various reasons, perhaps to petition the gods for the prevention of illness, to give thanks for their good health, or to seek a cure for whatever ailed them.[12] Visiting a temple for healing purposes required following certain preparatory rituals to ensure physical purity.[13] Sacrifice was an integral part of temple culture in ancient Greece, and it usually took the form of animal killings followed by a ritual meal. Before the slaughter, purified visitors made preliminary offerings to the god by laying cheesecakes, honey, bread, roasted meats, and fruits upon an aperture before the god's image. In many cases, after this ritual the supplicant would visit a healer, who would inquire into his or her condition, give instructions, and finally deliver a prognosis.[14]

Another important building for healing in ancient Greece was the *abaton*, a long and narrow building where patients slept and rested, with an open portico and oriented to the south. The supplicants lay on the ground, both inside the temple and outside, in the open air. The populous city of Epidauros, which was known for its healing features, had a huge hostel with about 180 rooms. The *abaton* in this city was located near a sacred well and next to a bathhouse facing east. As Epidauros grew, new temples were constructed in order to stage elaborate festivals, as well as new guest lodgings to accommodate the visitors.[15]

Following in the footsteps of the Greeks, the Roman Empire (753 BCE–476 CE) tried to promote public health through sanitation and hygiene not only in Rome but also in their colonies. Grasping the relationship between urban design and architecture on the one hand, and public health on the other, they commissioned infrastructural building projects that contributed to the public's physical and mental health. The constant growth of an imperial state and the development of sophisticated civil engineering, such as aqueducts, which ran through much of Rome by the second century CE, facilitated urban sanitation.[16] The popularity of bathhouses further promoted public health and hygiene, especially for wealthier citizens.

The legions of soldiers and slaves that greased the wheels of the empire likewise required the construction of military and slave infirmaries. In large estates, landowners sometimes built smaller facilities on site to care for sick slaves, although, in times of surplus, sick ones would be abandoned, likely to be either sold off in the marketplace or disposed for "healing" at a temple of Asclepius—the Greek god of healing, who was imported to Rome in 292 BCE.[17] In the event of a supply shortage of slave labor, however, an infirmary known as the *valetudinarium* was recognized as a means of extracting more labor out of existing slaves, prolonging their life and increasing their loyalty and productivity.[18] As the Roman agricultural writer Columella (60–65 CE) narrates: "Attention of this kind is a source of kind feelings and also obedience. Moreover, those who had recovered their health, after careful attention has been given them when they were ill, are eager to give more faithful service than before."[19] Little is known about the architecture of the slave *valetudinarium*; however, the military *valetudinarium* is described as a rectangular plan with four wings surrounding a central courtyard or garden.

Health and Architecture

Similarly, the Roman military infirmary was a refined amenity, with inpatient care and advanced medicine for the time administered by a corps of trained professionals and lay practitioners.[20] According to Risse:

> This inward focus provided relative closure to the street for privacy and rest. In some cases, the entrance to the building led to a large receiving room, the atrium, with rooms or cubicles arranged around the peristyle, with its adjacent latrines and courtyard. The number of rooms appears to have had a standard relationship to the number of legionaries stationed in a given fort.[21]

Like their Greek counterparts, Roman health practitioners advocated for personal hygiene, good dieting, and a healthy lifestyle. Some Romans viewed Greek medicine suspiciously, regarding it as overly hypothetical, especially in its prescription of complex drug recipes involving a multitude of ingredients. The tendency of Greek doctors to disagree about the causes of disease, or take a fee for their services, looked unprofessional from the Roman perspective. For most denizens of ancient Rome, treatment of illness remained within the family, with the head of the household maintaining responsibility for the health and fertility of his family members, slaves, and domestic animals. Therapies, which were applied topically, were mainly based on readily available materials, such as wool, eggs, cabbage, and bruised leaves. Depending on the severity of the disease, family members caring for their sick might accentuate the treatment with magic hymns or chants. If things worsened, it was always an option to plead for good health at the temple of the relevant god or goddess.[22]

The philosophies, tools, knowledge, and practices established in ancient civilizations, including but not limited to the Egyptians, Mesopotamians, Greeks, and Romans, laid the foundation for medical practices in the medieval age. While these regional traditions were developed in parallel, with corresponding transformations in practices in the Far East and the Americas, what distinguished them was the degree of intercultural exchange and confluences among them, especially between the Greeks and Romans in the West.

Medieval World

Europe

In the Byzantine Empire (330–1453 CE), the earliest hospitals or *xenon* (literally "house for strangers") began to develop in the fourth century. These health institutions, which were founded by emperors, clergymen, monks, and lay individuals, were often associated with monasteries and provided medical care, food, and shelter. The *xenon* is often said to resemble modern hospitals more than any other ancient medical institution. The first-known major *xenon* was built by St. Basil of Caesarea (*c.* 329–379) in present-day Anatolia in approximately 370 CE. It included a poorhouse, hospice, and hospital.[23] The concept spread throughout the Byzantine Empire in the following centuries.

The hospitals of the Middle Ages catered to four categories of users: the lepers, the poor, the sick, and the inhabitants of the almshouses. Around 580 CE, the first Spanish hospital, founded by the Catholic Visigoth Bishop Masona at Merida, was a *xenodochium*, a type of hospital built for travelers and pilgrims. This hospital was endowed with farms to feed its visitors and patients. In 650 CE, another hospital, Hotel-Dieu, was founded in Paris. This multipurpose institution, which is considered the oldest running hospital in the world, tended to the sick and poor.[24] Emperor Charlemagne (742–814) ordered each cathedral and monastery to have a hospital attached to it.[25]

In the mid-800s, some 160 charitable institutions operated across the Byzantine Empire, although most of them served more as hospices than hospitals. The most famous of these was the Hospital of the Pantocrator, built by Emperor John Commenos II (1087–1143) in Constantinople. According to its foundation charter, the hospital had five wards for inpatients, including a surgical ward and a women's ward, comprising a total of fifty to sixty beds, and an outpatient clinic. Unlike in other hospitals of the time, the administration provided proper heating, lighting, and bed linen, as well as bathing facilities and latrines. The patients were fed a carefully planned vegetarian diet and received an allowance for purchasing additional food and drink. A large and specialized staff of physicians, medical assistants, and orderlies ministered to the patients. The hospital's charter also refers to a medical school, although historians are unsure whether it was used for educational purposes.[26]

The Byzantine historian, Timothy Miller, indicates that by the eleventh and twelfth centuries it became common for the general population to receive specialized treatment and walk-in clinical services at *xenones*. Moreover, these hospitals provided medical instructions, in terms of both practice and theory, to students.[27] It should also be noted that, despite the existence of an advanced medical infrastructure in this era, many people still believed in the magic and chants of God-inspired men because of their aversion to the fees charged by medical practitioners and to the foul smells permeating the *xenones*. These holy-men healers would typically recommend alternatives to surgery and would always refer the sick to a specific doctor. In some cases, they discouraged patients from visiting hospitals altogether and instead persuaded them to seek the restorative power of hot springs. These incidents led to a certain level of hostility and antagonism between these two distinct approaches to the embodiment of disease.[28]

Christianity was largely responsible for institutionalizing and expanding charity efforts across the Byzantine Empire, providing various forms of care and shelter for the poor and the sick. After the legalization of Christianity in the fourth century, Bishop Leontius (344–58) founded many hostels. By the fifth and sixth centuries, such institutions became so widespread that a typical town would usually have at least one or two such hospitals.[29] These hospitals also acted as charities for the sick and the poor and for travelers as well. As historians Nicholas Orme and Margaret Webster write, some institutions perceived themselves as hospitable inns rather than as hospitals per se and turned away the sick or dying in fear that treatment of difficult illnesses would divert attention from worship.[30]

Moreover, what explains the dominance of medieval hospitals is that one of their primary functions was to increase the worship of God. Hence, most hospitals included a minimum of one clergyman, a chapel, and inmates who were expected to assist with prayers. Worship sometimes even appeared to take priority over medical care, serving as a way of reducing and mitigating the illnesses of the sick and, when relief was not possible, of ensuring their salvation.[31] In fact, the reality of medical practice during the Middle Ages revolved around worship and rites, not therapeutics.[32] For instance, St. John's Hospital in Canterbury (*c.* 1085), one of the earliest hospitals in medieval England, admitted paupers, poor scholars, and "corrodians" (pensioners who lived in monasteries or convents). This entity (an inchoate hospital) was seen as a source of employment and a refuge for the needy. The few who were admitted among a large pool of the poor and sick were chosen with great care, irrespective of the length of stay. Many believed that the patients were Christ's truest representatives, claiming that they were presumably respectable, and not of the very poorest stock. The occupants of this hospital were expected not only to take care of themselves but also to participate in communal religious activities in order to merit their superiors' good will and kindness.[33] This has led to a justifiable generalization that medieval hospitals were more like poorhouses and retirement homes built by a charitable person or organization.[34]

The historical evidence paints a clear picture of how hospitals in the medieval era functioned. For instance, the fifteenth-century Rule of the House within the Hospital of St. Nicholas de Bruille in Tournai in modern-day Belgium (founded approximately in 1230) gave full weight to the connection between treatment and health, with six Augustinian nurses and some trainees in charge of caregiving. This document explains how the sisters prepared food, fed the patients based on their infirmities and their preference, and how they took care of the patients until they regained their health.[35]

Nevertheless, accounts of medical care from the medieval period may have exaggerated the capabilities of healers, including surgeons, physicians, magicians, and holy men, to actually cure the sick. Medical healers of the medieval world focused more on prognosis, opining on what would happen with or without the use of medication. For instance, a recent synopsis of *Medicine in the English Middle Ages* by Faye Getz reveals that, in 1205, the personal physician to Archbishop Hubert Walter did nothing more than prognosticate about his illness. Rather than administer drugs or inspect urine, he advised the first confession, then the last rites.[36] Many medieval healers focused on diet as the main tool for preventing diseases. It was also commonplace for non-physicians to advise on matters of health. The lay approach to preserving health insisted on maintaining a correct emotional balance. It further suggested that concepts such as motion, rest, repletion and evacuation, sex, and good cheer belonged to medical procedure as much as dieting and regimen did.[37]

Monasteries later replaced these larger *xenones* in meeting the needs of the sick after they were shut down due to the loss in revenues following the death of Charlemagne. Monastery infirmaries often operated out of small houses, had a pharmacy and garden of medicinal plants, and provided the basics of food, shelter, and general nursing for the poor and lame. They were a haven for travelers and pilgrims. From the seventh century on, surgeries were performed in a variety of institutions and at varying levels of sophistication. The many names given to these institutions, including hospice, hostel, poorhouse, sick house, and hospital, reflected the diversity of these establishments, despite some overlap in their function. Developed under the auspices of the Church, the majority of these structures provided some form of welfare.[38]

By the tenth century, monasteries became an integral part of the healthcare system, as the care of sick members of the community became an important obligation within each monastery. Apart from an infirmary for the faithful, each monastery had a hospital in which physicians were cared for. By the eleventh century, some monasteries began training their physicians,[39] and monasteries soon became a central node of Christianity and medical care throughout Europe. Medieval medicine incorporated the monastic tradition of herbals and botany. All monastic gardens included medicinal plants, and the herbal medicine they produced became a mainstay of the treatments provided by monasteries. Monks often wrote treatises on herbal medicine that were frequently modified from one copy to the next, with drawings and notes added to the margins as the monks acquired more knowledge and experimented with the remedies and plants described in the books.

The rich body of literature, influencing this practice, consisted of translations of texts from classical antiquity, such as *Naturalis Historia* written by Pliny in 77–79 CE and *De Materia Medica* written by Dioscorides in 50–70 CE, and Greek medical texts.[40] The Arabic translations of classical Greek medical texts, translated by monks, allowed the ancient Hellenic world of medicine to help change the course of Western medicine in the Middle Ages.[41] As these texts quickly spread between schools or monasteries in neighboring regions, they hastened the rediscovery of ancient medical knowledge in Western Europe.[42] The medical practice in Europe was isolated geographically until after the military pilgrimages, aka crusades, that began in the late eleventh century when cultural encounter re-shaped the discursive and textual horizons across the Mediterranean.

Islamic World

The advent of Islam in the seventh century in Arabia accelerated the development of places of care in various forms across the Middle East, North Africa, and into the Iberian Peninsula. Emphasizing the importance of physical, mental, and social health, the Prophet Mohammed turned good health into an individual mandate while encouraging the wealthy to contribute to the cause of public health however they could. The earliest hospitals in the Islamic world were most probably designed based on Greco-Persian models in the pre-Islamic era, especially Jundi Shapur (Gundi Shapur), the Sassanian university hospital in modern-day southern Iran.[43]

As one of the most preeminent academic centers in the world between the sixth and eighth centuries CE, Jundi Shapur was a haven for many international scholars, especially Greek physicians exiled by the Byzantine Emperor Justinian.[44] It not only served as a model emulated by hospitals elsewhere in the Islamic world but also laid the foundations for the Renaissance age of Islamic science and medicine. The Prophet Mohammed's physician was a graduate of Jundi Shapur.[45] Furthermore, the Abbasid Caliph Abu Jafar Al-Mansour (r. 754–75) appointed the Nestorian chief of Jundi Shapur as his court physician. Later, Caliph Harun Al-Rashid (r. 786–809) invited his son to Baghdad to build the first *bimaristan* (hospital) in their new capital, Baghdad.[46]

Bimaristans in the Islamic world could be either fixed or mobile. While the former were built mostly in dense urban settings near other landmarks, such as mosques, madrasas, libraries, palaces, and bazaars, the latter followed the tent cities (*ordu*) that were erected for kings and rulers moving across regions.[47] In most tent cities, a separate tent or quarter was erected for the wounded or sick. With the elaboration of the concept of mobile hospitals, dispensaries with doctors and pharmacists would also eventually accompany the *ordu*.[48]

In contrast to medieval Europe, which struggled with major health issues, the medieval Islamic world experienced a blossoming in public health through the construction of new cities, amenities, and hospitals. Multiple factors explain this development. First and foremost, Islam encouraged people to use their charity funding, such as *zakat* and *sadaqa*, for health purposes and donate money for the construction of new hospitals and places of care, which were constructed as *waqf* (charity) properties.[49] Ironically, this construction boom occurred in parallel with increased reverence among ordinary people and healers for religious rituals, institutions, figures (e.g., sufis, imams, etc.), and Islamic buildings (e.g., shrines and mosques).[50] Moreover, the patronage networks for many urban projects, especially after the twelfth century, focused on initiatives that promoted health in an urban context through the construction of new urban amenities, such as water fountains and places of care, the implementation of more effective means of garbage collection, and the enforcement of sanitation and hygiene standards. Powerful political figures interested in securing a legacy for themselves would sponsor the construction of urban hospitals and healthier quarters for their subjects.[51] These hospitals signified growth, civilization, and scientific progress not only for newly founded cities such as Baghdad but also for cities invaded by Muslims after the eighth century.

The increasing political patronage by Muslim rulers, especially after the tenth century, resulted in the spread of science and medicine in the Islamic world, mass translation of manuscripts from Greek, Roman, Persian, and Indian,[52] and consequently the rise of a unique class of scientists and researchers who made huge contributions to science not only in the Islamic world but also beyond.[53] Benefiting from the largesse of political figures, these scientists mostly worked with the major schools and academies. For instance, the Persian physician, Ibn Sina, or Avicenna (980–1037), who has been also called the father of early modern medicine, wrote a medical encyclopedia, *The Canon of Medicine*, that served as a major reference in the Islamic world and in Europe until 1650. He is credited for major medical discoveries, some of which resulted in developments in hospital design such as the creation of quarantines.[54] The growth of science and medicine in the Islamic world also had to do with the extensive engagement of non-Muslims, especially Jews and Christians, in the medical field, whose expertise highly contributed to the development of medicine and hospitals in the Islamic world.

While the wealthy were traditionally treated within their own homes, hospitals received patients from all backgrounds, cutting across age, race, gender, and religion. The main mission of hospitals was to provide a shelter for the ill, but the historical records[55] refer to a wide range of typologies for places of care: general hospitals, hospices, mental asylums and psychiatric facilities, and specialized hospitals for specific diseases such as leprosy.[56] Many of these entities had close ties to universities, academies, and even administrative complexes that facilitated medical research. While the organization of these individual healthcare facilities of course varied, in general, the ones that were created after the fifteenth century included a more sophisticated plan that not only separated different types of patients and isolated contagious diseases but also incorporated natural elements including light, air, and water. Unfortunately, due mostly to major destructions caused by wars, the number of historic hospitals remaining in the Islamic world is a fraction of what it once was, and this explains why any research on hospitals in this region mostly relies on archival material. It should be noted again that the Greco-Roman practice along with the accomplishments of medical care in the Islamic world created an important triangulation that brought Europe into this body of knowledge centuries later.

Africa

Before the arrival of colonialists and missionaries, the places of healing in Africa were under the influence of local healing traditions, most of which were tribal in nature. According to their traditional religious belief systems, Africans believed in the omnipresent and eternal spirit of ancestors and their prayers and supplications were to be delivered through the medium of such ancestors with the help of traditional healers.[57] The healers' diversity in terms of specialty and training usually demonstrated the intricacies of tribal belief system. For example, in the Bapedi tribe in South Africa, the traditional healers included various groups: "dingaka" or "mangaka," who encompassed diviners and used bones and the spirits of the ancestors to diagnose and treat physiological, psychiatric, and spiritual conditions; the Sanusi (Sedupe) who served as both diviners and herbalists; and Babelegisi, who acted as traditional surgeons and birth attendants.[58]

Due to the spiritual, symbolic, and medical significance of plants in healing rituals in Africa, the forests were regarded as important components of health treatments.[59] The Africanist Georges Niangoran-Bouah notes that sacred groves not only housed the most important religious and ritual relics but also served as the site of ancestral burials and ritual healings. Moreover, most villagers found specific plant medicines in these sacred groves.[60] For instance, the Fang people in southern Cameroon had a "temple" at the foot of a large tree in a forest where medicinal plants grow. Signifying the forest which houses the body of god, this tree and the forest medicines are believed to be intermediaries for communicating with God.[61] Similarly, the Kom tribe in Cameroon performed healing rituals with rare medicinal plants in sacred forests.[62] In another tribe in Tanzania, the Buha, the families of individuals who contracted diseases were advised by diviners to make offerings to ancestors[63] in shrines that were made for the gods and ancestors close to the nearby sacred trees.[64]

These cases show not only the impact of plants and nature on healing procedures but also their central role in defining the places of care in traditional tribal life in Africa, prior to the arrival of missionaries. The healers not only used natural sites to conduct healing ceremonies but also conducted therapeutic ceremonies in huts. For instance, the Masai villagers in Kenya, who built their huts around a circular open yard, dedicated one of the huts to medical procedures. This hut was used as the setting to conduct healing procedures while keeping the patients separate from the rest of the tribe.

Asia

As in other regions, the history of healing and places of healing in Asia is rooted in indigenous practices and faith traditions, yet also influenced by cultures within and outside this region. In order to highlight the diversity and complexity of the development of places of healing and the impact of local political, cultural, and religious forces, here we discuss pre-colonial healing places in three countries: China, Japan, and India.

In China's early, pre-Han periods (approximately 1500–206 BCE), the concept of health and illness was animated by the idea that ailments were an accursed result of supernatural forces in the natural world or of the spirits of ancestors. Healing rituals were performed by healers well versed in local traditions, the patient's family history, and medical know-how. They first diagnosed the illness using divination and then treated it mainly with exorcism.[65] The responsibility of healing later fell into the hands of shamans and physicians. Physicians tended to be more educated and would travel from one patron to another for support.[66] The approach towards healing and medicine evolved during China's storied Han Dynasty (206 BCE–220 CE), during which healthcare consisted of "household remedies, superficial surgery, emergency medicine, demonic and spirit healing, therapeutic exercise, and sexual and breath cultivation."[67] Physicians during this period began to settle in permanent locations.[68] A few references from China's early periods discuss the concept of hospitals other than services provided by monks at Buddhist temples. The core Buddhist tenets of altruism and compassion advocated medical treatment for all and not just the wealthy and the powerful. Accordingly, Buddhist temples became places where charitable medical services were performed for the poor and medicines were distributed. Dao Xuan (596–667) of the Tang Dynasty (618–906) recorded medical supplies and books, while temples that contained a large stock of medicines occasionally served as hospitals that cared for impoverished individuals who were sick. As Buddhism spread during the Tang period, temples that acquired large plots of land established "compassionate field homes" to care for poor patients.[69] Additionally, influenced by the concept of curing diseases through bathing, an idea that originated in Buddhist scriptures, hot springs became more common during this age (Tang dynasty), many of which were funded and maintained by the government.[70]

The concept and institution of the hospital was shaped by the social reform made during the Song Dynasty (960–1279) as part of the creation of new institutions to deliver medical services.[71] During this period, local officials appear to have been more heavily involved in managing the public welfare. Su Shi (1036–1101), a Chinese official known for his literary and calligraphic works, founded a hospital for the poor in a Buddhist monastery. Within three years, the hospital was caring for more than a thousand patients. In 1098, the Song Court followed suit and required that poorhouses like the one operated by Su be established throughout its jurisdiction.[72] In addition, records indicated that the concept of quarantine was practiced during the Song Dynasty—at least one Song hospital housed patients in different wards to prevent the spread of some diseases.[73] This concept carried into the Ming (1368–1644) and Qing (1644–1911) dynasties, during which the spread of leprosy in southern China resulted in the establishment of institutions in the region for the sole purpose of quarantining the sick. These institutions began in town centers, but eventually moved beyond the city walls and into remote areas to protect the local population.[74]

As with practices in early imperial China, medical care in Japan was first provided by religious orders within their places of worship. In fact, it is believed that hospitals were introduced in Japan after the spread of Buddhism to the island around 552 CE, and official records and literary works depict Buddhist monks as proficient curers or protectors against disease.[75] At Shitennoh-ji, a large Buddhist temple completed in 593 CE in Osaka, a hospital was built adjacent to it along with a dispensary, an orphanage, and an almshouse.[76] According to the Japanese medical historian Shizu Sakai, the first official records of the existence of hospitals in Japan began in 724 CE with the founding of Seyaku-in (a no-cost dispensary) and Hiden-in (a sanitorium for the poor and orphaned) within Kofuku-ji, a Buddhist temple in the city of Nara.[77] During the Kamakura period (1192–1333), a large Buddhist hospital in Kamakura was said to have had the capacity of hospitalizing more than a thousand homeless and poor patients, providing medical and nursing care.[78] The provision of medical care in Japan changed after the arrival of Christian missionaries in the mid-sixteenth century. With the help of feudal lords and the local wealthy, the Portuguese surgeon Luis de Almeida founded a Western-style hospital in 1556 in Funai on the island of Kyushu in southern Japan. Later, Christian missionaries set up medical facilities in other cities, such as Kyoto. Initially serving the local poor, these hospitals attracted the rich and the famous from afar who sought better medical care.[79] The ban on Christianity by the Japanese government in 1618, however, resulted in the closure of these missionary-operated hospitals.

In India, there are not many traces of ancient hospitals; however, they are repeatedly mentioned in ancient texts. One of these early medical texts was Caraka-Samhita (CS), dating to the first century CE, which referred to the concept of the hospital as "a kind of infirmary," according to the physician-historian Gerrit Jan Meulenbeld.[80] Chapter 15 of CS (1.15.1–7) provides a vivid description of the construction, design, and program of hospitals:

> Thus, an expert in the science of building should first construct a worthy building. It should be strong, out of the wind, and part of it should be open to the air. It should be easy to get about in, and should not be in a depression. It should be out of the path of smoke, sunlight, water, or dust, as well as unwanted noise, feelings, tastes, sights, and smells. It should have a water supply, pestle and mortar, lavatory, bathing area, and a kitchen.[81]

Nevertheless, some historians, like Jayanta Bhattacharya, believe that in CS hospitals ought to become "an extension of home" for patients, as they ought not to be disconnected from their "domestic setting." Bhattacharya acknowledges that during that period (between the second century BCE and the third century CE)[82] the amenities offered by hospitals were intended for the wealthy and for the nobility.[83]

Centuries later in 690 CE, Xuanzang, a Chinese Buddhist monk who traveled to India, documented the concept of hospitals. Writing about many almshouses or hospices that rendered help to the poor, needy, and travelers by giving them free food and medicine,[84] Xuanzang wrote:

> The nobles and householders of this country have founded hospitals within the city, to which the poor of all countries, the destitute, cripples, and the diseased may repair. They receive every kind of requisite help gratuitously. Physicians inspect their diseases, and according to their cases order them food and drink, medicine or decoctions, everything in fact that may contribute to their ease.[85]

In parallel to the development of hospitals, Buddhists and Hindus built healing temples in South Asia and South-East Asia. One of these temples, which is fortunately well preserved, is the twelfth-century Neak Pean (or Neak Poan), a Buddhist healing temple in Siem Reap, Cambodia. It was built by the Khmer king Jayavarman VII, who has been credited with the construction of 102 hospitals during his reign.[86] This healing sanctuary was located on an island at the central pond, surrounded by four smaller ponds. Neak Pean was originally designed for medical purposes, as ancient Khmers believed that bathing in these pools would cure their diseases.[87] It is believed that the temple was in close proximity to a real hospital where patients could be cured while their kin prayed in Neak Pean, although no traces of that hospital remain.

While the operation of medical facilities during early medieval India was conducted through Brahmanical religious institutions,[88] the Indian hospitals of the twelfth century were in the midst of transition from being operated at religious facilities or dormitories to dedicated spaces of care.[89] Indian hospitals became more prevalent after the arrival of Muslims after the tenth century.[90] For instance, Muhammad bin Tughluq (r. 1325–52 CE) founded fixed and mobile hospitals and appointed skilled physicians for each of them.[91] Under the Bahamani king Zafar Khan (r. 1347–58 CE), a large hospital was constructed in South India. He not only endowed lands and used the income generated to provide medicine, food, and water for the sick, but also dispatched both Hindu and Muslim physicians to treat the patients.[92] This serves as an example of a ruler adopting different approaches to caring for the sick in medieval India before the start of the Mughal dynasty, which is widely credited for the construction of hospitals in India after the sixteenth century. The surviving structures and the miniature paintings depicting scenes of treatment demonstrate how Mughal rulers and nobles adopted and adapted ideas coming from the Persianate world to develop facilities for the treatment of the sick and the destitute.

Americas

Before the arrival of European explorers in 1492, the American continent was occupied by a diverse range of peoples and political systems. The major pre-colonial civilizations, including the Mayans, Aztecs, and Incas, demonstrated advances in urbanism, technology, science, and architecture. Although these civilizations were highly developed before the arrival of Spanish and Portuguese voyagers, there were ethnically indigenous groups living primitively in large parts of America, including the Amazon forest.

Most first nations in America (referred to as native or indigenous people) believed in a holistic path of health and well-being and that many illnesses were also connected to spiritual health.[93] Thus, faith healers, shamans, and priests were made responsible for healing the body and purifying the spirit of the afflicted; health and healing had a mystical or magical connotation for these Americans.[94] For instance, in the Mayan civilization, priests and shamans, professions whose membership numbers peaked between 400 and 700, were responsible for the practice of medicine.[95] Their collective knowledge was passed on through the generations.[96] On the other hand, in these pre-colonial traditions, people were familiar with the medicinal and spiritual properties of plants, flora, herbs, trees, and roots. For instance, in the Aztec Empire, the garden was the apothecary, and the gardener was thought of as an expert on preparing medications.[97]

The first nations across the Americas practiced local healing traditions in open spaces or tents. For instance, when Europeans first established contact with the Kamayura (Kamaiura) tribe in 1884, they observed that this tribe had combined the healing properties of plants with rituals concerning the power of spirit animals, demonstrating their beliefs in the unity of the cosmos—in which humans, animals, and nature were one.[98] In Brazil, to this day, the pajes use a ritual altar, called a "mesa," where diverse artifacts are displayed. Those artifacts originated from living creatures, plants, and/or rocks, and they are believed to have harnessed the power of cure and to permit the pajes to communicate with deities. These artifacts were used to summon the gods in order to guarantee full recovery of the ill. These artifacts and the act of summoning the gods were imperative, since it was believed that, in their absence, the botanical remedies themselves would have no healing effect. In another tribe in present-day Brazil, the Kariri-Xoco, religious healing rituals took place inside a tent built with fresh leaves from Ouricury palm trees, which were believed to be the actual manifestation of the Warakidza god. In what is known today as Argentina, the Guarani tribe performed their healing rituals outdoors, so that the entire village could participate.[99]

Although historians speak of the existence of botanical gardens and ritual tents among many ethnic groups, in the Mayan and Aztec civilizations, whether hospitals existed is mostly unknown.[100] A lack of hospitals might be explained by the common indigenous belief of cosmic unity,[101] according to which a specific place for healing was unnecessary, as nature and the open environment could actively facilitate the healing process.[102]

Early Modern Era

Coinciding with the emergence of three powerful empires in the Islamic world—the Ottomans, Safavids, and Mughals—the European Renaissance and, subsequently, the Enlightenment revolutionized Western medicine. Medical practices in Europe in the post-medieval age were based on translation projects and increased awareness of Islamicate practice, which in turn had already incorporated Greco-Roman anatomical treatment and bodily investigation and diagnosis. Furthermore, the burst of scientific inquiry and free thought during these eras reinvigorated scientific research in medical fields, leading to sweeping discoveries in the study of anatomy and diseases, as well as fruitful cross-cultural exchanges between physicians and healers. Simultaneously, as cities grew, putting greater stress on public health, sanitation took on a more prominent role in urban planning, while new kinds of hospitals were built to attend to the mental, social, and physical health of urban populations. As urban infrastructure now consciously addressed public health, cities became less susceptible to disease outbreaks and fundamentally more livable.

Along with connections with the Islamic world which opened Europe to new knowledge, the new discoveries catalyzed by the Renaissance also formed the bedrock of modern medical practices, characterized by greater accuracy, effectiveness, and comprehensiveness. Some of the key areas of innovations during this period included research into human anatomy by Andreas Vesalius (1514–64) and Leonardo Da Vinci (1452–1519), the study of blood circulation by William Harvey (1578–1657), pharmaceutical discoveries by Paracelsus (1493–1541), and advancements in surgical practices by Ambrose Paré (1510–90). While disease outbreaks and plague epidemics continued to occur during the Renaissance, hospitals moved toward greater specialization and secularization—and away from the domineering influence of the Catholic Church, which nonetheless remained an influential player.[103]

According to historian of the Renaissance John Henderson, hospitals in the Italian Renaissance were civic institutions that also played a religious role. In Florence, the center of the medical Renaissance, hospitals were regarded not only as important charities but also as crucial architectural monuments.[104] These hospitals were both more numerous and more diverse in size and typology compared to those in the medieval period.[105] And, unlike the hospitals of that age, which primarily served the clergy and their charges, those of the Renaissance focused their attentions on the infirm poor.[106] Architecturally, the Florentine Renaissance-era hospitals were known for their aesthetic qualities.[107] Several exterior features, such as frescoes, religious- and charitable-themed decorative elements, and loggia, distinguished them as city monuments, standing apart from other civic buildings. In fact, it has been suggested that, in addition to its aesthetic role, the loggia served as a buffer between the public (the street) and the private (the institution) while providing a waiting area for patients that also protected them from extreme weather.[108] Generally, Italian Renaissance hospitals possessed similar functional spaces: male and female wards, a pharmacy, cloisters and a church, kitchen and refectory, living quarters for the staff, and storage areas.[109] Some hospitals placed patients in separate sections according to their ailments, which in turn were arranged internally by gender.[110] In addition to the church, an altar was placed at the head of each of the wards (ward chapel) from which the chaplain would celebrate Mass with the patients. The presence of both functional and spiritual spatial elements at these hospitals affirmed their mission of healing both body and soul.[111]

In England, the Reformation in the 1530s and subsequent Dissolution of the Monasteries by Henry VIII (r. 1509–47) shuttered many of the hospitals run by monks for the poor and the sick.[112] Even before the Reformation, the growing power of laypeople gradually overshadowed that of the Church. At hospitals, the laity—as individuals and in guilds—began to assume responsibilities as founders and governing bodies. Although the involvement of the clergy in hospitals and almshouses decreased, the process of hospital secularization in England was complicated by the fact that many hospitals continued to gather alms associated with indulgences.[113] During the Reformation, English hospitals and almshouses varied considerably in size, age, and financial and physical condition. Some survived this period of change; others did not. London, for example, had lost five of its ancient hospitals by the 1560s[114] but acquired two new ones.[115]

In addition to hospitals that treated general ailments, specialized hospitals continued to exist and develop during the Renaissance period that confined those with commutable diseases. The proliferation of pox, which later was identified as syphilis, in Europe in the mid-1490s also facilitated the creation of specialized hospitals in Italy, Germany, and England, often situated away from densely populated areas.[116]

For instance, in Italy, the pesthouse, or *lazaretto*, was especially designed to treat individuals afflicted, or suspected of being afflicted, with plagues or other infectious diseases. The pesthouse traced its roots to the late medieval hospitals for housing sick or needy individuals. In 1423, Venice established its first permanent pesthouse in what used to be a hospice for pilgrims on the small island of Santa Maria de Nasova. Initially, only one or two physicians and three servants under the supervision of a prior ran the twenty-bed facility. Within a few years, the Venetian pesthouse expanded its staff to include a priest, male and female servants, boatmen, and gravediggers. By the end of the fifteenth century, pesthouses were needed to receive plague patients in many northern European cities, including Münster, Frankfurt, and Nürnberg in Germany. As Guenter B. Risse writes, the purpose of these institutions was "to guarantee physical separation between the healthy and those suspected of having or already afflicted with pestilence with simultaneously ensuring social control."[117] By the sixteenth century, the best-known Italian example of a permanent *lazaretto* was a structure in Milan. By then, the Milanese authorities believed the plague was transmitted by contact and not by wind or vapor. Each of the Milanese pesthouse's 280 units faced a central courtyard with a chapel and contained a bed, toilet, fireplace and chimney, and windows facing the courtyard and allowing for the flow of open air. It also featured guard towers, a moat repurposed as a sewer, and a separate canal system for laundry.[118] As the prevalence of plague gradually dwindled in the eighteenth century, some pesthouses were adapted to treat smallpox patients and, in the nineteenth century, sufferers of typhus and cholera. Others became prisons or military hospitals.[119]

The pox house, or *Blatternbaus*, was another type of specialized institution established during the Renaissance era. It provided isolation for treatment of victims of the pox. The first pox houses were established in southwest Germany. In 1495, one of the biggest community hospitals specializing in pox was founded in Augsburg. This typical *Blatternbaus* took the form of a townhouse with separate rooms for male and female patients as well as rooms for the perishing and the convalescents. It also had a unique feature called the *Holzstube*, or sauna room, where sweating was induced in the patients as part of their treatment.[120] This demonstrates how existing architectural infrastructure was utilized to address public health issues and to house patients.

While most European hospitals at the height of the Renaissance continued to serve charitable ends, such as providing shelter, food, and religious guidance, many large-scale hospitals began to focus more sharply on restoring their patients' physical health. This was primarily because of the shift in patient demographics, as greater numbers of younger workers regarded hospitals as the first line of help when they fell ill.[121] This trend continued in the seventeenth and eighteenth centuries in Europe, as economic growth, political stability, and medical discoveries resulted in improving public health, and led to policies to ensure urban health, ultimately establishing hospitals as a major building typology, and later exporting the concept of general and specialized hospitals to European colonies across the world.

Colonialism in Asia, Africa, and Americas

Despite diverse and multitudinous approaches to the design and construction of institutions containing diagnostic treatments in pre-colonial communities, the development of the established healthcare system is often attributed to Christian missionaries and colonialism in various parts of the world, which mostly initiated the delegitimization of earlier methods of treatment by using European models rather than creating a hybrid medical practice. What makes the study of medical design in the colonial era complicated is its complex chronology and dynamics in various contexts from the Americas to Southeast Asia. Scholars have contradictory opinions on the motivations behind the development of colonial medicine in Africa and beyond. For instance, the experts on African medicine Seggane Musisi and Nakanyike Musisi state that colonial medicine in Africa not only opened Africa for trade and exploitation but also enabled colonial powers to conquer, occupy, and "civilize" Africa by offering medical treatments to European explorers, missionaries, administrators and their families, and native Africans. Traditional medicines were "observed, but not studied," and often "ridiculed," "banned," and "demonized."[122] Unlike Musisis, some other scholars appear to take a more sympathetic view toward colonial medicine, seeing it as a tool that helped advance imperialism.

Emphasizing that European authorities had different ways of managing the variety of healing systems in their colonies, the medical anthropologist Cristiana Bastos explains that Portuguese colonialism was "more interactive, more humane, gentle and benign" than other forms of colonialism.[123] According to Bastos, borrowing from indigenous healing practices or combining both indigenous and European practices (hybridization) were acceptable in the Portuguese colonies at a time when European medicine was not dominant in those colonies and plans for establishing an empire on the continent had not yet matured.[124] An example is the suggestion made by Ferreira dos Santos, the director of the Mozambique Health Services, to construct hospital buildings like hut villages to reduce costs and increase Portugal's appeal to native Africans.[125] Bastos believes that this attention to the local context seems to be a pattern for the Portuguese: at the colonial medicine conference held in Lisbon in 1920, more than one of the Portuguese delegates presented their recommendations to use and adopt native medicine in medical practice in the African colonies.[126] That said, Bastos admits that, as the end of the nineteenth century approached and the desire for establishing an empire was cemented, adaptation of European medicine became a key tool of control.[127]

As noted, modern European healing traditions came to Africa first through religious missionaries. Although the first missionary contact with Africa traced back to the sixteenth century, "missionary medicine" as we know it began in the eighteenth and nineteenth centuries as the result of the Protestant evangelical movement.[128] In East Africa, for example, mission dispensaries, hospitals, and clinics began to be established in the interior from the 1880s onwards. The places of healing in these missionary organizations were founded in the growing theology of healing within an evangelical setting, the rise of the professional physician, and the emergence of colonial establishment and domination.[129] According to the Africanist Michael Jennings, for most of the early colonial era across sub-Saharan Africa, and among British colonies in particular, the majority of biomedical services offered to the natives were provided by missions. For instance, the first Western hospitals, clinics, and doctors in Tanganyika (modern-day Tanzania) were managed by missionaries.[130]

It should be noted that mission doctors and the British Colonial Medical Service worked closely together as partners. Historian Yolana Pringle explains the reasons behind such partnerships in the context of Uganda: some missionaries desired to broaden their outreach; some wanted to rise professionally; and some hoped to make more income beyond what they perceived as inadequate missionary allowances.[131] Such strategic partnerships might have also resulted due to the lack of resources on the part of the colonial governments. This issue was raised in a 1903 complaint by Robert Moffat, the principal medical officer in Uganda who indicated that government support to native hospitals was so dismal that no native hospitals could "be dignified by the name," and that hospitals with government support consisted "generally of small temporary sheds or huts in which a sick man can be sheltered."[132]

In most cases, medical reforms enacted in a colonizer's home county were subsequently introduced in their colonies. For example, in Indonesia, the concept of mental health facilities was introduced in the late nineteenth century by Dutch colonizers, who implemented their own reform of mental health care about thirty years prior. Accordingly, four mental health hospitals were established between 1882 and 1923. Two of these hospitals accepted both European and indigenous patients. However, inequality existed in their respective treatment: hospitals available to European patients included baths, bed, and open air; for indigenous patients, most males engaged in occupational (primarily agricultural) therapy.[133]

Especially after the eighteenth century, the expansion of European colonial power resulted in the construction of new hospitals and extensions of existing ones. Under the British authorities' direction, the Hong Kong Government Civil Hospital, which once operated in temporary buildings, was relocated to a two-story masonry building in 1880. Nine years later, a three-story building was built, bringing the hospital's capacity to receiving inpatients from 1,055 to 1,793.[134] The new building was a "Western-style" building in which "lighting and ventilation were optimized, creating favorable conditions for treating patients with infectious disease."[135] It was also noted that the spatial organization of this hospital, run by colonial authorities, was very different from that of other hospitals: based on the concepts of Western medicine, the hospital established a laboratory, a mortuary, a surgical room, and rooms for handling infectious diseases and conducting vaccinations. This stood in contrast to its Chinese counterparts, such as the Tungwah Hospital, the first hospital in Hong Kong that practiced Chinese medicine, and both spatial arrangements were put to the test during Hong Kong's plague epidemic in 1894. According to the colonial authorities, the Tungwah Hospital became "a hotbed of plague" due to its spatial arrangement and, specifically, the absence of a bacteriological laboratory, post-mortem room, and surgical room. It also lacked an isolation ward.[136] This case shows how colonizers saw a need to create a reform in healthcare design as a tool to enhance their power and protect their new subjects.

On the other side of the globe, scientific and geographical advances made by Europeans resulted in their so-called "discovery" of the New World.[137] Starting in 1492, a clash of cultures commenced in the Americas between colonizers and native inhabitants—whether between the Spanish and the Aztecs, or between the Portuguese and the Tupi-Guaranis in South America. The early colonizing efforts by the Spanish and Portuguese resulted in invasions, destructions, and the complete decimation of the native pre-colonial civilizations. Through the first three centuries of colonization, no formal health systems existed in the continent. The colonizers living in American lands had no preference in being treated by their fellow countrymen or by members of the first nations.[138] Even in the fifteenth century, and especially in Brazilian territory, the Portuguese would practice healing through witchcraft as they deemed fit.[139] This melting pot of healing techniques is depicted by the painter Jean Baptiste Debret in the painting *Boutique de barbier* (1821), in which black surgeons would have their offices on the sidewalks of local markets, offering free or low-cost treatment to patients who could not afford visits to a formal European doctor. In addition, Jesuit priests responsible for converting and educating indigenous people took responsibility for the act of healing by acquiring indigenous knowledge and gaining international acclaim with their medical innovation and efficacy. Since the Jesuits had access to both European and indigenous medicine, they became the link between these two very different universes.[140]

Marking the start of professional medicine, the first Santa Casa de Misericordia, or Holy Mercy House, was inaugurated in 1529 in Olinda, northeast of Brazil. The original Holy Mercy House was founded by Queen Leonor in Portugal in 1498. Its main purpose was to house the poor and the ill by catholic principles, but it also helped establish Portugal's colonial dominance overseas. However, there was no formal education for doctors or standards of performance criteria for hospitals.[141] Santa Casas, as they are commonly known, served as local hospitals for low-income communities and homeless individuals. The Holy Mercy House, also served by the Jesuits, is considered the first charity organization in the Americas.[142]

It was decades and even centuries after colonization that European hospitals were introduced in Central and South America. Some countries had a slower transition from their shaman-administered and indigenous medicine to European and scientific medicine. For instance, in Guatemala it was not until 1773 that the first Health Council was created, targeting the typhus outbreak at the time. Many health campaigns traced their origins to that council, especially the ones concerning cleanliness and disease epidemics.[143]

The dynamics of colonial hospital construction in Central and South America had to do with local politics. For instance, Brazil opened its first facility in 1852 upon the approval of a decree authorizing the construction of mental health hospitals.[144] It was a much-needed action since the "madmen and imbeciles,"[145] as they were called, would wander around the streets, be thrown in jail, or be mistreated by institutions such as the Santa Casas.[146] The first institute for the mentally ill was the Pedro II Hospice for the Alienated, which was located in Rio de Janeiro.[147] The French doctor Philippe-Marius Rey, who visited this facility in 1875, described it as being rectangular in shape with no external interruptions, apart from the hospital church. The building was two stories high with an exterior stairway that marked the main entrance and the central portion of the building, where the hospital administration, consultation room, kitchen, and dining hall were located. There was also access to a church, a food pantry, and a pharmacy across from the central portion of the building. Addressing the indigenous people's legacy and knowledge of the healing properties of plants, the kitchen and the pharmacy were connected through a herbal garden, which served as an area for food and medicine preparation.[148] Additionally, patients would have their artwork displayed in a room located on the second floor, as straw handcrafts and sewing were some of the therapies offered by the hospital.[149]

The left and right wings housed men and women, respectively. Both of the lateral wings of the hospital were symmetrical to one another and could be accessed from the central area of the building. Typical of buildings from the nineteenth century, the facility had the same divisions on the ground and second floors in order to ease the structural loads into the ground. However, the second floor also had laundry rooms, a library, and terraces for patients to enjoy. The ground floor was used to house mentally ill patients who were paranoid, had mobility constraints, or had epilepsy. It also housed violent patients who had committed crimes, with special asylum cells similar to those in Europe, where the exterior wall, made of wood, could be moved toward the other walls, limiting the size of the cells. The second floor housed patients who were calm in their demeanor and those with other different diagnoses.[150] The Pedro II Hospice for the Alienated was in use until 1944, at which point all the patients were relocated to different hospitals in the area.[151] This hospital is a very good example of nineteenth-century colonial hospitals outside Europe that were programmed, designed, and constructed purely based on advanced principles of hospital design in Europe with almost no major input from the local context.

Conclusion

This brief review of healthcare facilities in the pre-modern era highlights a few major points. First, the history of places of care shows two parallel movements, one having to do with so-called Western medicine, which itself is the byproduct of the progress of science and medicine in many countries across the world including non-Western countries; the other one having to do with a medical care system that was based on indigenous medical traditions across the world, which were not necessarily aligned with the development or discoveries of Western medicine. This chapter demonstrates how fluidly places of care were designed in vernacular traditions and how these places were perceived differently from the movement of hospital design established and evolved across geographies. Second, the historical development of healthcare facilities has been the result of complex intersections of factors, including local politics, cultural/social/religious contexts, and medical traditions. Third, the emergence of the specialized or so called modern hospital concept in the nineteenth century is indebted not only to the rapid and groundbreaking medical discoveries in this era but also to centuries of historical development of places of care since ancient times.[152] In other words, while the concepts of medical practice and physician are not modern, their hegemonic status is modern, as it is part of the "disciplinization" of the nineteenth century of sciences and even the humanities more generally. Fourth, while colonialism and missionaries are rightly blamed for their widespread major destructions and diminishments of regional civilizations and local communities, they should be credited for establishing a unified and homogeneous concept of the European hospital in various parts of the world, especially after the seventeenth century. This trend contributed in a major way to the unification of the concept of the hospital in various parts of the world before the establishment of the modern hospital in the nineteenth century, which is based on the concentration of medical knowledge, funding, and practitioner in one institutional context. Despite earlier nuanced approaches and multiple orientations to the body and its treatments in various contexts, the colonialism modernity initiated a process of exclusion and marginalization, this procedure is now being corrected, with the re-introduction of traditional, alternative, and holistic treatment methods into the presumably "Western" system of diagnosis and care.

Acknowledgment: I would like to thank my research assistants Naomi Wong Hemme and Jessica Freitas for their help with the preliminary research and my friend Heather Ferguson for reviewing the earlier draft of this chapter.

Notes

1. Cor Wagenaar, *Architecture of Hospitals* (Rotterdam: Netherlands Architecture Institute, 2006), 255.
2. For more about changes in medicine and hospitals, see Guenter B. Risse, *Mending Bodies, Saving Souls: A History of Hospitals* (New York: Oxford University Press, 1999); Mary Lindemann, *Medicine and Society in Early Modern Europe* (Cambridge: Cambridge University Press, 2010); Laurence I. Conrad et al., eds., *The Western Medical Tradition: 800 BC–1800 AD* (Cambridge: Cambridge University Press, 1995); John Henderson, *The Renaissance Hospital: Healing the Body and Healing the Soul* (New Haven: Yale University Press, 2006); Michel Foucault, "The Politics of Health in the Eighteenth Century," in *Power/Knowledge*, ed. Colin Gordon (New York: Pantheon Books, 1980), 166–82; Michel Foucault, *The Birth of the Clinic* (London: Routledge, 2003). On architectural changes in Western hospitals, see Harriet Richardson, ed., *English Hospitals, 1660–1948: A Survey of Their Architecture and Design* (Swindon: Royal Commission on the Historical Monuments of England, 1998); Jeanne Kisacky, *Rise of the Modern Hospital: An Architectural History of Health and Healing, 1870–1940* (Pittsburgh: University of Pittsburgh Press, 2017).
3. J. J. Mark, "Egyptian Medical Treatments," *Ancient History Encyclopedia*, accessed October 12, 2019. https://www.ancient.eu/article/51/egyptian-medical-treatments/
4. J. Barr, "Vascular Medicine and Surgery in Ancient Egypt," *Journal of Vascular Surgery* 60, no. 1 (July 2014): 260–3.
5. For more information on medicine in Ancient Egypt, please read the following: N. I. Ebeid, *Egyptian Medicine in the Days of the Pharaohs* (Cairo: General Egyptian Book Organization, 1999); J. W. Estes, *The Medical Skills of Ancient Egypt* (Canton, MA: Science History Publications, 1993).
6. Allen D. Spiegel, "Hammurabi's Managed Health Care—Circa 1700 B.C.," *Managed Care*, accessed January 29, 2019. https://www.managedcaremag.com/archives/1997/5/hammurabis-managed-health-care-circa-1700-bc.
7. C. F. Kleisiaris, C. Sfakianakis, and I. V. Papathanasiou, "Health Care Practices in Ancient Greece: The Hippocratic Ideal," *Journal of Medical Ethics and History of Medicine* 7, no. 6 (March 2014).
8. Charles Allison Behr, *Aelius Aristides and The Sacred Tales* (Amsterdam: A. M. Hakkert, 1968), 251.
9. According to historian Guenter Risse, water had a symbolic cleansing quality in ancient Greek culture. Hence, it was believed that springs had a prognostic power, since they combined the cleansing quality of water with the good spirits thought to reside in the mountains and olives tree groves that surrounded them (Risse, *Mending Bodies*, 22).
10. Kleisiaris et al., "Health Care Practices in Ancient Greece."
11. At some other locations, there were also smaller shrines at the outskirts devoted to other deities, such as sacred dogs and snakes; see Robert Garlands, *Introducing New Gods: The Politics of Athenian Religion* (Ithaca: Cornell University Press, 1992), 116–35.
12. Risse, *Mending Bodies*, 28.
13. Emma J. Edelstein, Ludwig Edelstein, and Gary B. Ferngren, *Asclepius: Collection and Interpretation of the Testimonies* (Baltimore: Johns Hopkins University Press, 1998), 164.
14. Risse, *Mending Bodies*, 29.
15. Alison Burford, *The Greek Temple Builders at Epidauros* (Liverpool: Liverpool University Press, 1969), 50.
16. Dorothy Porter, *Health, Civilization and the State: A History of Public Health from Ancient to Modern Times* (London: Routledge, 1999), 19.
17. Andrew T. Crislip, *From Monastery to Hospital: Christian Monasticism & the Transformation of Health Care in Late Antiquity* (Ann Arbor: University of Michigan Press, 2005), 125. Also see Risse, *Mending Bodies*, 46–7.

18. It is believed that the *valetudinarium* anticipated the Christian hospital (ibid., 50).
19. Lucius J. M. Columella, *On Agriculture (De Re Rustica)*, trans. H. Boyd Ash, vol. 3 (Cambridge, MA: Harvard University Press, 1960), 183.
20. Crislip, *From Monastery to Hospital*, 127.
21. Risse, *Mending Bodies*, 49.
22. Anonymous, "Household Medicine in Ancient Rome," *The British Medical Journal* 1, no. 2140 (1902): 39–40.
23. Risse, *Mending Bodies*, 76.
24. T. McHugh, "Establishing Medical Men at the Paris Hôtel-Dieu, 1500–1715," *Social History of Medicine* 19, no. 2 (2006): 209–24.
25. Kristen L. Mauk and Mary Hobus, *Nursing as Ministry* (Burlington, MA: Jones & Bartlett Learning, 2019), 11.
26. Peregrine Horden, *Hospitals and Healing from Antiquity to the Later Middle Ages* (Aldershot: Ashgate Variorum, 2008), 45–70.
27. Timothy S. Miller, *The Birth of the Hospital in the Byzantine Empire* (Baltimore: Johns Hopkins University Press, 1997), xi.
28. All those who carried out the instructions of the god-inspired man recovered their health while those who disobeyed him—through neglect, by resorting to doctors or by using a different treatment plan—did not.
29. Nigel Allen, "Hospice to Hospital in the Near East: An Instance of Continuity and Change in Late Antiquity," *Bulletin of the History of Medicine* 64, no. 3 (1990): 446–62.
30. Nicholas Orme and Margaret Elise Graham Webster, *The English Hospital 1070–1570* (New Haven: Yale University Press, 1995), 49.
31. Barbara S. Bowers, *The Medieval Hospital and Medical Practice* (London: Routledge, 2017), 79.
32. Miri Rubin, *Charity, and Community in Medieval Cambridge* (New York: Cambridge University Press, 1987), 184–92.
33. Marjorie K. McIntosh, *Autonomy and Community: The Royal Manor of Havering, 1200–1500* (Cambridge: Cambridge University Press, 1986), 239–40.
34. Tatjana Buklijaš, "Medicine and Society in the Medieval Hospital," *Croatian Medical Journal* 49, no. 2 (2008): 151–4.
35. Quoted from Carole Rawcliffe, "Hospital Nurses and their Work," in *Daily Life in the Middle Ages*, ed. Richard Britnell (Stroud: Sutton Publishing, 1998), 57.
36. Faye Getz, *Medicine in the English Middle Age* (Princeton: Princeton University Press), 3–4.
37. Peregrine Horden, "A Non-Natural Environment: Medicine Without Doctors and the Medieval European Hospital," in *The Medieval Hospital and Medical Practice*, ed. Barbara S. Bowers (London: Routledge, 2017), 139.
38. Porter, *Health, Civilization and the State*, 22.
39. Clifford Hugh Lawrence, *Medieval Monasticism: Forms of Religious Life in Western Europe in the Middle Ages*, 2nd ed. (London: Longman, 1989), 19–40.
40. Rachel Hajar, "The Air of History (Part II) Medicine in the Middle Ages," *Heart Views* 13, no. 4 (2012): 158–62.
41. David C. Lindberg, *The Beginnings of Western Science: The European Scientific Tradition in Philosophical, Religious, and Institutional Context, Prehistory to A.D. 1450*, 2nd ed. (Chicago: Chicago: University of Chicago Press, 2007), 327.
42. Charles H. Talbot, "Medicine," in *Science in the Middle Ages*, ed. David C. Lindberg (Chicago: University of Chicago Press, 1978), 403.
43. Andrew C. Miller, "Jundi-Shapur, Bimaristans, and the Rise of Academic Medical Centres," *Journal of the Royal Society of Medicine* 99, no. 12 (December 2006): 615.
44. Husain Nagamia, "Islamic Medicine History and Current Practice," *Journal for the International Society for the History of Islamic Medicine* 2 (2003): 19–30.
45. Harry Brewer, "Historical Perspectives on Health: Early Arabic Medicine," *Journal of Social Health* 124 (2004): 184–7.
46. Nagamia, "Islamic Medicine History," 21.
47. Miller, "Jundi-Shapur," 616.
48. Per Lunde and Christine Stone, "Early Islamic Hospitals: In the Hospital Bazaar," *Health and Social Service Journal* 91, no. 4777 (December 1981): 1548–51.
49. Emilie Savage-Smith, *A Brochure to Accompany an Exhibition in Celebration of the 900th Anniversary of the Oldest Arabic Medical Manuscript in the Collections of the National Library of Medicine* (Oxford: University of Oxford, 1994).
50. Ellen J. Amster, *Medicine and the Saints: Science, Islam, and the Colonial Encounter in Morocco, 1877–1956* (Austin: University of Texas Press, 2013), 17.
51. For more information, please refer to Ahmed Ragab, *The Medieval Islamic Hospital: Medicine, Religion, and Charity* (Cambridge: Cambridge University Press, 2015).

52. Peter E. Pormann and Emilie Savage-Smith, *Medieval Islamic Medicine* (Edinburgh: Edinburgh University Press, 2007), 23.
53. In 830 CE, Caliph Al-Mamun founded Bait-ul-Hikma (House of Wisdom). The Muslim scholar and bibliographer Ibn Nadim listed fifty-seven translators who were hired by this institution to contribute to a translation of many scientific manuscripts that were granted by the Byzantine emperor (Nagamia, "Islamic Medicine History," 22).
54. Moosavi Jamal, "The Place of Avicenna in the History of Medicine," *Avicenna Journal of Medican Biotechnology* 1, no. 1 (2009): 3–8.
55. For instance, the *waqf* document for the Mansuri Hospital in Cairo included the following statement: "The hospital shall keep all patients, men and women until they are completely recovered. All costs are to be borne by the hospital whether the people come from afar or near, whether they are residents or foreigners, strong or weak, low or high, rich or poor, employed or unemployed, blind or signed, physically or mentally ill, learned or illiterate. There are no conditions of consideration and payment, none is objected to or even indirectly hinted at for non-payment. The entire service is through the magnificence of Allah, the generous one." Quoted from Nagamia, "Islamic Medicine History," 25.
56. Joel Montague, "Hospitals in the Muslim Near East: A Historical Overview," in *Mimar* 14, ed. Hasan-Uddin Khan (1984): 20.
57. M. G. Mokgobi, "Understanding Traditional African Healing," *African Journal of Physical Health Education and Recreation Dance* 20, suppl. 2 (September 2014): 26.
58. Ibid., 28.
59. Julia Falconer, "The Use of Forest Resources in Traditional Medicine," *The Major Significance of "Minor" Forest Products: The Local Use and Value of Forests in the West African Humid Forest Zone*, ed. Carla R. S. Koppell (Rome: Food and Agriculture Organization of the United Nations, 1990).
60. George Niangoran-Bouah, "Le Silence dans les traditions de culture Africaine," *Revue Ivoirienne d'Anthropologie et de Sociologie* 3 (1983): 6–11.
61. J. Binet, "Drogue et mystique: le Bwiti de Fangs (Cameroon)," *Diogéne* 86 (1974): 34–57.
62. Walter Gam Nkwi, "The Sacred Forest and the Mythical Python: Ecology, Conservation, and Sustainability in Kom, Cameroon, c. 1700–2000," *Journal of Global Initiatives: Policy, Pedagogy, Perspective* 11, no. 2 (April 2017): 39.
63. Johan H. Scherer, "The Ha of Tanganyika," *Anthropos* 54, no. 5/6 (1959): 889.
64. Salvatory Stephen Nyanto, "Indigenous Beliefs and Healing in Historical Perspective: Experiences from Buha and Unyamwezi, Western Tanzania," *International Journal of Humanities and Social Science* 5, no. 10 (October 2015): 193.
65. Constance A. Cook, "The Pre-Han Period," in *Chinese Medicine and Healing: An Illustrated History*, ed. T. J. Hinrichs and Linda L. Barnes (Cambridge, MA: The Belknap Press of Harvard University Press, 2013), 5.
66. Ibid., 11.
67. Vivienne Lo, "The Han Period," in Hinrichs and Barnes, *Chinese Medicine and Healing: An Illustrated History*, 31.
68. Ibid., 40.
69. Fan Ka-wai, "The Period of Division and the Tang Period," in Hinrichs and Barnes, *Chinese Medicine and Healing: An Illustrated History*, 78–9.
70. Ibid., 80.
71. T. J. Hinrichs, "The Song and Jin Periods," in Hinrichs and Barnes, *Chinese Medicine and Healing: An Illustrated History*, 99.
72. Ibid., 101.
73. Ibid., 111.
74. Ibid., 156–7.
75. C. Kleine, "Buddhist Monks as Healers in Early and Medieval Japan," *Japanese Religions* 37, no. 1/2 (2012): 19–23.
76. Kiyoshi Iwasa, "Hospitals of Japan: History and Present Situation," *Medical Care* 4, no. 4 (October–December 1966): 241.
77. Shizu Sakai, "History of Medical Care at Inpatient Facilities in Japan," *The Journal of the Japan Medical Association* 54, no. 6 (2011): 351.
78. Iwasa, "Hospitals of Japan," 241.
79. Sakai, "History of Medical Care," 351.
80. G. Jan Meulenbeld, *A History of Indian Medical Literature*, vol. 1A (Groningen: Egbert Forsten, 1999), 17.
81. Dominik Wujastyk, *The Roots of Ayruveda: Selections from Sanskrit Medical Writings* (New Delhi: Penguin, 2003), 36.
82. Some scholars put the date of CS between third or second centuries BCE and the period of Gupta Dynasty (CE 320–420), while others placed the date between 100 BCE and CE 150–200.

83. Jayanta Bhattacharya, "The Hospital Transcends into Hospital Medicine: A Brief Journey through Ancient, Medieval and Colonial India," *Indian Journal of History of Science* 52, no. 1 (2017): 30.
84. *The Great Tang Dynasty Record of the Western Regions*, trans. Li Ronxi (Berkeley: Numata Center for Buddhist Translation and Research, 1996), 113.
85. Xuanzang, *Si-Yu-Ki: Buddhist Records of the Western World*, trans. Samuel Beal, vol. 1 (London: Trubner & Co., 1884), lvii.
86. Charles Higham, *The Civilization of Angkor* (London: Weidenfeld & Nicolson, 2001), 127.
87. Ibid., 124–5.
88. Bhattacharya, "The Hospital Transcends into Hospital Medicine," 33.
89. "Dominik Wujastyk," *Academia*, unpublished paper, accessed May 16, 2019. https://ualberta.academia.edu/DominikWujastyk/talks
90. Fabrizio Speziale, "Introduction," in *Hospitals in Iran and India, 1500–1950s*, ed. Fabrizio Speziale (Leiden: Brill, 2012), 2.
91. R. L. Verma, "The Growth of Greco-Arabian Medicine in Medieval India," *India Journal of History of Science* 5, no. 2 (1970): 351.
92. Ghulam Yazdani, *Bidar: Its History and Monuments* (Oxford: Oxford University Press, 1944), 130.
93. "Moctezuma," *Aztec History*, accessed April 9, 2019. http://www.aztec-history.com/moctezuma.html.
94. On Line Editora, ed., *Guia Segredos Do Império 03—O Povo Asteca*, March 22, 2017.
95. Mary Koithan and Cynthia Farrell, "Indigenous Native American Healing Traditions," *The Journal for Nurse Practitioners* 6, no. 6 (2010): 477.
96. Carlos Rivera Williams, "Historia de la medicina y cirugía en América: La Civilización Maya," in *Revista Medica Hondureña* 75, no. 3 (July/August 2007): 152.
97. *Guia Segredos Do Império 03—O Povo Asteca*, March 22, 2017.
98. "Kamaiurá," *Kamaiurá—Povos Indígenas No Brasil*, accessed April 9, 2019. https://pib.socioambiental.org/pt/Povo:Kamaiurá.
99. Clarice Novaes da Mota and Rodrigo de Azeredo, *Os filhos de jurema na floresta dos espíritos: ritual e cura entre dois grupos indígenas do nordeste Brasileiro* (Maceió, Brazil: EDUFAL, 2007), 165.
100. For more information, please refer to F. J. Carod and C. Vazquez-Cabrera, "Pensamiento mágico y epilepsia en la medicina tradicional indígena," *Revista de Neurologia* 26, no. 154 (1998): 1064–8.
101. On Line Editora, *Guia segredos do império Maia: os senhores da Mesoamérica*.
102. An example of this was found among indigenous women from the Tupinamba tribe, also inhabitants of Brazilian territory. When these women were in labor, they would lie down on a wood plank or on the ground of their village, during which all of the women there would gather and help deliver her baby, supporting the idea of their perception of cosmic connection (Carlos Alberto Cunha Miranda, *A arte de curar nos tempos da colônia: limites e espaços da cura* (Recife: Editora Universitária UFPE, 2011), 237).
103. Steven E. Barkan, *Health, Illness, and Society: An Introduction to Medical Sociology* (Lanham: Rowman & Littlefield Publishers, 2016), 22.
104. John Henderson, *The Renaissance Hospital* (New Haven and London: Yale University Press, 2006), 14.
105. Ibid., 50.
106. Ibid., 15–17, 25.
107. Ibid., 70.
108. Ibid., 72, 76–7.
109. Ibid., 85.
110. Sharon Strocchia, "Caring for the 'Incurable' in Renaissance Pox Hospitals," in *Hospital Life: Theory and Practice from the Medieval to the Modern*, ed. Laurinda Abreu and Sally Sheard (Bern: Peter Lang, 2013), 72.
111. Henderson, *The Renaissance Hospital*, 87–8.
112. Arthur Salusbury MacNalty, *The Renaissance and its Influence on English Medicine, Surgery and Public Health* (London: Christopher Johnson, 1946), 17.
113. Orme and Webster, *The English Hospital*, 146.
114. John Stow, *A Survey of London. Reprinted from the Text of 1603*, ed. C. L. Kingsford (Oxford, 1908), 185, British History Online, accessed January 6, 2021. http://www.british-history.ac.uk/no-series/survey-of-london-stow/1603; A. B. Emden, *A Biographical Register of the University of Oxford, A.D. 1501 to 1540* (Oxford: Clarendon Press, 1974), 321.

115. Orme and Webster, *The English Hospital*, 161.
116. Strocchia, "Caring for the 'Incurable,'" 67–8.
117. Risse, *Mending Bodies*, 203.
118. Ibid., 204.
119. Andrew B. Appleby, "The Disappearance of Plague: A Continuing Puzzle," *Economic History Review* 33 (1980): 161–73; Paul Slack, "The Disappearance of Plague: An Alternative View," *Economic History Review* 34 (1981): 469–76.
120. Ibid., 215.
121. Risse, *Mending Bodies*, 214.
122. Seggane Musisi and Nakanyika Musisi, "The Legacies of Colonialism in African Medicine," Lecture, "The Impact of Decolonization and the End of Cold War on Health Development in Africa," Kenya, Nairobi (February 6, 2007), accessed October 21, 2018. https://www.who.int/global_health_histories/seminars/nairobi02.pdf?ua=1.
123. Cristiana Bastos, "Medical Hybridisms and Social Boundaries: Aspects of Portuguese Colonialism in Africa and India in the Nineteenth Century," *Journal of Southern African Studies* 33, no. 4 (December 2007): 768.
124. Ibid., 774.
125. Ibid., 781.
126. F. Ferreira dos Santos, "Assistência médica aos Indígenas e processos práticos da sua hospitalização," *Revista Médica de Angola* 2, no. 4 (1924): special issue dedicated to the First West Africa Tropical Medicine Conference, 51–71; J. Firmino Sant'Anna, "O problema da assistência médico-sanitária ao indígena em Africa," *Revista Médica de Angola* 2, no. 4 (1924): 73–200.
127. Ibid., 774.
128. Michael Jennings, "Healing of Bodies, Salvation of Souls: Missionary Medicine in Colonial Tanganyika, 1870s–1939," *Journal of Religion in Africa* 38, Fasc. 1 (2008): 29.
129. Ibid., 30.
130. Ibid., 28.
131. Yolana Pringle, "Crossing the Divide: Medical Missionaries and Government Service in Uganda, 1897–1940," *Beyond the State: The Colonial Medical Service in British Africa*, ed. Anna Greenwood (Manchester: Manchester University Press, 2016), 19.
132. Ibid., 21.
133. H. Pols, "The Development of Psychiatry in Indonesia: From Colonial to Modern Times," *International Review of Psychiatry* 18, no. 4 (August 2006): 363–4.
134. Kyu-hwan Sihn, "Reorganizing Hospital Space: The 1894 Plague Epidemic in Hong Kong and the Germ Theory," *Korean Journal of Medical History* 26, no. 1 (2017): 75.
135. Ibid., 73–4.
136. Ibid., 84.
137. Carmen Junqueira, "Pajés e feiticeiros," *Estudos Avançados* 18, no. 52 (2004): 289–302.
138. Miranda, *A arte de curar nos tempos da colônia*, 237.
139. Flávio Edler and M. R. F. da Fonseca, "Saber erudito e saber popular na medicina colonial," *Cadernos da ABEM* 2 (2006): 8–9.
140. Miranda, *A arte de curar nos tempos da colônia*, 237.
141. Edler and Da Foncesa, "Saber erudito e saber popular na medicina colonial," 6.
142. Renato Júnio Franco, "O modelo luso de assistência e a dinâmica das Santas Casas de Misericórdia na América portuguesa," *Revista Estudos Históricos* 27, no. 53 (2014): 5–25.
143. Élfego Rolando López Garcia, "Historia de la farmacia en Guatemala" (MA thesis, Universidad Complutense de Madrid Facultad De Farmacia, 2012), 31.
144. Ibid.
145. Galdini Raimundo Oda, Ana Maria, and Paulo Dalgalarrondo, "História das primeiras Instituições para Alienados no Brasil," *História, Ciências, Saúde—Manguinhos, Rio De Janeiro* 12, no. 3 (September–November 2005): 992.
146. Ibid., 991.
147. Ibid., 985. José Francisco Xavier Sigaud, "Reflexões sobre o trânsito livre dos doidos pelas ruas da cidade do Rio de Janeiro," *Revista Latinoamericana de Psicopatologia Fundamental* 8, no. 3 (2005): 559–62.
148. Philippe-Marius Rey, "O Hospício de Pedro II e os Alienados no Brasil (1875)," *Revista Latinoamericana de Psicopatologia Fundamental* 15, no. 2 (2012): 385.

149. Ibid., 383.
150. Ibid., 387.
151. Antonio E. Nardi, Adriana Cardoso Silva, Jaime E. Hallak, and José A. Crippa, "A Humanistic Gift from the Brazilian Emperor D. Pedro II (1825–1891) to the Brazilian Nation: The First Lunatic Asylum in Latin America," *Arquivos de Neuro-Psiquiatria* 71, no. 2 (2013): 126.
152. George Weisz, "The Emergence of Medical Specialization in the Nineteenth Century," *Bulletin of the History of Medicine* 77, no. 3 (2003): 536–75.

PART I
RELIGIOSITY: HEALTHCARE IN RELIGIOUS CONTEXT

CHAPTER 2
THE HOSPITAL DESIGN IN HISTORY
THE DICHOTOMY OF RELIGIOUS AND SECULAR CONTEXTS
Guenter B. Risse

In the introduction to his monumental *History of Architecture*, Spiro Kostof stressed the need for interpreting the full scale of building production. Since all structures reflect the societal values and aspirations of the people involved in their creation, searching for contexts in the constructed world offers valuable information about meaning and purpose. Design not only mirrors but also in return shapes culture.[1] In fact, history reveals that architecture has managed to encode a wide and often diverse spectrum of beliefs based on community needs and economic imperatives. According to first-century BCE Roman author and engineer Marcus Vitruvius, design not only satisfies symbolic and aesthetic concerns but also responds to contemporary pragmatic purposes and wants.[2]

Since the birth of the Western hospital, institutional space and design were never conceived in a void but closely followed function.[3] Together, they performed a key human task: dealing with both the physical and emotional impact of illness or preparing inmates for death. "Reading" hospital buildings, therefore, allows us to detect and illuminate shifting notions of sickness, relief, and restoration.[4] Under such circumstances, room for solemn religious rituals, compassionate nursing, and medical care left their indelible marks on a variety of buildings around the world. Their typology has been recently inventoried by employing Google Earth as a tool to locate and photograph surviving hospital structures. Indeed, the chronologically arranged collection allows access to a virtual tour of such institutions from antiquity to the present.[5]

Architectural styles should not be divorced from the physical, social, and cultural milieu in which they were conceived. A panoramic historical review of important pre-modern buildings devoted to caring for sick people discloses and confirms a gamut of beliefs about illness and strategies developed to counter and perhaps mitigate its effects.[6] In fact, hospitals have been recently included among structures said to exemplify "Quadralectic Architecture," a novel reframing of the entire field based on instinctive spatial perception and a penchant for selecting square or rectangular structures for stability and balance, ostensibly reflecting humankind's upright position and movements on a horizontal ground.[7]

Since early times, injuries and sickness with their associated disabilities have tended to disrupt peoples' ordinary lives. Pain and dysfunction triggered concern, alarm, frustration, and denial, often turning into fear and terror if symptoms persisted or worsened. Vulnerable and frequently shunned, those who became ill suddenly found themselves cast outside the realm of normal tribal foraging routines. In spite of family or community displays of empathy, individual suffering tended to impact a close-knit clan, engendering misgivings and spreading anxiety. Those afflicted and their relatives frequently entered into relationships with recognized healing experts or institutions expected to provide assistance: indeed, the ill became "patients."[8]

As with all other life experiences, sufferers and their societies eagerly searched for meaning, seeking coherent explanations for their distress. Although there are multiple definitions, most people agree that religion is an organized set of cultural beliefs, practices, and institutions that evolved in early human societies in tandem with their biological and social evolution. Since that time, explanations for the existence of life, sickness, and death have been indispensable for perceiving and interpreting causality. Events were believed to occur as a blending or balance of universal supernatural forces or particular divinities, notions that not only provided agency but also allowed for reassurance, adaptation, and meaning.[9]

Health and Architecture

As confirmed by anthropological studies of contemporary hunter-gatherers, illness during most ancient times was frequently perceived within specific supernatural contexts: a range of sacred forces and personalities governing the world. Myths based on their magical powers and alleged interventions were products of early human imagination and language. In time, elaborate doctrines came to identify particular divine agents capable of inflicting disease and thereby punishing individual failings or communal morality violations. Believed to be acting as intermediaries between humanity and the holy, especially selected tribal members, often called shamans, interpreted illness as demonic invasions for violations of social taboos. Under such circumstances, the ill were frequently held responsible for alleged misdeeds and subjected to elaborate purification ceremonies staged to appease angry and vengeful gods.[10]

Since wellness remained a uniquely personal experience based on habits, role, occupation, and emotional circumstances, sufferers also explored non-religious, empirical dimensions of their troubling situation. Trauma, discomfort and pain, mobility issues, and selective organ dysfunctions urgently demanded succor. Self-help was the first choice for therapeutic relief, based on traditional, proven domestic measures. Rest seemed intuitively essential. All means known to lessen suffering and escape mortality were considered: dietary routines could be halted, popular and available plant- and animal-based remedies tried.[11] Since our bodies are genetically programmed for recovery of functional integrity, most episodes of illness remained limited.[12]

Following frequent migrations, and the gradual rise of agriculture around 8000 BCE, expanding populations established the early civilizations in the fertile Middle East crescent. Their urban centers came to experience a growing burden of infectious disease, notably through the proliferation of lethal epidemics. Such unexpected and widespread disasters prompted increased social solidarity, cooperation, and greater attention to human suffering and provision of care.[13] Patienthood constructed as punishment for presumed personal misdeeds due to moral failing remained a widely accepted cultural view still persisting into the present day. Such entrenched religious doctrines offered possibilities for redemption and recovery through divine assistance.

As early as 4000 BCE, empires in the Ancient Near and Far East, notably Mesopotamia, Egypt, India, and China, gave greater meaning to suffering. With exploding populations ravaged by epidemic disease, these cultures offered the sick a measure of solace. Healing, therefore, changed dramatically in scope as organized religions with their elaborate pantheons of gods and goddesses came to provide anxious sufferers with a complex system of divination and magic to account for the appearance of sickness. Staging elaborate rituals in monumental temples, the authorities sought to accept their transgressions and instill a measure of faith and hope.[14] In many countries, specific individuals from the official priesthood were identified as possessing shamanistic healing skills, such as ancient Mesopotamia's magical expert, the *ashipu*, Egypt's priest *wabw*, India's exorcist, and China's *wu*, diviner and wizard.[15] In addition, both ancient Mesopotamia and Egypt staged special and communal rituals in splendid temples specially dedicated to gods of healing such as the Babylonian goddess Gula and the Egyptian Sekhmet.

In their most elementary form, all religious healing ceremonies primarily targeted the emotional aspects of experiencing sickness. They attempted to manipulate key cultural symbols and offered social support as well as opportunities for prayer, rest, and contemplation. Such efforts were designed to restore a sense of personal wholeness, control, and hope for a possible recovery. Indeed, most early societies' health notions were heavily permeated with religious and moral symbolism. Among the most enduring actions observed in ancient healing rituals was communication with the sacred and identification of causal agents—both divine and natural. With the help of family, friends, and other caregivers, as well as the mobilization of entire communities, confession as well as both spiritual and bodily purification followed.[16] Moreover, the sick could supplement their efforts by employing known domestic medicinal herbal preparations as well as consulting a cadre of lay healers and surgeons, emphasizing their empirically acquired skills.[17]

Whether religious, secular, or both, the ultimate goal was the restoration of a person's physical and spiritual balance, allowing sufferers to return and reoccupy their previous social and economic niche. With the help of powerful symbols and dramatic performances, combined with the administration of certain drugs, increasingly complex healing ceremonies evolved, supported by an assembly of buildings, including sanctuaries, shelters, eateries, and theaters. The intention was to identify and legitimate a number of distinct and divine authorities capable of punishing individuals and larger populations by sending sickness and also empathic healing agents capable of mitigating the negative effects of illness if correctly propitiated.[18]

To be successful, these pageants required special settings and structures capable of eliciting strong human feelings and enforcing a prescribed social behavior. In fact, from the earliest times, the architectural design of monumental temples with hideaway sanctuaries or chapels featuring statues of divinities linked to healing sought to impress anxious sufferers. Such impressive buildings and ceremonies arose in response to shifting ecologies of disease and human needs as well as novel interpretations to reframe health and illness. Faith was deemed an optimal vehicle for reassurance, hope, and possible recovery. Massive walls and vast courtyards allowed the participation of large crowds of sufferers who made their individual or collective pilgrimages in search of relief. While inspiring awe and reverence, the imposing buildings also offered protection, fellowship, and solidarity.

In ancient Greece, for example, a mythical and deified physician, Asclepius, became the center of a popular healing cult during the fifth century BCE that survived throughout the eastern Mediterranean for more than half a millennium.[19] Located in valleys near springs or caves and designed to impress visitors, numerous monumental temple complexes dedicated to this god and displaying his effigy became famous places of refuge and worship. Sacred springs provided for spiritual and physical cleansing. Statues of Asclepius and the public display of votive offerings gifted by previously recovering pilgrims as testament of the god's efficacy were designed to solidify the visitor's expectations for miraculous cures. Hostels or *katagogion* allowed for overnight rest and opportunities for highly suggestive dreaming experiences centering on Asclepius' divine visitations and medical advice.[20] Coincidentally, a somewhat similar cult appeared during the 26th dynasty (*c.* 400 BCE) in Hellenized Egypt, which focused on Imhotep, a legendary official and now deified sage. Originally located near the capital of Memphis in Sakkara—presumably near his original burial place—Imhotep's shrine became a popular destination for those who sought divine intervention and life-enhancing blessings. Aided by specially designed structures such as chapels and storage tunnels for votive offerings, such cults epitomized the growing faith in ritualism and magic, especially among lower levels of society.[21] Given their precarious social and economic existence in congested and unhealthy urban slums, such cults became convenient and inexpensive means for securing sympathy, reassurance, and assistance.

In the classical Greek example, Asclepius' priesthood sponsored purification rites, prayer, penance, and sacrifice, as well as suggesting and creating conditions for visitors to experience healing dreams. Submerged in an atmosphere of divine power and hope, crowds of supplicants sought advice for their health problems. Indeed, most visitors expected to have a personal and magical contact with the divinity through the medium of a vision that promised relief and restoration. Besides prayer, prescription of dietary and pharmacologically active compounds recommended by priests could follow. Later, during Roman times, the frequent staging of elaborate festivals and processions, musical contests, theatrical performances, poetry readings, and athletic competitions provided collective distraction and relaxation, putting ill visitors at ease and lifting their spirits and hope for eventual recovery. Bonds of mutual understanding and support contributed to the quest for such healing.[22]

At the same time, secular concerns about fitness and health of members belonging to the imperial Roman Army inspired the creation of a special institution in the first century CE for sick and wounded legionaries: the *valetudinarium*. Based on the use of shelters and dormitories for slaves working on large estates, these quarters were constructed within a string of fortresses built to defend the northern Roman frontier along the Rhine and Danube rivers. The building's design, a hollow rectangle symmetrically surrounded by small rooms with vestibules, opened into a central corridor circling around the entire building. In some instances, the entrance to the compound led to a larger receiving room and administrative facilities. With origins in ancient Persia, Egypt, and the Orient, and imported into ancient Greece during Hellenistic times, this popular courtyard design displayed a notable inward focus, a common feature of single or multi-story Roman town buildings. The *valetudinarium*'s spatial fragmentation prevented excessive noise and acted as a barrier to contagion, offering privacy and facilitating rest and recovery of its sick and wounded inmates.[23]

With its ideology of benevolence and salvation, the advent and spread of Christianity in the Eastern Roman Empire in the early centuries after Christ primarily targeted the urban homeless and sick poor. Adopting ancient Egyptian and Jewish models of social welfare, Church leaders acknowledged and legitimized their charitable obligations. Christ had linked an obligation to visit the sick to the essential good works necessary for earning eternal salvation. Such calls came to include gifts, food provisions, and the performance of basic caring chores. Moreover, aid was gradually extended further to offer shelter and lodging to the dispossessed. By the fourth century CE, such philanthropic efforts and a growing respect for the power of medicine in urban centers led to the creation of institutions capable of sheltering and tending to a growing number of sick brethren.[24]

The image of Christ as the Great Physician replaced the altar and statues of Asclepius and other popular pagan deities. Side by side with the establishment of ornate churches and monasteries, the early Christian clergy came to sponsor and operate a variety of simple guest houses, or *xenones*, for those who were sick and in need of shelter, food, and medicine. Primarily considered religious spaces and initially located mostly within the confines of the Byzantine Empire, these institutions facilitated the staging of ceremonies and routines intended to affirm the Christian faith and thus save the souls of gravely ill sufferers expected to die.[25]

The basic early Christian refuge or lodge sought to protect inmates from harmful outside events, a defensive posture adopted in a world still populated by hostile pagans. All such facilities stressed "*hospitalitas*."[26] The term came to be linked to the display of Christian receptiveness and kindness in hosting as well as protecting sojourners in search of sanctuary, rest, and nourishment. Their reaffirmation of spiritual beliefs offered other benefits, including recovery from illness.

Architecturally, these early hospitals followed a consistent and recognizable courtyard archetype.[27] Indeed, the lodges, large or small, consisted of square or rectangular structures featuring windowless rooms. Surrounded by a covered arcade, these secure chambers were arranged around a similarly shaped open central courtyard, often transformed into a garden or even a chapel. Once again connecting all chambers, this colonnade was primarily designed to allow light and air into the rooms while offering a path for the circulation of staff and patients. Moreover, the portico also protected guests and caregivers from sun, rain, and inclement weather, an arrangement that created an exposed core space, often converted into a park for direct contact with nature.[28]

Courtyards were traditionally considered an oasis, retreats away from the pressures of rapid urbanization. Previously, in fact, Roman villas had adopted such a scheme centuries earlier, adding pools and fountains, trees, shrubs, and flowers to their central enclosures, as well as designing pathways for internal promenades. Such spaces could be havens for privacy or focal points for socializing. Their restorative role came to be widely recognized. Soothing or invigorating, outdoor places were ideal for prayer and reflection, as well as spiritual and physical transformations. Later, the planting of juniper trees or other evergreens in such landscapes came to symbolize the Tree of Life from Genesis.[29]

Makeshift early Byzantine *xenones* or shelters were viewed as communities of the faithful, temporarily assembled in a house of God. A famous example was a complex consisting of a church, administrative residence, soup kitchen, quarters for caring personnel, and a series of lodges established in the city of Caesarea on the Mediterranean coast around 370 CE by Basil, its current bishop. The *Basileiados* was simultaneously conceived as a religious space, soup kitchen, hospice, and, at times, *nosokomeion*, a place where hired physicians managed those who were sick. Such fluid boundaries between the various tasks performed in hospitals continued throughout the Middle Ages until the Renaissance, when a new vision of man and novel social and economic conditions prompted further medicalization. Caregiving services, including medical interventions, were universally provided to all inmates, including ill religious and lay staff members, pilgrims, and the local poor.[30]

As in other regions of the medieval world, care of the sick remained a fundamental task and opportunity for the exercise of piety and reaffirmation of faith. The practice of healing sick brethren in spirit and flesh endured, performed in monasteries large and small, distributed throughout the Christian world. Establishments in the Latin West, notably those operating under the rule of Benedict of Nursia (480–547), eagerly sought to replicate the multipurpose single rectangular room format. Called the *infirmarium*, it was divided by pillars and opened directly to the chapel. Beds were arranged at right angles to the walls. Numerous arrangements and relationships between a central large hall or shelter and a chapel or church came to prevail. Although often quite small, they were all considered religious spaces with an average capacity of 4–10 beds.[31]

Hospital designs reflected both the culture and needs of society as well as the nature of individual sick persons housed in them. Strict separation of the sexes was enforced. While allowed to withdraw and rest, inmates in Christian hospitals were encouraged to fully participate in all daily religious ceremonies. Meditation and reflection were considered proper coping mechanisms for sinners. Proximity of the church or chapel allowed direct access to pageants. The rites were intended to encourage contemplation and provide spiritual solace and personal security with marginal attention paid to the physical components of their suffering. Prayer and song as well as the reception of holy sacraments would ensure eternal life or perhaps facilitate recovery. As houses of redemption, the infirmary's paramount objective was to save the souls of the sick; death was ubiquitous and thus preparations to ensure eternal life were urgent and proper.[32]

Following the devastating Black Death, the periodic presence of epidemic or endemic disease in European urban settings began to threaten entire communities, demanding stricter segregation practices and confinement. While religious symbolism, agendas, and ceremonies played a pivotal role in molding institutional communities of faith, epidemiological notions of contagion now increasingly demanded the strict separation of sick individuals from the rest of society. By the fifteenth century, therefore, in an effort to cope with new calamities like leprosy and further plague outbreaks, some Christian shelters morphed into isolated leprosaria and lazarettos. To protect the healthy, towns threatened by these scourges quarantined those presumed to suffer from these diseases.[33] Some establishments built by municipalities—often called "general hospitals" —turned out to be veritable welfare warehouses safeguarding the poor, sick, foundlings, and orphans, as well as the mad, young, and aged.[34]

Because of the demographic explosion and urbanization in Western Europe after the twelfth century, Christian hospitals began to grow in size, notably in the city-states of Italy. Guided by new aesthetic views, architects elaborated on previous hospital plans, supported by the charitable goals and aspirations of their royal, municipal, and private founders. Many "Hostels of God" came to display impressive entry gates, decorated beams, elaborate stairwells, and tiled floors. Cross-shaped, they offered four square or rectangular arms with a central altar almost always facing east, although site constraints affected orientation. The crossing often featured a tower or dome. Nestled among the transepts were several courtyards. Made of leaded glass, the high windows were decorated and stained, in sharp contrast to colorless lower ones located near the ground to provide more light and ventilation.

Nevertheless, like before, the religious purpose remained paramount: shelter a larger number of inmates and allow them to witness religious ceremonies from their beds. Prayer, chant, and the daily provision of sacramental offerings such as communion and last rites remained pivotal. To create a larger reverberation in buildings of greater volume, designers and builders recognized the need for sound-reflective and amplifying surfaces or "live" spaces through the generous use of marble, ceramic tile, and mosaics.

While the hospital's traditional religious goal was to restore faith in divine intervention, design now also was forced to address a series of practical issues emanating from the fact that ever-larger groups of distressed poor and homeless people in need of aid had successfully obtained admission, expecting to find favorable conditions that would allow their bodies to rest and replenish. The purpose was to minister to self-sustaining inmate communities sometimes numbering in the thousands. Toilets and kitchens, storage rooms for food and clothing, as well as occasional communal dining facilities were necessary. Nearby burial of deceased patients came to require adjacent cemeteries. Outwardly, the sheer monumentality of these hospital facilities came to project the enhanced wealth and power of their patrons as well as the civic identity and pride of the cities hosting them.

To further increase institutional capacity during the Italian Renaissance, some proposed two cross-like wards, one for each sex, separated by a large rectangular courtyard with a chapel at its center. Planners argued that such double-cross-shaped hospitals would allow the placement of more beds while retaining easy access to the altar, with the ceremonious center preferably oriented toward the east. In many buildings, the cross elements were combined with outer quadrangular enclosures housing staff personnel. Some church-like complexes were surrounded by an outer enclosure, allowing for rectangular courtyards and elaborate gardens endowed with fountains. Such was the case of the massive Ospedale Maggiore in Milan, designed in Renaissance style by the architect Antonio Filarete with an arched brick facade. A small-domed, square church was constructed across the entrance. Partially opened in 1458, the very large building—a consolidation of thirty smaller institutions—was eventually completed four centuries later.[35]

Perhaps the most prominent and emblematic Renaissance hospital was the Santa Maria Nuova in Florence, founded in 1288 at the site of an earlier convent. Originally arranged like a cross-shaped Christian basilica, this institution became a blueprint for contemporary cities in Italy and Europe planning similar establishments. The primacy of prayer and hopes for redemption still guided design. With the nave oriented along an east–west axis and the altar prominently located at the central rotunda, this arrangement allowed inmates direct participation in religious rituals. Devotional imagery, including commissioned frescoes, paintings, and statuary, played religious and aesthetic roles for spiritual inspiration and comfort.[36] Over the next few centuries, however, fueled by subsequent bequests and public funding, the institution experienced a fundamental shift. Local leaders, private donors, and their successors sponsored new buildings—a male infirmary in 1313 and a female one in 1376—as well as a dispensary with a "*ricettario*," or collection of about a thousand remedies prescribed by a team of house physicians. In fact, by the sixteenth century, patients were arriving voluntarily to seek treatment.[37]

After a destructive fire in 1471, the crumbling Ospedale di Santo Spirito in Sassia, an ancient shelter for Anglo-Saxon pilgrims since the seventh century, was rebuilt. Located near the Vatican, the project, headed by Pope Sixtus IV, featured a single-story and large rectangular infirmary as well as a colonnaded brick courtyard. With an octagonal dome rising midway, the Sistine Ward became at the time the largest unit of its kind in Europe, capable of housing nearly three hundred patients. Two centuries later, an additional perpendicular hall was added, creating a T-shaped building that contributed to the separation of the sexes. Like its Florentine model, the new Santo Spirito soon acquired a reputation as an excellent medical institution.[38]

To preserve a degree of geographic isolation while enforcing the segregation of patients, establishments like the Santa Maria Nuova and Santo Spirito traditionally functioned as gated communities. Zealous porters guarded the entrances, screening arrivals and restricting access to designated times of the day and week. Upon admission, a change of clothing and a soothing bath were persistent rites of passage toward hospital patienthood. This ceremonial practice had started centuries earlier as part of a set of required physical cleansing steps that sought to supplement the desired spiritual purification through prayers, confession, and communion. Once cleansed, hospital patients were escorted to the wards, selected according to gender, social class, and, later, medical criteria and disease classifications.[39]

The notion of the pre-modern hospital as a stage for the performance of healing rituals can be useful. Since their inception, "God's hostels" effectively combined the characteristics of temple, shelter, church, palace, and residence. Hospitals remained powerful places, rich in religious, aesthetic, and moral meanings. They had been purposely designed to restore identity, stability, order, and continuity—all qualities deemed essential to counteract the bewildering chaos produced by sickness and promote patient recovery.

Recent insights into the effects of space on "behavior setting" can further enlighten our understanding of the impact of past hospital interiors on its occupants' mental and physical status. Each building and community shapes its own environment, creating unique atmospheres and distinctive personalities.[40] Since hospitals were places intended for penance and captivity for the sinful ill, immersion into a sacred institutional environment commanded awe and attention.[41] Good hospital architecture required stimulation of the senses to elevate the mood of those who came to dwell in them. The visual perception of horizontal lines suggested restfulness; vertical lines implied aspiration and assertiveness, while diagonals conveyed dynamic action. More importantly, benefactors provided statuary with images of the Holy Family and saints. Notable artists decorated the inner brick walls with frescoes depicting biblical acts of mercy. Under Pope Sixtus's rule, the Ospedale di Santo Spirito featured scenes of papal patronage and Boticelli's painting regarding the cleansing of a leper.[42]

As the size of the buildings expanded over time, bed capacity and ward placement became detrimental for the patient's physical recovery. In typical medieval monastic shelters, communal living and sleeping had simply taken place in a central dormitory filled with large mattresses arranged at right angles to the walls. Arrivals were assigned to specific, numbered pads routinely occupied by one or more bedmates. Indeed, sick people historically shared a cot with two or three other individuals seeking refuge in a new and strange environment, an uncomfortable albeit reassuring intimacy symbolizing Christian brotherhood. Eschewing ventilation, the decorated windows located high up the walls were designed to only filter heavenly light, often creating a somewhat somber and stale habitat. Although initially intended as a source of human closeness and physical warmth, these arrangements tended to favor the transmission of new infectious diseases in a time of increased urbanization and frequent epidemic outbreaks.

Indeed, the effects of pre-modern hospitalization in multiple crowded wards during the late medieval and early Renaissance periods deserve further attention. In a world increasingly afflicted with easily transmissible conditions, contemporary architectural hospital designs failed to provide sufficient cross-ventilation, thus favoring institutional contagion, a much-dreaded complication that, during subsequent centuries, converted majestic establishments into notorious "death traps." Another early source of exposure was the practice of creating a direct access to the wards from the street through large doors. These entrances, of which the Ospedale di Santo Spirito had two, allowed high-ranking church authorities and prominent private donors and their corteges to visit patients and attend special celebrations.

From the start, indoor hospital space defined and structured a full range of human experiences and responses. Despite a bathing requirement upon admission, low priority was given to personal hygiene and institutional sanitation, and there remained little privacy. Because of their majestic design, some early hospitals were also quite cold and difficult to heat. Since the central dome often functioned as the sole ventilation mechanism, the premises could get polluted. Spacious wards by their very nature were hard to keep clean;

latrines were insufficient and distant, causing night pots to overflow. A disagreeable stench composed of perspiration, urine, feces, vomit, and sick breath must have permeated the premises. With continuous use, straw and seaweed mattresses became damp and saturated with bodily fluids. Only convalescent patients, eager to catch fresh air and sunlight, could leave and head for the open spaces.

Partitions and curtains were added for protection against cold drafts and noxious smells as well as to carve out a minimum amount of space for individual patients. Narrowly subdivided corridors ran around the wards for the sick to walk and reach the latrines. This arrangement allowed for a measure of privacy and greater social control, while shrouding the upheaval caused by frequent sounds and signs of institutional suffering and dying. Paradoxically, the subsequent partitioning into smaller units impeded circulation, creating favorable conditions for the transmission of airborne diseases. Often influenced by design, insufficient space around beds hampered visits from relatives and hospital personnel, including caregiving nurses and an ever-expanding medical staff.

Interactions between the sick and their caregivers always took place in environments reflective and supportive of institutional goals. With larger buildings and a growing number of inmates, control as well as expanding caring routines demanded expansions of the caregiving staff. Inspired by the work of St. Vincent de Paul, religious nursing orders like the Sisters of Charity in the seventeenth century filled the gap. Even more important was the growing presence of lay physicians and surgeons, a product of the gradual emphasis directed toward medical diagnosis and treatment. Such secular goals—notably greater emphasis on surgical and pharmaceutical interventions—tended to displace traditional religious aims. Tensions involving patrons, administrators, and staff concerning the shifting needs of the sick often fostered confusion, although the intent remained to provide reassurance and solidarity.

While subtle, fellowship was extremely important. Disoriented and crammed together, inmates longed for divine confirmation; authentication of their human sufferings was essential for rebuilding confidence and building hope for a possible recovery. Bodily exposures created a climate of intimacy. Admitted for weeks, months, and even years, sufferers had ample time to share their life stories as well as swap illness narratives. Witnesses of personal suffering and redemption, inmates tended to commiserate with each other and form close social groups. They prayed for each other, and together followed the daily ceremonies, sharing the sacraments and attending funerals.[43]

As already noted, placed for ultimate environmental effect, hospital buildings were historically conceived to receive, protect, and facilitate the recovery of sick people. To this day, the architectural design of a hospital remains an integral part of the in-house treatment and outcome of patients brought into such an establishment. Since the late 1970s, consumerism and environmentalism, combined with a progressive patients' rights movement, have continued to seek changes in the architectural design and spatial organization of hospitals.[44] Dominated by secular goals based on the premises of scientific medicine, wellness and consumer-driven participation have allowed for a resurgence of humanitarian concerns arguing for friendly, non-threatening surroundings to overcome the emotional sterility of current institutions. There is also greater awareness of the important role of human spirituality and the persistence of traditional religious beliefs regarding disease causality.[45]

History is prelude. Shaped for several millennia by both religious and secular strategies, hospital architecture managed to create and redefine the spaces selected for dealing with both the emotional and physical aspects of human sickness and healing. This evolutionary process from private homes to temples, monastic shelters and isolated pesthouses to majestic God's Hostels, was accomplished by fulfilling one of architecture's most important functions: creating favorable spaces for efforts to deal with the perennial challenge of human sickness and healing. Above all else, design and institutional routines became important factors in controlling and bringing order into patients' troubled lives. In doing so, hospital design fulfilled Vitruvius's notions of utility and material and aesthetic quality.

Notes

1. Spiro Kostof, "The History of Architecture," in *A History of Architecture: Settings and Rituals*, 2nd ed. (New York: Oxford University Press, 1995), 3–19.
2. For more details, see Ingrid Rowland, *Vitruvius: Ten Books of Architecture* (Cambridge: Cambridge University Press, 2001).
3. The best panoramic treatment of the subject remains John D. Thompson and Grace Goldin, *The Hospital: A Social and Architectural History* (New Haven: Yale University Press, 1975). A useful summary is Nikolaus Pevsner, "Hospitals," in *A History of Building Types*, ed. Nikolaus Pevsner (London: Thames & Hudson, 1976), 139–58.
4. More details can be found in Dankwart Leistikow, *Ten Centuries of European Hospital Architecture*, trans. O. Hill (Ingelheim: Böhringer, 1967).
5. Quim Bonastra and Gerard Jori, "El uso de Google Earth para el estudio de la arquitectura hospitalaria, (i) de los asclepiones a los hospitales medievales," *Ar@cne, Revista Electronica de Recursos en Internet sobre Geografia y Ciencias Sociales Universidad de Barcelona* 122, accessed July 1, 2009. http://www.ub.es/geocrit/aracne/aracne-122.
6. L. Prior, "The Local Space of Medical Discourse: Disease, Illness, and Hospital Architecture," in *The Social Construction of Illness*, ed. J. Lachmund and G. Stollberg (Stuttgart: F. Steiner Verlag, 1992), 67–84. For an evolutionary view of hospital history, consult Guenter B. Risse, *Mending Bodies, Saving Souls: A History of Hospitals* (New York: Oxford University Press, 1999). Another useful collection of essays on the subject is Lindsay Granshaw and Roy Porter, eds., *The Hospital in History* (London: Routledge, 1989).
7. Marten Kuilman, *Quadralectic Architecture: A Panoramic Review*, August 2013, accessed December 31, 2020. https://quadralectics.wordpress.com
8. Guenter B. Risse, "Patients: Historical Perspectives." (unpublished paper, updated November 2015). https://ucsf.academia.edu/GuenterRisse/papers
9. For details, Robert N. Bellah, *Religion in Human Evolution: From the Paleolithic to the Axial Age* (Cambridge, MA: Belknap Press, 2011), 1–44.
10. For a brief summary, see Guenter B. Risse, "Shamanism: The Dawn of a Healing Profession," *Wisconsin Medical Journal* 71 (1972): 18–23. The classical work on this topic is Mircea Eliade, *Shamanism: Archaic Techniques of Ecstasy*, trans. W. R. Trask (Princeton: Princeton University Press, 1964).
11. Lorna Tilley, "Introducing the Bioarcheology of Care," in *Theory and Practice in the Bioarcheology of Care* (Cham: Springer, 2015), 1–11. See also Lorna Tilley, ed., *New Developments in the Bioarcheology of Care* (Cham: Springer, 2017).
12. Albert Zink et al., "Possible Evidence for Care and Treatment in the Tyrolean Iceman," *International Journal of Paleopathology* 25 (2018).
13. James C. Scott, "Zoonoses: A Perfect Epidemiological Storm," in *Against the Grain: A Deep History of the Earliest States* (New Haven, CT: Yale University Press, 2017), 93–115.
14. For a recent perspective, Stephen K. Sanderson, *Religious Evolution and the Axial Age: From Shamans to Priests to Prophets* (London: Bloomsbury Academic, 2019).
15. Details in E. K. Ritter, "Magical Expert (*ashipu*) and Physician (*asu*). Note on Two Complementary Professions in Babylonian Medicine," *Assyriological Studies* 16 (1965): 299–321; Paul U. Unschuld, *Medicine in China: A History of Ideas* (Berkeley: University of California Press, 1985).
16. For more information, Michael Winkelman, *Shamanism: A Biopsychological Paradigm of Consciousness and Healing* (Santa Barbara, CA: Praeger, 2010).
17. For details, see Joshua J. Mark, "Health Care in Ancient Mesopotamia," in *Ancient History Encyclopedia*, accessed December 31, 2020. https://www.ancient.eu/article/687/health-care-in-ancient-mesopotamia; Anu Sini, "Physicians of Ancient India," *Journal of Family Medicine and Primary Care* 5 (2010): 254–8.
18. Guenter B. Risse, "The Healing Framework," in "Medical Care," *Companion Encyclopedia of the History of Medicine*, ed. W. F. Bynum and Roy Porter (London: Routledge, 1993), vol. 1, 45–77.
19. Michael T. Compton, "The Union of Religion and Health in Ancient Asklepieia," *Journal of Religion and Health* 37, no. 4 (1998): 201–12.
20. Alison Burford, *The Greek Temple Builders at Epidauros: A Social and Economic Study of Building in the Asklepian Sanctuary* (Liverpool: Liverpool University Press, 1969). See also Guenter B. Risse, "Dreaming of Asclepius: Ancient Greek Temple Healing," in *Mending Bodies, Saving Souls: A History of Hospitals* (New York: Oxford University Press), 15–38.

21. Guenter B. Risse, "Imhotep and Medicine: A Reevaluation," *The Western Journal of Medicine* 144 (1986): 622–4.
22. Guenter B. Risse, "Asclepius at Epidauros: The Divine Power of Healing Dreams" (unpublished Lecture, May 13, 2008), accessed December 21, 2020. https://ucsf.academia.edu/GuenterRisse/papers
23. Risse, "Collective Care of Soldiers and Slaves: Roman *Valetudinaria*," in Risse, *Mending Bodies, Saving Souls*, 38–59.
24. Risse, "Early Christianity? A New Vision of the Sick," in Risse, *Mending Bodies, Saving Souls*, 69–87. For more details and recent analysis, Gary B. Ferngren, *Medicine and Health Care in Early Christianity* (Baltimore: Johns Hopkins University Press), 2009.
25. For details, Timothy S. Miller, *The Birth of the Hospital in the Byzantine Empire* (Baltimore: Johns Hopkins University Press, 1997).
26. R. Greer, "Hospitality in the First Five Centuries of the Church," *Medieval Studies* 10 (1974): 29–48.
27. For details, consult L. Michael White, *The Social Organization of Christian Architecture* (Valley Forge: Trinity Press, 1996).
28. Clare Cooper Marcus and Marni Barnes, *Gardens in Health Care Facilities: Uses, Therapeutic Benefits and Design Recommendations* (Concord, CA: Center for Health Design, 1995).
29. Check the contributions in Michel Conan, ed., *Middle East Gardens: Traditions, Unity and Diversity* (Washington, DC: Dumbarton Oaks, 2007).
30. Peregrine Horden, "How Medicalized Were Byzantine Hospitals?" *Medicina e Storia* 10 (2008): 45–74. See also Guenter B. Risse, "Medicalization: Hospitals Become Sites of Medical Care and Learning" (unpublished paper, 2004).
31. A typical example was the Abby of St. Gall. See W. Vogler, "Historical Sketch of the Abbey of St. Gall," in *The Culture of the Abbey of St. Gall. An Overview*, ed. J. C. King and P. W. Tax (Stuttgart: Belser Verlag 1991), 9–23.
32. T. S. Miller, "From Poorhouse to Hospital," *Christian History* 101 (2011). Reprinted online: https://christianhistoryinstitute.org/magazine/article/from-poorhouse-to-hospital.
33. Risse, "Hospitals as Segregation and Confinement Tools," in Risse, *Mending Bodies, Saving Souls*, 167–229.
34. See, for example, Karka Keyvanian, *Hospitals and Urbanism in Rome 1200–1500* (Leiden: Brill, 2016), 339–83.
35. D. Jetter, "Das Mailänder Ospedale Maggiore und der kreuzförmige Krankenhausgrundriss," *Sudhoffs Archiv* 44 (1960): 64–75.
36. K. Park and J. Henderson, "The First Hospital among Christians: The Ospedale di Santa Maria Nuova in Early Sixteenth-Century Florence," *Medical History* 35 (1991): 164–88.
37. For details, John Henderson, *The Renaissance Hospital: Healing the Body and Healing the Soul* (New Haven: Yale University Press, 2006). For a review, G. B. Risse, *Medical History* 51 (2007): 352–3.
38. Silvia Mattoni et al., "From a Pope's Nightmare, A Great Public Health Institution: The Santo Spirito in Saxia Hospital in Rome," *Italian Journal of Public Health* 7, no. 2 (2010): 115–17. See also Charlotte Graham, "The Hospital of Santo Spirito in Sassia" (University of Washington Libraries, Seattle, 1975).
39. More details can be found in Nancy G. Siraisi, *Medieval and Early Renaissance Medicine: An Introduction to Knowledge and Practice* (Chicago: University of Chicago Press, 1990).
40. H. M. Proshansky, W. H. Ittelson, and L. G. Rivlin, eds., *Environmental Psychology: People and their Physical Settings* (New York: Holt, Rinehart & Winston, 1970), especially part VII, "The Built Environment," 433–89. See also Pierre Bourdieu, "Social Space and Symbolic Power," *Social Theory* 7 (1989): 14–25.
41. Katherine Park, "Healing the Poor: Hospitals and Medicine in Renaissance Florence," in *Medicine and Charity*, ed. J. Barry and C. Jones (London: Routledge, 1991), 26–45.
42. For more details, Eunice D. Howe, *The Hospital of Santo Spirito and Pope Sixtus* (New York: Garland Publishing, 1978).
43. For a more recent discussion of cross-shaped hospital examples, Neil Kellman, "History of Healthcare Environments," in *Innovations in Healthcare Design*, ed. Sara O. Marberry (New York: John Wiley & Sons, 1995), 38–47.
44. Marberry, *Innovations in Healthcare Design*.
45. For more information, see an international study of the relationship between hospital architecture and the health of patients, based on a project sponsored by the University Medical Center of Groningen, Cor Wagenaar, ed., *The Architecture of Hospitals* (Rotterdam: NAi Booksellers, 2006).

CHAPTER 3
A PLAN FOR THE KING AND THE SICK
PORTUGUESE HOSPITAL ARCHITECTURE DURING THE AGE OF EXPLORATION
Danielle Abdon

Starting in the fifteenth century, governmental bodies throughout Europe began reorganizing charitable networks, reforming and taking control of systems of public health and social welfare for the sick and poor.[1] This chapter addresses one phenomenon of this broader reformation of charity, and specifically healthcare, in early modern cities: the appearance and dissemination of an architectural typology exclusive to hospitals. Characterized by a cruciform design, this architectural development promoted medical and sanitary innovations, including triage, separation of the sick and poor, isolation, and sewage disposal, among other novelties (Figure 3.1). The plan, which originated in northern Italy, became so successful that it quickly spread to other regions, finding an especially receptive audience in Portugal and Spain. Focusing on the port city of Lisbon, the first global metropolis of early modern Europe, this study explores the adoption of the cruciform plan for hospitals in a period when the Portuguese monarchy moved to control public health and social welfare as sanitary and social pressures became increasingly critical due to intensified maritime activity during the Age of Exploration (*c.* 1400–1700).

Scholarship on the importance of the cruciform plan as a typology for hospital architecture first emerged in the 1930s as a result of studies of the Ospedale Maggiore (1456), the general hospital commissioned by Duke Francesco Sforza (r. 1450–66) and Duchess Bianca Maria (1425–68) for the city of Milan (Figures 3.1 and 3.2). Since then, architectural historians have addressed several aspects of the design, including the charitable reform that promoted the plan; its symbolism and associated medical innovations; the origins of the design, whether in central or northern Italy; and the impact of Tuscan hospitals on this Lombard development.[2] These studies often mention the rapid spread of the cruciform plan to other European regions, particularly Spain. This focus on the Spanish context stems from the historical, though now refuted, association of three hospitals with the architect Enrique Egas (1455–1534).[3] Yet, these publications merely list occurrences of the plan as evidence of the success of the Italian model, consequently framing the adoption of the design outside of Italy as a passive diffusion and disregarding the resulting hospitals as relevant developments themselves.[4] In comparison to Spanish hospitals, the Hospital Real de Todos-os-Santos (1492) in Lisbon remains particularly neglected despite its earlier date and significant structural developments, emphasizing the peripheral position of Portugal within scholarship on Iberia and the western Renaissance (Figure 3.3).[5] As a result, discussions of the cruciform design support the traditional framework of centers and peripheries that has long dominated studies of Renaissance art and architecture, overlooking the potential contributions of case studies in the so-called art historical periphery.[6]

This chapter proposes an alternative approach to the Iberian adoption of the cruciform plan, moving away from the implications of "influence" and the assumption that importation indicates cultural weakness.[7] Rather, it aims to portray a different view of fifteenth- and sixteenth-century Lisbon as a city that actively imported the latest fashions from various regions, creating a palimpsest in which Italian and Northern European artists and traditions clashed and blended with local styles, objects, and materials from Africa, Asia, and Brazil. Recent studies have emphasized this international environment, which was echoed in contemporary descriptions

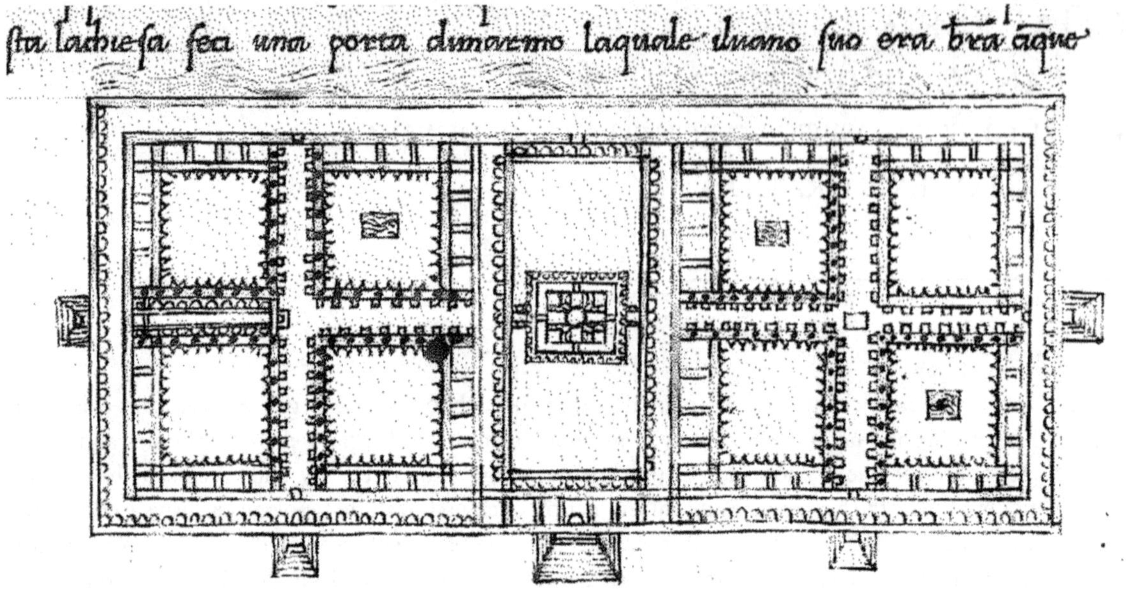

Health and Architecture

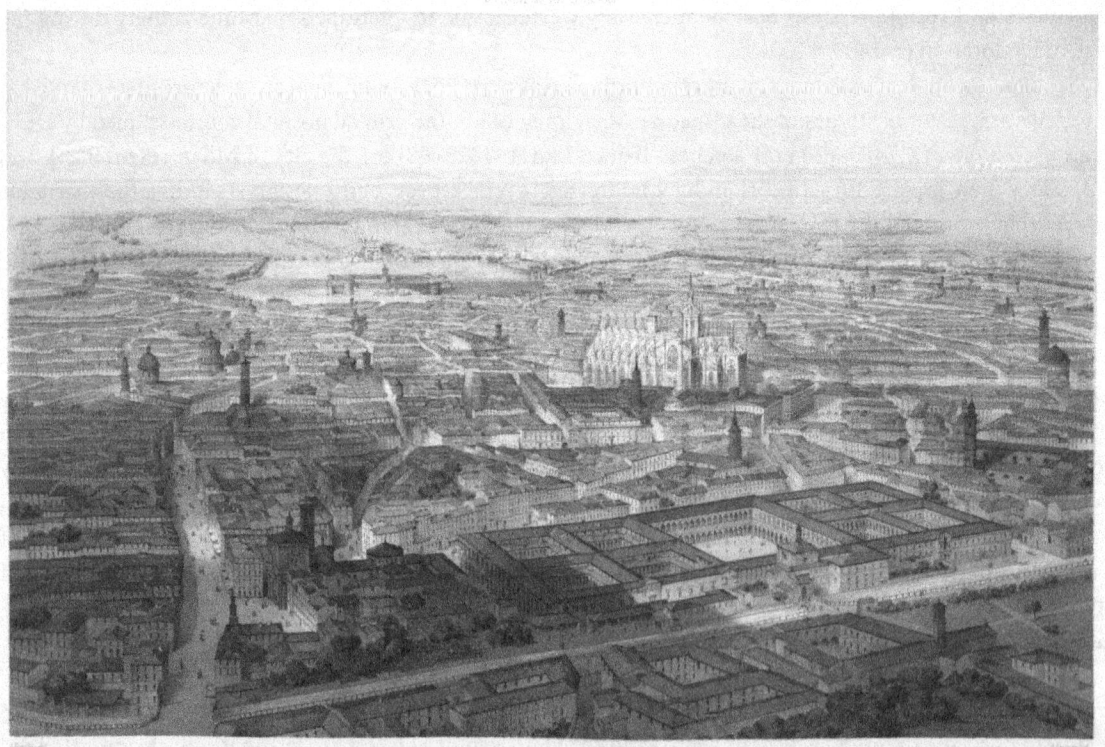

Figure 3.1 Antonio Averlino (il Filarete), *Treatise on Architecture*, c. 1461–4. Source: Spencer 1965, facsimile edition of *Treatise on Architecture*, Book XI, fol. 82v

Figure 3.2 Alfred Guesdon, *View of Milan*, lithograph, c. 1850. Source: Österreichische Nationalbibliothek—Austrian National Library

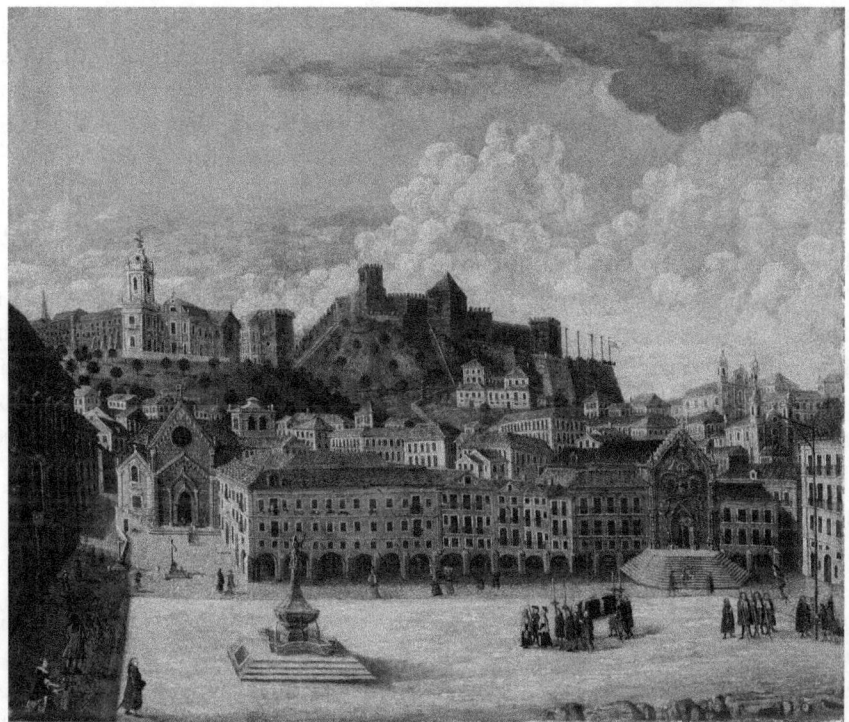

Figure 3.3 Anonymous, possibly Portuguese, *Hospital Real de Todos-os-Santos (View of Rossio)*, eighteenth century, oil on canvas, 39 × 59 cm. Courtesy of Álvaro Roquette and Pedro Aguiar Branco, Antiquary. Photo by Onshot / Rui Carvalho

of Lisbon and perhaps best illustrated by the 1581 travel account of Venetians Vicenzo Tron and Girolamo Lippomano, who recorded a common saying in the city that "you haven't seen anything good until you've seen Lisbon."[8] In this context, Portuguese importation of an Italian plan for hospitals, then the most up-to-date European development in the architecture of healing spaces, appears as part of a larger initiative that reflected the Portuguese monarchy's agency to achieve cultural enrichment and embodied their wish for its capital to reflect the Crown's expanding international network. Further, this importation also marked a shift in the royal approach to hospital architecture: from improvised to purposefully designed buildings that echoed contemporaneous advancements in Italy while tending to and incorporating local needs.

Social Reform in Northern Italy

As is the case today, poverty and disease were often connected in the early modern period. Different from modern-day hospitals, however, fifteenth- and sixteenth-century institutions aimed to address both issues. Already in the Middle Ages, hospitals for the most part functioned as shelters for the sick and poor, places where one could find spiritual and physical comfort. Derived from ecclesiastical and monastic architecture, these institutions were traditionally small structures with one long ward for patients and an altar, oratory, or chapel at the end. In many cases, they also existed in repurposed buildings not originally designed as hospitals. Their patronage could stem from religious, private, or even state donations, but in general, medieval hospitals offered care with a strong religious component.[9]

The reorganization of healthcare that began in fifteenth-century Europe marked a transitional period in the history of charity. This reform varied across cities, but three main aspects remained common to most locations: an increased governmental involvement in the administration of hospitals, an amplification of the medical care provided by these institutions, and the appearance of specialized establishments for specific categories of the needy, such as abandoned children or syphilitic patients.[10] Traditionally, early modern cities promoted reform in two distinct ways, following either the Florentine or Milanese model. In Florence, this reorganization strengthened the medieval system of healthcare by increasing the physical and service capacity of existing hospitals and establishing new institutions specializing in the treatment of particular groups of the needy.[11] The Milanese model, on the other hand, amalgamated several previously distinct medieval hospitals under one main institution, an *ospedale grande* or general hospital.[12] These models coexisted in Italy, and both promoted the appearance of a true architectural typology for hospitals through the planning and construction of new structures purposefully designed as healing spaces.[13] These buildings provided large facilities necessary to expand existing charitable systems and functioned as monumental symbols of civic pride, visually augmenting the magnificence of their cities and patrons. Most important for the history of medicine, however, their architecture developed hand-in-hand with the increasing medicalization of hospitals.

Innovations in Hospital Architecture and their Circulation

In this context of reform and innovations in hospital architecture, the cruciform plan for hospitals first appeared in Lombardy, quickly spreading across Southern Europe. The plan emerged with the Ospedale di San Matteo (1449), the general hospital of Pavia, and achieved its full potential and monumentality with the Ospedale Maggiore in Milan, designed by the Florentine architect Antonio Averlino (c. 1440–69), best known as Filarete (see Figures 3.1 and 3.2).[14] Yet, in the period between 1440 and 1480, many of the developments associated with the plan appeared simultaneously at several northern Italian institutions and contemporary textual sources, as exemplified by the architectural treatises of Filarete himself and of architect and theorist Leon Battista Alberti (1404–72).[15] Therefore, attributing a unique source for these novelties can oversimplify a more complex scenario.

Common characteristics of cruciform structures began with their site, chosen based on the salubriousness and connectivity of the location, key for the transportation of building materials and later hospital supplies.[16] Ideally situated outside the center but still inside city walls, the site was typically selected based on proximity to a body of water, natural or artificially created, for guaranteed water supply. The cruciform plan formed four arms departing from a core structure, allowing for the creation of long and tall infirmaries with beds placed perpendicularly against the wall and the separation of women and men in different arms of the cross (see Figure 3.1).[17] Wood was used in a shallow-sloped roof to facilitate insulation, and windows near the roof illuminated the wards and promoted airflow.[18] The crossing served a religious and organizational purpose: while it often housed an altar, so the sick could participate in liturgy from their beds, it also created a central viewpoint for the monitoring of patients in the infirmaries. Further, the insertion of the cross within a square structure created four courtyards around the wards, guaranteeing patients' access to the exterior but keeping them removed from street noise and, most importantly, the healthy. This square structure also created crucial peripheral spaces to house service areas, such as kitchens and laundry facilities. Finally, the design of these hospitals as crosses filled them with religious symbolism.[19] In a period when the suffering of the needy was often compared to that of Jesus, the cruciform plan could have served as a powerful metaphor for Christ on the cross.[20]

Attention to the health of a healing site was not new to the Renaissance but dated back to the classical period. In his *Ten Books on Architecture* (30–20 BCE), Roman architect and engineer Vitruvius (c. 80/70–15 BCE) explained the importance of water supply for the shrines of gods associated with health and curing the sick. In this case, the author perceived water as facilitating recovery. Proximity to swamps, however, was to be avoided, "for when the morning breezes enter the town with the rising sun, whatever mists have formed overnight are joined with them. Their gusts spew the poisonous exhalations of the swamp animals, which have been mixed in with the mist, at the bodies of the inhabitants, and these will make the place pestilent." For Vitruvius, based on water, one could determine whether a place was naturally healthful or pestilent.[21]

In the Renaissance, the concern for water supply, airflow, and natural light in hospital structures strongly aligned them with contemporary medical thinking, which also had classical origins. In the fifteenth century, medicine followed a Galenic view based on humoral theory, according to which health consisted of a balance of four bodily humors. Quality of air was particularly important since it was believed that noxious airs contained miasmatic particles that could poison the lungs and disturb proper humoral balance, leading to disease.[22] Treatments aimed at re-balancing the humors through medical intervention, but the regulation of six physical and environmental factors, called non-naturals, was also key in healing and preventive care.[23] These factors included air, sleep, food and drink, evacuation and repletion, motion and rest, and passions and emotions.[24] Consideration of these aspects was already part of ancient medicine, as indicated by the Greek physician Hippocrates' (c. 460–370 BCE) treatise *Airs, Waters, and Places* (c. 400 BCE). Among non-naturals, the concern for air quality and water supply were particularly relevant in a hospital context.

In hospitals, water was necessary for the kitchen, laundry, and cleaning, while airflow and sunlight prevented the presence of noxious fumes or stagnant or damp air, both of which continued to be considered harmful during the early modern period.[25] Writing in 1478, Italian humanist Marsilio Ficino (1433–99) had warned against the dangers of enclosed and humid air not renewed or purged by the sun with dry wind.[26] Alberti expressed similar concerns, claiming that the ancients only built hospitals "in healthy places, with wholesome breezes and the purest water, so that the rate of recovery would be enhanced by a combination of divine assistance and local benefits."[27] For him, the ideal location for a hospital "would be dry, stony, and fanned by continual breezes … since damp encourages decay."[28] Preoccupations regarding water supply and salubriousness, particularly provided by airflow and sunlight, thus were present simultaneously in literature and architecture.[29]

The most advanced ideas of the time came together with Filarete's design for the Ospedale Maggiore, a building that marked the reform of the healthcare system of Milan with the unification of medieval hospitals under this institution.[30] Filarete extensively described his plan for the hospital in his *Treatise on Architecture* (1460–4), which also included drawings of the ground plan and elevation (see Figures 3.1 and 3.4). The former shows a longitudinal structure divided into three sections. The central courtyard houses a church, while each flanking symmetrical structure features a Greek cross. Lavishly ornamented, the elevation shows prominent staircases, towers, domes, and spires, an impressive display of the architect's creativity and competence.[31]

In his *Treatise*, Filarete initially praised the location selected by the duke for the Ospedale as "beautiful and admirably suited" for a hospital. He explained that the structure would fulfill the needs of the sick particularly through a sewer system, or *destri*, which allowed for "convenience and cleanliness."[32] In this system, latrine openings on the infirmary walls next to patients' beds connected the wards to the *destri* through small pipes for the disposal of excrements. The building's location allowed Filarete to divert water from a nearby canal to flow through the structure in vaulted conduits in its foundation (Figure 3.5). The water exited at the other side of the hospital into a small lake, or *laghetto*, that emptied back into the canal. This flow kept the *destri* clean, avoiding the formation of stagnant and putrid waters. Moreover, large terracotta pipes built inside structural piers rose from the *destri* to the roofs, exhausting potential noxious fumes. These pipes also served as gutters, admitting rainwater into the *destri* to flush the entire system. Filarete's sewer system alone highlights the

Health and Architecture

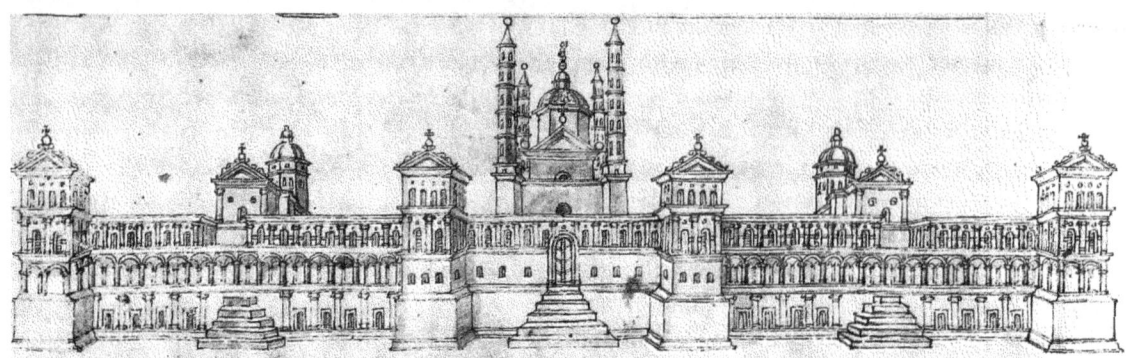

Figure 3.4 Antonio Averlino (il Filarete), *Treatise on Architecture*, c. 1461–4. Source: Spencer 1965, facsimile edition of *Treatise on Architecture*, Book XI, fol. 83v

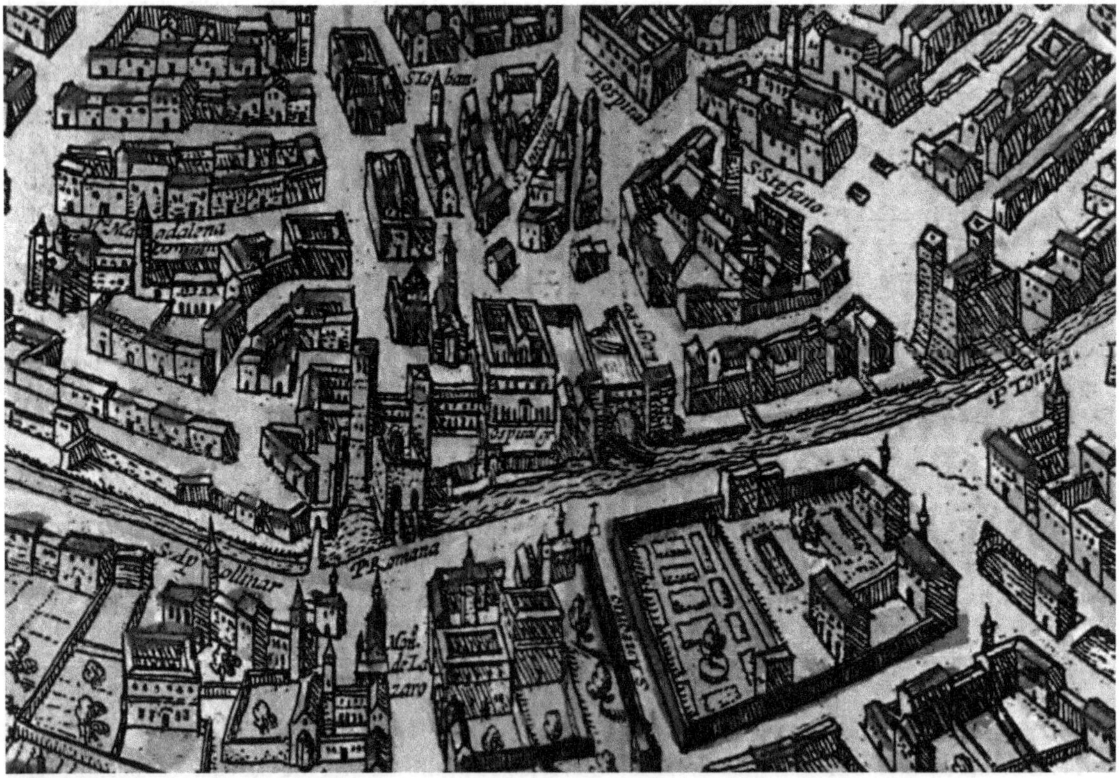

Figure 3.5 Georg Braun and Frans Hogenberg, Detail of *Milan*, *Civitates Orbis Terrarum*, vol. 1, 1572. Source: Library of Congress, https://www.loc.gov/resource/g3200m.gct00128a/?sp=96 (accessed September 18, 2020)

importance of water access and the concern for quality of air in a hospital setting, but the architect also boasted that his design sent water to many other areas of the building, "which will be very useful to the hospital."[33] These structural innovations, alongside the monumentality of the building and its lavish decoration, have been responsible for the reputation of the Ospedale Maggiore as a model Renaissance hospital.[34]

Despite Filarete's extensive description of the Milanese institution in his *Treatise* and the appearance of similar structures soon after in Spain and Portugal, scholars have not yet pinpointed the ways through which the exportation of the architect's design innovations occurred. Aside from the actual cruciform buildings in northern Italy, which travelers could have experienced in person, the *Treatise* would have been the most straightforward textual and visual source for other patrons and architects. Specialists on hospital architecture tend to assume that Filarete's manuscript circulated widely in the fifteenth and sixteenth centuries, explaining the diffusion of the cruciform plan to Iberia. Yet, architectural historians remain skeptical of the *Treatise*'s reach, arguing for a very limited circulation of the manuscript since it was not printed until modern times.[35]

Filarete wrote his *Treatise* between 1460 and 1464 while in Milan, dedicating it to Duke Francesco Sforza.[36] In 1465, due to political disputes that culminated with his removal from the hospital project, the architect left the city and returned to Florence. In an attempt to gain favor with the ruling Medici family, he rededicated a second copy of the *Treatise*, known as the *Codex Magliabechiano*, to Piero de' Medici (r. 1464–9).[37] While the Milanese version constituted either the original manuscript or the first copy of a now lost original that remained in Filarete's possession, a scribe created the *Codex Magliabechiano*, working under the architect's supervision to add drawings that included the designs of the Ospedale Maggiore associated with Filarete today. Housed in the Medici Library, the *Codex Magliabechiano* was lent on occasion, such as in 1482, when the manuscript was sent to Rome so another copy could be made for Alfonso, Duke of Calabria (1448–95) and co-regent of Naples with his father, King Ferrante (r. 1458–94).[38] Additionally, in 1488, a copy of the manuscript was translated into Latin at the court of King Matthias Corvinus (r. 1458–90) of Hungary, leading to further dissemination of the work.[39] By the end of the fifteenth century, there were at least three copies of the manuscript in Italy as well as a Latin version in Hungary—all of them in considerably international courts. Therefore, the treatise might have been accessible to artists and architects outside of Italy in the fifteenth and sixteenth centuries. Yet, the reluctance expressed by scholars regarding the circulation of Filarete's *Treatise*, and therefore of his cruciform design for hospitals, hinders our understanding of the exchange of medical, technological, and architectural knowledge during the period. In the face of this issue, what can the adoption of the cruciform plan in a "peripheral" city tell us about the broader circulation of the design and its associated innovations?

Crisis and Healthcare Reform in Iberia

As the main port city in Portugal and Iberia during the Age of Exploration, Lisbon suffered incomparable social and sanitary pressures in the late fifteenth and sixteenth centuries. Studies of Renaissance ports have shown that, through expansionist activity, cities such as Lisbon and Seville engaged in unprecedented systems of exchange, resulting in a constant flux of people and goods. This dynamic environment generated many benefits, such as a high flow of information, intellectual exchanges, and technological developments, but there were also negative consequences to this scenario—such as urban overcrowding, unstable economies, and especially the constant arrival of foreign ships and transient groups—that put the population of these hubs at higher risk for poverty and disease.[40]

As Laurinda Abreu has explained, "fear of epidemics at a time of intense migration, which was of particular concern when spurred on by poverty, legitimised the intervention of central government," and, in the case of early modern Portugal, the Crown interfered by moving to reform its capital's existing healthcare system.[41] In August, 1479, Prince and future King of Portugal Dom João II (r. 1477/81–95) received papal permission to merge medieval hospitals in Lisbon under one main institution—the Hospital Real de Todos-os-Santos.[42] At that time, the city had almost seventy hospitals, forty-three of which were incorporated into the royal institution.[43] While some of these hospitals dated to the thirteenth and fourteenth centuries, approximately thirty-three of them had been founded in the fifteenth century. Through this measure, the Crown clearly rejected the earlier, inefficient system of support in favor of its new hospital, which reflected the monarchic control of social and health issues in Lisbon.

A 1427 census indicates that Lisbon had a population of 60,000–65,000 people.[44] Prior to the construction of the Hospital Real, the existing hospitals in the city were smaller, featuring a maximum of twenty-five beds. The average, however, was of five beds per institution, a ratio of approximately one bed per 263 inhabitants.[45] Documents from the period between 1440 and 1490 reveal serious issues with these medieval hospitals, including administrative negligence, disregard for hospitals' statutes and the testaments of founders who had endowed the institutions, and extreme deterioration of hospital structures or unauthorized repurposing for other functions.[46] With the intensification of seafaring activity, the population of Lisbon continued to increase, reaching 100,000 by the mid-sixteenth century.[47] This population growth, especially through the arrival of Jews expelled from Spain in 1492 and an increase in transient populations connected to the explorations, combined with famines and constant plague outbreaks served to validate governmental intervention in the social welfare and public health systems of the still medieval city.[48]

In this context, considering the Iberian adoption of a typology specific to hospitals offers three main benefits in studies of their architecture. First, an examination of a major port's strategies for handling social and sanitary crises and the way hospital design fits into broader measures of public health and social welfare increases our knowledge of why the plan was deemed successful. Further, since the resulting Portuguese hospital was not only a monumental structure but, based on ideas of symmetry and order, one of the first Renaissance buildings in Lisbon, this institution provides crucial evidence for understanding hospitals as sites of exchange between Italy and Iberia.[49] Finally, considering the role of Lisbon as a major port and gateway to Africa, the Indies, and the New World, this line of inquiry ultimately offers more nuanced insight into the Renaissance as a global phenomenon and the process of "globalization of the hospital."[50]

The Hospital Real de Todos-os-Santos

Building of the Hospital Real de Todos-os-Santos began on May 15, 1492.[51] During the twenty-three years between the 1479 papal bull authorizing construction of the hospital and the opening of the institution in 1502, the unwavering support of the Portuguese Crown created a bureaucratic machine to fund the construction of the Hospital Real. As indicated by royal measures from the period, this official engine encompassed three main approaches. The first, already mentioned, included the amalgamation of medieval institutions, which started as early as 1484.[52]

The second strategy began in 1493, when King Dom João ordered the donation to the hospital of properties of mosques in Lisbon, presumably to be sold for profit.[53] With the monarch's death in 1495 and the ascension of his nephew, Dom Manuel (r. 1495–1521), to the Portuguese throne, the new king ordered further measures against Muslims and Jews as part of his broader goal to stabilize Portugal's relationship with Spain, whose monarchs had already taken forceful actions against those two religious groups.[54] As such, royal decrees from the period of 1497–1502 included the appropriation of synagogues and mosques as well as properties from Jews and New Christians who had left the Portuguese kingdom without permission—all to benefit the hospital.[55] This orchestration culminated in June 1501, when Dom Manuel determined that the Hospital Real would take control of all properties left in the Jewish and Moorish communes and those in their cemeteries.[56] Through the latter, the king authorized the use of tombstones as construction materials for the hospital, essentially performing a religious cleanse of the city.[57]

The third strategy for funding the Hospital Real encompassed royal donations, which had both a national and international aspect.[58] In his will from 1495, Dom João had ordered the purchase of croplands to generate

A Plan for the King and the Sick

funds for the institution.⁵⁹ While acquisition was underway, financial support for the hospital was to come from the revenue of São Jorge da Mina, the first Portuguese base in Africa, whose extensive profits stemmed from gold mining at Costa da Mina (present-day Ghana). Further income would come from the patronage of royal churches (Padroados das Igrejas da Coroa), and both Dom João and Dom Manuel donated lands in Lisbon and Portugal to the hospital.⁶⁰ As Portuguese maritime expansion increased, however, profits from colonialism began to endow the institution. For example, a royal measure from 1501 guaranteed the donation of sugar from the Madeira Islands to be sold by the hospital for profit.⁶¹

In his will, Dom João mentioned the dedication of the Hospital Real to All Saints and emphasized its role to care for the sick and poor of Lisbon. He further instructed that construction of the hospital should continue following the original design, and his executor, Dom Manuel, was assigned its governance. Dom João also wished that the administration of the institution "more or less followed the regiment that they have in Florence and Siena."⁶² This passage likely referred to the well-known large hospitals of Santa Maria Nuova (1288) in Florence and Santa Maria della Scala (1090) in Siena, considered model medieval institutions.⁶³ Thus, his will indicates an awareness of the functioning and administration of Tuscan hospitals—an attentiveness to international trends that mirrors the knowledge and adoption of the northern Italian cruciform plan for the Portuguese hospital.

The Hospital Real was demolished in the 1770s after significant damage following the 1755 earthquake and subsequent fire that destroyed most of Lisbon. Built in the wide and ample area known as Rossio, in a garden formerly owned by the adjacent Dominican convent of São Domingos (1242) on the northern side, the hospital occupied most of present-day Praça da Figueira, originally established as an open market following eighteenth-century plans to rebuild the city. Despite the destruction of the hospital, primary sources, contemporary depictions of Lisbon and the Rossio, survey measurements of the area, and excavation campaigns from 1960 and 1999–2001 provide extensive knowledge of the original institution, an irregular complex built with a cruciform building at its core and surrounded by supporting structures (Figure 3.6).⁶⁴ While located inside the fourteenth-century city walls, Rossio remained a transitional space between the developing commercial center of Lisbon on the riverside area of Ribeira and the rural regions surrounding the

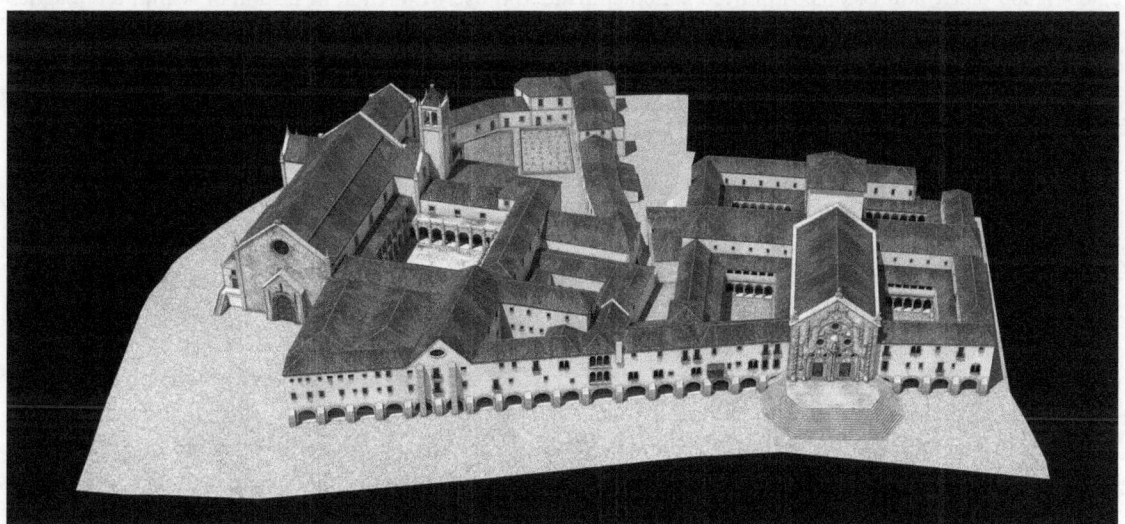

Figure 3.6 Reconstruction of hospital complex in 1755. Colecção do Museu de Lisboa / Câmara Municipal de Lisboa–EGEAC

city.⁶⁵ Urbanization of this open plot had begun with construction of the Paço dos Estaus (1434), a residence for noblemen and foreign ambassadors who came to court, but the Hospital Real definitively changed the site with its horizontal facade.⁶⁶ The hospital complex regularized the shape of the square, making Rossio the only revitalized area of the city further inland, and facilitated the creation of a new, north–south commercial axis for Lisbon, embodied by the Rua Nova d'El Rey, the main street connecting Rossio in the north to the bustling Ribeira in the south.⁶⁷

In his 1552 *Grandeza e Abastança da Cidade de Lisboa*, sixteenth-century writer João Brandão extensively described the Hospital Real de Todos-os-Santos. The author began with the prominent facade of the institution, facing the Rossio and characterized by an extensive arcade and staircase leading to the striking front of the hospital church (see Figure 3.3).⁶⁸ Different from most northern Italian hospitals, which either had a separate church or a chapel with an altar at the crossing, the plan for the Hospital Real placed the church in one arm of the cruciform structure—a similar arrangement to that found at the general hospitals built in Mantua (early 1460s) and Parma (1476) (see Figure 3.6).⁶⁹ In this way, the church functioned as a transitional space between the healthy and the sick but also connected the hospital to city life through its public use.⁷⁰ Despite this adaptation, at the Hospital Real, the chancel of the church occupied the crossing of the hospital structure, allowing patients from all three infirmaries to participate in the liturgy.

In terms of areas destined for the treatment of the sick and the day-to-day functioning of the hospital, the first ward, to the south of the complex, was the infirmary of São Vicente for clinical male patients, the so-called men with fevers. Surgical male patients, or wounded men, received treatment in the northern infirmary of São Cosme. Finally, the third infirmary, dedicated to Santa Clara, served women, either wounded or with fevers, and occupied the eastern arm opposite to the church. According to Brandão, in the interior of the wards, doors beside each bed led to a hallway where sick patients could attend to bathroom needs and waste matter could be removed. Further, church and infirmaries occupied the second story of the complex, guaranteeing better aeration and sun exposure. The shape of the institution also created four surrounding courtyards and several annexes for service areas located at the corners of the complex.⁷¹ As evident in Brandão's description, the Hospital Real echoed medical preoccupations and advice of the period reflected in northern Italian hospital architecture. At the time Brandão wrote in 1552, the hospital had over 130 patients in its care, with 2,500–3,000 yearly admissions. Admitted patients included those who fell ill in Lisbon or within ten leagues of the city, travelers who arrived from maritime trips, and the foreign or local poor who could not receive treatment elsewhere.⁷²

As one of the first high-profile projects in a port city whose urbanscape would significantly evolve in the following years with the rise of structures to support Portuguese maritime expansion, the hospital appears centrally in several views of Rossio and Lisbon from the sixteenth century onwards. These representations highlight the facade, which extended from the monumental portal of the church to the northern side of the square, encompassing a cluster of hospital structures up to the Convent of São Domingos (see Figures 3.3 and 3.6). With the exception of the church portal, the building matched the architecture typical of mid-fifteenth-century Portugal and associated with the limited economic conditions of Dom João's reign—a style marked by smooth walls, lacking decoration, and often whitewashed or showing stonework.⁷³ Yet, with Dom João's death in 1495 and continuation of construction under Dom Manuel, the highly ornamented portal of the hospital church reflects the opulent Manueline style of sixteenth-century Portuguese architecture. This shift in power is evident in the church facade, which features the coats-of-arms of both monarchs, the pelican linked to Dom João and the armillary sphere associated with Dom Manuel. Hence, the facade reveals not only a transition in institutional patronage but primarily the uninterrupted monarchic control of social welfare and public health under both kings, embodied by the hospital itself.⁷⁴

Contributions from the "Periphery"

The Hospital Real exemplifies how knowledge of the northern Italian cruciform design for hospitals rapidly reached other European areas. This knowledge went well beyond a formal understanding of hospital architecture, encompassing awareness of structural innovations as well as familiarity with reform systems and the administration of charitable institutions. However, the means through which this knowledge disseminated remain unclear. It is possible that travelers might have accessed hospitals in northern Italy and carried that knowledge to Iberia, and the Portuguese monarchy's strong ties with Italy have also been established, representing another potential way of communication.[75] For example, architect Andrea Sansovino (c. 1467–1529) was sent to Portugal by the Medici family in c. 1492 following a request by Dom João, and scholars have noted the participation of Portuguese patrons in the Florentine book market.[76] Both connections could have led to knowledge of Filarete's *Treatise* through the *Codex Magliabechiano*, then in Florence under Medici possession. Yet, the accessibility and circulation of the cruciform design through the manuscript, even into the sixteenth century, continue to be questioned. While the following discussion does not attempt to resolve this issue or to claim a direct connection between the *Treatise* and the Hospital Real in Lisbon, it hopes to bring to light overlooked evidence of the circulation of the plan in the sixteenth century through an investigation of representations of the Portuguese hospital during the period. The implications, if any, of this evidence for the Portuguese adoption of the plan in the fifteenth century remain to be determined, especially since knowledge of the cruciform design then could have been disseminated by travelers. Rather, by demonstrating the international circulation of Filarete's plan in the sixteenth century, this chapter calls attention to the need to reevaluate the reach of the *Treatise* in the late 1400s, particularly as it relates to the global spread of a new architectural typology for hospitals.

As illustrated in the *Hospital Real de Todos-os-Santos* (View of Rossio) (eighteenth century) by an anonymous Portuguese artist, historical representations of the Hospital Real and surrounding area frequently highlight the facade of the institutional church, particularly its prominent staircase (see Figure 3.3). In strong contrast, depictions of the Portuguese institution in panoramic views of Lisbon from the river tend to emphasize the design of the hospital complex.[77] This latter trend began with one of the earliest depictions of the hospital, an illuminated miniature in a folio of the lavishly decorated chronicle *Genealogy of the Royal Houses of Spain and Portugal* (1530–4) (Figure 3.7). Attributed to António de Holanda (1480–1571), Flemish court artist for King Dom Manuel, the miniature shows the hospital complex with a central church and flanked by two asymmetrical, rectangular structures, each forming a courtyard. The monumental staircase leading into the hospital church appears prominently, as does a spiral lantern marking the crossing. A visible extension behind the church suggests the presence of a cruciform design, creating a structure that closely resembles the proposed reconstructions of the hospital today.

Despite this initial representation, subsequent depictions of the Hospital Real show an unusual development. This transition began with the *View of Lisbon* (c. 1565), created by an anonymous artist for the *Civitates orbis terrarium*, a collection of city views created by geographer Georg Braun (1541–1622) and engraver Franz Hogenberg (1535–90), whose first volume was published in Cologne and Antwerp in 1572 (Figure 3.8).[78] Similar to Holanda's illumination, the *Civitates* engraving of Lisbon as seen from the Tagus River shows the royal institution with a central church flanked by two rectangular structures. The prominent staircase of the hospital church remains, as does the characteristic spiral lantern, but closer examination shows the precise symmetry of the structures to the right and left of the hospital church. Most significantly, each rectangular building features a cruciform design inside, giving the hospital complex a total of eight courtyards.[79]

Health and Architecture

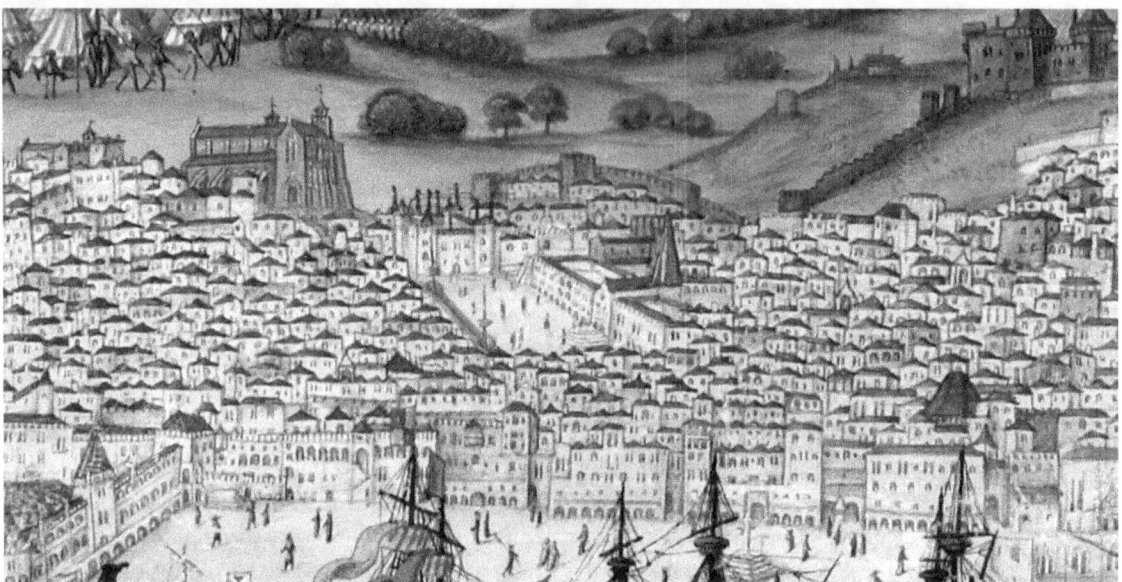

Figure 3.7 António de Holanda, Detail of *Genealogical Tree of the Kings and Queens of Portugal from Alfonso Enriquez to Alfonso II*, fol. 7, in *Genealogy of the Royal Houses of Spain and Portugal* (Ms. Add. 12531), *c.* 1530–4. © The British Library Board

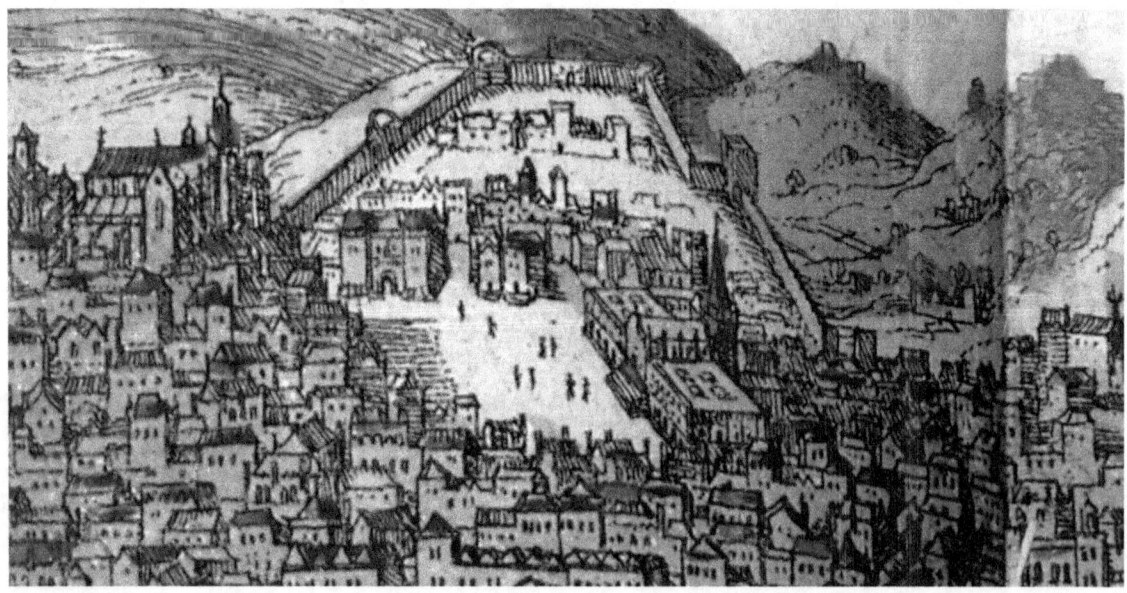

Figure 3.8 Georg Braun and Frans Hogenberg, Detail of *Lisbon*, *Civitates Orbis Terrarum*, vol. 1, 1572. Source: Library of Congress. https://www.loc.gov/resource/g3200m.gct00128a/?sp=14 (accessed September 18, 2020)

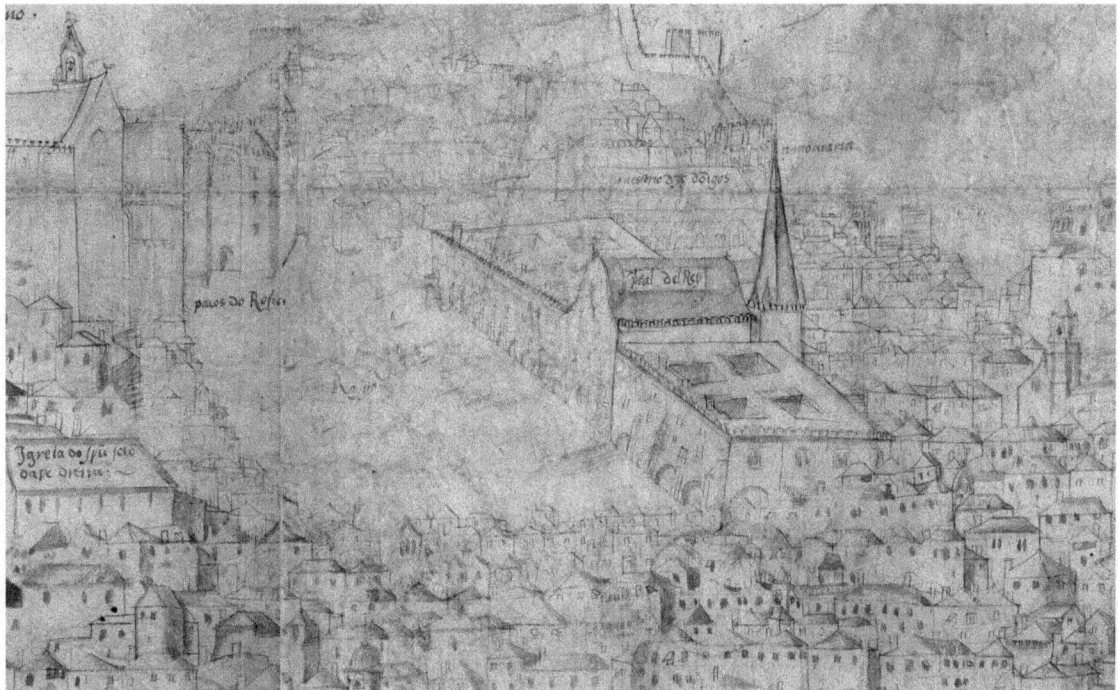

Figure 3.9 Anonymous artist (Flemish or Spanish), Detail of *Panoramic View of Lisbon*, c. 1570–80. Source: Leiden University Library, Leiden

A similar representation of the hospital appears in a drawing of Lisbon from *c.* 1570–80, likely created by a Spanish or Flemish artist and currently at the Library of the University of Leiden (Figure 3.9).[80] Despite missing at least three sheets and having suffered significant damage on the left-hand side, the drawing shows the royal institution as a symmetrical structure with a central church flanked by two rectangular buildings. The prominent staircase leading into the church is barely visible, and the spiral lantern persists as an important marker of the institution. Again, each of the rectangular structures features its own cruciform building. The plan is clearer in the southern cross, but faint outlines indicate that the left side of the hospital mirrored the right, once again creating eight courtyards inside the complex.

Scholars have commented on the unusual appearance of the Hospital Real in these representations, and a close resemblance to the Ospedale Maggiore has been noted even in Holanda's miniature, but no in-depth analysis of this tendency has followed.[81] Especially curious is the view of Lisbon for the *Civitates*, since the volume also included a view of Milan, allowing comparisons between the Hospital Real and the Ospedale Maggiore (see Figures 3.5 and 3.8). The depiction of the Lombard city shows the Milanese institution near a canal, with labels indicating both the hospital and *laghetto*.[82] The depicted hospital, however, does not resemble in any way the magnificent structure envisioned by Filarete or the finished building. By the end of the sixteenth century, only one cross of the double-cross plan had been built, and the view precisely reflects this delay in construction. The central church, a key point in Filarete's design, was never built and is also accurately absent from the rendering.[83] Since construction of the second cross did not begin until 1624, the hospital existed as a single-cross structure throughout the 1500s, when the *Civitates* was published, and the view of Milan in the volume mirrors the contemporary building.

Health and Architecture

This delay in construction and departure from original design indicate that the Ospedale Maggiore itself could not have been the source for the sixteenth-century representations of the Hospital Real de Todos-os-Santos. The Ospedale was also the only cruciform hospital envisioned as a double cross, making it unlikely that the artists who depicted the Portuguese institution used other northern Italian hospitals as inspiration.[84] Nevertheless, the two unusual representations of the Portuguese hospital reveal a striking similarity to the design for the Ospedale depicted by Filarete in his *Treatise* (see Figures 3.1, 3.8, and 3.9). In this case, the prominent staircase and church spiral remain the only residues of Holanda's illuminated miniature and perhaps the actual hospital complex (see Figures 3.7, 3.8, and 3.9). Otherwise, the Hospital Real was replaced by a completely different building.

According to architectural historian Philip Foster's milestone study of the Ospedale Maggiore, the cruciform plan appeared in northern Italy in the fifteenth century but spread widely in the 1500s—the period when the two representations of Lisbon were created. This dissemination started with Cesare Cesariano's edition of Vitruvius's *Ten Books* from 1521, which compared the Ospedale Maggiore to an ancient *oecus* (house) and featured an illustration of a single-cross building.[85] Foster further claimed that a drawing attributed to architect Antonio da Sangallo the Younger highlights the prominence of the Ospedale Maggiore's design during this period.[86] The drawing sketches a ground plan similar to Filarete's double-cross design for the hospital, which, due to the construction delays previously mentioned, Sangallo could only have seen in a copy of the treatise. For Foster, this pervasive awareness of the plan culminated with a discussion of the Ospedale Maggiore in Giorgio Vasari's *Lives of the Artists* (1550, 1568), which lacked an image of Filarete's original plan but described the double-cross design of the hospital. Sangallo's and Vasari's knowledge of the design likely stemmed from the *Codex Magliabechiano* at the Medici Library.[87]

Recent hospital studies continue to examine the propagation of these sources, which suggests a general knowledge of the cruciform typology.[88] Yet, what do they tell us about contemporary awareness of Filarete's original design for the Ospedale as featured in the *Treatise*, and what was their actual role in the dissemination of the plan? Of the sources proposed by Foster, only Sangallo and Vasari could have had a solid impact on the dispersal of Filarete's double-cross design for the Milanese hospital—the former through his drawings and the latter his writings, making the dating and accessibility of these works crucial. Following Sangallo's death in 1546, most of his drawings remained in the possession of his heirs or collectors until 1574, when the Grand Dukes of Tuscany began acquiring the works. It has been noted that, until that time, the circulation and accessibility of the drawings were limited.[89] While Filarete was included in the 1550 version of Vasari's *Lives*, only the 1568 edition featured a description of and praise for the Ospedale Maggiore.[90] This chronology suggests that Filarete's treatise and original plan for the hospital only began circulating more widely on the Italian Peninsula around the last quarter of the sixteenth century, with a *post quem* date of 1568.

This suggestion, however, conflicts with contemporary representations of the Hospital Real. Considering the established uniqueness of Filarete's double-cross, symmetrical plan with a central church, the artists responsible for the *Civitates* and Leiden views of Lisbon must have seen the original plan for the Ospedale Maggiore as depicted in the *Treatise*. Yet, based on the later impact of Sangallo's drawing and Vasari's *Lives*, this knowledge likely did not come from these two sources. As evidenced by the two representations of the Portuguese institution, contrary to what has been assumed, Filarete's plan began circulating before the last quarter of the sixteenth century. By that point, the design had already attained an international reach.

Conclusion

While it remains unclear whether the artists of the *Civitates* and Leiden views of Lisbon saw a copy of Filarete's *Treatise* in Portugal, Italy, or their place of origin, the evidence presented here refutes the assumption that

Filarete's *Treatise* remained obscure and inaccessible until the late sixteenth century; rather, by the 1570s, the design was already internationally known. Regardless of the source, these artists' knowledge of the plan sheds light on our understanding of the design in different ways. While scholars today consider Filarete's plan for the Ospedale Maggiore as the prime example of a Renaissance hospital, these depictions serve as visual evidence that, less than a century after Filarete wrote his *Treatise*, the design became the definitive symbol, the "architectural image," of monumental hospital architecture in Italy and beyond.[91] However, these views also advanced the plan as the model design for Renaissance hospitals, increasing its prominence. Not only did this happen around the same time, or perhaps even earlier, as through the assumed Italian sources, but their reach, particularly in the case of the *Civitates*, was much broader.[92] Although a direct connection between the manuscript and the Hospital Real cannot be established for the fifteenth century, the evidence presented calls for a reconsideration and more careful study of the immediate impact and accessibility of Filarete's *Treatise* in an international context. Finally, it is crucial to highlight that depictions of the Hospital Real as the Ospedale Maggiore further promoted the view of Lisbon as a global metropolis where one could find the best of everything and, significantly for the period, that included innovations in the architecture of hospitals.

As mentioned above, the exportation of the cruciform plan from Italy and its adoption in Iberia has been under-analyzed in scholarship, as if the resulting buildings simply represented the success and conventional repetition of an Italian model. This trend is particularly neglectful when it comes to the Hospital Real de Todos-os-Santos, which has remained either omitted in studies of the cruciform design or mentioned as an appendix to Spanish hospitals. Yet, this analysis of the Portuguese institution suggests a more complex scenario. Strategically, the Portuguese monarchy embraced a range of innovations from Italy prior to their arrival in Spain but combined them with local developments to suit the needs of a burgeoning port city. Seeking to reform healthcare in their capital, Portugal opted for the so-called Milanese model, amalgamating medieval hospitals under one large institution. This reform helped partially fund their royal hospital, but it took years to actually yield financial results. In the meantime, the bulk of resources stemmed from royal measures, either in the form of land donations, the appropriation of former Jewish and Moorish properties, or profits from colonial goods. The latter two strategies, in particular, demonstrate the resourceful ways through which the Portuguese monarchy endowed its hospital by profiting from Lisbon's increasingly global status.

As for the functioning of the institution, the Tuscan hospitals of Florence and Siena offered the initial model, and the plan itself was imported from northern Italy. Yet, the location and structure both demonstrate incorporation of local needs. By building the hospital on Rossio, the monarchy promoted the urbanization of a then transitional space, creating a new commercial axis for the city that also facilitated access to the hospital from the Ribeira, the city's port and main arrival area. Structurally, the institution moved away from the ornamentation typically associated with the northern Italian Renaissance, and especially Filarete's design for the Ospedale Maggiore, but kept its monumentality, which allowed for the treatment of a large number of patients. The hospital also appears to have featured a similar system of latrines, crucial for preventing the formation of bad airs inside the building.[93] Adjusted to fit the property, the plan varied with the incorporation of the church into an arm of the cross, a strategy seen at hospitals in Mantua and Parma, serving as a transitional space between the healthy and the sick and retaining its public function, which increased the civic prominence of the institution. Finally, the magnificent church facade reflected the royal patronage of the hospital, framing the Hospital Real as symbolic of the Portuguese monarchy's move for control of social welfare and public health in the increasingly wealthy, yet critically overloaded port city.

Acknowledgment: This chapter stems from my dissertation, "Poverty, Disease, and Port Cities: Global Exchanges in Hospital Architecture during the Age of Exploration" (Temple University, 2020). I am most grateful to Marlise G. Brown, Tracy E. Cooper, and Kimberly L. Dennis for their comments and suggestions.

Health and Architecture

This research benefited from funding support from the Bibliotheca Hertziana-Max Planck Institute for Art History, the Getty Foundation, and Temple University.

Notes

1. On the social and economic pressures in this transitional period from the Middle Ages to the early modern period, see Thomas Max Safley's "Introduction" in *Reformation of Charity: The Secular and Religious in Early Modern Poor Relief*, ed. Thomas Max Safley (Boston: Brill, 2003), 1–9, which also includes a summary of the historiography of charity. A more recent overview of this historiography, particularly in relationship to charitable institutions, appears in Nicholas Terpstra's "Introduction" to his *Cultures of Charity: Women, Politics, and the Reform of Poor Relief in Renaissance Italy* (Cambridge, MA: Harvard University Press, 2013), 1–18.
2. Laura Baini provides an overview of the historiography on the cruciform plan in "Ipotesi sull'origine della tipologia cruciforme per gli ospedali del XV secolo" in *Processi accumulativi, forme e funzioni: Saggi sull'architettura lombarda del Quattrocento*, ed. Luisa Giordano (Florence: La Nuova Italia Editrice, 1996), 65–8. John Henderson summarizes the debate and evidence against the Florentine primacy in *The Renaissance Hospital: Healing the Body and Healing the Soul* (New Haven: Yale University Press, 2006), 149–53.
3. See, for example, Nikolaus Pevsner, *A History of Building Types* (Princeton: Princeton University Press, 1976), 144–5, and Catherine Wilkinson, *The Hospital of Cardinal Tavera in Toledo* (New York: Garland Publishing, 1977), 6–10. The three hospitals historically associated with Egas are the Hospital Real de Santiago de Compostela (1501), the Hospital de la Santa Cruz (1504) in Toledo, and the Hospital Real (1504) in Granada. Today, it is known that the architect was only involved with the first one. It has also been established that the Hospital dels Folls (1493) in Valencia and the Hospital de Nuestra Señora de Gracia (1496, destroyed in 1808) in Zaragoza were the first cruciform hospitals in Spain, post-dating the Portuguese institution. See Fernando Marías, "Arquitectura y Sistema hospitalario en Toledo en el siglo XVI," in *Tolède et l'expansion urbaine en Espagne, 1450–1650: actes du colloque organisé par la Junta de Comunidades de Castilla-La Mancha et la Casa de Velázquez, Tolède-Madrid, 21–23 mars 1988* (Madrid: Recontres de la Casa de Velázquez, 1991), 54.
4. Besides Portugal and Spain, the plan later appeared in France and England. See Pevsner, *History of Building Types*, 143–7.
5. Rafael Moreira argues that, while the hospital has been extensively studied by Portuguese scholars, the lack of attention to the architecture of the Hospital Real, particularly its cruciform plan, is common even in local scholarship. See Rafael Moreira, "O Hospital Real de Todos-os-Santos e o Italianismo de D. João II" in *Hospital Real de Todos-os-Santos: Séculos XV a XVIII*, ed. Paulo Pereira (Lisbon: Museu Rafael Bordalo Pinheiro, 1993), 24. Studies of Spanish cruciform hospitals tend to neglect the Portuguese institution altogether.
6. For a recent discussion of artistic centers and peripheries in the Renaissance, the issues associated with this model, and potential alternatives, see Stephen J. Campbell, "Artistic Geographies," in *The Cambridge Companion to the Italian Renaissance*, ed. Michael Wyatt (Cambridge: Cambridge University Press, 2014), 17–39.
7. My methodology is based on the concept of world cities, which stems from the field of sociology and the World System Theory developed by Immanuel Wallerstein in the late 1970s. Nicolas Bock first applied the concept to art historical studies, using this methodology in his analysis of fourteenth- and fifteenth-century Naples. According to this framework, world cities imported artists, media, and materials in order to gain cultural, political, or economic centrality. On the other hand, there were cities considered cultural producers, such as fifteenth-century Florence, which ideologically incorporated a patrimony created abroad—for example, through the exportation of art and architectural styles and their practitioners—as part of their identity. Cultural producers and world cities coexisted, exchanged, and legitimated each other, but while the former gained their centrality through exportation (of people, ideas, materials, etc.), world cities fashioned themselves as having only the best offered by cultural producers. See Immanuel Wallerstein, *The Modern World System: Capitalist Agriculture and the Origins of the European World Economy in the Sixteenth Century* (New York: Academic Press, 1974); Nicolas Bock, "Patronage, Standards, and *Transfert Culturel*: Naples between Art History and Social Science Theory," *Art History* 31 (2008): 594–7, 601–2; and Campbell, "Artistic Geographies," 25–7.
8. This trend has culminated with *The Global City: On the Streets of Renaissance Lisbon*, ed. Annemarie Jordan Gschwend and Kate Lowe (London: Paul Holberton Publishing, 2015), and the 2017 exhibition and catalog *A Cidade Global:*

Lisboa no Renascimento / The Global City: Lisbon in the Renaissance (Lisbon: Museu Nacional de Arte Antiga, 2017). The original expression recorded by the Venetians was "Chi no vee Lisboa, non vee cosa boa." Cited and translated in Kate Lowe, "Foreign Descriptions of the Global City: Renaissance Lisbon from the Outside," in *On the Streets*, 39.

9. Francesco Bianchi and Marek Słoń, "Le riforme ospedaliere del Quattrocento in Italia e nell'Europa centrale," *Ricerche di storia sociale e religiosa* 35 (2006): 15–17.
10. Bianchi and Słoń, "Le riforme ospedaliere," 15–16.
11. Henderson, *Renaissance Hospital*, 90–1, and Bianchi and Słoń, "Le riforme ospedaliere," 28–31.
12. However, Milan was not the first city to implement this reorganization of charity. See Bianchi and Słoń, "Le riforme ospedaliere," 20–8.
13. In many cities, this development gained further importance in architectural history due to its association with important fifteenth-century architects, such as Brunelleschi and Michelozzo in Florence and Filarete in Milan. Bianchi and Słoń, "Le riforme ospedaliere," 17–19.
14. As established by Philip Foster in "Per il disegno dell'Ospedale di Milano," *Arte Lombarda* 18 (1973): 1–12.
15. See Raffaella Gorini, "Gli ospedali Lombardi del XV secolo. Documenti per la loro storia," in *Processi accumulativi*, 11–58 for a comprehensive discussion of the architectural histories of several northern Italian hospitals, particularly as they relate to the cruciform plan. For English translations of Alberti's and Filarete's treatises, see Leon Battista Alberti, *On the Art of Building in Ten Books*, trans. Joseph Rykwert, Neil Leach, and Robert Tavernor (Cambridge, MA: MIT Press, 1998), and Filarete, *Treatise on Architecture; Being the Treatise by Antonio di Piero Averlino, Known as Filarete*, trans. John R. Spencer, 2 vols. (New Haven: Yale University Press, 1965). Alberti's treatise was written in *c*. 1450 but only published in 1486, while Filarete wrote his treatise in 1460–4. The latter, however, was partially published in 1890 and only became fully available in print in English in 1965 and in Italian in 1972.
16. Lucio Franchini, "Introduzione," in *Spedali Lombardi del Quattrocento: Fondazione, trasformazioni, restauri*, ed. Lucio Franchini (Como: Edizioni New Press, 1995), 46–52 offers a comprehensive examination of cruciform structures, including their commonalities and variations.
17. Baini, "Ipotesi," 68, and Franchini, "Introduzione," 34. In the case of the Ospedale Maggiore, this separation happened through the dedication of a cross for women and another for men, while in Mantua different stories were used for men and women.
18. Franchini, "Introduzione," 48–9. Information on windows remains limited, but evidence suggests that some could be opened using ropes. See Henderson, *Renaissance Hospital*, 159–60, and Eva Maria Herrmann et al., *Enclose | Build: Walls, Facade, Roof*, ed. Alexander Reichel and Kerstin Schultz (Basel: Birkhäuser, 2015), 104.
19. For an overview of the historiography on the cruciform plan as it relates to religious symbolism and metaphors, see Franchini, "Introduzione," 35–6.
20. Franchini, "Introduzione," 35.
21. Vitruvius, *Ten Books*, 26–7. The author also discusses the importance of wholesome food when determining the healthiness of a site.
22. Renzo Baldasso, "Function and Epidemiology in Filarete's Ospedale Maggiore," in *The Medieval Hospital and Medical Practice*, ed. Barbara S. Bowers (Burlington, VT: Ashgate, 2007), 114. In an attempt to correct the condition, the body would form buboes to expel the poison.
23. Henderson, *Renaissance Hospital*, xxix–xxx.
24. Sandra Cavallo and Tessa Storey, *Healthy Living in Late Renaissance Italy* (Oxford: Oxford University Press, 2013), 5, and Ken Albala, *Eating Right in the Renaissance* (Berkeley: University of California Press, 2002), 115–16.
25. Henderson, *Renaissance Hospital*, 158; Cavallo and Storey, *Healthy Living*, 81.
26. Marsilio Ficino, *Consiglio contra la pestilenzia* (Florence: San Jacopo a Ripoli, 1481), 63. Cited in Henderson, *Renaissance Hospital*, 159.
27. Alberti, *On the Art of Building*, 129–30.
28. Alberti, *On the Art of Building*, 130.
29. These fifteenth-century developments should not be surprising since advice regarding healthy sites dates back to the classical period. Particularly relevant was the information found in Vitruvius' *Ten Books on Architecture*. Cavallo and Storey, *Healthy Living*, 80–1.
30. Unification was authorized in 1459 through a bull by Pope Pius II. For the welfare reform in Milan, see Evelyn Welch, *Art and Authority in Renaissance Milan* (New Haven: Yale University Press, 1995), 136–43. This amalgamation of medieval hospitals was not new in northern Italy and had already happened in several cities between 1437 and 1459.

See Sandra Cavallo, *Charity and Power in Early Modern Italy: Benefactors and their Motives in Turin, 1541–1789* (Cambridge: Cambridge University Press, 1995), 32.

31. On Filarete's use of the *Treatise* to gain favor with his patrons, see Valentina Vulpi, "Finding Filarete: The Two Versions of the Libro architettonico," in *Raising the Eyebrow: John Onians and World Art Studies: An Album Amicorum in his Honour*, ed. Lauren Golden (Oxford: Archaeopress, 2001), 329–39.
32. For the description of the hospital by the Florentine architect, see Filarete, *Treatise on Architecture*, vol. 1, 137–46. Baldasso addresses the *destri* in detail in "Function and Epidemiology," 115–20. The system and the Ospedale are both praised by Giorgio Vasari in his Life of Filarete. See Giorgio Vasari, *Le vite de' più eccellenti pittori, scultori ed architettori*, 9 vols., ed. Gaetano Milanesi (Florence: G. C. Sansoni, 1878–85), vol. 2, 455–7.
33. Filarete, *Treatise on Architecture*, vol. 1, 140.
34. Welch, *Art and Authority*, 152.
35. A partial edition was published in 1896, but complete versions only appeared with an English translation in 1965 and an Italian edition in 1972. John Spencer argues that "we still do not know the accessibility of the treatise," although he believes that it did have an impact on contemporary architecture. Luisa Giordano claims that the narrative format of the work, combined with "the patchy treatment of architectural theory, made the treatise of little interest to later generations," as illustrated by Giorgio Vasari's dismissive comments in the 1568 edition of the *Lives*. Mario Carpo believes that the treatise was not unknown, but the manuscript format made it difficult to consult. Valentina Vulpi hypothesizes that the ultimate reason for the "long oblivion" of the *Treatise* was the architect's "inability to transcend a strictly personal patronage relationship," failing to appeal to a broader audience and not rising above local specificity. See John Spencer, review of *Antonio Averlino detto il Filarete. Trattato di Architettura*, by Anna Maria Finoli and Liliana Grassi, *Art Bulletin* 57 (1975): 131–3; Luisa Giordano, "On Filarete's *Libro Architettonico*," in *Paper Palaces: The Rise of the Renaissance Architectural Treatise*, ed. Vaughan Hart and Peter Hicks (New Haven: Yale University Press, 1998), 53; Mario Carpo, *Architecture in the Age of Printing: Orality, Writing, Typograph, and Printed Images in the History of Architectural Theory*, trans. Sarah Benson (Cambridge, MA: MIT Press, 2001), 135; and Vulpi, "Finding Filarete," 339. For Vasari's comments, see *Le vite*, vol. 2, 457–8.
36. This copy, known as the *Codex Trivulziano* (Ms. 863), had been housed in the Biblioteca Trivulziana in Milan prior to its destruction in 1944 as a result of aerial bombing of the city.
37. For a summarized history of the copies of Filarete's original manuscript, see Spencer, "Introduction," in *Treatise on Architecture*, vol. 1, xvii–xviii. For details on each copy, see Anna Maria Finoli, "Nota al testo," in Filarete, *Trattato di architettura*, 2 vols., ed. Anna Maria Finoli and Liliana Grassi (Milan: Edizioni Il Polifilo, 1972), vol. 2, cvii–cxxix.
38. Georgia Clarke, "Vitruvian Paradigms," *Papers of the British School at Rome* 70 (2002): 327–8, and Tammaro de Marinis, *La biblioteca napoletana dei re d'Aragona*, 2 vols. (Verona: Stamperia Valdonega, 1969), 50–1. This copy, now lost and known as the *Codex Valencianus* (Ms. 837), was ordered by Cardinal Giovanni of Aragon (1456–85) and eventually made its way to Valencia as part of the Royal Library of Naples. The manuscript was likely inaccessible until 1523, and in 1546 the copy was donated to the Monastery of San Miguel de los Reys. See Wilkinson, *The Hospital of Cardinal Tavera*, 248, n. 50, and Finoli, "Nota al testo," cviii–cix.
39. Pavel Kalina, "European Diplomacy, Family Strategies, and the Origins of Renaissance Architecture in Central and Eastern Europe," *Artibus et Historiae* 30 (2009): 175.
40. On the benefits and difficulties faced by port cities, see Cátia Antunes, "Early Modern Ports, 1500–1750," *European History Online (EGO)* (2010): n.p.
41. Laurinda Abreu, *Political and Social Dynamics of Poverty, Poor Relief and Health Care in Early-Modern Portugal* (New York: Routledge, 2016), 14.
42. Permission given through the papal bull *Ex debito solicitudinis office pastoralis*, issued by Pope Sixtus IV. For a history of this healthcare reform in Portugal, see Abreu, *Political and Social Dynamics*, 25–34.
43. Anastásia Mestrinho Salgado, *O Hospital de Todos-os-Santos: Assistência à pobreza em Portugal no século XVI; A irradiação da assistência médica para o Brasil, Índia e Japão* (Lisbon: By the Book, 2015), 38–52 and 193–202 lists these institutions and includes a map with their location.
44. Irisalva Moita, "A imagem e a vida da cidade," in *Lisboa quinhentista: A imagem e a vida da cidade*, ed. Irisalva Moita (Lisbon: Câmara Municipal de Lisboa, 1983), 14.
45. Salgado, *Assistência à pobreza*, 60.
46. Paulo Drumond Braga, "A crise dos estabelecimentos de assistência aos pobres nos finais da idade média," *Revista Portuguesa de História* 26 (1991): 175–87.

47. Moita, "A imagem e a vida," 15. Moita argues that this population increase would have been more significant had it not been for the impact of plague outbreaks, deaths caused by shipwrecks, voluntary migrations to conquered areas, and wars to support these new domains. Salgado points out that, by being the capital, Lisbon also attracted people on personal business at important organs, such as the Casa do Cível or the Casa da Suplicação. See Salgado, *Assistência à pobreza*, 85
48. In Fernando da Silva Correia, *Subsídios para a história da saúde pública portuguesa do Século XV a 1822* (Oporto: n.p., 1958), 6, the author lists at least twelve outbreaks in the fifteenth century, which happened in the years of 1423, 1432, 1435, 1438 (leading to the death of then King Dom Duarte, r. 1433–38), 1458, 1464, 1465, 1467, 1469, 1477, 1490, and 1496. Augusto da Silva Carvalho, *Crónica do Hospital de Todos-os-Santos* (Lisbon: n.p., 1949), 18 argues that the situation became particularly critical between 1480–7 and after 1490.
49. Cruciform hospitals have also been considered the earliest Renaissance buildings in Spain. See Wilkinson, *The Hospital of Cardinal Tavera*, 6.
50. This gap in the history of colonial hospitals and the phenomenon of the globalization of the hospital are emphasized by John Henderson, Peregrine Horden, and Alessandro Pastore in their "Introduction. The World of the Hospital: Comparisons and Continuities," in *The Impact of Hospitals, 300–1200*, ed. John Henderson, Peregrine Horden, and Alessandro Pastore (Oxford: Peter Lang, 2007), 27–31.
51. Until the celebration of the 500th anniversary of the Hospital Real in 1992, the two main monographs on the institution were Carvalho, *Crónica do Hospital*, and Mario Carmona, *O Hospital Real de Todos-os-Santos da Cidade de Lisboa* (Lisbon: n.p., 1954). These publications include extensive archival research on the hospital and still remain relevant, but the most recent study of the institution is *Hospital Real de Todos-os-Santos: Séculos XV a XVIII*.
52. See Carmona, *Hospital Real*, 53–4 for a summary of documents indicating that a treasurer and clerk had already been appointed by 1484.
53. Carmona, *Hospital Real*, 54.
54. These measures began in December 1496, when Dom Manuel ordered all Jews and Muslims to leave his kingdom in the following ten months. Those who did not follow the king's orders would face the death penalty and loss of their properties. While it has been traditionally assumed that Dom Manuel's measures against Jews resulted from his marriage to Princess Isabel, the eldest daughter of Spanish monarchs Isabel of Castile (r. 1474–1504) and Ferdinand of Aragon (r. 1479–1516), who had expelled Jews from their territories in 1492, experts now believe that these measures were fueled by Dom Manuel's desires to finance a voyage to India and launch a new crusade against Muslims in Morocco, both of which required an enduring peace with the Spanish monarchy. See François Soyer, *The Persecution of the Jews and Muslims of Portugal: King Manuel I and the End of Religious Tolerance (1496–7)* (Leiden: Brill, 2007), 1–8.
55. Nuno Daupiás outlines these measures in *Cartas de Privilégio, Padrões, Doações e Mercês Régias ao Hospital Real de Todos-os-Santos (1492–1775): Subsídios para a sua história* (Lisbon: Imprensa Portuguesa, 1959), 18–21. See also Carmona, *Hospital Real*, 54–6.
56. Daupiás, *Cartas*, 20.
57. Dom Manuel had first ordered this measure in 1497, but the Chamber of Lisbon protested, leading to the 1501 decree reinforcing the initial order. This issue had to be eventually resolved in court. On the archaeological evidence of the decree, see Irisalva Moita, "As escavações de 1960 que puseram a descoberto parte das ruínas do Hospital Real de Todos-os-Santos," in *Hospital Real de Todos-os-Santos: Séculos XV a XVIII*, 22, n. 4. On the dispute, see Carvalho, *Crónica do Hospital*, 41.
58. As Carmona argues, royal support represented the main source of income for the Hospital Real while the reorganization of hospitals was underway. The author believes that the hospital only started receiving funds from medieval institutions in 1501. See Carmona, *Hospital Real*, 187–8.
59. See Carmona, *Hospital Real*, 14–15 for a transcription of Dom João's will as it pertains to the hospital.
60. Carmona, *Hospital Real*, 188. The Padroado was an agreement between the Holy See and the Portuguese monarchy granting the latter autonomy in the administration of local churches.
61. Salgado, *Assistência à pobreza*, 81. Initially, the amount was 70 *arrobas*, the equivalent of approximately 1,029 kilograms. By 1517, the donation amount had reached 700 *arrobas* or 10,290 kilograms. Salgado addresses further measures on pp. 78–83.
62. Carmona, *Hospital Real*, 14–15.
63. Scholars of the Portuguese hospital have debated how closely its statute actually reflected those of Florence and Siena since the Hospital Real had already been functioning for two years by the time the document was created. Ana

Cristina Leite believes that there were very few similarities, and Laurinda Abreu acknowledges the difficulties in addressing the issue and offers a more encompassing comparison. See Ana Cristina Leite, "Hospital Real de Todos-os-Santos. Uma Obra Moderna," in *Omnia Sanctorum. Histórias da História do Hospital Real de Todos-os-Santos e seus sucessores*, ed. Jorge Penedo (Lisbon: By the Book, 2012), 31, and Laurinda Abreu, "O que nos ensinam os regimentos hospitalares? Um estudo comparativo entre os Hospitais das Misericórdias de Lisboa e do Porto (séculos XVI e XVII)," in *A Solidariedade nos Séculos: A Confraternidade e as Obras*, ed. Santa Casa da Misericórdia do Porto (Porto: Santa Casa da Misericórdia do Porto e Alêtheia Editores, 2009), esp. 268–74. For the statute of the Hospital Real de Todos-os-Santos, see *Regimento do Hospital de Todos-os-Santos (Edição Fac-Similada)*, ed. Abílio José Salgado and Anastásia Mestrinho Salgado (Lisbon: Comissão Organizadora do V Centenário da Fundação do Hospital de Todos-os-Santos, 1992).

64. For the 1960 excavation campaign, see Irisalva Moita, "Hospital Real de Todos-os-Santos (relatório das escavações a que mandou proceder a CML de 22 de agosto a 24 de setembro 1960)," *Revista Municipal* 101–11 (1964–6). A summary of the excavation campaign appeared in Moita, "As escavações de 1960," in *Hospital Real de Todos-os-Santos: Séculos XV a XVIII*, 20–2. Records of the 1999–2001 excavation campaign are still being processed and have not been published. I would like to thank Rodrigo Banha da Silva, the archaeologist in charge of the campaign, for his generosity in sharing the initial findings with me.
65. Renata de Araújo, *Lisboa: A Cidade e o Espetáculo na Época dos Descobrimentos* (Lisbon: Livros Horizontes, 1993), 62; Moita, "A imagem e a vida," 9. The move of the commercial center of the city toward the Ribeira happened in the mid-fourteenth century, when Portuguese maritime activities began under King Dom Diniz (r. 1279–1325). This wall, the Muralha Fernandina, was built by King Dom Fernando (r. 1367–83) in 1373 to include the Alfama, a neighborhood village that had appeared outside the previously existing wall ordered by Dom Diniz to protect the then quickly increasing population of the Baixa area of Lisbon.
66. Araújo, *A Cidade e o Espetáculo*, 62–3, and Moita, "A imagem e a vida," 14. In the mid-sixteenth century, the Paço dos Estaus became the Palace of the Inquisition. For the history of this building, see Delminda Maria Miguéns Rijo, "Palácio dos Estaus de Hospedaria Real a Palácio da Inquisição e Tribunal do Santo Ofício," *Cadernos do Arquivo Municipal* 5 (2016): 19–49.
67. The Rua Nova d'El Rey was perpendicular to the Rua Nova dos Mercadores, which constituted the east–west commercial axis of Lisbon. Araújo, *A Cidade e o Espetáculo*, 59.
68. This contemporary account appears in João Brandão de Buarcos, *Grandeza e Abastança de Lisboa em 1552*, ed. José da Felicidade Alves (Lisbon: Livros Horizontes, 1990), 123–30. See also Ana Cristina Leite, "O Hospital Real de Todos-os-Santos," 7–12, and Irisalva Moita, "O Hospital Real de Todos-os-Santos: Enfermarias—Aposentadorias—Serviços," 40–7 in *Hospita Real de Todos-os-Santos: Séculos XV a XVIII* for detailed descriptions of the hospital complex.
69. Franchini, "Introduzione," 35, 50.
70. Leite highlights the use of the hospital church for public events, such as the coronation of Cardinal Dom Henrique in 1578. She argues that the number of celebrations at the church might have led to the closing of the infirmary openings in 1617. See Leite, "O Hospital Real de Todos-os-Santos," 10.
71. Among these structures was the Casa das Boubas with two isolated wards for men and women with syphilis. These areas also included apartments for hospital staff, since many had to live on site, a ward for convalescents, an infirmary for Capuchin friars, the hospital kitchen, a pharmacy, a refectory, a house for abandoned children, as well as an admissions and triage area. Moreover, on the ground floor facing the Rossio, the Casa dos Pedintes Andantes temporarily sheltered beggars. See Leite, "O Hospital Real de Todos-os-Santos," 8.
72. Leite, "Uma obra moderna," 33. Incurable patients, which in this case refers to those with leprosy, were initially not admitted, although that restriction was removed later on.
73. Leite, "O Hospital Real de Todos-os-Santos," 13.
74. Scholars have interpreted the portal as a political monument, a symbol of the centralization of hospitals and royal power and propaganda. See, for example, Leite, "O Hospital Real de Todos-os-Santos," 14.
75. There was also an Italian community living in Lisbon. See *Cultural Links between Portugal and Italy in the Renaissance*, ed. Kate Lowe (Oxford: Oxford University Press, 2000) for several examples of these connections.
76. Vasari claimed that Lorenzo de' Medici's agency guaranteed Sansovino the position, but Lorenzo had been already been dead for eight months when the Florentine artist signed a contract on December 9, 1492. See Vasari, *Le vite*, vol. 4, 513, and Janez Höfler, "New Light on Andrea Sansovino's Journey to Portugal," *The Burlington Magazine* 134 (1992): 234–8, particularly p. 236 for the Portuguese interest in and connections with Italy. Albinia de la Mare has highlighted several instances in which Portuguese patrons commissioned or acquired books in the Florentine book

trade during this period. These patrons included Dom Manuel, who while prince in 1494 used an agent to commission manuscripts from two scribes who had also worked for King Matthias Corvinus of Hungary, the Cardinal of Aragon, as well as Lorenzo and Piero de' Medici. All of these patrons either owned or commissioned copies of Filarete's *Treatise* at some point in the late fifteenth century. This does not indicate that the Portuguese monarchy necessarily had a copy of the *Treatise*, but, as de la Mare has suggested, it certainly highlights the role of the monarchy in the Florentine book trade and its preference for manuscripts rather than printed books. See Albinia de la Mare, "Notes of the Portuguese Patrons of the Florentine Book Trade in the Fifteenth Century," in *Cultural Links*, 167–81.
77. Created in their majority by foreign artists, many of these city views have not survived. See Annemarie Jordan Gschwend and Kate Lowe, "Princess of the Seas, Queen of Empire: Configuring the City and Port of Renaissance Lisbon," in *On the Streets*, 12–35 for a discussion of views of Renaissance Lisbon.
78. Jessica Robey offers a brief overview of the *Civitates* in "From the City Witnessed to the Community Dreamed: The *Civitates Orbis Terrarum* and the Circle of Abraham Ortelius and Joris Hoefnagel" (Ph.D. diss., University of California, Santa Barbara, 2006), 25–30.
79. A later view of Lisbon, published in 1598 as part of the fifth volume of the *Civitates*, includes a depiction of the Hospital Real that perhaps more closely resembles the actual structure. This view is often mistaken for the 1572 one, but it is important to emphasize that it is indeed a later creation. This confusion with the date appears in, for example, Annemarie Jordan Gschwend and Kate Lowe, "Sítios globais da Lisboa renascentista," in *A Cidade Global*, 36–8.
80. The watermarks on the paper date to 1560. See Gshwend and Lowe, "Sítios globais," 32–4, 36.
81. Leite, "Uma obra moderna," 37, n. 16.
82. Labeled "ospital gr" and "lageto."
83. For a chronology of the Ospedale Maggiore, see Liliana Grassi, *Lo 'Spedale di Poveri' del Filarete: Storia e restauro* (Milan: Università degli Studi di Milano, 1972), 43–74.
84. Half of the plan for the Escorial, also featured in the 1572 volume of *Civitates*, strongly resembles Filarete's design for the Ospedale Maggiore.
85. Cesare Cesariano, *Di Lucio Vitruvio Pollione de Architectura libri dece*, 10 vols. (Como: 1521), vol. 6, fol. icix v. As Fernando Marías has highlighted, Cesariano's reference was to cruciform hospitals in Italy, which he understood as existing in Florence, Siena, Rome, and Milan. As such, he was not referring specifically to Filarete's design for the Ospedale Maggiore, and in this case it is crucial not to conflate a single-cross plan with Filarete's double-cross design. See Marías, "Arquitectura y Sistema," 58.
86. Foster, "Per il disegno," 11, 18. Foster does not include a date for the Sangallo drawing, which is not addressed at length by Gustavo Giovannoni in his study of Sangallo or in the main recent publication on Sangallo's works at the Gabinetto dei Disegni e delle Stampe delle Gallerie degli Uffizi. See Gustavo Giovannoni, *Antonio da Sangallo il Giovane*, 2 vols. (Rome: Tipografia Regionale, 1959), vol. 1, 21, and *The Architectural Drawings of Antonio da Sangallo and His Circle*, ed. Christoph L. Frommel and Nicholas Adams, 2 vols. (Cambridge, MA: MIT Press, 1994–2000).
87. When criticizing the *Treatise*, Vasari specifically says that it was dedicated in 1464 to Piero di Cosimo de' Medici and later in the possession of Duke Cosimo, suggesting that he indeed accessed the Medici copy. See Vasari, *Le vite*, vol. 2, 457.
88. As an example, see Bernardo Santos Dias, "A História na medida do Presente. O Ospedale della Misericordia di Parma" (MA thesis, Universidade do Porto, 2015–16), 58–9.
89. Christoph L. Frommel, "Introduction: The Drawings of Antonio da Sangallo the Younger: History, Evolution, Method, Function," in *Architectural Drawings*, 1, 5.
90. Vasari, *Le vite*, vol. 2, 455–7.
91. Wilkinson had already called attention to Filarete's role in creating the "architectural image" of a general hospital, though she did not believe that the *Treatise* had any direct impact on later architecture. See Wilkinson, *The Hospital of Cardinal Tavera*, 14–15.
92. The popularity and success of the *Civitates* is attested by its continuous publication in a total of six volumes. While the volumes targeted the wealthy, individual prints of cities were sold separately, reaching a more popular and general audience. See Robey, "From the City Witnessed to the Community Dreamed," 34–41.
93. I explore this topic in a chapter of my dissertation. See Danielle Abdon, "Poverty, Disease, and Port Cities: Global Exchanges in Hospital Architecture during the Age of Exploration" (Temple University, 2020), chapter 3.

CHAPTER 4
HEALING OF THE POOR
THE HOSPITAL OF OUR LADY OF POTTERIE IN BRUGES AND THE MIRACLE BOOK (*c.* 1520–1)
Miyako Sugiyama

The Hospital of Our Lady of Potterie in Bruges is home to a small manuscript known as the *Miracle Book of Our Lady of Potterie*.[1] The hospital has attracted many pilgrims for centuries, as it preserves the miraculous statue of the Virgin Mary (Figure 4.1), which is the subject of the miracle book. Although no document concerning the author or purpose of the book is preserved, it is generally accepted that the book was created around 1520–1, which corresponds to the period when devotion of the Virgin reached its peak in the hospital. The book records the various miracles performed by the statue of the Virgin that was venerated by the patients in the hospital. This book is unique among many books recording miracles performed by the Virgin or saints,

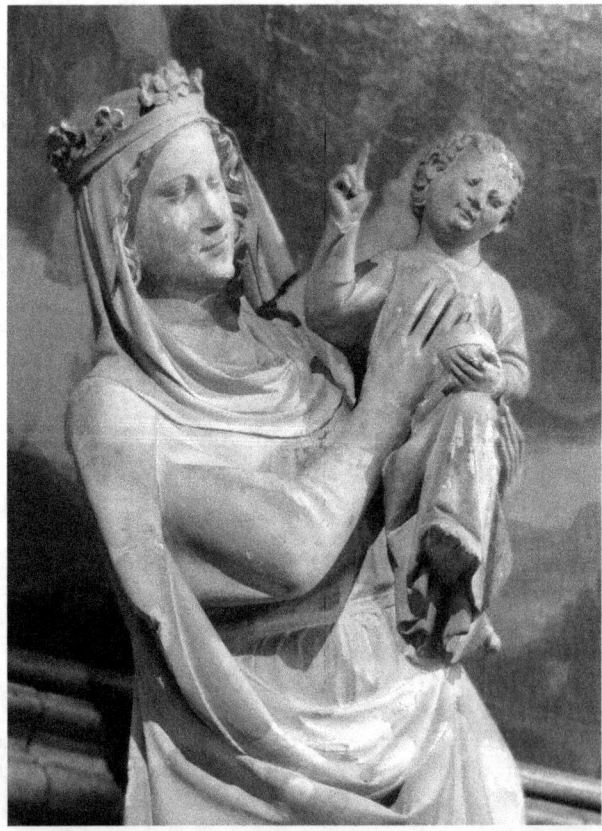

Figure 4.1 Miraculous statue of Our Lady of Potterie, *c.* 1270–80, white stone, 160 cm, Museum Onze-Lieve-Vrouwter-Potterie. Musea Brugge, www.artinflanders.be, photo: Hugo Maertens

as it not only tells stories of miracles but also visualizes them with rich illustrations that were, to some extent, intended to assist those who could not read in conveying the importance of faith and the power of the church.

This chapter considers the sacred and profane in a pre-modern hospital through this case study of the *Miracle Book of Our Lady of Potterie*. Previous research on the miracle book has focused primarily on the series of miracles attributed to Our Lady of Potterie. The present study shifts the focus from the sacred presence performing these miracles to the beneficiaries of these sacred acts. For the first time, the miracle book will be considered not just in terms of these miraculous events but also as a book depicting "the poor" and the community's support for them. Importantly, this dual focus also brings to light the developing social welfare mission of the local hospital.

To understand the mission of a pre-modern hospital, a broader understanding of the poor and how they were perceived by others during this period is critical. In the sections that follow, a brief survey of the architecture and history of the hospital is provided, including the genesis and story of the miraculous statue of the Virgin. This expanded portrayal of the poor will then be considered in light of the *De Subventione Pauperum* ("On the Relief of the Poor"), an academic report written in 1526 by Juan Luis Vives (1492–1540) for the Senate of Bruges. Notably, this treatise presents a decidedly more sympathetic view of the indigent, as well as the changing environment for social welfare in early sixteenth-century Bruges, home to the Hospital of Our Lady of Potterie. On the basis of Vives's view of the poor as encompassing people facing a range of challenges (both physical and circumstantial), those represented in the miracle book are also viewed in this light and analyzed in detail. Finally, the study of these two different perspectives, religious and academic, will reveal that the poor represented in the miracle book were not only receivers of heavenly grace but also receivers of earthly support.

Architecture and History of the Hospital

The city of Bruges, in the Belgian province of West Flanders, established itself as one of the economic, cultural, and international trade centers of Europe in the twelfth century.[2] International merchants and travelers came from all over Europe to the city center via the Reie River. It was along this river, in an area called Potterierei where many pot bakers (*pottenbakkers*) had settled, that a hospital was founded in the thirteenth century to provide shelter for travelers and the sick. The hospital was known as the Hospital of Our Lady of Potterie. Renovated in 1881, it was subsequently converted into a hospital museum.[3]

As a result of renovations and extensions in the nineteenth and twentieth centuries, it is difficult to reconstruct the original architectural design. When it still functioned as a hospital, the structure included a ward, church, kitchen, laundry, bakery, brewery, cowsheds, and mill.[4] The facade of the hospital is composed of two anchored pointed gables and a spout gable on saddleback roofs.[5] All three parts show pointed-arch windows with traceries. The composition was a result of the 1881 renovation by architect Karel Verschelde (1842–81), who intended to restore the facade to its original form.[6] The left section of the hospital ward now serves as the central area of the hospital museum. A fireplace with a chimney was once installed at the front of the ward to warm the space. Entering a rounded-arch door framed with limestones, visitors today can see a large number of liturgical objects and artworks commissioned by those who lived and worked there. Although the hospital ward is now divided by walls from the hospital church, these two parts were originally united: the former provided space for physical rest for those who stayed in the hospital, and the latter served as a space to purify their spirits by celebrating mass. Even those unable to leave their beds could follow the mass, as there was no barrier between the ward and the church that impeded their ability to listen to prayers.

The entrance to the central part of the complex consists of a sculpture of the Holy Spirit and a pointed-arch door that leads into the hospital church, consecrated in the mid-fourteenth century. The north side of the church was originally connected to the hospital ward. After the two parts of the structure were separated by a door, a room called "the front hospital" (*het voorhospitaal*) provided additional shelter. In the seventeenth century, a new chapel dedicated to the Virgin Mary was built to enlarge the church, which is situated in the right part of the architectural complex. The space of the former church is called the Gothic wing and that of the new chapel (*Mariakapel*) is known as the Virgin wing.[7]

The earliest document referencing the Hospital of Our Lady of Potterie dates back to 1276 when the chapter of St. Donatian's in Bruges asked the bishop of Tournai (Doornik) to grant his approval for an institution called *Spietaal van Onser Vrouw*.[8] The bishop's official consent for the construction of a church with a churchyard and for the making of bells was also sought and granted in 1289.[9] The first chapel of the hospital was completed in 1292.[10] Shortly thereafter, the hospital began attracting local patrons, including Alardus Lam, who founded a perpetual chaplaincy in the chapel in honor of Our Lady of Potterie on November 13, 1302. A hospital ward was built at the beginning of the fourteenth century, converting the building into a functional *hospitaal*.[11]

In fourteenth-century Bruges (and throughout the two centuries that followed), the term *hospitaal* in Flemish, or *hospitalis* in Latin, was mainly used to denote a place that gave shelter to those in need. Thus, a hospital commonly catered to the sick, the elderly, travelers, and those who were physically and/or mentally weak.[12] As will be discussed in greater detail in this chapter, those who sought the services of a hospital were often referred to as "the poor" (*pauperes* in Latin; *arme mensen* in Flemish); in this light, a medieval hospital became synonymous as place for a range of individuals who sought assistance of one kind or another. Similarly, the Hospital of Our Lady of Potterie originally functioned as a shelter for travelers and the sick. The charitable community consisted of lay sisters and two or three commanders (chaplain, magister, and receptor).[13] They offered food, drink, and lodging to patients. A priest was appointed to the hospital so that it could function as an independent parish.[14]

Due to financial challenges in the early fourteenth century, the hospital merged with the Holy Ghost God House (*Heilige Geest Godshuis*), a charitable institution that offered help to invalids, located on de Goezeputstraat in Bruges.[15] The Holy Ghost God House was run by brothers, and their daily work was supervised by the city magistrate. From 1319, the Hospital of Our Lady of the Potterie and the Holy Ghost God House together served as a unified charitable institution operated by lay brothers and sisters who typically came from middle-class families. A "master," who was responsible for managing and controlling the properties of the institution, supervised the brothers,[16] while a "mistress" took responsibility for the sisters, the household, and the daily care of patients. The Bruges city magistrate appointed two guardians to supervise the administrative and financial functions of the hospital.

When the hospital was structurally joined with the Holy Ghost God House, it was also renovated and enlarged; similarly, the chapel of Our Lady of Potterie was enlarged and a new church was consecrated on April 7, 1359.[17] Three altars were placed in the church: one in the choir and two under the choir screen. As in the case of many other medieval hospitals, no wall existed between the hospital ward and the church, which made it possible for bed-ridden patients to attend masses celebrated in the church. Before a wall was built between the ward and church in 1529, this inner structure of the hospital formed the foundation for the spiritual treatment of those confined to the hospital.[18]

In approximately 1410, the hospital opened its doors to the elderly, travelers, and the sick.[19] Around the same time, the lay community of brothers and sisters took monastic vows, pledging to follow the religious rules developed by St. Augustine (354–430), thus anointing themselves the Third Order of St. Augustine. The monastery for the hospital staff was built next to the hospital ward around 1470. Marcus Gerarts (1521–1604) recorded this architectural complex in a famous city map in 1562. In 1538, the last brother took his vows. After that no new brothers joined the community and by the end of the sixteenth century all the brothers had left the hospital. From then on the sisters managed all duties in the hospital on their own. In

1625, a new chapel known as the Virgin Chapel and dedicated to the miraculous statue of the Virgin Mary was built to enlarge the church. This chapel still treasures the miraculous statue, which has been venerated for centuries for its purported power to cure people affected by various ailments and predicaments. It is this miraculous statue that turned the hospital into one of the most important pilgrimage sites in the southern Netherlands.

The Miraculous Statue and Miracle Book

The history of the hospital cannot be told without describing what many have considered to be the miraculous statue of Our Lady of Potterie, which is today preserved on the altar of the Virgin Chapel in the hospital church. The statue is made of white stone and was initially gilded and polychromed. Heavily damaged during the First World War, the statue was eventually restored following the war, but its original color was lost. On the basis of its style, the statue is generally dated around 1270–80, making it one of the oldest stone statues in Bruges. Stylistically, the Virgin holds the Child in her left arm and supports his chest with her right hand. She wears a crown and a thick mantle over a long dress. The Christ Child is shown giving a blessing with his right hand and holding a globe in his left hand.

The statue was originally placed in a niche behind bars at the left side of the church entrance, where it could be seen from the street.[20] At a certain point at the end of the fifteenth century or the beginning of the sixteenth century the statue was moved into the church, as miracles attributed to it had begun to increase and it needed to be protected and decorated in a proper way. In the hospital church, the miraculous statue was positioned on an altar dedicated to the Virgin and placed under the choir screen.[21] The shrine was at that time owned by a group of pot bakers, and later the ownership was passed to a community of free sailors.[22]

Detailed information on the miracles associated with the statue of the Virgin is provided in a small manuscript, the so-called *Miracle Book of Our Lady of Potterie*. The manuscript (pen, ink on paper, 215 × 140 mm) shows a watermark consisting of a sacramental wine jug.[23] The same watermark appears on an account book of the hospital dated 1520–1, which provides a *terminus post quem* of the production of the book. Several blank pages preceding the original part were added, possibly in the first quarter of the seventeenth century. The text on the first of these added pages mentions that the earliest-recorded miracle occurred on the first day of November 1009, stating that the statue stood on the altar in "the god-house of the pottery." However, as will be discussed later in this chapter, the anonymous author of this text seems to have misread the date noted in the miracle book. The text refers to an *ex-vote* (votive gift) donated by Nicolaus de Schietere, Mayor of Bruges, on August 24, 1605. The entire text was cited and published by Heribertus Rosweydus in 1623; thus, the text added later must have been written between 1605 and 1623.[24]

The miracle book has attracted the interest of historians and art historians for centuries, as each page includes not only an eight-line verse but also a drawing portraying a miracle associated with the statue. This structure is unusual for a miracle book, more generally called the "Lives of Saints," which tends to list and describe saintly miracles with text to, in a sense, publicize what might be possible for Christian believers. In contrast, the combination of text and image is generally found in miracle paintings (*mirakelschilderijen*), which were largely created in the southern part of the Netherlands throughout the Counter-Reformation period. In a similar manner to the miracle paintings, the illustrations of this particular book are designed to assist readers in understanding the conditions by which they could receive heavenly grace. The first detailed analysis of the miracle book was made in 1666 by Philippus Taisne, a Jesuit priest who noted that the miraculous statue was originally placed in a niche to the left of the entrance of the hospital church so that it could be venerated from the street.[25] Nothing is known, however, about the book's author and artist, or its original intent. Octave Delepierre, an archivist and historian in Bruges, attributed the book

Health and Architecture

to Margareta van Eyck, the younger sister of the celebrated painter Jan van Eyck (*c.* 1390–1441).[26] Given Delepierre's failure to substantiate this claim, however, this attribution is generally not accepted today. As for its intent, historian Dieter Harmening considered the book to be a work of devotional propaganda featuring the miraculous statue in the hospital.[27] In the late 1970s, art historian Charlotte Pannier argued that the miracle book served as both a historical record for descendants and as a manual for clergy to produce their sermons.[28] Recently, art historian Marlies Nijkamp provided detailed information on the condition of the book and reconsidered its original function.[29] According to her account, it was created to represent miracle paintings that had been lost or endangered during a church renovation project in the 1520s. Although many different theories have been proposed, decisive evidence has yet to be brought forward that certifies its true history and intent.

What we do know is that the book records sixteen miracles attributed to the statue of Our Lady of Potterie, with an introductory and concluding folio. According to the verse on the introductory folio, the first miracle

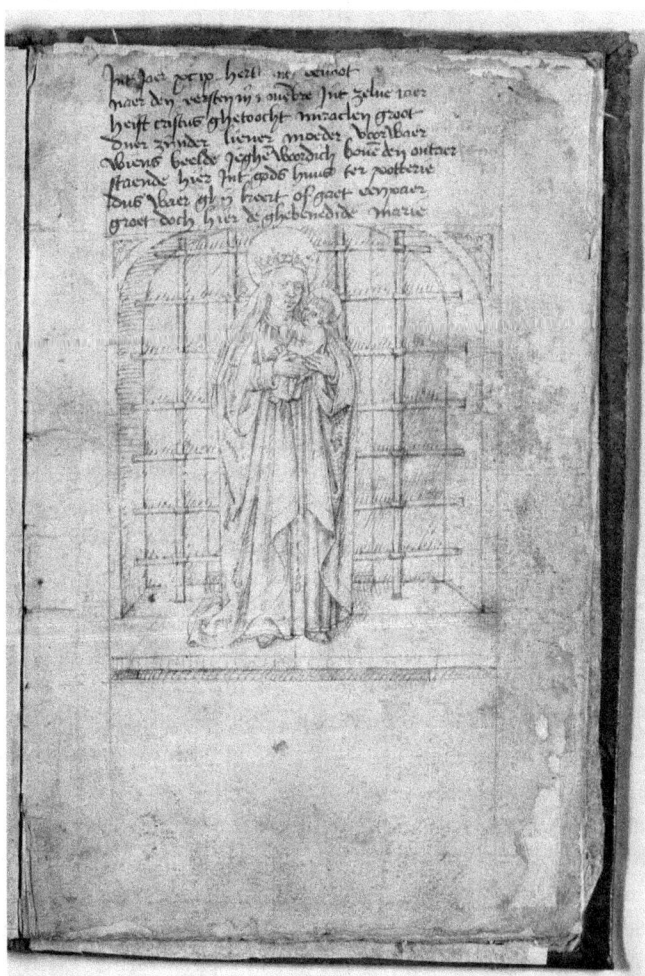

Figure 4.2 Virgin and Child, *The Miracle Book of Our Lady of Potterie*, *c.* 1520–1, pen, ink, on paper, originally fol. 2r, currently fol. 5r, 21.7 × 14.2 cm, Museum Onze-Lieve-Vrouw-ter-Potterie. Musea Brugge, www.artinflanders.be

occurred on the first day of November "in the year XCIC" when the statue of the Virgin was positioned on the altar in the church of the hospital (Figure 4.2).³⁰ Rosweydus (1623) and Taisne (1666), who wrote chronicles of the hospital, interpreted that number as 10 times 10 and 9, thus 1009. Alfons Maertens (1937), who was a priest and historian, later suggested that it be read literally as 99; Maertens also asserted that since the book is dated *terminus post quem* 1520–1, it is reasonable to conclude that 99 means 1499.³¹ One should recall, however, that the statue itself is dated between 1270 and 1280, which means that that first miracle could also have taken place much earlier, say in 1299 or 1399.

The first drawing shows the Virgin looking at the Child held in her left arm. She is standing in front of a niche covered with bars, which most likely reflects the original location of the statue. The later placement of the statue is represented on the concluding folio (Figure 4.3). The drawing shows the Virgin and Child

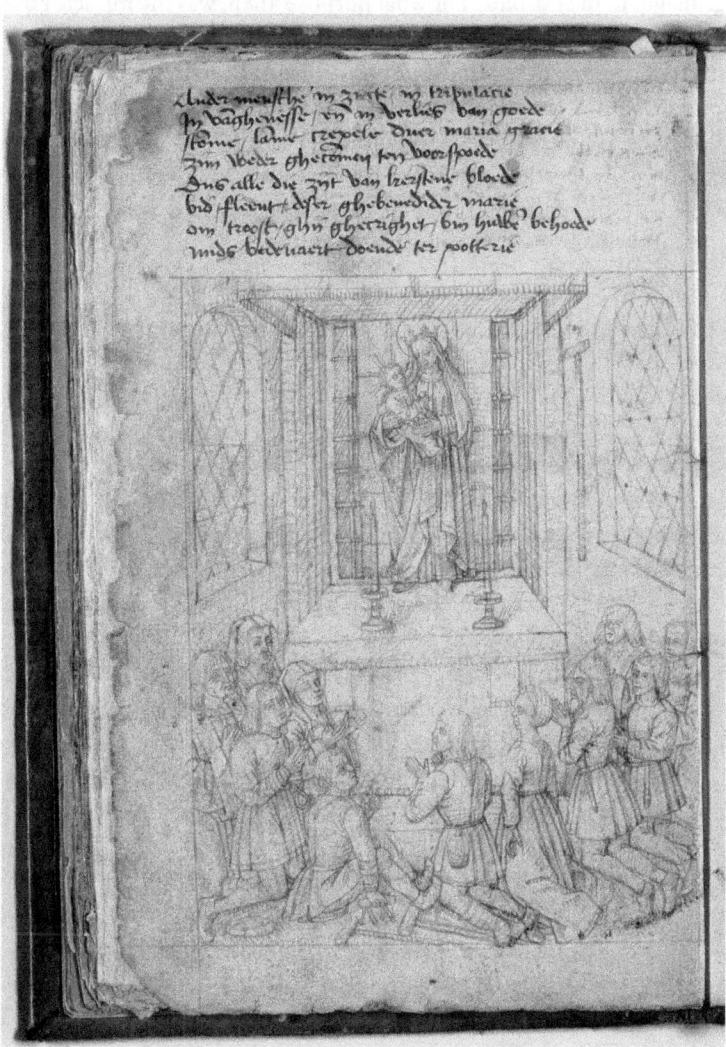

Figure 4.3 Virgin Potterie helped those who venerated her, *The Miracle Book of Our Lady of Potterie*, originally fol. 11v, currently fol. 14v. Musea Brugge, www.artinflanders.be

on an altar decorated with a canopy, curtains, antependium, and two lit candles. In front of the altar are eleven people, including a crippled man, a woman whose arms are turned backward, and a blind woman. Two crutches are placed on the floor, and an object similar to crutches is hung on the wall to the right of the Virgin, which may suggest an *ex-vote* dedicated to the Virgin after a crippled man was cured. As mentioned in the verse of the first drawing of the book, the scene most likely reflects the way in which the statue was venerated in the church when the book was written. According to the verse above the image, those who were sick, foolish, lame, or crippled could receive heavenly grace if they made a pilgrimage to Our Lady of Potterie.[32]

The contrast between the two images is striking. In the first image (Figure 4.2), the miraculous living statue of the Virgin is placed outside the hospital building and thus could be seen and venerated by a large audience. After the initial miracle, the statue was moved into the church, as shown in the latter image (Figure 4.3), meaning that privileged opportunities to venerate the statue were chiefly available to those who lived in or made pilgrimages to the hospital. For what purpose, then, was the miracle book made? What kind of message does it text and images seek to convey? It is highly possible that, as mentioned in the last folio, the book was created to encourage donations and pilgrimages to the hospital, which actually did become one of the most important sacred sites in Bruges. The book, however, has an additional, more benevolent function. As will be detailed herein, each illustration of the miracle book advocates support for the poor and how they should be perceived by others, which is not always explained in the accompanying text. This uniqueness is likely related to the mission of the hospital and increasing concern for the poor during the period in question.

The Hospital and the Environment of Social Welfare: The Poor in *De Subventione Pauperum*

In the 1520s, around the time when the miracle book was made, social welfare emerged as a great concern among humanists in Europe.[33] Socioeconomic challenges and continuing population growth from the mid-fifteenth century onwards led to serious poverty and vagrancy in urban locales. Contemporary humanists were conscious of the dismal quality of urban life and the growing social inequities, but asserted that municipal governments, not the Church, should address problems of social welfare.[34] Nonetheless, individuals who faced financial, physical, or mental problems still turned to the church and nearby or adjoining hospitals run by monastic foundations for help and shelter. Such was the case for the Hospital of Our Lady of Potterie.

By this era, several cities in Northern Europe, especially in Germany, had devised a civic welfare system that included various charitable activities; however, such a system had not yet been established in Bruges. Among many humanists who proposed strategies for creating a new social welfare system, Juan Luis Vives (1492–1540) played a crucial role in efforts to improve the lot of the less fortunate in Bruges, having published the first academic report on a new welfare system that could help the poor in the city.[35] Born in Valencia, he studied in Paris between 1509 and 1512 and moved to Bruges in 1514. In 1517, Vives settled in Leuven, where he held an academic position teaching at the Collegium Trilingue and wrote several moralistic and theological reports. Between 1523 and 1528, Vives traveled frequently between England and Bruges. In England, he held an academic position at Corpus Christi College, Oxford.[36] In the early 1520s, Vives wrote a number of moralistic reports, including reports on the education of women (*De institutione feminae Christianae*) and human ethics (*Introductio ad sapientiam*).[37] In the summer of 1524, Vives moved back to Bruges to be married, a city he referred to as "home."[38] It was there that Vives formed his ideas and developed his interests in the relief of the poor, culminating in the treatise he wrote in 1526 for the Senate of Bruges, *De Subventione Pauperum*.

The overarching idea behind this treatise is the notion that God's love and grace will bond Christians in a community dedicated to pursuing mutual well-being and charity for others (*caritas*):

> It is not possible for things which relate to some of us to remain absolutely alien to others. This is because Christian grace unites us all, binding us with the strongest cement.[39]
>
> Above all, there is the love of people for others, which is marked by the mutual exchange of welfare, done straightforwardly, with simplicity and without a backward glance. Surpassing all, there is the heavenly reward, which we have shown is destined for the alms which spring from charity.[40]

While mutual support and concern for others are essential to maintaining the solidarity of the Christian community, they are also fundamental tenets in caring for the sick and indigent. The first part of Vives's treatise provides theoretical and moralistic observations about "the poor," while in the second part he proposes a new system for alleviating urban poverty. One of the innovative aspects of Vives's work is that rather than dismissing the poor as beggars and vagrants, he offers radical methodical solutions such as employment and educational programs supported by municipal governments.[41]

Vives's objective is clear: to emphasize how the support of the Christian community can comfort and assist the poor, and not just those who lack money but also those who are poor in spirit. As Vives notes,

> We are not fed by money or bread, which anyway will never be lacking for those who are the sort of poor that Jesus loves: simple, pure, humble and friendly. He does not call every poor person blessed, but those whose spirit is poor—that is, moderate and pious—those who do not give way to greed or the love of money.[42]

Vives categorizes the poor into two groups. The first group includes those who lack the ability to function on a daily basis, including those suffering from physical (and, presumably, mental) illness ("[V]arious things could happen. Some people were unable to work because of physical illness and fell into poverty because they were placed under an obligation to spend their money without receiving any more").[43] The second group includes those who had lost something of value through misfortune ("The same thing happened to those that lost their goods through war or in some other great calamity, an inevitable part of living in this unpredictable world, such as fires, floods, ruin or shipwreck").[44] Vives emphasizes the moral imperative of accepting people regardless of their circumstances and offering support in whatever form is needed, be it financial, material, emotional, or physical. Vives sees this ideal vision in the hospital. Accordingly, the hospital played a critical role in this multifaceted objective, where, according to Vives, "sick people are nursed and cared for, where a certain number of needy people are maintained, where boys and girls are educated, where children are brought up, where mad people are detained and where blind people pass their lives."[45]

As defined by Vives, a hospital represented a multidimensional charitable community that provided support for poor people in physical and/or mental distress, including the sick (the first category), as well as the recently impoverished who might have fell victim to calamitous events—fires, floods, financial ruin, shipwreck, and so on (the second category). Vives clearly considers the plight of the poor, stressing that rather than casting them aside they should be united by love within the Christian community and their needs addressed directly and proactively, which he encourages in his treatise. It is the idea of charity and kind attitude toward the poor that connects Vives's treatise and the miracle book, even though the former is an academic report and the latter is a religious document. In an analogous way, the poor and the importance of supporting them are represented in striking ways within *The Miracle Book of Our Lady of Potterie*, which was created in Bruges shortly before Vives constructed his treatise.

Health and Architecture

Miracles for the Poor

Along with the introductory and concluding folios already noted (see Figures 4.2 and 4.3), sixteen miracles performed for the poor by Our Lady of the Potterie are recorded. Similar to how Vives presented an expanded view of those needing social assistance in his academic treatise, the miracle book also classifies the poor in much broader terms. Specifically, they are either sick, disabled, and injured (those suffering from water sickness, blindness, paralysis, cancer, madness, a tumor, falls, a cut, or infertility), or befalling some calamitous event such as a shipwreck, a poor fishing catch, or some form of malfeasance such as theft. Demonstrating how the poor are represented in the miracle book can best be accomplished by describing the miracles, not in chronological order, but according to the categories of people for whom the miracles occurred. The poor in the first category are depicted in twelve of the miracles described. They can be further subcategorized into the physically and mentally ill, handicapped, injured, and sterile. Physically sick patients are represented in the first, fifth, eighth, thirteenth, and fourteenth miracles. The first miracle was granted to a woman who had been suffering from water sickness for ten weeks (Figure 4.4). After she invoked the help of the Virgin of Potterie, the water exited her body through her mouth and she was cured.[46] Note that although the Virgin and Child, surrounded by a halo, are represented on a small scale in the upper-right corner, the focus of the drawing is on the patient who is vomiting water with the support of a young woman standing behind her, who is not mentioned in the text.

Those caring for or observing the patients depicted in these representations are important elements in the miracle book, as these secondary characters suggest earthly support for the poor as well. According to the verse associated with the thirteenth miracle, Bruges resident Kateline Smids, who lived on de Balgestraat, suffered from a sore throat for two months, likely the result of an abscess. She invoked the Virgin's help and was completely cured.[47] In the drawing, Kateline is in bed being cared for by a young woman shown serving food or administering medicine with a spoon while another woman, in front of the bed, looks on. Both figures, who are again unmentioned in the text, suggest the patient was not alone but nursed by her family or friends. A very similar composition can be found in the drawing of the fourteenth miracle, which was granted to another Bruges resident, Marje Scermers. She was lame, confined to bed for half a year, and only able to move her tongue. She invoked the help of the Virgin who cured her lameness, inspiring Marje to promise to undertake a pilgrimage.[48] As with the previous drawing, a young woman positioned at the front of the bed appears to be keeping the patient company. While the miracle is certainly remarkable in and of itself, the artist also emphasizes the presence of those who offer support to the suffering, embodying the idea of human charity.

In contrast to the aforementioned drawings, the fifth and eighth miracle drawings depict patients in the presence of individuals showing repugnance or hesitation in dealing with their malodorous charge. These depictions can be best understood as criticizing those who choose not to embody the Christian principles of charity and love. Specifically, the fifth miracle involves Victor Carre, who was born in Ieper and was suffering from smallpox (variola). He was confined to bed over an extended period, devoid of energy, and prayed to the Blessed Virgin to help him.[49] According to the verse, his abdomen was open, giving off a terrible stench. This unfortunate condition is implied in the drawing, which shows a young woman standing by his bed holding her nose so as not to inhale the smell. Yet again we find the images of the Virgin and Child, but also that of a young man—possibly the cured Victor himself who is looking up at the Virgin, praying. A similar story can be found in connection with the eighth miracle. Andries Bootaert, a merchant from Rotcheele, was suffering from a cancerous foot that emitted a terrible odor. As a result, few took pity on him. However, after promising the Virgin that he would donate a vat of wine to the church he was cured.[50] In the drawing he is accompanied by two men, one pointing to Andries' leg and the other holding his nose to avoid the smell. On the right is a

Healing of the Poor

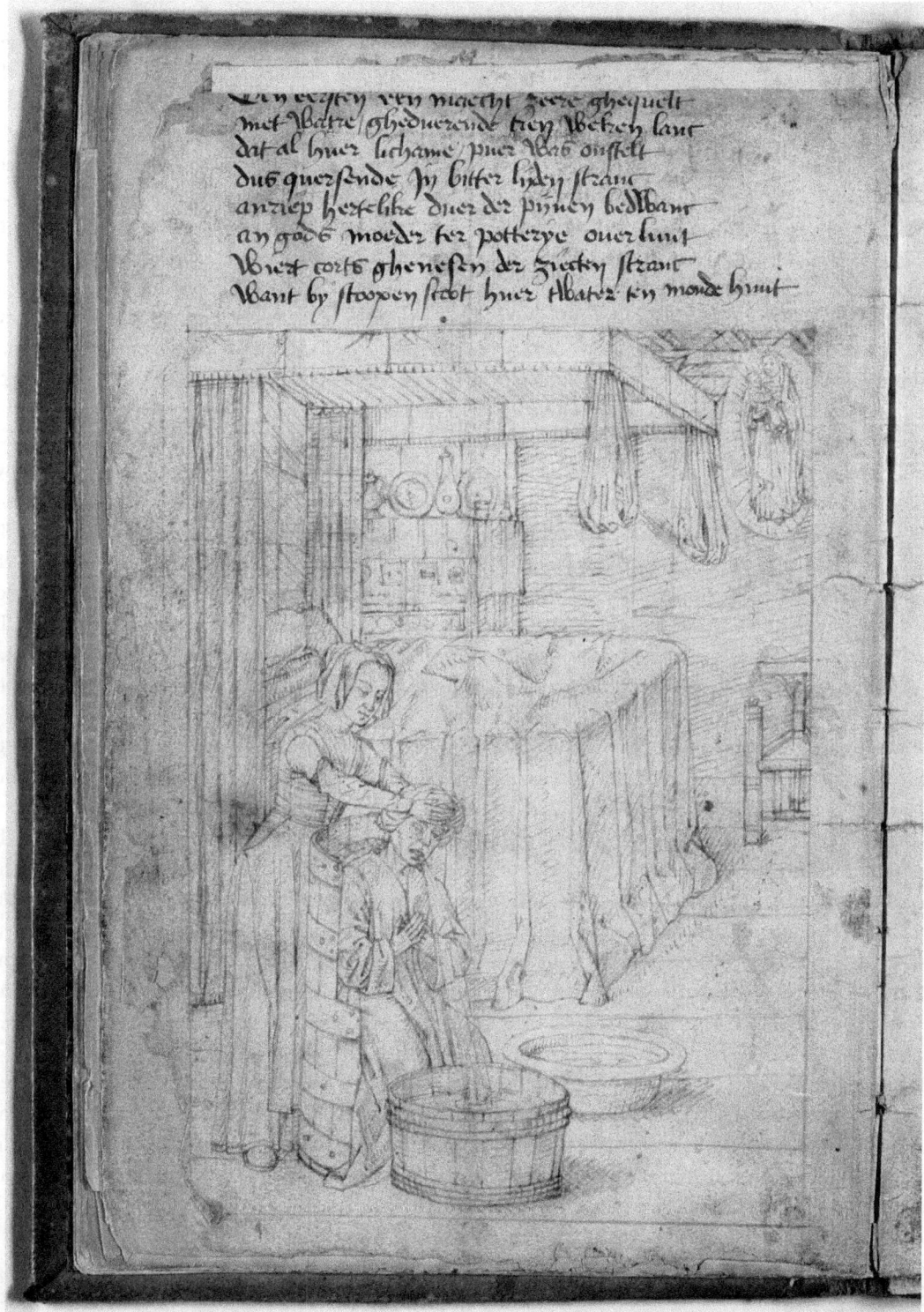

Figure 4.4 Woman cured from water sickness, originally fol. 2v, currently fol. 5r. Musea Brugge, www.artinflanders.be

gate through which we can see a ship and a man looking up and praying to the Virgin in the sky above. At his foot is a wooden barrel; the man is most likely Andries himself in his healed state after his offering of wine.

Mental illness is also mentioned in the miracle book. During the period concerned, it was believed that physical illness was caused by sin, and those who had mental issues were often thought to be possessed by a devil. This is why those who wished to be taken care of in the hospital had to confess their sins to a priest before entering the hospital, as the confession allowed them to purify their spirit, and this was the first step in the healing process, followed by the celebration of mass.[51] According to the verse associated with the sixth miracle, the wife of Jacob van Snijders had been possessed by a devil for three years. As represented in the drawing, she was in a terrible state as she was deranged, danced spontaneously, sprang about, wished to drown, and tore at her clothing. After undertaking multiple pilgrimages and offering goods and money, she was cured.[52] In the background of the drawing once can see a man, most likely her husband, kneeling in prayer to the Virgin and Child on behalf of his wife, who are represented as small figures in the upper-right corner.

Those with physical handicaps were also cured by the Virgin, as depicted in the second, third, and eleventh miracles. The second miracle concerns a child whose arms and hands were badly deformed and who was extremely weak. The Virgin cured the child after the parents invoked her help.[53] The third miracle involved a blind woman, the daughter of Clays Pierssoens, possibly from Bruges ("here at the city"). Her eyesight was restored after she brought offerings and prayed to the Virgin.[54] In the drawing, the patient is supported by another young woman, both of whom are walking in the countryside, presumably on the way to the hospital to make a pilgrimage and offerings to the Virgin. A similar story is conveyed in the eleventh miracle. Celie, a woman who lived on Speilmansstraat in Bruges, was completely blind for half a year, but was given sight after seeking the Virgin's help.[55] Sterility is also introduced as a physical disability in the miracle book. The sixteenth miracle mentions women in and around Bruges who had difficulty conceiving children (Figure 4.5). The accompanying drawing shows several women, possibly midwives, caring for and bathing newborn babies, implying that the Virgin had helped many such women,.[56]

The miracle book also tells the story of two people injured in accidents, both of whom were saved by the Virgin. The verse of the seventh miracle concerns the five-month-old child of Andries Laurens, who lived near the Carmelite cloister, who was severely injured from having fallen from a high place. The drawing suggests that the child fell down a flight of stairs. The parents invoked the Virgin's help and the child was cured.[57] The fifteenth miracle involves the two-year-old child of Loy van der Rake from Coolkerke. The child's throat had suffered a serious cut during the barley harvest from what would appear in the drawing to be a small sickle. The child slipped into a coma, but was saved after the parents prayed to the Virgin.[58]

As noted earlier, Vives makes a distinction between the poor who suffer from some physical or emotional challenge, and those who experience misfortune of a different nature. Four miracles (the fourth, ninth, tenth, and twelfth) pertain to this second group of unfortunates. In particular, the fourth miracle concerns sailor Pieter Adriaens from Spain (Figure 4.6), who found himself battling heavy seas as he approached the coast of England with two ships. One ship sank, but the Virgin of Potterie protected the other and brought Pieter and his crew safely to the harbor of Vlissingen.[59] The ninth miracle aided the fisherman Pieter Brant Stierman from Sluus. For eight weeks he was unable to locate any fish in the North Sea area where he had been fishing; three days after praying to the Virgin, he came upon a great number of fish in the open sea.[60] The tenth miracle also concerns a fisherman, this one from Oostende, who had sailed into a storm in rough water and lost his rudder. The Virgin mercifully appeared to the fearful fisherman and calmed him, leading him to safety.[61] In each of the three drawings of these events, the beneficiary of the miracle is accompanied by his crew, praying together to the Virgin. The twelfth miracle is exceptional among the other miracles in that it depicts the victim and the perpetrator, rather than family or friends of the poor. This miracle tells the story of Kateline Strompers in Bruges, whose tinworks had been stolen. Suffering from terrible grief, she begged the Virgin for help, and

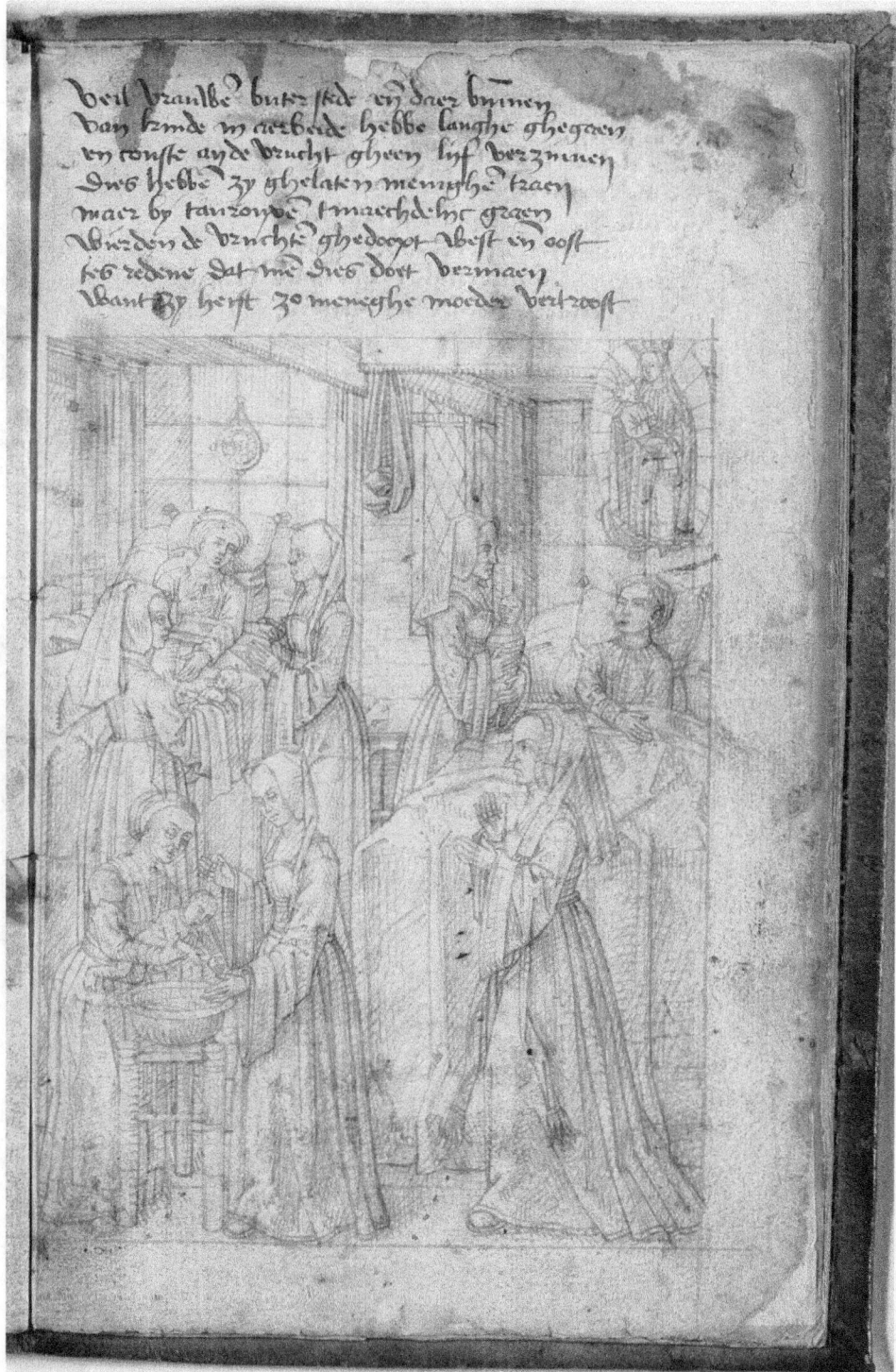

Figure 4.5 The Virgin helped women who had difficulties in becoming pregnant, *The Miracle Book of Our Lady of Potterie*, originally fol. 11r, currently fol. 14r. Musea Brugge, www.artinflanders.be

Health and Architecture

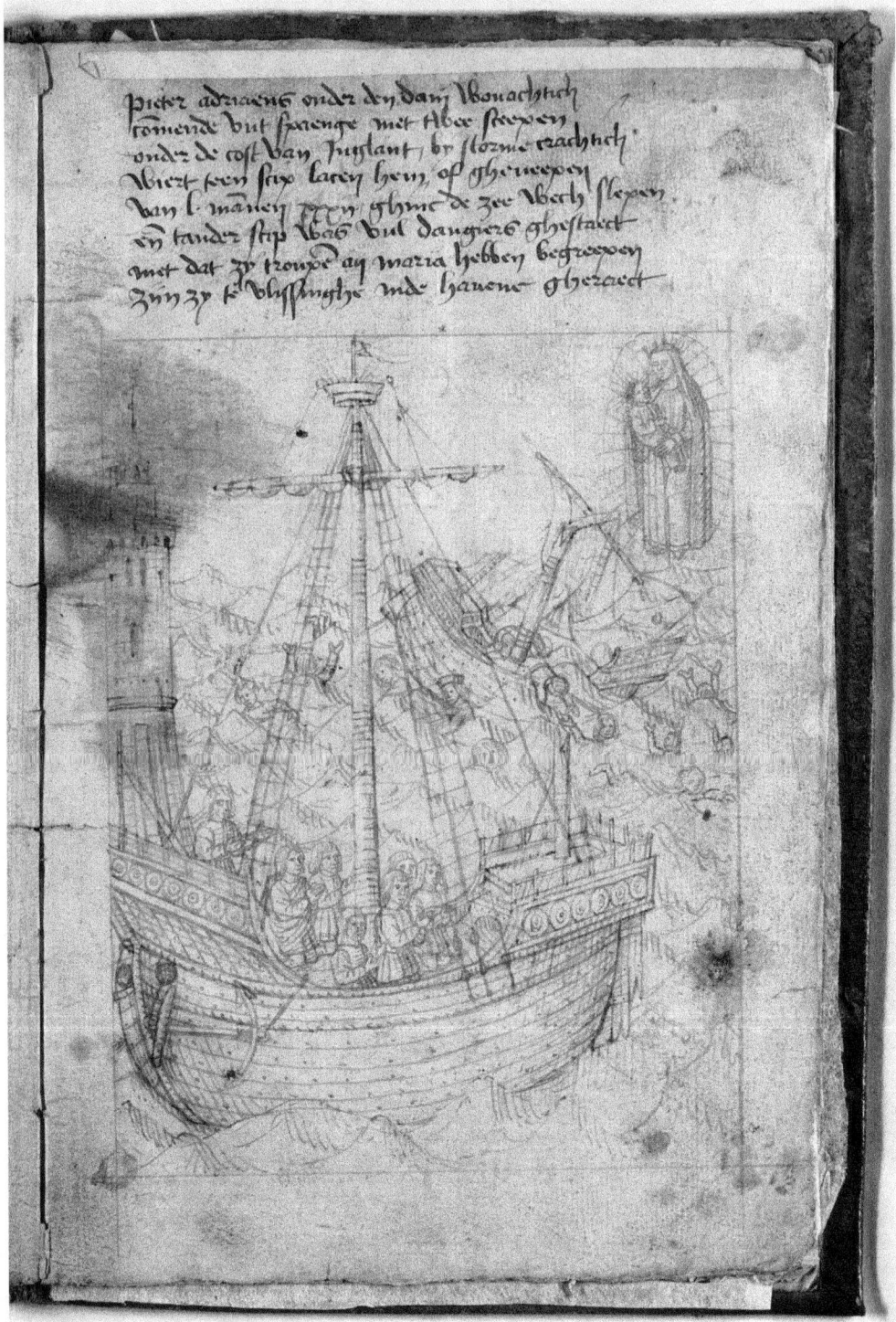

Figure 4.6 Pieter Adriaens escaped from a storm in England, *The Miracle Book of Our Lady of Potterie*, originally fol. 4r, currently fol. 7r. Musea Brugge, www.artinflanders.be

upon arriving home she discovered that the stolen tinworks had been returned, as represented on the right side.[62] Perhaps surprisingly, the thief himself is represented on the left side of the drawing.

It is striking that the visual depictions of these miracles, with the exception of the first and last drawings (see Figures 4.2 and 4.3) illustrating the initial and subsequent location of the miraculous statue, focus distinctly less on envisaging the Virgin of Potterie and instead on those who had suffered illness or misfortune and subsequently received their heavenly reward.[63] Moreover, the beneficiaries of these miracles are not represented as solitary figures, but rather are shown in the company of others who are offering support or praying for them. *The Miracle Book of Our Lady of Potterie*, therefore, shows us two different but interrelated ways to receive heavenly grace. The first, as mentioned in several folios, is through donations and pilgrimages by the poor to the Virgin of Potterie. The second way, as represented in the illustrations, is by directly assisting the poor or unfortunate or by praying on behalf of the individual. This selfless support calls to mind the interaction between the living and the dead, as prayers of the living had the ability to ease the suffering of the dead in purgatory.[64] On the basis of these two perspectives, it can be concluded that the book serves two purposes. The first, and perhaps most utilitarian, is to assist in magnifying the potential influence of the Virgin of Potterie by soliciting donations and increasing pilgrimage visits to the site. The second and more nuanced message that we can draw from the miracle book pertains to the importance of support, both physical and mental, to ease the suffering of the poor. It is clear that the miracle book is not simply about the sixteen miracles attributed to the statue of Our Lady of Potterie. Instead, to a great extent it is about the Christian community's obligation to care of the poor, who occupy more space in the drawings than the Virgin herself.

Conclusion

The Miracle Book of Our Lady of Potterie records, as we have seen, what kind of heavenly grace was performed by the Virgin to various poor people. It tells not only the story of the miraculous statue of the Virgin, which is still venerated in the hospital chapel, but it also reflects the charitable activity and attitude toward the poor in the hospital. The importance of the miracle book to the hospital and chapel has since grown beyond its original intentions, as representations of the miraculous statue and the poor it aided have been replicated in various ways within the hospital itself. On the upper-left side of the chapel of the Virgin are a series of tapestries from the seventeenth century; on the upper-right side are a series of stained-glass windows from the nineteenth century.[65] It is clear that the design of both the tapestries and the stained-glass windows were inspired by drawings from the miracle book. Next to the altar on which the miraculous statue is placed are many *ex-votes* dedicated to the Virgin and a means to invoke her help or offer her gratitude. It is truly impressive to witness how a series of images stimulated the creation of other representations and inspired various devotional acts over the centuries. Indeed, the healing space is replete with layers of images and objects glorifying the Virgin's help for the poor.

As a follow-on study, it would be interesting to further investigate the degree to which the poor and those who were represented with them within the miracle book (and who later inspired the creation of tapestries and stained glass) were able to further encourage the charitable works performed by the sisters and brothers in the hospital. Just as the poor receiving heavenly grace were supported by others on earth, a great many nameless ill-fated people were helped by the hospital staff with commensurate work and dedication. With this support, the hospital staff offered not only physical treatment but also mental care, mostly through confession and celebrating mass, to various poor people. Moreover, they preserved the miraculous statue of the Virgin, which had power to cure those praying, donating, or making pilgrimages to her. These devotional practices by the poor might also have contributed to their recuperation, both physical and spiritual, by washing their sin to become spiritually healthy. The celestial and terrestrial support in the hospital must have given strong hope to poor people. This double healing system supported by the hospital staff and the miraculous statue was, however, unique to this hospital, and a more organized, effective welfare system was needed to help the poor in other cities. Indeed, shortly after the miracle book was created, Vives brought forward his then-revolutionary ideas about a more formalized social welfare system in Bruges designed to help a broader swath of local residents. Although undocumented, he may have had an opportunity to visit the hospital of Our Lady of Potterie and interact with the staff and the indigent there. Both the miracle book and *De Subventione Pauperum* focus on the poor, although from very different approaches. While Vives viewed the poor with a judicious, yet sympathetic, eye with the goal of establishing an efficient and systematic way to help them, the miracle book recorded a series of miraculous events that alleviated the often-wretched circumstances of the poor and indigent. The latter, it must be noted, also had a more utilitarian goal of conveying the purported power of faith to a popular audience, some of whom were illiterate and relied on illustrations to convey information. Nonetheless, the two books still share the common idea that the poor should not be abandoned, but instead should be supported by and welcomed into the Christian community. By examining and comparing these two works of literature—one academic and the other religious—we can glean new insights into the attitudes toward the poor in the early sixteenth century.

Notes

1. Musea Brugge, O. L. V. ter Potterie; inventory number 0.OTP0016.II, pen and ink, on paper, 21.7 × 14.2 cm.
2. On medieval Bruges, see Andrew Brown, *Civic Ceremony and Religion in Medieval Bruges c. 1300–1520* (Cambridge: Cambridge University Press, 2011); Andrew Brown and Jan Dumolyn, eds., *Medieval Bruges, c. 850–1550* (Cambridge: Cambridge University Press, 2018).
3. From 1925, the hospital museum was managed by the civic cultural sector (COO). In 1932, under Alfons Maertens, pastor and author of a history of the hospital, the museum was renovated. Under the Public Center for Social Welfare, the museum reopened in 1982. In 1990, the Municipal Museums of Bruges (Musea Brugge) took over management of the museum. Matthias Depoorter, *The Hospital Museum, Bruges* (Ludion: Antwerp, 2016), 117.
4. On development of the building complex between the thirteenth and sixteenth centuries, see Alfons J. Maertens, *Onze Lieve Vrouw van de Potterie* (Brussels: St. Pietersabdij, 1937), 208–15.
5. On the facade, see Maertens, *Onze Lieve Vrouw van de Potterie*, 204–8; Depoorter, *The Hospital Museum*, 119.
6. On the restoration by Karel Verschelde, see A. Duclos, "M. Verschelde's werk aan de Potterie," *Rond den Heerd* 17, no. 7 (1882): 49–53.
7. In the Gothic wing, Blessed Idesbald, Abbot of the Abbey of the Dunes in Koksijde between 1155 and 1156, is venerated. On Idesbald devotion, see Depoorter, *The Hospital Museum*, 124–5.
8. Maertens, *Onze Lieve Vrouw der Potterie*, 4.
9. Marlies Nijkamp, "Mijrakelen van onse lieue vrauwe te potterije: Studie naar de functie van een zestiende-eeuws Brugs manuscript" (MA thesis, Rijksuniversiteit Groningen, 2014), 8.
10. Ibid., 8.
11. Maertens, *Onze Lieve Vrouw der Potterie*, 48.
12. Ibid., 4.
13. Ibid., 23.
14. Nijkamp, "Mijrakelen," 8.
15. Ibid., 9.
16. Depoorter, *The Hospital Museum*, 117.
17. On February 13, 1354, an indulgence letter was issued in Avignon to confirm a forty-day indulgence for those who helped build the new church. This indulgence must have contributed to attracting local devotees and to collecting money to complete the church. On the indulgence letter, see Maertens, *Onze Lieve Vrouw der Potterie*, 417–20.
18. Nijkamp, "Mijrakelen," 9.
19. Ibid., 9.

20. Philippus Taisne, "Onse Lieve Vrauwe van Potterye toevlucht der sondaeren, en van alle behoeftighe menschen, het oudste mirakeleus beeldt van ons Nederlant, door veel jonsten vermaert, ende te Brugghe besonderlyk vereert," 1666, Bruges, reprinted in Jean Meulemeester et al., eds., *Van Blindekens naar de Potterie: een eeuwenoude Brugse belofte* (Bruges: Jong Kristen Onthaal voor toerisme, 1980), 156–97, 165.
21. Ibid., 50, assumed that the statue was also venerated in the church and could be seen both from the street (the front side of the statue) and from the inside of the church (the back side of the statue). This theory is implausible to the author and generally not accepted.
22. A group of free sailors owned the chapel, at the latest, in 1586-7 ("ontfaen van de vrije veerlieden, van dat zij ghebruucken onse-vrouw capelle omme huer lieden dienst te doen staende onder den doxael binnen deze godshuuse die over de jaeren verschenen alf ougst 1586–87"). Charlotte Pannier, "De mirakeltekeningen van Onze-Lieve-Vrouw van de Potterie te Brugge. Hun situering ten opzichte van XVIe en XVIIe eeuwse Westvlaamse mirakelvoorstellingen van Onze-Lieve-Vrouw. Schilderijen en wandtapijten" (MA thesis, Ghent University, 1978), 54.
23. The watermark is reproduced in Nijkamp, "Mijrakelen," 77, 81, 85, 89.
24. Heribertus Rosweydus, "Kerckeliicke historie van Nederlandt," in *Generale kerckelycke historie van de gheboorte onses H. Iesu Christi tot het Iaer MDCXXIV*, ed. Caesar Baronius (Antwerp: Jan Cnobbaert, 1623), part 2, 99.
25. Taisne, "Onse Lieve Vrauwe van Potterye," reprinted in Jean Meulemeester et al., eds., *Van Blindekens naar de Potterie: een eeuwenoude Brugse belofte* (Bruges: Jong Kristen Onthaal voor toerisme, 1980), 156–97.
26. Octave Delepierre, *Guide indispensable dans la ville de Bruges ou description des monuments curieux et objets d'art que renferme cette ville* (Bruges: Bogaert, 1847), 128.
27. Dieter Harmening, "Mirakelbildzyklen—Formen und Tendenzen von Kultpropaganda," *Bayerisches Jahrbuch für Volkskunde* (1976/7): 53–6.
28. For example, a book on the miracles of the Virgin was published in Leiden in 1503; a book on the miracles of St. Alena was printed in Brussels in 1518. Several examples are mentioned by Charlotte Pannier, "De mirakeltekeningen," 106.
29. Nijkamp, "Mijrakelen."
30. "Int jaer XCIX hert[eke]ns deuoot / naer den eersten in Noue[m]bre int zelue iaer / heift christus ghetoocht miraclen groot / duer zijnder lieuer moeder voorwaer / wiens beelde jeghe[n]woordich boue[n] den outaer / staende hier int gods huus ter potterie / dus waer ghij keert of gaet eenpaer / groet doch hier de ghebenedide marie." Transcription cited from Nijkamp, "Mijrakelen," 20.
31. Maertens, *Onze Lieve Vrouw der Potterie*, 46.
32. "Ander mensche[n] in zieckte, in tribulancie / In va[n]ghenesse, en in verlies van goede / Stom[m]e, lam[m]e, crepele duer maria gracie / zij weder ghecom[m])en ten voorspoede / dus alle die zijt van kerstene bloede / bid, fleent, deser ghebenedider marie / om troost, ghij ghecrighet, bin huwe[n] behoede / mids bedeuaert doende ter potterie." Nijkamp, "Mijrakelen," 38.
33. On social welfare in medieval and late medieval Europe, see Griet Maréchal, *De sociale en politieke gebondenheid van het Brugse hospitaalwezen in de middeleeuwen* (Kortelijk-Heule: UGA, 1978); Robert Jütte, "Poor Relief and Social Discipline in Sixteenth-Century Europe," *European Studies Reviews* 11 (1981): 25–52; Atsushi Kawahara, "Imaging Medieval Charity: Social Ritual and Poor Relief in Late Medieval Ghent," *Journal of Social Sciences and Humanities* 257 (1995): 1–32; Ole Grell and Andrew Cunningham, *Health Care and Poor Relief in Protestant Europe 1500–1700* (London: Routledge, 1997).
34. Jütte, "Poor Relief and Social Discipline," 25–7.
35. On Vives's life and *De subventione pauperum*, see Juan Luis Vives, *Concerning the Relief of the Poor or Concerning Human Need, a Letter Addressed to the Senate of Bruges by Juan-Luis Vivès January 6, 1526*, trans. Margaret Sherwood (New York: The New York School of Philanthropy, 1917); A. Travill, "Juan Luis Vives: A Humanistic Medical Educator," *Canadian Bulletin of Medical History* 4, no. 1 (1987): 53–76; A. Travill, "Juan Luis Vives: The *De Subventione Pauperum*," *Canadian Bulletin of Medical History* 4, no. 2 (1987): 165–81; Charles Fantazzi, ed., *A Companion to Juan Luis Vives* (Boston and Leiden: Brill, 2008); Gilbert Tournoy, "Towards the Roots of Social Welfare: Joan Lluís Vives's *De subventione pauperum*," *City* 8, no. 2 (2004): 266–73. Latin texts cited in this chapter are from Juan Luis Vives, *De subventione pauperum sive de humanis necessitatibus, libri II. Introduction, Critical Edition, Translation and Notes*, ed. and trans. Constant Matheeussen and Charles Fantazzi (Leiden: Brill, 2002) (hereafter *J. L. Vives*). English translations are from Paul Spicker, ed. and trans., *The Origins of Modern Welfare: Juan Luis Vives, De subventine pauperum, and City of Ypres, Forma Subventionis Pauperum* (Oxford: Peter Lang, 2010).
36. Spicker, *The Origins of Modern Welfare*, xi.

37. Enrique G. González, "Fame and Oblivion," in *A Companion to Juan Luis Vives*, ed. Charles Fantazzi (Leiden: Brill, 2008), 365. Also see Frederik C. Ljungqvist, "Female Shame, Male Honor: The Chastity of Code in Juan Luis Vives' De institutione feminae Christianae," *Journal of Family History* 37, no. 2 (2012): 139–54.
38. Matheeussen and Fantazzi, *J. L. Vives*, 2, 4.
39. "quamquam neque naturae lex alienum ab homine quicquam sinit esse quod sit hominum et Christi gratia velut tenacissimum glutinum homines omnes inter se copulavit." Latin text from Matheeussen and Fantazzi, *J. L. Vives*, 2. English translation from Spicker, *The Origins of Modern Welfare*, 3.
40. "Verum omnia superat incrementum mutui amoris quod fiet communicandis ultro et citro beneficiis, candide ac simpliciter, sine suspicione indignitatis; et hinc praemium illud caeleste quod paratum esse ostendimus eleemosynis, quae ex caritate proficiscuntur." Latin text from Matheeussen and Fantazzi, *J. L. Vives*, 142. English translation from Spicker, *The Origins of Modern Welfare*, 100.
41. Tournoy, "Towards the Roots of Social Welfare," 272.
42. "Non enim pecunia est quae nos alit aut panis, minime defuturus iis qui vere se tales pauperes praebuerint quales ipse diligit: simplices, puros, verecundos, amabiles. Neque enim ille omnes pauperes vocat beatos, sed eos in quibus est pauper spiritus (id est: modicus et pius) et in quem pecuniae nec cupiditas nec amor penetrant." Latin text from Matheeussen and Fantazzi, *J. L. Vives*, 34. English translation from Spicker, *The Origins of Modern Welfare*, 27.
43. "Verum multi casus interveniunt. Alii aegritudine corporum ab opere cessantes, expendendis et non accipiendis pecuniis in egestatem recidunt." Latin text from Matheeussen and Fantazzi, *J. L. Vives*, 12. English translation from Spicker, *The Origins of Modern Welfare*, 12.
44. "Idem iis accidit qui bello aut aliqua ingenti calamitate sua perdiderunt, cuiusmodi permultas in hoc turbulento orbi positis necesse est contingere, velut incendia, eluviones, ruinas, naufragia." Latin text from Matheeussen and Fantazzi, *J. L. Vives*, 12. English translation from Spicker, *The Origins of Modern Welfare*, 12. Vives mentions these two categories again in a later part of the book: "Nec succurrendum modo pauperibus qui iis carent quae in diem ad vitam pertinent, sed illis etiam quibus subitus aliquis casus ingruit, velut captivitas in bello, carcer ob debita, incendium, naufragium, eluvies, multa morborum genera, denique innumera fortuita quae honestas affligunt domos" (we should not only try to relieve poor people who lack what they need on a daily basis but also those who find themselves suddenly in great distress. Examples include prisoners of war, imprisonment for debt, fire, shipwreck, flood, the many kinds of disease, and the countless events which afflict honest households and families). Latin text from Matheeussen and Fantazzi, *J. L. Vives*, 122. English translation from Spicker, *The Origins of Modern Welfare*, 88.
45. "Ex pauperibus alii vivunt in iis quae vulgo hospitalia dicuntur, Graece ptochotrophia, sed notiore illo utendum erit; alii publice mendicant; alii ferunt, ut possunt, domi quisque suae suas necessitates. Hospitalia voco, ubi aegri aluntur et curantur et ubi certus inopum numerus sustentatur et ubi pueri ac puellae educantur et ubi expositi infantes nutriuntur et ubi mente capti continentur et ubi caeci degunt." Latin text from Matheeussen and Fantazzi, *J. L. Vives*, 96. English translation from Spicker, *The Origins of Modern Welfare*, 70.
46. "Ten eersten een macht zeer ghequelt / met water gheduerende tien weken lang / dat al heur lichame puer was onstelt / dus quersende in bitter lydens stranc / anriep hertelyke duer der pynen bedwanc / an gods moeder ter potterije overluut / wierd corts ghenesen der ziekens tranc / want bij stoopen stoot huer t water ten monde huut." The verse is transcribed in Nijkamp, "Mijrakelen," 21–2.
47. "Hier binne brugghe in de baelige strate / een kateline smids bekent al daer / hadde twee maenden ghelegghen in scamelen state / inde kele, van eender aposteme swear / onder heur sacrame[n]ten, zo dat me[n] heur laefde daer / met eender pen[n]e maer ouer godes gracie / en duer tanroupe[n] zijnder moeder eenpaer / es ghenesen der zwaerder apostumacie." Nijkamp, "Mijrakelen," 34.
48. "Marje scermers te brugghe de weste[n] vleeschuusse by / een alf jaer te bedde lach zeer onzochte / van groter lam[m]icheit, niet hebbende vry / meer dan huer tonghe, diese roere[n] mochte / van dat maria qua[m] in huer ghedochte / mids bedeuaert huer beloue[n]de by desen / de goddelijcke gracie in huer zo wrochte / ter stont wiert van der lamheit genesen." Nijkamp, "Mijrakelen," 35.
49. "Victor carre van yper ghebooren / Vande[n] felle pocken lach menighe[n] dach / hebbende de cracht van zyn lede[n] verloren / zijn inghewandt inde buuc me[(n] spelen zach / zeer fellijk stinckende, maer zonder verdrach / beloofde maria te verzouckene in zijn lijnen cleet / duert welke dat lieuelijc ooghe vp slach / heift an huere[n] zone he[m] ghezonde bereet." Nijkamp, "Mijrakelen," 26.
50. "Andries bootaert coopma van rotcheele ghebooren / van eenen quaden beene lach meneghen dach / hebbende vanden meesters den trost verloren, / want men den cancker daer in speelen zach / zeer fellijc stinckende maer zonder verdrach / beloofde maria een vat wijns te gheuen / dus duer dat lieuelijc oghe up slach / heeft hy ghesonde en[de[) troost besceuen." Nijkamp, "Mijrakelen," 29.

51. The same obligation can be seen in other hospitals in Bruges, including St. John's hospital. Barbara G. Lane, *Hans Memling: Master Painter in Fifteenth-Century Bruges* (Turnhout: Brepols, 2009), 175–8.
52. "Twijf iacop uan snijders ter sluus barbie r/ was vande[n] viand drie jaer ghequelt, / angaende tgheloue, in zwaer dangier / zo dat al huer leden puer waren ontstelt / dansende, springhende, dicwijl gheqelt / om huer verdrincken, huer cleeder scuerende / veel pelgrimage[n] doende met goet ghelt / duer maria es huer hier eerst ghesonde ghebuerende." Nijkamp, "Mijrakelen," 27.
53. "Een kindeken wies armen en handen stonden / en langhe ghestaen hadde overzyde / zo dat 't kint es onmachteloos vonden / dies vader en moeder tot elken tyde / waren vul drux maer de ghebenedide / gods moeder maria hoochst gheresen / midts bede thuerwaers wyde en zyde / heift dit kindt weder ghenesen." Nijkamp, "Mijrakelen," 23.
54. "Van leffinghe clays pierssoens dochter bekent / vul lijdens, vul drux, in zwaerder onlede / vp erderijc, wesende steke blent / dies zou anroupende was hier ter stede / gods moeder de welke huer gracie dede / midts dat zou huer quam offerande beweghen / lancx den wech com[m]ende, doende huer ghebede / heift duer maria huer geseichte ghecreghen." Nijkamp, "Mijrakelen," 24.
55. "Een vrouwe te brugghe gheheeten celie / in 't speelmansstrate gods moeder di mijn / maria de ghebenedide zuver lelye / heift wel dezer vrauwe troost ghezyn / want een half iaer in groot ghepyn / heift blent ghezyn in bede huer oghen / maer duer tbetrau up tmoederlyc schyn / heift willen huer maechdelyke gratie toughen." Nijkamp, "Mijrakelen," 32.
56. "Veile vrouwe buter stede en daer binnen / van kinde in aerbeide hebbe langhe ghegaen / en conste aen de vrucht geen lyf verzinnen / dies hebbe zy ghelaten menighe traen / maer by taenroepe tmaechdelic graen / wierden de vruchten ghedoopt west en oost / ter reden dat me dies doet vermaen / want zy heeft zo meneghe moeder vertroost." Nijkamp, "Mijrakelen," 37.
57. "Andries laurens by tcarmers cloostre / hadde een kijndt vijf maenden houdt / god was hem duer zijn moeder een troostre / want tkindekin viel by der fortune[n] ghewont / van eene[n] hoghe[n] steegher dies menich vondt / an maria wiert roupende om troost confoort / want deuocie es beter dan zeluer of goudt / dies maria heift huerlieder bede ghehoort." Nijkamp, "Mijrakelen," 28.
58. "Loy van der rake in coolkerke elc macht weten / en zijn wyf in den oust elc gheerste sneet / hadde een kint van ii jare by hem ghezeten / een haertien stoot in zyne kele zo elc weet / tkint viel neder ter doot bereyt / de moeder dit ziende vp bede huer knien / anroupende maria verre en breet / dies zach men t'kynd daer ghezonde ghescien." Nijkamp, "Mijrakelen," 36.
59. "Pieter adriaens onder den dam wonachtich, / Com[m]ende vut spaenge met twee sceepen / onder de cost van inglant, by storme crachtich. / wiert teen scip lacen hein of gheneepen / van l. man[n]en xxxij ghinc de zee wech slepen. / en[d] tander scip was vul dangiers ghestaect / met dat zy troupe[n] an maria hebben begreepen / zijn zy te vlissinghe in de havene gheraect." Nijkamp, "Mijrakelen," 24–5.
60. "Pieter brant stierman ter Sluus wonachtich / ligghende inde noortzee met eene[n] scepe / viij weken zonder yet te vanghen dits warachtich / was van grooten drucke gheneepe / maer hy heeft zulken troost an maria begrepen / datty bin[n]) drie daghen zünde inde wilde zee / vinc zo vele vissch met houcken met slepen / datty verzoutte tzestich hoet zouts of meer." Nijkamp, "Mijrakelen," 30.
61. "Een visscher van Oostende in de wilde zee, / hadde by tempeeste zijn roer verloren / van zijne schepe in een bitter wee / dinckende: ic zal hier moete versmooren / maria ter potterije quam hem vooren / de welcke hem poochde met trooste te lavene / daer zijn hertelycke groote devotieus oorboren / quam onghequetst t' oostende inde havene." Nijkamp, "Mijrakelen," 31.
62. "Kateline strompers tware scade verholen / wonnachtich in brugghe warachtich ghesciet / vp een tiit was al huer tinwerc ghestolen / Dies zou int therte hadde groot verdriet / maria zou niet te biddene liet / en[d] heeft deuotelijc huer hier verzocht / met datse thuus comt en[d] inwaert ziet / was al huer tinwerc weder thuus ghebrocht." Nijkamp, "Mijrakelen," 33.
63. This characteristic is common for various miracle paintings produced in the late sixteenth and early seventeenth centuries, and the miracle book is one of the earliest surviving examples that apply this structure (although it is not a painting).
64. James B. Gould, *Understanding Prayer for the Dead: Its Foundation in History and Logic* (Cambridge: The Lutterworth Press, 2017).
65. The tapestries are described by Pannier, "De mirakeltekeningen," 121–37. Further research on the tapestries and stained glass will be carried out in a subsequent investigation.

CHAPTER 5
"THE LOVE OF FRIENDS MADE THIS IN THE CAUSE OF HUMANITY"
THERAPEUTIC ENVIRONMENT IN QUAKER ASYLUM DESIGN AT THE YORK RETREAT

Ann-Marie Akehurst

The architectural typology "hospital" includes space for a very broad range of conditions: from the positive health state of childbirth, through acute problems of accidental trauma, to the control of endemic disease and epidemics. Common to addressing these conditions is their impact on the human body and an increasing understanding of the need for specialized spaces and equipment to tackle them. Mental illness is different: its diagnosis has often been colored by social constructs of normal and aberrant behavior; while some sufferers are physically incapacitated, others are not only fit, but may exhibit extraordinary strength. Consequently, the construction of places where mentally ill or impaired people might be contained—for the protection of the sufferers themselves and society in general—responded to a different set of desiderata from those of infirmaries.

The treatment of mentally ill people has often been influenced by a public order imperative to contain and control responses to varying degrees of altruistic motives. The French philosopher Michel Foucault observed medieval sufferers from leprosy were socially ostracized and physically marginalized from communities, arguing that, with the decline of leprosy, mad people filled the social vacuum. Across Europe from the Renaissance on, mentally ill people found themselves confined. From the seventeenth century, René Descartes's *cogito, ergo sum* formulation placed sufferers on the wrong side of the definition of human, validating their treatment as animals. With the rise of the late eighteenth-century culture of sentiment, however, a more humane approach developed, foregrounding care over containment, and England's ancient city of York became a laboratory for notions of how to care—and indeed cure—those suffering mental illness.

The Retreat Asylum was founded by the Religious Society of Friends (Quakers) near the city of York in the UK. The Retreat has been regarded as a groundbreaking psychiatric institution because its regime represented a new, humane attitude toward mentally ill people; affording patients dignity, encouraging them to pet animals, to engage in social events, and partake in what we now call Occupational Therapy. Early modern Europe saw the evolution of hospitals from places of *care*, to spaces limiting the spread of disease and facilitating *cure*. The Retreat's holistic approach to care *and* cure has led it to be cited as an early example of a therapeutic environment, but the focus of the literature—informed by the hospital's extensive archives—overlooks the notion of architecture as an agent of cure; the extent to which that architecture was shaped by the distinctive religious beliefs of its founders; and the relationship between the two.

The substantial clinically focused literature from the History of Psychiatry and of Social Policy only superficially addresses its Quaker origins in discussing the therapy.[1] Conversely, Quaker apologists stress the theological underpinnings of the Retreat's regime but ignore its architecture.[2] Since it was surrounded by gardens, historians identify their debt to elite gardening fashions but uncritically accept the concept of a therapeutic environment.[3] This chapter examines how we might understand the Retreat as a therapeutic environment and explores to what extent this innovative hospital embodied a particular religious ideology. To do this requires setting broad research parameters, locating the institution in the context of hospital typology and Quaker theological culture, and critically examining the notion of the therapeutic environment. Since

Quakers shunned writing about architectural design until after the Retreat's success, there is no account of their aesthetic approach. This chapter addresses that lacuna by locating the Retreat in the English Puritan tradition of self-discipline, restraint, and simplicity.

Few scholars have unpacked what the term *therapeutic environment* specifically denotes, but one taxonomy of restorative space comes from the cultural geographer Wilbert M. Gesler, who hoped in *Healing Places* (2003) to influence twenty-first-century hospital design by distilling empirical evidence from historical wisdom to argue "place matters to health."[4] His broad interpretation of healing, outside the biomedical paradigm of Western medicine, includes faith- and dream-based healing. Gesler used historical case studies of Epidauros in Greece and Bath in England, combined with a first-hand ethnographic study of Lourdes in France, to uncover their constituent elements, aiming to produce qualitative sociological observations to nuance analysis of quantitative clinical outcomes. This holistic approach conditions the necessary complexity of healing spaces. While acknowledging his approach disregarded historical and cultural specificity, Gesler distilled generalities and hypothesized that therapeutic places are an emergent property of the interaction of four types of environment: the built, the natural, the social, and the symbolic. Despite historiographical naiveté, these four simple categories offer a useful framework for discussing the Retreat that largely satisfies Gesler's test for therapeutic environments. Moreover, Gesler's only general architectural historical knowledge resonates with the Quakers, who embodied non-academic responses to architectural forms across the longue durée.

The goal of this chapter is to synthesize all these ideas by contextualizing Samuel Tuke's famous *Description of the Retreat: An Institution Near York* (1813), which describes the establishment of his grandfather William's asylum, together with foundation documents and religious writing, and by testing Gesler's categories against what is recovered. After briefly tracing the evolution of the European hospital I will discuss the construction and use of this particular institution, arguing that only by locating the Retreat in the theological context from which it emerged can we grasp the distinctive praxis and aesthetics conceptualized as agents of healing for a specific group sharing idiosyncratic knowledge.

The Rise of Scientific Medicine in Europe

To appreciate the singularity of the Retreat we must first address previous changes in hospital design and practice that highlight why it was regarded as so exceptional. In early modern Europe, the term "hospital"—derived from the Latin *hospes*, meaning guest and host—embraced a wide range of institutions. Bodily and spiritual care had remained central in the medieval era when the Christian injunction to enact corporal works of mercy concentrated a variety of spaces for social care in monastic institutions. Alms were provided for poor people, and the care for sick patients, lodged in multiple-occupation beds, drew on spirituality. Medieval hospital wards focused on murals and altarpieces; one that remains is *The Last Judgment* commissioned in 1443 from Rogier Van der Weyden (c. 1400–64) for the Hôtel-Dieu de Beaune in France by the Chancellor of the Duchy of Burgundy. That large polyptych altarpiece was positioned on the high altar, within view of the beds of immobile patients, and, since illness could be considered as divine punishment, was intended to remind the dying of their faith, review their life choices, and direct their thoughts toward the afterlife. When closed, healing—represented by Saints Sebastian and Anthony—reassured dying people by their intercessions. On opening, Van der Weyden's expansive Last Judgement represented Christ seated behind Archangel Michael who dispassionately weighs naked souls while advancing to judge the viewer. The alternatives were clear: Heaven and salvation, or Hell and damnation. A gilded church suggests the way to Heaven, its gate resembling that of the Beaune hospital. Unusually, the hellscape conveys inner rather than external torment.

Between 1660 and 1820 across Europe, hospitals evolved from religious foundations—caring for sick poor people—to increasingly specialized, purpose-built machines for cure.[5] Responding to the late seventeenth-century scientific revolution, shaped by the local religio-political climate, the operating table replaced the altar, the surgeon replaced the priest, and architecture demonstrated faith in science rather than faith in God. However, it is important not to overstate the degree of secularization; while the medical sciences drew on rationalist approaches, post-Reformation culture remained Christian, nuanced by position on the Catholic-Protestant continuum.

Following the mediaeval episcopal practice of building hospitals near cathedrals, from the thirteenth century, new hospitals became located in urban as well as monastic settings, and by the late seventeenth century many towns had a foundation based on Quattrocento Italian models. In form, the palace-type hospital comprised three elements: the cruciform ground plan, the colonnaded court, and the loggia exemplified by the loggia facade of the Florentine Ospedale degli Innocenti (1419–26) by Filippo Brunelleschi (1377–1446), and by Milan's Ospedale Maggiore (c. 1456) by Filarete (c. 1400–c. 1469).[6] Filarete's pair of cross-within-square plans produced intersecting wings forming eight courts surrounded by colonnades, flanking a prominent central church.[7] An altar in the center of each cross, sited under a cupola, like the cruciform plan itself, reflected the continued centrality of Christian spirituality to the healing process, while the symmetrical design lent itself to separation of the sexes. Such flexibly rational and religiously symbolic designs had great longevity in Catholic Europe until the end of the eighteenth century.

In Northern Europe, the Protestant Reformation impacted those charitable activities that were formerly administered by the Catholic Church. Community-organized voluntary relief for poor people replaced monastic almsgiving and generated alternative spaces for social care. The cultural fault line followed religious rather than national borders. So, for example, in German-speaking Catholic Bavaria and Austria cruciform and centralized plans continued in use, whereas to the north new domestically derived forms developed.

For a while, architectural primacy and epistemic advance gave France the lead, and, despite political conflict, new ideas circulated through the Republic of Letters, internationally informing new designs. General hospitals—called Hôtels-Dieu—balanced Catholic tradition and new thinking. While not abandoning the cloistral quadrilateral and the cross plan, awareness was growing of the prevalence of plague, epidemics in coastal areas imported by mariners, and the risk of infectious disease among large populations housed in institutions. Air contaminated with vapors called miasmata was then believed to transmit disease, and the importance of good ventilation came to the fore.

These understandings were reflected in architectural planning: in the late seventeenth century, the hospital at Lyon (1652–63) was relocated from the town to benefit from fresh air, and new ventilation systems were installed there in 1737. Windows opposing across a range permitted salubrious cross-ventilation, and the arrangement of wings around a *cour d'honneur* allowed circulation of air. The sanitary U-plan, as it has since been called, was exemplified at the Hôpital Saint-Jacques in Besançon (1686–1703). Climate conditions in some places resulted in the U-plan combining with the Southern European loggia facade as at Marseille (1757–81). Across early modern France, religious and private hospital ownership, combined with rationalist philosophical positions, conferred little economic and creative freedom and halted French innovation. In Paris, the Hôtel-Dieu retained its medieval buildings until a fire in 1772. The subsequent protracted debate about its replacement produced more than two hundred plans and forty architectural projections: a discourse in which the nature of the hospital—by then characterized as an agent of cure—was thoroughly aired.

London's Bethlem Hospital: A Paradigmatic Asylum

Hospital provision in England was exceptionally poor. After the suppression of the monastic infirmaries in the 1530s, five were transferred to the authority of the City of London and remained the only such institutions in England for the following two centuries. After 1660, the restored monarchy invested in ostentatious charitable foundations that placed care of the body central to public life. Simultaneously, the establishment of the Royal Society supported a critical mass of scientifically and empirically engaged architects, physicians, and surgeons. This created a forum where new understandings of the etiology and progress of disease could be discussed, stimulating demand for, and informing the design of, specialized spaces.

By the early eighteenth century, increasing urbanization prompted population growth and the concomitant epidemiology created demand for hospital beds. In 1697 the political arithmetician Gregory King (1648–1712) compiled a national survey of almshouses and hospitals that aided government analysis of poor relief.[8] In 1714, the political economist and Quaker John Bellers (1654–1725) enumerated medical uses for the public good, and the following year the religious writer and philanthropist Robert Nelson (1656–1715) set out an agenda of public projects for the wealthy to support.[9] A public subscription was opened in 1719 for England's first voluntary hospital—the Westminster Infirmary—and from that point the voluntary hospital movement stimulated the foundation of hospitals across England, corporately funded by public subscriptions and designed variously and collaboratively by doctors, architects, and scientists.

One such example was Europe's oldest psychiatric hospital, the medieval foundation dedicated to the care of "lunatics," as disordered people were then called. Bethlem Hospital, one of the few metropolitan hospitals to survive the Dissolution of the Monasteries physically intact, was jointly administered by the Crown and the City of London authority. In 1676, it was handsomely rebuilt at Moorfields, backing on to London City Wall and facing open gardens, to designs by Dr. Robert Hooke, then Surveyor to the City of London.[10] Bethlem's palatial facade, over 500 feet long, strung out between three stone-fronted pavilions, enriched with swags and a Corinthian order, was in part intended to attract the wealthy and stimulate donations. Additionally, its narrow form—a single-pile structure, open to light and air—was designed with therapeutic efficacy in mind.[11] The site was deliberately chosen "for health and Aire" and Hooke, the Royal Society's Curator of Experiments, alongside Robert Boyle and Sir Christopher Wren, had experimentally endeavored to understand the importance of air to life. On the principal stories of each wing, behind iron grilles, two 193-yard-long exercise galleries, intended as day rooms, fronted patients' cells, that might be understood as a Northern European interpretation of the loggia. The windows of the cells remained unglazed, guarding against overheated brains that were regarded as potentially injurious to sanity. The hospital governors claimed they provided every "Lunatick … with a Room in a good Air, proper Physick, and Diet gratis."[12] Bethlem became an architectural model for two hundred years; as the architectural historian Christine Stevenson observed, it evoked "magnificent beauty, charitable hospitality, good and healthful order."[13] The concern for physical well-being manifested at Bethlem reflected the more general concern regarding the prevalence of endemic disease among confined populations, as in prisons and aboard ships. In that respect, though a purposely salubrious place, Bethlem cannot be regarded as a therapeutic environment since it aimed to prevent disease, rather than to heal it.

In the rest of England, the story was less optimistic. Since diagnosis and efficacious treatment were in the future, psychiatric disorder was regarded as much in terms of public order as ill health.[14] Some mentally ill people were cared for at home, but if there were public order concerns, the Vagrancy Act of 1744 stipulated violently insane people were to be restrained for the common good, and incarcerated in Bridewells alongside local miscreants.[15] Wealthier families might take advantage of private madhouses, but by the early 1760s anxieties about the vested financial interests of the medical profession, the motives of confining sane people to the madhouse, and their subsequent maltreatment there, prompted the establishment of the cross-party government Select Committee of 1763. Bills regulating private madhouses and safeguarding against illegal detention were finally passed in 1773 and 1774.

While the legal framework determined when and how hospitals were founded and funded, their architecture, and what it denoted, was complex. Situated at the intersection between Christian charity and natural philosophical empiricism, and framing encounters between impoverished patients and their

Health and Architecture

benefactors, hospital—and especially asylum—architecture became an aesthetic battleground. Bethlem had been satirized as a palace for lunatics, and debates regarding decorum influenced attitudes toward asylum appearance. London's second asylum, St. Luke's, with its blind walls, was consequently austerely utilitarian.[16]

The debate spread nationally, and the case study that forms the rest of this chapter is based on a hospital in northern England. Yorkshire—England's most extensive region—is bounded to the north by the River Tees, to the east by the North Sea, to the south by the Humber Estuary and rivers Don and Sheaf, and stretching almost to the Irish Sea in the west. These limits contain mountains, coastline, fertile plains, moorland, and, in the eighteenth century, bourgeoning cities like Leeds and Sheffield that were powerhouses of Britain's Industrial Revolution. It was divided into three administrative counties, one of which alone comprised England's largest county. This physical and economic dominance, and its persistent centrality to political events, combined with York's historic role as England's second city to generate a powerful and independent regional identity.

York Lunatic Asylum—a public psychiatric hospital serving all of Yorkshire—was planned while Parliament was debating private madhouse regulation. Eight members of its founding committee held a parliamentary

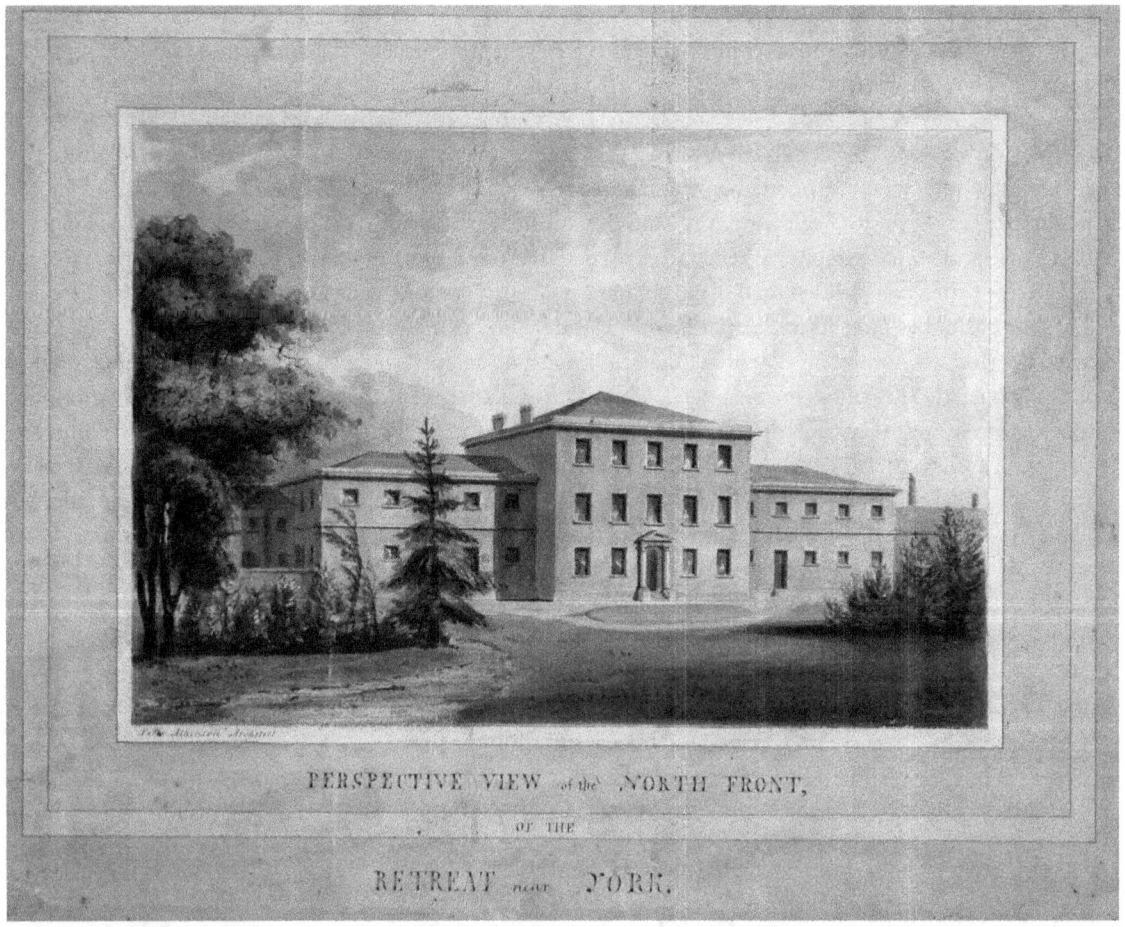

Figure 5.1 Peter Atkinson the Younger, *Perspective View of the North Front of the Retreat near York*, 1812 (BIA RET 2/1/2/1), subsequently published in Samuel Tuke, *Description of the Retreat: An Institution Near York, for Insane Persons of the Society of Friends* (York, 1813). Source: Borthwick Institute, University of York

seat for a Yorkshire constituency, so the asylum's establishment responded to an awareness among the political class of the unsatisfactory nature of these institutions. John Carr (1723–1821), northern England's principal designer, and the only regional architect to be elected to the London Architects' Club, had recently completed Leeds General Infirmary; he was consequently invited to design the York Asylum, which opened in 1777.[17] Like the London asylums, it too was subject to scrutiny, and its resemblance to a country house invited criticism as ostentatiously wasting public money, provoking the founding of the York Retreat in 1792 by the Religious Society of Friends for mentally ill co-religionists. The Friends distilled the spiritual, empirical, and a non-academic aesthetic in an innovative space that some have argued is an early example of a completely designed "therapeutic environment," that is, a modern, semi-medicalized construct for elite cultural practice dating back to antiquity (Figure 5.1). The modest Retreat appears to stand in mute criticism of the York Asylum and the rest of this chapter will discuss its appearance, and broader significance with regard to its garden setting, therapeutic regime, and its role in furthering social reform in England.[18]

Samuel Tuke's *Description of the Retreat* (1813)

Much scholarly ink has been spilled in understanding York Friends' Retreat relying on Samuel Tuke's *Description of the Retreat*. It is an excellent—if problematic—source; Samuel's lucid prose, architectural plans, and picturesque views combined with his shrewd PR sense produced an ürtext in the History of Psychiatry, securing the asylum's international reputation, spawning, among others, America's first purpose-built psychiatric institution, the Philadelphia Friends' Hospital at Frankford (Figure 5.2).[19]

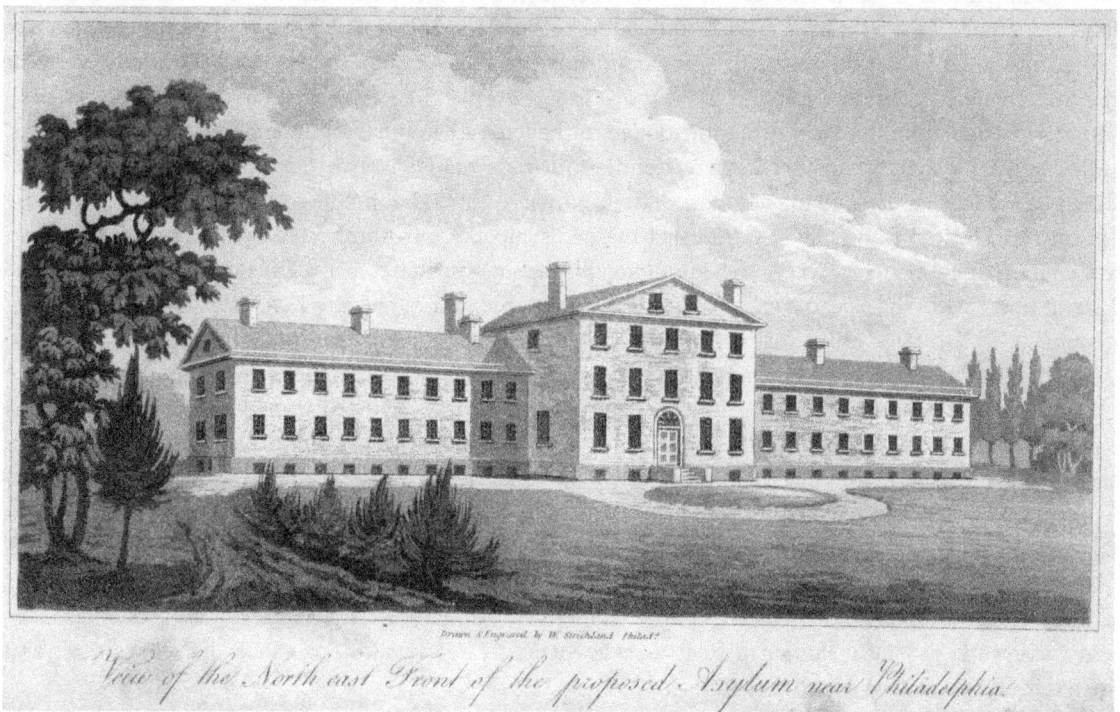

Figure 5.2 W. Strickland, *View of the North East Front of the Proposed Asylum near Philadelphia* (1814). Source: The Library Company of Philadelphia

The book was published in York by family member William Alexander (1768–1841), dedicated to Samuel's grandfather, and distributed in the important Quaker cities of London and Bristol. Though superficially parochial, the book pointed to French therapeutic innovation, and was to command international influence. It was published and circulated during debates in the British parliament concerning the provision for treatment of insane persons when there was considerable interest in legislation. The Select Committee to Enquire into the State of Criminal and Pauper Lunatics in England informed the County Asylum Act of 1808.[20] Responding to requests for such a work, Tuke's timely volume aimed, "in the interests of humanity and science," to help others planning similar institutions by throwing light on the Retreat's distinctive method of housing and caring for disordered people. He confirmed that, despite its modest size, the establishment had "met the approbation of many judicious persons who have had the opportunity of inspecting its internal economy and management," some reports of which were reproduced in the appendix.[21]

In the preface, Tuke cites the French alienist and father of modern psychiatry, Philippe Pinel (1745–1826), who had argued

> He who cultivates the science of medicine, as a branch of natural history, pursues a more frank and open system of conduct; nor seeks to conceal the obstacles which he meets with in his course. What he discovers, he feels no reluctance to show; and the difficulties which he cannot master, he leaves with the impression of his hand upon them, for the benefit of his successors in the same route.[22]

Pinel—an atypical French doctor—supported the French Revolution and adopted a humane approach to treatment of mental disorder, now called *moral therapy*, at l'Hôpital Bicêtre in Paris and the Hospice de la Salpêtrière where he was chief physician from 1795. Pinel's *Memoir on Madness* had been read to the Society for Natural History in Paris on December 11, 1794, soon after the fall of the Jacobin dictatorship and, it has been argued, is a political appeal to the Revolutionary government to build asylums where mentally ill patients could be decently treated.[23] It is important not to overstate Pinel's significance; his gesture of removing patients' chains at Bicêtre in 1797, and at la Salpêtrière, three years later, has been demonstrated to be partly hagiographical.[24] Pinel is not mentioned in the Retreat's foundation documents, and my argument is the Retreat's distinctive approach emerged independently from Quaker theological culture. Nevertheless, Pinel's empiricist approach, unorthodox anti-authoritarianism, and political campaigning for humane treatment resonated with Quaker values that meshed sympathy for incarcerated people and a profoundly anti-authoritarian mentality with radical thinking; by aligning the Retreat with Pinel, Samuel positioned the Retreat in the wider European context of humane psychiatric reform and the *Description* as a campaigning document.

In England, the reporting of medical success by physicians was not generally replicated in the area of mental health. Like Pinel, Samuel's book reflected the scientific method, giving objective descriptions validated through the first-hand witnessing of third parties, some of whose endorsements were attached in the appendix. Furthermore, while advertising "the discoveries we make, or the failures which happen to us, in a pursuit so intimately connected with the happiness of our species," he aimed through a comparative method to elicit general laws and "infer the most probable means of rescuing or relieving the unhappy victims of this disease."[25] Using archival material, the book addresses institutional history, fundraising, appointment of non-clinical staff, and summarizes financial reports. It describes the building's design, the domestic establishment and therapeutic regime including patient assessment and categorization, methods of (self-)control and coercion, and promotion of patient comfort.

Partly because of Tuke's *Description*, the Retreat has been regarded as a groundbreaking psychiatric institution because its therapeutic regime represented a new humane attitude toward psychiatric patients.

However, only by locating the Retreat in the theological context from which it emerged can we grasp the distinctive praxis and aesthetics conceptualized as agents of healing for this specific group sharing idiosyncratic knowledge.

Built Environment: Design Process

The Religious Society of Friends were originally a left-wing puritan sect of the 1640s. Despite a distinctive spirituality, their culture of restraint and austerity retained many puritan characteristics since seventeenth-century radicalism shaping the Society chimed with late eighteenth-century radicals.[26] Quakers routinely refused to conform to many social norms and developed instead a comprehensive culture of prescribed behaviors. The York Retreat project—process and product—was deemed "right ordered," that is, built according to Quaker norms of financial transparency and collaboration. This "right ordering" and the asylum's subsequent success reformed Quaker attitudes toward the practice of architecture as a vehicle for God's work.[27] It was funded through a subscription among the Society across England; Philadelphian Lindley Murray (1745–1826) was its most generous benefactor, and William Tuke donated thirty years of his time.[28] It was designed by Tuke, the London Quaker builder John Bevans, and the York architect Peter Atkinson the Elder (1735–1805) as executant on the ground. Its form emerged from the interplay between that trio and the Quaker community in Yorkshire. Local monthly meetings afforded opportunities for members to deliberate and report their views. The Society's pragmatic open-mindedness to innovation was anchored by established best practice. Tuke sent ideas to Bevans, requesting a plan "for Friends different ideas to be well considered, for we must expect diversity of Opinions."[29] Correspondence and drawings modified with pencil lines testify to Friends' detailed engagement; they rejected some aspects, concerned that the asylum should not have a "melancholy appearance," and patients' views should not be obstructed (Figure 5.3).[30] The prospect from the hospital was regarded as essential to patients' welfare, suggesting regard for their humanity and the importance to Quaker thought of light as an agent of divine inspiration.

In his study, Will Gesler cites Florence Nightingale regarding the importance to patients of lower densities, circulation of fresh air, adequate light, good drainage, clean laundry rooms, and kitchen.[31] As we now understand, this was received wisdom established from the seventeenth century. Satisfying the Quaker requirement to consider best current practice, Tuke and Bevans visited St. Luke's Asylum in London, designed by George Dance, the Younger (1741–1825), that had opened just a few years before in 1787. St. Luke's was widely admired and used as a model of asylum planning by seven provincial English asylums in the second half of the eighteenth century.[32] They read appraisals of European and British hospitals by John Howard (c. 1726–90) who admired the Quakers.[33]

Howard—the High Sheriff of Bedfordshire, and a social reformer—had spent the 1770s and 1780s traveling in Britain, inspecting prisons with regard to the conditions in which the inmates were housed to establish norms of safety and hygiene, and to advertise places failing to meet his standards. He subsequently broadened his interests to asylums in Britain and abroad, composing *An Account of the Principal Lazarettos of Europe* (1789). Howard died in Russia the following year, becoming the first civilian honored by a statue in St. Paul's Cathedral. England's most modern asylum was described by Howard as a "noble hospital."[34] Howard's preferred plan comprised a central block, with single-loaded wings containing a gallery, evoking Hooke's Bethlem. General consensus suggested provision of individual patient cells for safety.[35] Bevans's Retreat planning followed Howard, though concerns about gallery width resulted in doubled-loaded airing galleries with vaulted rooms protected against those perennial asylum hazards of patient assault and fire.[36]

Health and Architecture

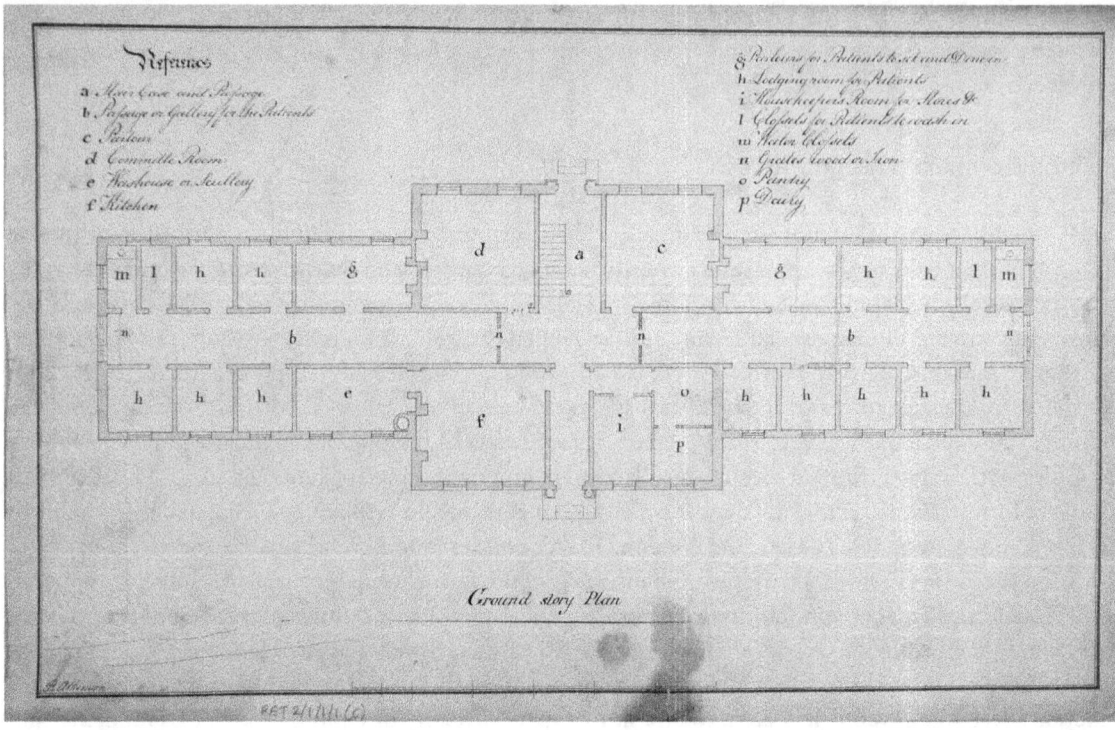

Figure 5.3 The Retreat: Ground Story Plan showing pencil revisions (BIA RET 2/1/1/1(c)). Source: Borthwick Institute, University of York

Built Environment: Plan and Appearance

Gesler's category of the built environment is predicated on fusing an assumption of a sensory response to architecture with an intellectual knowledge of institutional history, conferring a sense of security. He argues that impressively ordered and built space generates, by extension, patients' confidence in therapy. In this context his specific observations are of limited value. Despite the seventeenth-century belief in architecture as embodying history, the Retreat was a new type of institution without genealogy, counteracted, as I argue below, by Samuel Tuke's *Description* that generated a powerful creation myth.

The low-lying city of York sits at the confluence of two rivers. Early modern engravings reveal that for miles around, across the floodplain, viewers could behold the circuit of magnesian limestone city walls, and a skyline punctuated by medieval church steeples surrounding the unmistakable silhouette of Northern Europe's largest gothic cathedral, York Minster. The Retreat was built on Lamel Hill, a mile southeast of the center of York, its salubrious location described by Thomas Wilkinson (1751–1836), the Quaker gardener of Yanwith and friend of poet William Wordsworth (1770–1850), in a contemporary verse:

> On a fair hill, where York in prospect lies
> Her towers and steeples pointing to the skies,
> A goodly structure rears its modest head;
> Thither my walk the worthy founder led.[37]

This hilltop location coupled with the asylum's plan of long wings and opposing windows dispelled "vitiated" or "spent" air. Individual rooms with ingenious windows offered salubrious ventilation while bars concealed in the muntins did not obstruct the view. Service apartments were repositioned to avoid giving patients "a nauseous view." Objects of contemplation in hospitals were of course traditional, as we have seen, but in the Protestant context of the Quaker Retreat, Nature was the subject, and sitting rooms for the intended thirty patients all had garden outlooks. Modern empirical evidence, cited by Gesler, suggests better outcomes for recovering patients who could see trees,[38] though the original Retreat patients—who were Quakers— would have experienced Nature in a different way, as we shall see.

Eighteenth-century Quaker theology was informed by ideas from Cambridge Platonism, with which founding member William Penn (1644–1718) had been linked.[39] John Smith (1618–52), was credited with developing a deeply rational Christian philosophy that was both open to the new science, and yet directed to the practical goal of living a religious life: Reason was "the candle of the Lord." In this theology, Reality was known not by physical sensation alone, but by intuition of the intelligible Forms that exist behind the material world of everyday perception. Abundant light flooded Quaker spaces, signifying God's agency in luminous interiors of bare boards and white walls.[40] The design historian David Brett has proposed the evolution of an abstract aesthetics, tracing the disappearance of the figurative from puritan culture in which "plainness and perspicuity" was the objective.[41] This shift from pictorial—through symbolic—to abstract memory, founded a type of utopianism. The iconic function of the picture became displaced onto workmanship and materials, creating an aesthetic in which unadorned plain stone, timber, and plaster, and space and light itself embodied the numinous. Such abstraction facilitated control over inner life—a self-discipline that Quakers deemed essential. Moreover, since in Quaker theology, Scripture was interpreted through an auditory channel through which God spoke, expectant waiting was silent.[42] The Retreat's removal from the city conferred that necessary peace.

The Retreat's design team comprised a Quaker elder (Tuke) and builder (Bevans), and the local community, combined with the local architect Peter Atkinson, the business partner of John Carr (Figure 5.4). This combination meant Quaker norms and ideas were filtered through the professional practice of a local architect. The Society's preference for employing people from within their own community meant that most of their buildings were constructed by local builders in a vernacular style, using local materials and traditional techniques in a functional rather than ornamental way.[43] "Vernacular" architecture is often opposed to "polite" or "academic," but that is not the sense here: in linguistics, "vernacular" denotes demotic, everyday language and this use of the metaphor in architectural discourse is entirely appropriate for speech and its absence were foregrounded in Quaker culture where plain speech and denial of ostentatious status markers were reflected in their counter-rhetorical design. The Quaker preference for vernacular elevations, then, might be understood as intentionally resisting architectural loquacity: articulating instead locational decorum, speaking in the local dialect that was sometimes well informed, at others uneducated. Early modern York was a major center for architectural practice and had seen the construction of many classical town houses, meaning that a subdued classicism became the local urban vernacular.

While the style of the Retreat was local vernacular, the composition and setting were also classical (Figure 5.5). Italian Humanist villas embodying personal moderation, withdrawal, and *santa agricoltura* (holy agriculture), as extolled by Venetian nobleman Alvise Cornaro (*c.* 1467–1566), were well known in the eighteenth century.[44] The original Renaissance villas of the Venetian *terraferma* and the Brenta Canal emerged from the farms and dwellings of the Veneto.[45] They offered twin architectural models: the better-known *casa di villa* (proprietor's house) would—via the works of Andrea Palladio (1508–80)—inform grandiloquent eighteenth-century English country houses; the second model was the modestly utilitarian working farmhouse with flanking *barchessa* (barn) wings, constructed of brick and stucco that settled in to the countryside. In such villa planning, the farmhouse was flanked with wings housing agricultural services. As an architect, Peter Atkinson could apply academic architectural knowledge to the Retreat design. The essentially conservative

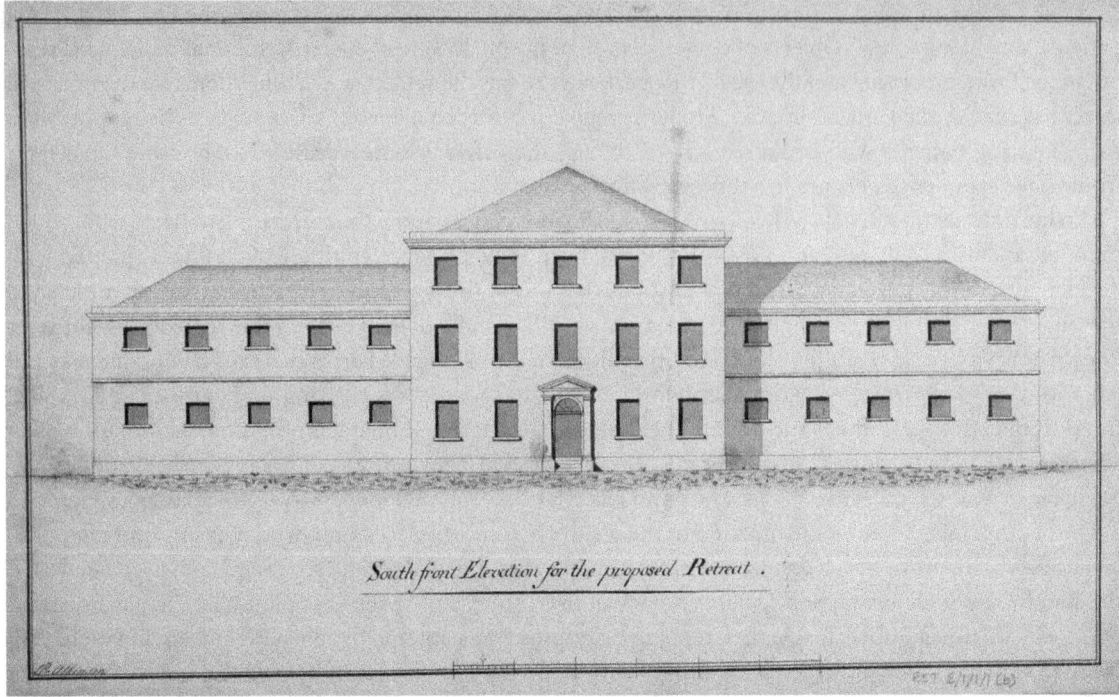

Figure 5.4 South front elevation for the proposed Retreat, consultation drawing (BIA RET 2/1/1/1(b)). Source: Borthwick Institute, University of York

nature of Renaissance villa life chimed with the backwards-looking aspects of Quaker culture, counterpoising the modern influences of new asylum design. Furthermore, the application of classical models—albeit in a pared-down way—dignified the inhabitants of the asylum: both the patients and those who cared for them. Its central block, capped with a pyramidal roof, was rigorously symmetrical, flanked by wings housing an airing galley and patients' rooms.

The Retreat's classicism articulated Quakerly restraint in the York local vernacular, while its location, a mile outside the city walls, meant its farmhouse typology was entirely appropriate. In this way the asylum fused therapeutic innovation and the traditional salubrity of rural life. Underlining its humane philanthropy and quiet classicism, the foundation stone was inscribed in Latin: *Hoc fecit amicorum caritas in humanitatis argumentum* ("The love of Friends made this [building] in the cause of humanity").[46]

The central block resembled farmhouse planning—substituting public offices with a dairy, parlor, and kitchen, comparable with the plan of a Yorkshire farmhouse.[47] The kitchen, which in contemporary medical institutions occupied the building's periphery as at the London Hospital, was central.[48] Supervision was aided by axially aligned doors as Howard recommended. The closeness of patients to domestic activity manifested belief in hard work and discipline as a means of aiding redemption and cure, while facilitating surveillance. It appeared as a farm, not a prison, and was interpreted as such at the time. In 1798, soon after opening, Charles-Gaspard de la Rive (1770–1834), a Genevan physician specializing in the treatment of mental illness, visited the asylum and observed: "Cette maison est située à un mille de York au mileau d'une campagne fertile et riante: ce n'est point l'idée d'une prison qu'elle fait naître, mais plutôt celle d'une grande ferme rustique, elle est entourée d'une jardin fermé" ("This house is situated a mile from York, in the midst of a fertile and cheerful country; it presents not the idea of a prison, but rather a large rural farm. It is surrounded by a garden").[49]

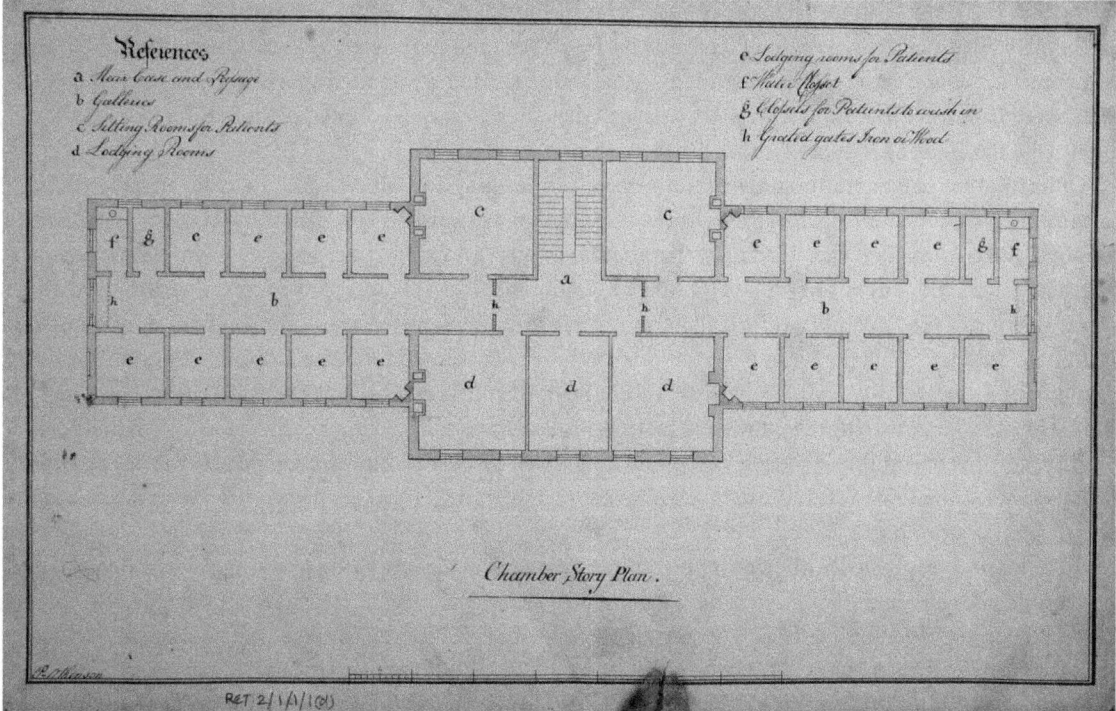

Figure 5.5 Chamber Story Plan of the Retreat, consultation drawing (BIA RET 2/1/1/1(d)). Source: Borthwick Institute, University of York

This comment would have delighted the founders because it confirmed they had achieved their aesthetic objective. Perhaps with George Dance's forbidding cyclopean Newgate Prison (1769–77) in mind, the Retreat design correspondence reveals the sole articulated aesthetic consideration was that the asylum shouldn't resemble a prison, because "if the outside appears heavy and prison-like it has a considerable effect upon the imagination."[50] Contrary to other asylums, here patients inhabited a "room" not a "cell."[51] Surveillance was, of course, essential; Howard's admiration for the Constantinople asylum was associated with safety.[52] While reconnecting with God, Retreat patients were protectively watched. The lavishly fenestrated annular *Panopticon* recently published by Jeremy Bentham (1748–1832), extended "the principle of omnipresence" as an agent of control.[53] Yet despite its rationalism, Bentham's model was not adopted since it reflected a penitentiary philosophy with which Quakers—whose published *Sufferings* recalled the era of imprisonment—could not have sympathized.

Natural Environment: God's Handiwork and Puritan Paradise

Gesler's Natural Environment combines a seemingly universal belief in Nature's regenerative powers with the assumption that an aesthetic response to the natural environment confers pleasure, and total removal from society into Nature is beneficial.[54] As with the built environment, Quaker engagement with Nature fused ancient and contemporary beliefs and aesthetics with their distinctively religious contemplative dimension. Gesler's observation that "looking at or working in Gardens is also considered to have a therapeutic effect" finds support in this case.[55] The Retreat's eleven-acre hilltop location, "in an airy situation," commanded views over a rolling pastoral landscape; York's picturesque ancient skyline presented an unparalleled eye-catcher. Detailed planting, within a concealed ha-ha rather than perimeter wall, took place before building commenced.[56] Plant variety, including many American specimens, supplied year-round interest and color; there were fruit trees, but the gardens were designed as much for quiet contemplation as for provisioning.[57] Eventually the building sheltered under broadleaves and conifers.[58]

Quakers were permitted to study useful Natural Philosophy for education, medicine, and recreation.[59] Inward Light was balanced against the Natural, informed by outward senses. Visual and sensory appreciation of God's work stimulated the search for truth and was an agent of recuperation. Puritans saw gardens as a *type* of Eden, and gardening—modeled first by Adam and Eve—an acceptable recreation through which contemplation of God's natural world and harmony between Humanity, Nature, and God were re-established and Eden remade.[60] William Penn, Pennsylvania's founder who aimed to create utopia in America, idealized rural life in *Some Fruits of Solitude* (1693).[61] In England, the puritan John Milton's widely read *Paradise Lost* had associated Satan with the monumental metropolis Pandemonium, while Eden evoked sylvan landscapes. Prompted by his friend the Quaker Thomas Ellwood (1639–1714), Milton had composed *Paradise Regained*, which demonstrated Eden's recapture through rejecting materiality. Quakers developed a botanical aesthetic connecting Nature with its Creator.[62]

These notions resonated with late eighteenth-century radical ideas and the prevailing classical taste; ideal Roman life had, of course, balanced *Otium* against *Negotium*; Pliny's villa retreats were published in Robert Castell's *Villas of the Ancients* (1728),[63] and many eighteenth-century English hospitals were ideologically classical villas, such as St. George's, Hyde Park Corner (1733), York County Hospital (1740), and Gloucester Infirmary (1757–61). William Tuke's obituary recorded his retaining "a lively recollection of some passages of Vergil's *Georgics* in old age." Vergil's picture of frugal and austere rural life was harmonious with nature and the divine scheme of things, based on morally satisfying hard work, and was rewarded by peace and contentment.[64] Responding to this, and to Romantic aesthetics that conceptualized Nature as a locus for bodily and spiritual restoration, some, like the wealthy Goldney family in Bristol, created fashionable gardens.[65]

Gesler emphasized the role of faith and pilgrimage in the healing process, in which the patient's liminal state gives way to new relationships. In the case of the Retreat, that pilgrimage was an interior one, conditioned by the persisting eschatological mindset of what the literary historian M. H. Abrams called "left-wing Inner Light Protestants" in the Revolutionary era of late eighteenth- and early nineteenth-century England.[66] For radicals like the Quakers, as Wordsworth observed, "the grand store-house of enthusiastic and meditative Imagination … is the prophetic and lyrical parts of the holy Scriptures, and the works of Milton."[67] In the 1970s, Abrams established the circuit journey of pilgrims and prodigals that was essentially "the assimilation of a historical religion to a timeless Neoplatonised Christianity."[68] The individual soul and its one source becomes "the parable of an internal spiritual journey in a quest of a lost home." In this schema, sin is regarded as a falling away from God and redemption a process of reintegration. Christian history is conceived as a great circle; a structure manifest in the arts and philosophy, epitomized in the biblical parable of the Prodigal Son, and exemplified in the life of man in a peregrination toward New Jerusalem, such as in John Bunyan's allegory *Pilgrim's Progress* (1678). An 1828 plan of the Retreat shows gardens with circular walks, which offered a space where patients might perform a peregrination, enacting a puritan circuit pilgrimage, disclosing the inner self, where sensory botanical appreciation became a channel for God's grace. This contemporary Quaker association between gardens and prayer is reflected in the 1782 poem of Friend John Scott (1730–83):[69]

> But might thy genius, Friend, an Eden frame,
> Profuse of beauty, and secure from blame; …
> There love's sweet song adown the echoing dale,

To beauty's ear conveys the tender tale;
And there Devotion lifts his brow to Heaven,
With grateful thanks for many a blessing given.[70]

Mindful contemplation in the garden was spiritually restorative; it enabled introspection, contemplation of God's work and the performance of a puritan pilgrimage. In the context of the Retreat, however, despite a name that articulated the benefits of withdrawal, it was in the distinctive social aspects that the hospital was most efficacious.[71]

Social Environment: Quaker Social Culture

Gesler argued the best therapeutic outcomes were those where social relations were equal rather than hierarchical, within a constructed supportive therapeutic community with shared values.[72] This element is especially pronounced at the Retreat where Quaker theological culture underpinned the values of patients and caregivers alike. Friends aimed to be *in* society but not *of* it: a complex and shifting relation, partly shaped by the Society's origins. During England's 1650s Commonwealth, Messianic hope had fueled radical activism; Quakers were regarded as sowers of sedition, hostile to the Anglican Church, and supportive of poor people. The charismatic founder, George Fox (1624–91), advocated a telling transformation: repurposing monastic, ecclesiastical, and government buildings as almshouses.[73]

By the eighteenth century, the tension of being *in* the world but not *of* it was increasingly expressed visually through outward signs, discussed above. "Plaining," as it has been called, was "the creation of a symbolic order *vis-à-vis* the apostate church they defined themselves against."[74] Having accommodated to living in the Meantime (that is, until the Second Coming of the Messiah), a quietist period characterized by "retreat from the world and the self" saw radical individualism meld into self-abnegation, privileging domestic settings on the one hand, and broad social humanitarianism on the other.[75] These distinctive foci are expressed in the Retreat's dedicatory inscription: "The love of Friends made this [building] in the cause of humanity," and in its conception as a sequestered family home for sick members of the Religious Society of Friends.[76]

Dana Arnold has recently observed the domestic origins of some civic hospitals and stressed the interchangeability of residential and medical institutional space.[77] Setting English hospitals in the broader context of European hospitals, however, we observe a return—after the Reformation in the Protestant north and western regions—to domestic models to reinvent a typology formerly associated with the Catholic Church. In this respect, the Retreat's domesticity reflects religiously reformed social behavior as much as the strong Quaker domestic ethos.

Withdrawal from wider society for contemplation was another traditional notion chiming with Quaker separatism of rural life. The Retreat was expressly intended for "the care of those with whom they [patients] are connected in Religious Society." Gesler's assertion that healing is a social activity involving interactions between the people adopting social roles is supported by the inauguration of the asylum by the Quaker community as a whole.[78] Friends across England financially supported their co-religionists. Their shared theology was embodied in an asylum originally excluding those of confessional differences or suffering mental impairment who might not share it.[79] In Quaker mystical theology mental disorder was understood as an alternative, transient, and crucially curable psychological mode where patients were temporarily incapable of hearing God's voice. Social withdrawal—or retreat—to reconnect with God was therefore therapeutic. Patients were simply temporarily incapable social equals. During remission, it was assumed they would be happier surrounded by like-minded individuals, so class identity was retained. Artisans brought their tools and practiced their skills; working people farmed the land; socially elevated patients—perhaps like H. Bass who copied Peter Atkinson's 1812 *View* in 1831, and the architect-patient E. S. K. whose plans and drawings remain in the archives—were lodged in larger rooms with fires, enjoyed accommodation for their servants, and dined with the Superintendent; and lower-class patients were housed in the wings.[80]

In Gesler's characterization, conventional biomedicine is dispensed in hierarchical and controlling situations that may stimulate patient resistance. His observations, based on modern notions of hospitals and their social structures, need amplifying in this case, for the Retreat's contrast with early modern hospital hierarchies was even more pronounced.[81] Quakerism challenged the status quo, rejecting signs of rank and professional hierarchy. The patient-carer power-relation was paternalistic, not medical; there were no offices designed for professionals and the spaces conventionally dedicated to physicians, apothecaries, or surgeons were given over to the domestic. Rather, the asylum was conceptualized as a home, its ethos reflected in describing the institution as "a retired habitation," "Friends Lunatic House," and the residents as "the family": it was a *domus familia*—a domestic religious space.[82] The inscription on its foundation stone emphasizes its genesis in communal love. Its paternalistic regime, eventually characterized as Moral Management, was intended to support the individual on return to society by fostering self-discipline and self-esteem.

Symbolic Environment: The Power of Reputation

Superficially, Gelser's Symbolic Environment is least useful in this context. He stresses the importance of symbolic meaning embodied in rituals and physical objects invested with meaning by the users. As has been discussed, idiosyncratic rejection of much received belief and behaviors became the distinctive hallmark of Quaker theological culture, the withdrawn nature of which generated particularized understandings. Consequently, Gesler's belief in the powerful impression of a classical portico, the physician's white coat "associated with purity or honesty," and high-tech equipment symbolizing "the power of biomedicine" are irrelevant in this context where meditative worship and disavowal of social norms were commonplace.[83] More salient is his discussion of myths—described as symbolic stories—used to alter attitudes to physical states.[84]

Mythologizing narratives of place arguably can trigger what we now know to be the placebo effect and that may have been the case regarding the reputation of the Retreat. When writing his influential *Description*, Samuel Tuke was prosecuting a campaign for reform at the nearby York Asylum. He opened his account with the case of a Quaker patient who died there without the consolation of visits from her co-religionists. But there is no reference to her death in the archival foundation account where we can see that an additional handwritten statement was added at an unknown date (Figure 5.6).[85] This oppositional narrative of a helpless Quaker woman, left to perish alone in the hostile Asylum, persuasively animated Samuel's reforming agenda.

The *Description* deserves consideration for what it tells us of the early nineteenth-century regime, and because it was directly influential on international psychiatric care. It was not only the novelty of such a volume detailing the workings of an asylum that made it such a success; it balances a scientific approach with classical, biblical, and contemporary scholarship. Its account of the founding, building, and furnishing of the institution is based on archival material and its detail and comprehensiveness are supplemented by the endorsement of international visitors whose enthusiastic opinions were recorded.[86] In the early years, the advertised visits of the Genevan Dr. de la Rive, Dr. Naudi from Malta, the architect William Stark from Glasgow, and Philadelphian Thomas Scattergood were supplemented by those recorded in the Visiter's Book (*sic*) of Dr. Duncan from Dublin, three parties from the Russian royal family, and three First Nation Americans.[87]

"The Love of Friends Made This in the Cause of Humanity"

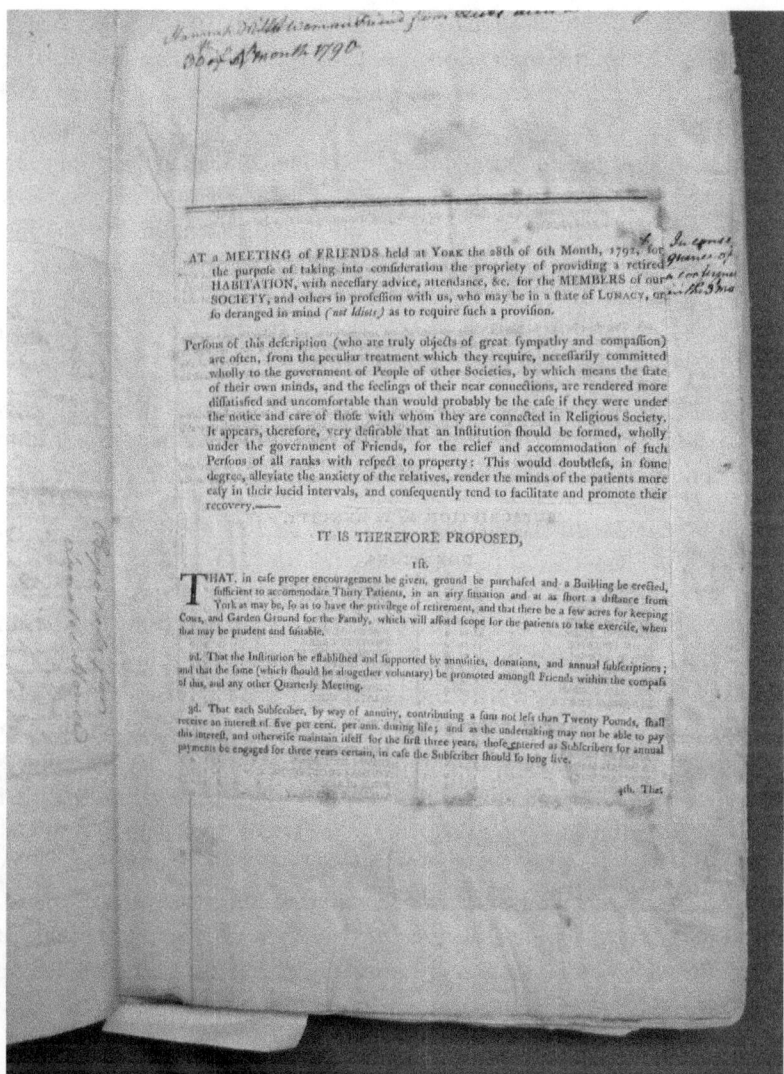

Figure 5.6 The Retreat Directors' Minute Book showing original subscription appeal in print and handwritten addition regarding Hannah Mills (BIA RET 1/1/1/1/, fol. 1r). Source: Borthwick Institute, University of York

As argued above, Tuke aligned his account with the late eighteenth-century radical French thinking of Pinel, but the *Description* also sits in the context of nineteenth-century English asylum reform. The social and economic historian Anne Digby argued its publication in the midst of the political controversy regarding financial cupidity and patient abuse at the York Asylum triggered

> a series of events exposing a marked contrast in the treatment of the insane at the Retreat and the asylum … Local reformers found contemporary parallels between the battlefield of Waterloo and their own hard-won victory in successfully reforming the asylum: Higgins was likened to Blucher and Best to Napoleon. The historian would assign the role of Wellington to Samuel Tuke who achieved overall victory.[88]

Health and Architecture

Thanks to this *cause célèbre* and the publication of the *Description*, Samuel was called to give evidence to the House of Commons Select Committee on Madhouses of 1814–16.[89] Within a few years of its publication, Samuel Tuke was regarded as a national authority on ethical asylum design, publishing several architectural treatises that enabled Quakers to embrace architectural practice. The Retreat convinced members of the Society of Friends that large-scale institutions required professional design and proved the process could be consultative and well informed. Friends had created a large semi-public space where their wider humanitarian projects might be furthered; campaigns for improved conditions for patients and for the abolition of slavery were conducted from the Retreat. It was a space that was thus invested with a moral weight partly because it was "right-ordered" in its design process and its end result, and partly because it made possible the pursuit of a national agenda of social reform. Therapeutic environments may be characterized by specificity, and certainly the Retreat originally emerged from and was intended for a very particular social group, its success predicated on a shared semiotic field of reference and cultural praxis—every element was a repository for meaning apprehended by the Quaker community. The symbolism evoked in the Retreat's powerful foundation myth then contributed to the positive expectations and associations of patients and caregivers alike.

Conclusion

During a discussion in 2009 regarding the power of religion in the public sphere, the Canadian philosopher Charles Taylor argued for a radical redefinition of secularism.[90] Though public institutions necessarily exclude overtly religious language from public discourse, on the grounds that it is based on a set of specific *a priori* not shared by non-believers, Taylor argues that does not necessarily mean that people automatically reject religious thought as lacking insight. The rise of European scientific medicine is generally set in the context of the growth of religious skepticism and concomitant secularism. Certainly, from the Enlightenment era, the application of medico-scientific knowledge regarding the genesis, spread, and treatment of disease met with greater success than the previous, spiritually engaged model. Yet the dominance of secularism in the Enlightenment narrative should not be overstated. Though new surgical procedures and therapies were increasingly grounded in the benefits of the scientific method, general hospitals continued to be built with chapels, and "spital sermons"—intended to stimulate charitable donations—were delivered in elite churches. While the institutions were increasingly secular, the patients and those who cared for them, whether pious or not, still inhabited a Christian culture.

Taylor aims to debunk the myth that Reason alone underpinned the Enlightenment by suggesting epistemic distinctions between rational and religious thought are unhelpful. As we have seen, Taylor's argument, that no such distinction obtained, finds support in the case of the York Retreat where the early Religious Society of Friends embraced complementary epistemic economies: the Outward and the Inward, foregrounded in their innovative hospital design. It demonstrates the caution with which we should accept such grand narratives. The Retreat's founders rejected the inclusion in the design of both modern professional offices and a traditional chapel, yet this denoted neither a rejection of the past nor the present. The asylum they created embodied wisdom reaching back to Antiquity fused with scientifically informed best practice and a profound, distinctive spirituality. It was a *domus familia* emerging from, and intended for, a social group with idiosyncratic knowledge, and excluding those not sharing its embodied theology.[91] Their collective semiotic field of reference and cultural praxis meant that, in creating the space, every element became a repository for meaning apprehended by the community. It was a space charged with religious significance, optimizing the circumstances in which God's voice might be heard and his Light might illuminate the soul; religious contemplation had a long history in hospitals, and even in 1792 it had not gone away. Indeed, a century later, one Cambridge Quaker paleographer reiterated, the "theory of the detachment of science and religion from one another *never has* been a working theory of the universe; the two areas must overlap and blend, or we are lost."[92]

Notes

1. Andrew Scull, *The Most Solitary of Afflictions: Madness and Society in Britain 1700–1900* (New Haven and London: Yale University Press, 1993), ch. 2. See also Harold Capper Hunt, *A Retired Habitation: A History of the Retreat at York* (London: H. K. Lewis and Co., 1932); Roy Porter, *Madmen: A Social History of Madhouses, Mad-Doctors and Lunatics* (Stroud: Tempus, 2004).
2. Mary R. Glover, *The Retreat, York: An Early Experiment in the Treatment of Mental Illness* (York: William Sessions, 1984); William Kaye Sessions, *The Tukes of York in the Seventeenth, Eighteenth and Nineteenth Centuries* (London: Friends Home Service Committee, 1971); Sheila Wright, *Friends in York: The Dynamics of Quaker Revival 1780–1860* (Keele: Keele University Press, 1995).
3. Sarah Rutherford, "Landscapes for the Mind: English Asylum designers, 1845–1914," *Garden History* 33, no. 1 (Summer 2005): 61–86, at 62. Clare Hickman supports the notion that the early modern asylum consciously constructed a therapeutic environment in "The Picturesque at Brislington House, Bristol: The Role of Landscape in Relation to the Treatment of Mental Illness in the Early Nineteenth-Century Asylum" *Garden History* 33, no. 1 (Summer, 2005): 47–60. See also Clare Cooper Marcus and Marni Barnes, eds., *Healing Gardens: Therapeutic Benefits and Design Recommendations* (Chichester: John Wiley & Sons, 1999): 236–7; Nancy Gerlach-Spriggs, Richard Enoch Kaufman, and Sam Bass Warner, Jnr., *Restorative Gardens: The Healing Landscape* (New Haven, CT: Yale University Press 1998).
4. Wilbert M. Gesler, *Healing Places* (Lanham, Boulder, New York, and Oxford: Rowman and Littlefield, 2003).
5. Dankwart Leistikow, *Ten Centuries of European Hospital Architecture: A Contribution to the History of Hospital Architecture* (Ingelheim-am-Rhein: C. H. Boehringer Sohn, 1967). Nikolaus Pevsner, *A History of Building Types* (Princeton: Princeton University Press, 1976) remains the most concise, informed, and well-illustrated account of the evolution of hospital and asylum form related to social context. John D. Thompson and Grace Goldin, *The Hospital: A Social and Architectural History* (New Haven and London: Yale University Press, 1975) considered ward morphology, and Harriet Richardson, ed., *English Hospitals and their Design 1660–1948* (Swindon: Royal Commission on the Historical Monuments of England, 1998) categorized hospitals by clinical specialism. Jean Imbert, ed., *Histoire des Hôpitaux en France* (Toulouse: Privat, c.1982) located French hospitals in their precise socio-cultural and politico-economic contexts, as did Guenter B. Risse, *Hospital Life in Enlightenment Scotland* (Cambridge: Cambridge University Press, 1986). Jonathan Barry and Colin Jones, eds., *Medicine and Charity before the Welfare State* (London and New York: Routledge, 1991) draws case studies from across Europe from the medieval period to the twentieth century. See also Guenter B. Risse, *Mending Bodies, Saving Souls: A History of Hospitals* (Oxford: Oxford University Press, 1999).
6. Leistikow, *Hospital*, 61–4; John Henderson, *The Renaissance Hospital: Healing the Body and Healing the Soul* (New Haven and London: Yale University Press, 2008), ch. 3.
7. Filarete, *Codex Magliabechianus*, Tractate on Architecture (1456), Book XI, fol. 79r.
8. Julian Hoppit, "King, Gregory (1648–1712), Herald and Political Economist," *Oxford Dictionary of National Biography* (September 23, 2004), accessed January 6, 2021. https://www-oxforddnb-com.sheffield.idm.oclc.org/view/10.1093/ref:odnb/9780198614128.001.0001/odnb-9780198614128-e-15563.
9. John Bellers, *An Essay Toward the Improvement of Physick* (London: J. Sowle, 1714); Robert Nelson, *Address to Persons of Quality and Estate* (London: G. James, 1715).
10. Christine Stevenson, "Robert Hooke's Bethlem," *Journal of the Society of Architectural Historians* 55 (1996): 254–75.
11. Ibid., 255.
12. Ibid., 264.
13. Ibid., 269.
14. Porter, *Madmen*, 117–72.
15. For a detailed account of the terms, see Kathleen Jones, *Lunacy, Law and Conscience 1744–1845: The Social History of the Care of the Insane* (London: Routledge and Kegan Paul, 1955), 28–9.
16. For a concise discussion of European hospitals, see Ann-Marie Akehurst, "'The Body Natural as well as the Body Politic stands indebted': The Hospital—Foundation, Funding and Form," in *Architectural Theory and Practice, Companion to*

Architecture in the Age of the Enlightenment, vol. 2, ed. Caroline van Eck and Sigrid de Jong (Chichester: John Wiley & Sons, 2017), ch. 11. For an account of early modern asylums, see Pevsner, *Building Type*, 148–50. For Bethlem's architecture in its socio-cultural context, see Christine Stevenson, *Medicine and Magnificence: Hospital and Asylum Architecture 1660–1820* (New Haven and London: Yale University Press, 2000), 89–97, and Christine Stevenson, *The City and the King: Architecture and Politics in Restoration London* (New Haven and London: Yale University Press, 2013), ch. 8.

17. Howard Colvin, *A Biographical Dictionary of British Architects:1600–1840* (New Haven and London: Yale University Press, 2008), 221.
18. For gardens, see Marcus and Barnes, *Healing Gardens*, 236–7; for York Asylum, see Ann-Marie Akehurst, "Architecture and Philanthropy: Building Hospitals in Eighteenth-Century York" (Ph.D. diss., University of York, 2009), ch. 3.
19. For the Philadelphian hospital, see Robert Waln, Jnr., *An Account of the Asylum for the Insane Established by the Society of Friends Near Frankford, in the Vicinity of Philadelphia* (Philadelphia: Benjamin and Thomas Kite, 1825), 23. For the US listing of Frankford hospital, see https://npgallery.nps.gov/pdfhost/docs/NRHP/Text/99000629.pdf (accessed January 4, 2020).
20. Jones, *Lunacy*, 72–3.
21. Samuel Tuke, *Description of the Retreat: An Institution Near York, for Insane Persons of the Society of Friends* (York: W. Alexander, 1813), appendix, 221–7.
22. Ibid., Preface, ix–x.
23. D. B. Weiner, "Philippe Pinel's 'Memoir on Madness' of December 11, 1794: A Fundamental Text of Modern Psychiatry," *American Journal of Psychiatry* 149, no. 6 (June 1992): 725–32.
24. D. B. Weiner, "'Le Geste de Pinel': The History of a Psychiatric Myth," in Mark Micale and Roy Porter (eds.), *Discovering the History of Psychiatry* (Oxford: Oxford University Press, 1994), 232–47.
25. Tuke, *Description*, Preface, viii, ix.
26. For a detailed discussion of Quaker theology, see Ben Pink Dandelion, *An Introduction to Quakerism* (Cambridge: Cambridge University Press, 2007); also, Douglas Van Steere, ed., *Quaker Spirituality: Selected Writings* (London: SPCK, 1984), 46–54. My discussion of Quaker architecture and its relation to puritan theology and Neoplatonism will be published as "'Inward Light': Taking Architecture Seriously with the Early Religious Society of Friends," in *Places of Worship in Britain and Ireland, 1689–1840*, ed. Paul Barnwell and Mark Smith, Rewley House Studies in the Historic Environment (Donington: Shaun Tyas, forthcoming).
27. Ann-Marie Akehurst, "The York Retreat, 'a Vernacular of Equality,'" in *Built from Below: British Architecture and the Vernacular*, ed. Peter Guillery (London and New York: Routledge, 2010), 73–98, at 92–3.
28. Anne Digby, "Tuke, William (1732–1822), Philanthropist and Founder of the York Retreat," *Oxford Dictionary of National Biography* (September 23, 2004), accessed January 6, 2021. https://www-oxforddnb-com.sheffield.idm.oclc.org/view/10.1093/ref:odnb/9780198614128.001.0001/odnb-9780198614128-e-27810.
29. BIA RET, 2/2/1/1, Building of the Retreat, Correspondence, Letter 8, William Tuke to John Bevans Application to Bevans for a plan, n.d.
30. BIA RET 2/2/1/1, Building of the Retreat, Correspondence, Letter 17, William Proud to William Tuke, April 3, 1794.
31. Gesler, *Healing Places*, 11.
32. Stevenson, *Medicine*, 254, n. 55, and her "Carsten Anker Dines with the Younger George Dance, and Visits St Luke's Hospital for the Insane," *Architectural History* 44, *Essays in Architectural History, Presented to John Newman* (2001) 153–61, at 155, fig. 2.
33. BIA RET 2/2/1/1, Building of the Retreat, Correspondence, Letter 12, John Bevans to William Tuke, December 20, 1794. See also John Aikin, *A View of the Life, Travels, and Philanthropic Labors of the late John Howard, Esquire L.L.D. F.R.S.* (Philadelphia: John Ormrod, 1794), 39.
34. John Howard, *An account of the Principal Lazarettos in Europe; with various papers relative to the plague: Together with Further Observations on Some Foreign Prisons and Hospitals* (London: Johnson, Dilly and Cadell, 1791), 139–40.
35. John Aikin, *Hospitals, Thoughts on Hospitals* (London: Joseph Johnson, 1771), 71; Jeremy Bentham, *Panopticon: or, the Inspection-House* (Dublin: Thomas Byrne, 1791), 97.
36. BIA RET 2/1/1/1/(3 & 4), Ground Story Plan for the Proposed Retreat, 1794.
37. Thomas Wilkinson, cited in Jones, *Lunacy*, 60. For an account of Wilkinson, see https://www.bl.uk/eblj/1982articles/pdf/article9.pdf (accessed January 4, 2020).
38. Gesler, *Healing Places*, 11.

39. There is no doubt that time spent with Quaker leaders when they were formulating theology and praxis must have been influential, and there are common ideological links between Platonism and Quaker thought. Penn was a friend of Anne Conway, Viscountess Conway (née Finch) (1631–79), the Cambridge Platonist who converted to Quakerism at the end of her life. Robert Barclay spent much time with Quaker schismatic and Church of England clergyman, George Keith (c. 1638–1716), the first in the region to publish an apology for Quakerism, *Immediate Revelation* (1668). On traveling to London, Keith encountered William Penn, George Whitehead, and George Fox, and they developed a close working relationship for two decades. He was also part of the circle of Anne Conway at Ragley, and spent time there with Francis Mercury von Helmont, the German philosopher-mystic. Keith traveled with Fox, Penn, and Barclay to the Netherlands and Germany. In the early 1680s Keith was master of the Quaker school at Waltham Abbey. Keith (who was appointed Surveyor-General of the colony of East Jersey under the governorship of William Penn) eventually repudiated Quakerism in the 1690s, having argued with Philadelphia Quakers. David Brett argues for Quaker origins in the *devotio moderna* and the secretive Family of Love, connected with the highest levels of intellectual culture and poetical influence in the Elizabethan court in David Brett, *The Plain Style* (Cambridge: The Lutterworth Press, 2004), 133.
40. Fringes, valances, and curtains were condemned as "superfluous." Joseph Pike insisted on removing such fripperies and replacing them with "useful, plain woodwork," see *Life of Joseph Pike* cited in Frederick B. Tolles, "'of the Best Sort but Plain': The Quaker Esthetic," *American Quarterly* 11, no. 4 (Winter 1959): 484–502.
41. Brett hypothesizes the removal of images from public life after England's Dissolution had consequences for "the inner space of 'private' experience and habits of visualization," amounting to "a cognitive and affective revolution in which knowledge is redefined and identity put on a new basis," Brett, *The Plain Style*, 49, 70, 73.
42. Geoffrey Cantor, "The Bible, the Creation and Inward Light: Tensions within Quaker Science,," 3, accessed January 4, 2020. http://fundacionorotava.org/media/web/files/page147__10_ing_Cantor_QuakerScience.pdf. For Quaker-founder Margaret Fell's interpretive strategy, see Jane Donawerth, "Women's Reading Practices in Seventeenth-Century England: Margaret Fell's 'Women's Speaking Justified,'" *The Sixteenth Century Journal* 37, no. 4 (Winter 2006): 985–1005.
43. David M. Butler, *Quaker Meeting Houses of the Lake Counties*. (London: Friends Historical Society, 1978), iv.
44. Alvise Cornaro, *Discorsi della Vita Sobria*, trans. Robert Urie (Glasgow, 1770). Cornaro extols the benefits of living long and well with sober moderation. His discourses were widely republished in translation; Addison declared them written "with such a spirit of cheerfulness, religion and good sense, as are the natural concomitants of temperance and sobriety," see Joseph Addison, *The Spectator*, 195, October 13, 1711, accessed January 4, 2020. https://en.wikisource.org/wiki/Page:EB1911_-_Volume_07.djvu/180.
45. James S. Ackerman, *The Villa: Form and Ideology of Country Houses* (Thames & Hudson: London, 1990), 89–107.
46. Jones, *Lunacy*, 60. Translation by Alex Akehurst.
47. Robert Morris, *Rural Architecture: Consisting of Regular Designs of Plans and Elevations for Buildings in the Country* (London: printed for the author, 1750), pl. 33; Susanna Wade Martins, *The English Model Farm: Building the Agricultural Ideal, 1700–1914* (Macclesfield: Windgather Press, 2002), fig. 31. The contemporary farmhouse Ellenthorpe Hall was designed by John Carr, Atkinson's partner, for himself, see Brian Wragg and Giles Worsley, *The Life and Works of John Carr* (York: Oblong Press, 2000), 140, fig. 137.
48. For the London Hospital plan, see Stevenson, *Medicine*, 145, pl. 58. For meetinghouse kitchens, see Hubert Lidbetter, *The Friends Meetinghouse* (York: William Sessions, 1979), 65, figs. 15, 16, 17, and 18.
49. Tuke, *Description*, 222–3, translated by Tuke from the French.
50. BIA RET 2/2/1/1, Building of the Retreat, Correspondence, Letter 16, John Bevans to William Tuke, February 26, 1795.
51. For the etymology of hospital cells and their relation to biological cells, see Stevenson, *Medicine*, 54–60.
52. Howard, *Prisons and Lazarettos*, 64.
53. Bentham, *Panopticon*, 96–8.
54. Gesler argues: "many if not most, societies around the world believed that nature has healing powers … Many people feel they contain physical, mental and spiritual healing simply by spending time out of doors or seeking remote or isolated places where they can get away from it all, surrounded by undisturbed nature." Gesler, *Healing Places*, 8.
55. Ibid., 9.
56. BIA RET 1/1/1/1, Retreat Directors' Minute Book 1792–1841, fol. 1r; BIA RET 2/2/1/1, Building of the Retreat, Document 10, Minutes of Committee Meeting, n.d.

57. BIA RET 1/1/1/1, Retreat Directors' Minute Book 1792–1841, fol. 16r. There were more than 1,500 trees and shrubs in addition to acres of hedging materials. Planting had taken place by April 4, 1794.
58. BIA RET 2/1/2/1.
59. Arthur Raistrick, *Quakers in Science and Industry* (York: Sessions, 1993; 1st ed. 1950), 243–77.
60. For a discussion of seventeenth-century puritan circuitous journeys and their influence upon late eighteenth-century radical thought, see M. H. Abrams, *Natural Supernaturalism: Tradition and Revolution in Romantic Literature* (New York and London: W. W. Norton, 1973).
61. BIA RET 1/1/1/1, Retreat Directors' Minute Book 1792–1841, fol. 7r. William Penn, *Some Fruits of Solitude, in Reflections and Maxims Relating to the Conduct of Human Life* (London, 1702), 73–4.
62. Donald Brooks Kelley, "'A Tender Regard to the Whole Creation': Anthony Benezet and the Emergence of an Eighteenth-Century Quaker Ecology," *The Pennsylvania Magazine of History and Biography* 106, no. 1 (1982): 69–88; Geoffrey Cantor, "Aesthetics in Science, as Practiced by Quakers in the Eighteenth and Nineteenth Centuries," *Quaker Studies* 4 (1999): 1–20.
63. Robert Castell, *Villas of the Ancients Illustrated* (London, 1728).
64. Vergil, *Georgics*, II, 459–69, accessed October 23, 2018. http://sabidius.com/index.php/prolegomenon/item/1326-virgil-georgics-book-ii.
65. Marcus and Barnes, *Healing Gardens*, 238; Robert J. G. Savage, "Natural History of the Goldney Garden Grotto, Clifton, Bristol," *Garden History* 17, no. 1 (Spring 1989): 1–40, at 2–3.
66. Abrams, *Natural Supernaturalism*, 51.
67. William Wordsworth, Preface to Poems 1815, Paragraph 29, accessed October 23, 2018. https://en.wikisource.org/wiki/Poems_(Wordsworth,_1815)/Volume_1#vii.
68. Abrams, *Natural Supernaturalism*, 151.
69. Anne McWhir, "Scott, John (1730–1783), Poet and Writer," *Oxford Dictionary of National Biography* (September 23, 2004), accessed January 6, 2021. https://www-oxforddnb-com.sheffield.idm.oclc.org/view/10.1093/ref:odnb/9780198614128.001.0001/odnb-9780198614128-e-24891.
70. John Scott, "Epistle I, The Garden: To a Friend," *Poetical Works* (London: J. Buckland, 1782), 262–5.
71. Botany was part of the curriculum at Ackworth Quaker School. Apothecary Joseph Gurney Bevan viewed "earthly things" as a "source of religious inspiration enabling the Inward Light to see beyond the creation and gain a flickering sense of its Creator," see Cantor, "Bible," 14.
72. Gesler, *Healing Places*, 14–15.
73. George Fox, *To the Parliament of the Common-wealth of England* (London: Simmons, 1659), 5–9.
74. Dandelion, *Quakerism*, 66–7.
75. Ibid., 59. For an account of Commonwealth Quakers' political stance, see Christopher Hill, *The World Turned Upside Down: Radical Ideas During the English Revolution* (London: Penguin, 1991), 234.
76. See n. 62 above.
77. Dana Arnold, *The Spaces of the Hospital: Spatiality and Urban Change in London 1680–1820* (London: Routledge, 2013), 58.
78. Gesler, *Healing Places*, 15.
79. BIA RET 1/1/1/1/p. 1. The foundation instrument expressly excluded "idiots," i.e., those suffering congenital mental impairments.
80. BIA RET 1/2/7/2, Plan of the Retreat and Estate by patient ESK, 1841; Peter Atkinson's 1812 *View* as copied by Retreat patient H. Bass in 1831.
81. Gesler, *Healing Places*, 15.
82. BIA RET 1/1/1/1, Retreat Directors' Minute Book 1792–1841, fol. 4r. For a discussion of the relation between language, place, and health, see Robin A. Kearns and W. M. Gesler, *Culture/Place/Health* (London: Routledge, 2001), 86–90. Phenomenologists stress the effects of the home as a key to individual well-being, see Gaston Bachelard, *The Poetics of Space*, trans. Maria Jolas (Boston: Beacon Press, 1964), ch. 1; and Juhanni Pallasmaa, *The Embodied Image: Imagination and Imagery in Architecture* (Chichester: John Wiley & Sons, 2011), 125.
83. Gesler, *Healing Places*, 13.
84. Ibid., 14.
85. BIA RET 1/1/1/1, Retreat Directors' Minute Book 1792–1841.
86. Tuke, *Description*, 221–7, appendix.
87. BIA RET 1/4/1/1, Visitors' Report Book 1815–67.

88. Anne Digby, "Changes in the Asylum: The Case of York, 1777–1815," *Economic History Review* 36, no. 2 (May 1983): 218–39, at 225.
89. Sydney Smith cited in Daniel Hack Tuke, "The Early History of the Retreat York," *Journal of Mental Science*, n.s. 38, no. 125 (July 1892): 352.
90. Eduardo Mendieta and Jonathan Vanantwerpen, eds., *The Power of Religion in the Public Sphere* (New York: Columbia University Press, 2011), 34–59. His discussants were Judith Butler, Cornel West, and Jürgen Habermas.
91. For "the care of those with whom they are connected in Religious Society": BIA RET 1/1/1/1/p. 1. The foundation instrument expressly excluded "idiots," i.e., those suffering congenital mental impairments. Friends across England financially supported their co-religionists. Opinions were invited regarding the design as shown in correspondence and modified drawings.
92. J. Rendel Harris, "The Attitudes of the Society of Friends towards Modern Thought," in *Report of the Proceedings of the Conference of Members of the Society of Friends, Held, by Direction of the Yearly Meeting, in Manchester from Eleventh to the Fifteenth of Eleventh Month, 1895* (London: Headley Brothers, 1896), 219, cited in Cantor, "Bible," 17.

PART II
POLITY: PUBLIC HEALTH AND POLITICS

CHAPTER 6
DAR AL-SHIFA' OR *BIMARISTAN*? ISLAMIC HOSPITALS OF DAMASCUS, SIVAS, AND CAIRO IN THE TWELFTH AND THIRTEENTH CENTURIES
Richard Piran McClary

The concept of alms giving or charity (*sadaqa*) was a fundamental component of religious belief and ethics in the medieval Islamic world.[1] In 1184 the Andalusian geographer and traveler Ibn Jubayr (1145–1217) wrote that hospitals were among the highest glories of Islam.[2] Founded in large numbers in urban centers across the medieval Islamic world, they provided free care to all Muslims, regardless of background or social status. Hospitals are known to have been built across the Islamic world since at least the eighth century, but it was during the twelfth and thirteenth centuries that some of the largest and best-documented structures were built, including the earliest surviving structures. The Islamic approach to health and healing grew out of the late antiquity traditions of medicine: the translation of key works by important classical scholars such as Galen formed the foundation of medical advances that took place in the medieval period.[3]

The combination of piety and politics resulted, among other things, in the construction of hospitals across the wider region, with the idea of a hospital emerging as an essential element of urban development during the tenth to eleventh centuries. However, while this royal custom of building and endowing hospitals was common in the Islamic world, it can be viewed as a regional[4] as much as an Islamic practice, with Christian Armenian kings, including Thoros I (r. 1100–29) and Leo II (r. 1198–1219) endowing such buildings in Sis.[5] One of the earliest attested hospitals in the Islamic world was built in al-Qatta'i', now part of Cairo, by Ibn Tulun, the Abbasid governor of Egypt, between 872 and 875, according to the fifteenth-century Egyptian historian al-Maqrizi (d. c. 1442).[6] The first hospital built in the new Abbasid capital of Baghdad was founded by al-Mansur in Karkh, southwest of the walled city, and it went on to become the cradle of the Baghdad school of medicine.[7] However, the most famous hospital was the one built in Baghdad for the Buyid Sultan 'Adud al-Dawla in 982.[8] All these structures are now lost, but a number of textual sources provide details on their location, staffing, and functions over time. Although evidence of specific structures is sparse, the building of hospitals was quite common. In a text from 1160, for example, the Jewish traveler Benjamin of Tuleda wrote that there were sixty medical institutions in Baghdad alone.[9]

The aim here is to give as clear a sense as is possible, with the limited surviving evidence, of both the form and the function of medieval Islamic hospitals. It will be shown, through the direct evidence of one of the three case studies, that the layout of hospitals is closely related to earlier palatial residential architecture, with extensive use of courtyards, fountains, and pools.[10] The surviving evidence is also used to show that these buildings were responding to specific needs within society, and reflect the increase in medical knowledge and understanding.

This chapter begins with an overview of the terminology and some of the textual sources that describe early, but now lost, Islamic hospitals.[11] Following this are three main case studies that demonstrate the particulars of individual monuments, examine the possible motivations of their patrons, and illustrate the range of approaches to the same basic typology from the middle of the twelfth century to the end of the thirteenth century. The first hospital to be studied, built for the Zangid ruler Nur al-Din in Damascus in 1154, laid the foundation for what was to come after, while the second, built for the Rum Seljuq sultan 'Izz al-Din Kay Kawus I in Sivas in 1217–18, is by far the largest surviving hospital in Anatolia, and one of the only extant structures with a surviving *waqf*[12] document.[13] The third case study, the al-Mansur Hospital, built for the Mamluk sultan al-Mansur Qalawun in Cairo as part of a larger complex in 1284, can be seen as the final flowering of the medieval Islamic hospital. Each of the buildings studied here exemplifies the type of hospital that elite patrons across the medieval Islamic world built from at least the tenth century onwards.

The Issue of Terminology

The first issue to clarify is that of terminology. An array of different terms is found both in the inscriptions on the buildings and the, albeit limited, surviving *waqf* (pl. *awqaf*) endowment documents, and other primary written sources, such as histories and travelers' accounts. The Persian term *bimaristan* is commonly used in the Islamic world as a general term for hospital. Although the term has been translated as meaning "a place for sick people,"[14] it can more accurately be translated as "place of health," with the antonym *maristan* being "place of illness," and it was the latter which was used to describe the hospital of Qalawun in Cairo.[15] The same term is seen at the end of the first line on a marble inscription panel on the portal of the hospital founded in Kayseri by Gevher Nesibe in 602/1205–6.[16] In addition, in Iraq the Persian term *khastakhana* (infirmary) was sometimes used.[17]

The word *bimaristan* occurs in a rare surviving *waqf* document of a lost Qarakhanid hospital in Samarkand dated 1065–6.[18] However, the same text also uses a more specific Arabic definition of the hospital, founded by the Qarakhanid ruler Ibrahim ibn Nasr: *dar li-'l-marda* (a house to serve the sick). The intermingling of Arabic and Persian, as well as the use of Arabic in predominantly non-Arabic speaking regions, can be seen in Anatolia in the thirteenth century, with the Sivas hospital of 'Izz al-Din Kay Kawus I in Sivas being referred to as *dar al-sihha* (house of health) in the inscription band over the doorway of the main entrance portal, while another nearby hospital in Divriği is referred to as *dar al-shifa'* (house of healing/cure).[19] In addition, the Ilkhanid *waqfiyya* of the charitable foundation of Rashid al-Din Tabib in Tabriz does not use the word *bimaristan*, but instead uses the phrases *darukhana* and *bayt al-adwiya*, both of which mean "house of medicines."[20]

Function and Facilities

The primary role of hospitals was to provide a place for rest and recuperation, with the drugs and food served being part of a single continuum.[21] The importance of food to the treatment of the sick cannot be underestimated in the context of Islamic medicine in the medieval period, which was based on the Galenic theory of the humors, which had been passed down from the Greeks.[22] The eleventh-century *waqf* document of a Qarakhanid hospital in Samarkand clearly states that it had to combine both curing and caring, and outlines the staff to be paid for from the endowment income. It provides for one physician, one expert on bloodletting, cooks, and a servant (*khadim*)[23]—much smaller in scale compared to the number of staff at major hospitals like the one founded by Qalawun in Cairo, discussed below. The surviving structures, as well as the information provided in the various *waqf* documents, show that alongside the open iwans,[24] which could have been used for a wide array of services, there were also functionally specific spaces in medieval Islamic hospitals, such as hammams, latrines, kitchens, and separate areas for treating and confining the mentally ill.

The famous doctor and former chief physician of Egypt, Ibn al-Nafis (d. 1288), donated both his library and his house to the hospital founded in Cairo by the Mamluk sultan al-Mansur Qalawun, further augmenting the collection of books available to the medical staff in that institution.[25] In addition to the hospitals themselves, many libraries had dedicated sections on medicine, with lists of all the manuscripts in the section to make searching easier. The Ashrafiya Library in Damascus had a classification system in its thirteenth-century inventory[26] that grouped together manuscripts on pharmacology, medicine, and veterinary medicine.[27]

Sources commonly use the terms *tabib* and *hakim* to refer to the clinical staff of hospitals, and although they are generally translated as "medical doctor" or "physician," in some cases they should perhaps be understood more as pharmacists, as in many cases their primary role consisted of preparing drugs.[28] However, sometimes more specific terms are used, including *al-aṭibbaʾ* and *al-tabaʾiyah* (physicians), *al-kahhalin* (ophthalmologists) and *al-jaraʾihiyah* (surgeons),[29] which suggests that the larger and more advanced institutions had a far greater degree of medical specialization than the hospitals of smaller towns and cities.

The al-Nuri Hospital, Damascus (1184)

As the construction of hospitals became a potent symbol of power for rulers by the twelfth century, the Zangid ruler Nur al-Din Mahmud founded his first hospital in Aleppo. While little survives of that structure, his later hospital project in Damascus is far better preserved. When the traveler ibn Jubayr visited the city in Rabiʾ II 580 (July–August 1184), he noted the existence of two hospitals: the al-Nuri, with a daily revenue of fifteen gold dinars, and, near the Great Mosque, an older one, which may have been founded by the Umayyad Caliph al-Walid in 706–7.[30] Damascus was Nur al-Din's capital from 1154–74, and the hospital was the first building he had erected in the city.[31] It is located in the quarter of Hajar al-Dhahab, southwest of the citadel. The lower portions of the building are constructed using large ashlars, most likely salvaged from an antique monument, while the upper sections consist of smaller ashlars cut specifically for the hospital.[32] Based on an inscription during his reign, the Mamluk sultan al-Mansur Qalawun (d. 1290) is thought to have repaired and embellished the al-Nuri Hospital in 1283[33] with the addition of a fountain to the right of the entrance to the hospital,[34] as well as the marble revetments and mihrab in the southern iwan.

The four-iwan plan of the hospital consists of three iwans of equal height and width to the north, south, and west, and a far larger eastern iwan, featuring the foundation inscription, opposite the entrance. This has two large niches in the back that were used for the storage of the numerous medical volumes provided by Nur al-Din, according to the thirteenth-century physician and historian of medicine Ibn Abi Usaybiʿah (d. 1290).[35] In addition to the four iwans, there are four large rooms in the corners of the courtyard with cross vaults and two small rooms on either side of the north and south iwans (Figure 6.1).[36] Unlike the two later hospitals discussed below, the original *waqfiyya* for the al-Nuri did not survive and as a result the specific functional role of each individual space within the building is largely unclear. However, the stepped pool in the center of the courtyard with circular niches in each corner is likely to have served a therapeutic function, as a person could have been seated in the water with ease. The introduction of pools of this type was to become a signature element of subsequent hospitals across the region. The only other space within the complex for which a specific purpose is clearly stated is the large east iwan, opposite the entrance on the other side of the courtyard.

The content of the Qurʾanic inscriptions on the dado of the east iwan, which make reference to remedies and cures, has been interpreted as evidence that it was a consulting room for the physicians,[37] but there is more compelling evidence showing that it was actually the library and lecture hall of the hospital, where groups of doctors would engage in medical discussions, according to Ibn Abi Usaybiʿah.[38]

Health and Architecture

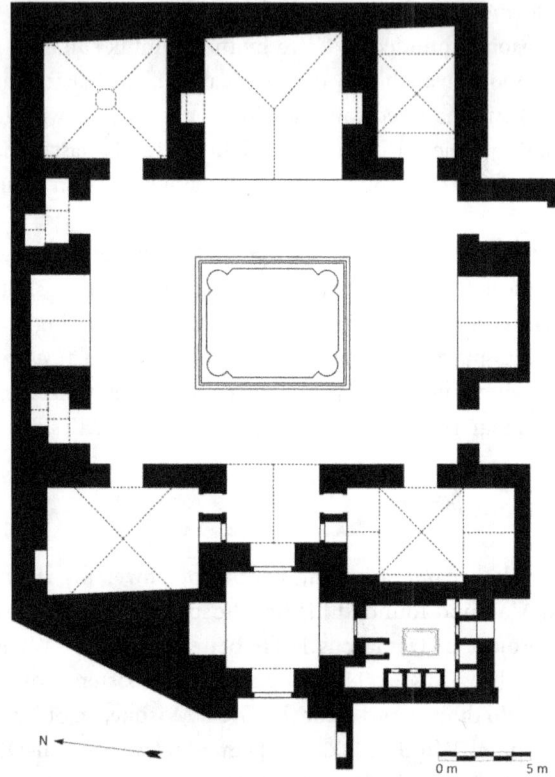

Figure 6.1 Plan of the al-Nuri Hospital, Damascus. Image: Richard Piran McClary

The shallow muqarnas over the entrance to the hospital makes it one of the earliest known portals of its type anywhere in the Islamic world, and although it is in stucco and attached to the masonry by way of wooden dowels, it acted as a prototype for the stone examples built later in the twelfth century in Aleppo and across Anatolia.[39] The entire composition was intended to be framed by a geometric strapwork pattern, but only a small section, at the upper left, appears to have been executed. Built by the Damascene engineer Abu-l-Fadl Muhammad al-Harithi, the brass-sheathed and -studded door is original. Its design is based on a triangular grid, with the primary unit being a six-pointed star inscribed within a hexagon.[40] The pediment over the doorway (Figure 6.2), in combination with the shallow muqarnas hood and the studded, brass-covered doors, has been argued to be one of the most successful examples of spolia in medieval Islamic architecture.[41] This combination of what was a relatively new form of decoration above the entrance with an ancient pediment on the main entrance to the building may be seen as a physical manifestation of the type of medicine practiced within, combining as it did the latest practices with the ancient Galenic theories of medicine. In later hospitals, more overtly apotropaic symbols, such as snakes and lions, were applied to the portals, but these are totally absent from the Damascus hospital of Nur al-Din. Despite this absence, the existence of at least two magic-medicinal bowls made for Nur al-Din in the late twelfth century is indicative of the combination of beliefs in Greek-based humoral theory and in the magical and occult properties of substances (*khawass*) popular in the wider society at the time the hospital was built.[42]

There is a large muqarnas dome over the vestibule next to the entrance portal, which is thought to be the second earliest in the region.[43] In the room to the right of the vestibule was an area with a series of cells and a

Dar al-shifa' or Bimaristan?

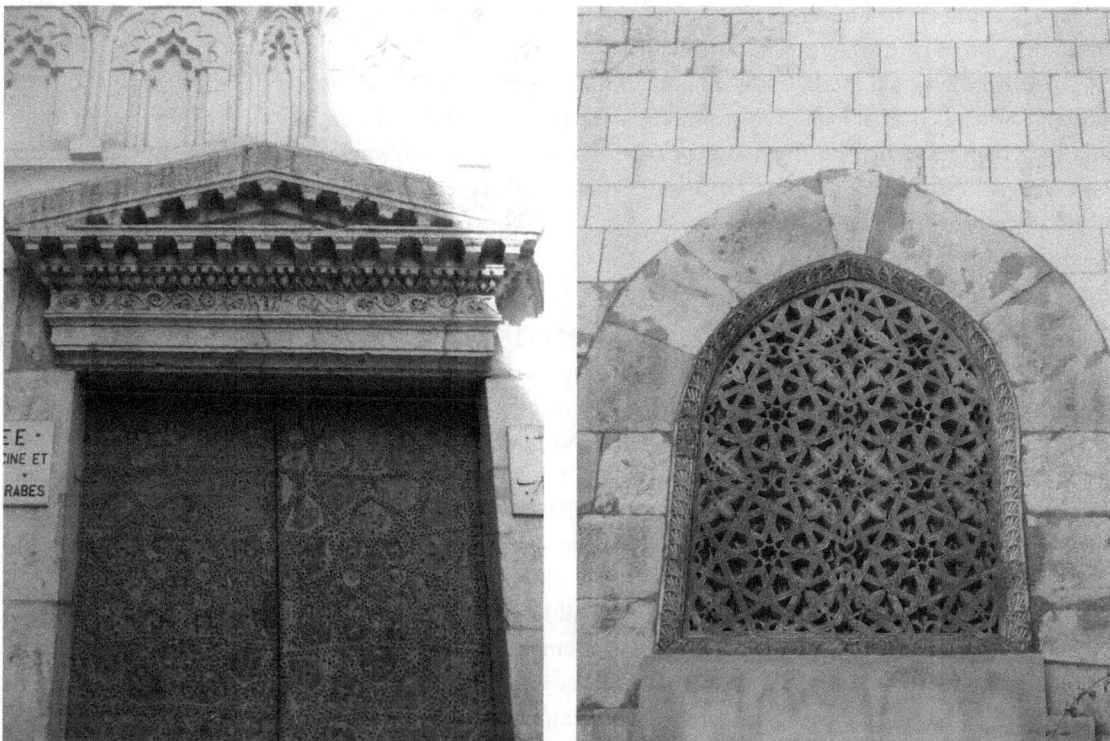

Figure 6.2 Decorative elements of the al-Nuri Hospital, Damascus. Image: Richard Piran McClary

central pool, but it appears to have been destroyed in the 1970s, possibly during the restoration of the complex and its conversion into a medical museum. The central pool was similar to the one in the main courtyard, but considerably smaller, and there were a series of chambers on three sides (see Figure 6.1). It has been argued that these chambers were the latrines for the hospital, and originally had another entrance to the south, which either faced the street or another lost courtyard.[44] However, Ibn Abi Usaybi'ah mentions the *qa'ah* (hall) of the *mamrurin* (fools) in the al-Nuri Hospital and notes that opium in barley water was successfully used to treat one of the patients.[45] Given the similarities in the plans of the area referred to as the latrines in Damascus and the two larger sections known to have been used for the treatment and confinement of the insane at the later al-Mansur Hospital in Cairo, it is quite likely that the lost section to the right of the atrium in Damascus was the area reserved for the insane in the al-Nuri Hospital.[46]

Aside from the doors, muqarnas hood, and muqarnas dome, the building in its original state appears to have been fairly plain and devoid of ornament. Apart from the *nashki* inscriptions in the east iwan, the only other major decorative elements datable to the initial phase of construction, rather than the later Mamluk additions of the late thirteenth century, are the two stucco window screens in the southwest corner of the courtyard, one of which is shown in Figure 6.2. The main compositional unit of the stucco screens is an eight-pointed star inscribed within a circle of arabesque scrolls, and it is framed with a pattern reminiscent of an acanthus leaf. The marble screens in the Umayyad great mosque have similar patterns, but without the vegetal elements. However, in both the hospital and the mosque the surface of the geometric bands features double line incisions, suggesting that the design of the stucco screens was directly inspired by the earlier marble ones.[47] As with the antique pediment on the portal, this appears to be a conscious attempt to connect the building with the prestigious architectural heritage of the city and place it within the continuum of royal Damascene patronage.

The al-Nuri Hospital marks the beginning of the adoption of the four-iwan plan for hospitals and is the earliest surviving co-axial four-iwan-planned Islamic building outside of Iran, as well as being the first stone-built four-iwan building, and the first hospital to use such a plan anywhere in the Islamic world.[48] Thus, it marks a watershed moment in the history of Syrian architecture,[49] and significantly influenced the layout of subsequent medical establishments across a far wider region, including the ones in both Sivas and Cairo, discussed below.

The 'Izz al-Din Kay Kawus I Hospital, Sivas (1217–18)

There are known to have been at least twenty-five hospitals built across the Rum Seljuq Empire,[50] but only four survive, in Kayseri, Amasya, Divriği, and Sivas. Sitting at the crossroads where the north-to-south trade in timber and slaves from the Black Sea coast to Egypt met the east-to-west trade from Iran to the Byzantine Empire and beyond, Sivas was the commercial capital of the Rum Seljuq Empire and the site of several important foundations built throughout the thirteenth century, the largest of which was the hospital and tomb complex.[51]

Like the Damascus hospital of Nur al-Din, the building founded in Sivas by 'Izz al-Din Kay Kawus I was built a short distance from the citadel, and is not far from the existing Great Mosque in the city, constructed by the Danişmendids in the late twelfth century.[52] Smaller in scale but similar in conception to the later Cairene foundation of Qalawun, the Sivas complex is an example of a new stage in the development of Sultanic patronage of hospitals in the Islamic world, as it included a tomb for the patron and a medical madrasa, as well as the hospital (Figure 6.3). It follows the basic overall form of the Çifte Madrasa in Kayseri, the earliest known hospital in Anatolia, which was built just a few years earlier in 1205–6 at the behest of Gevher Nesibe, the daughter of the Rum Seljuq sultan Kılıç Arslan II.[53]

In terms of proportion, the arrangement of the four iwans in the Sivas hospital clearly draws on the plan used for the hospital of Nur al-Din in Damascus, with a small entrance iwan opposite a larger east iwan, and smaller iwans on the north and south sides of the courtyard. In both cases the southern iwan became a place of devotion, featuring a mihrab, although in the case of the Sivas structure it had a specifically funerary role, as it was the tomb of the patron. The larger scale of the Sivas complex, as well as the addition of a *riwaq*, makes for a far more imposing structure, with many more rooms arranged around the courtyard. It also involved a far wider range of building materials, with a predominantly lithic exterior, but with extensive use of brick for the upper structure and the north iwan arch inside, as well as numerous examples of glazed tile inscriptions and decoration around the courtyard and in the north iwan (Figure 6.4).

The building as it currently stands only consists of the tomb and the hospital, with the madrasa, which may have formed almost half of the original structure, having been lost prior to the nineteenth century.[54] It has an even more imposing portal (Figure 6.5), which has a true sterotomic stone muqarnas hood, rather than the shallow stucco variant seen in Damascus, as well as a far more sophisticated series of framing bands of geometric ornament and a greater degree of articulation.[55]

The spandrels of the arch around the muqarnas hood feature fragmentary remains of zoomorphic sculpture. Although damaged, they appear to be a pair of affronted lions. Lion sculptures can be found on earlier Rum Seljuq portals, including a fragmentary single lion on the west portal of the hospital of Gevher Nesibe in Kayseri. The right-hand sculpture on the Sivas portal is more intact, but has less surviving surface decoration than the one on the left, although there are incised lines on the rump that appear to indicate fur. The outer rear

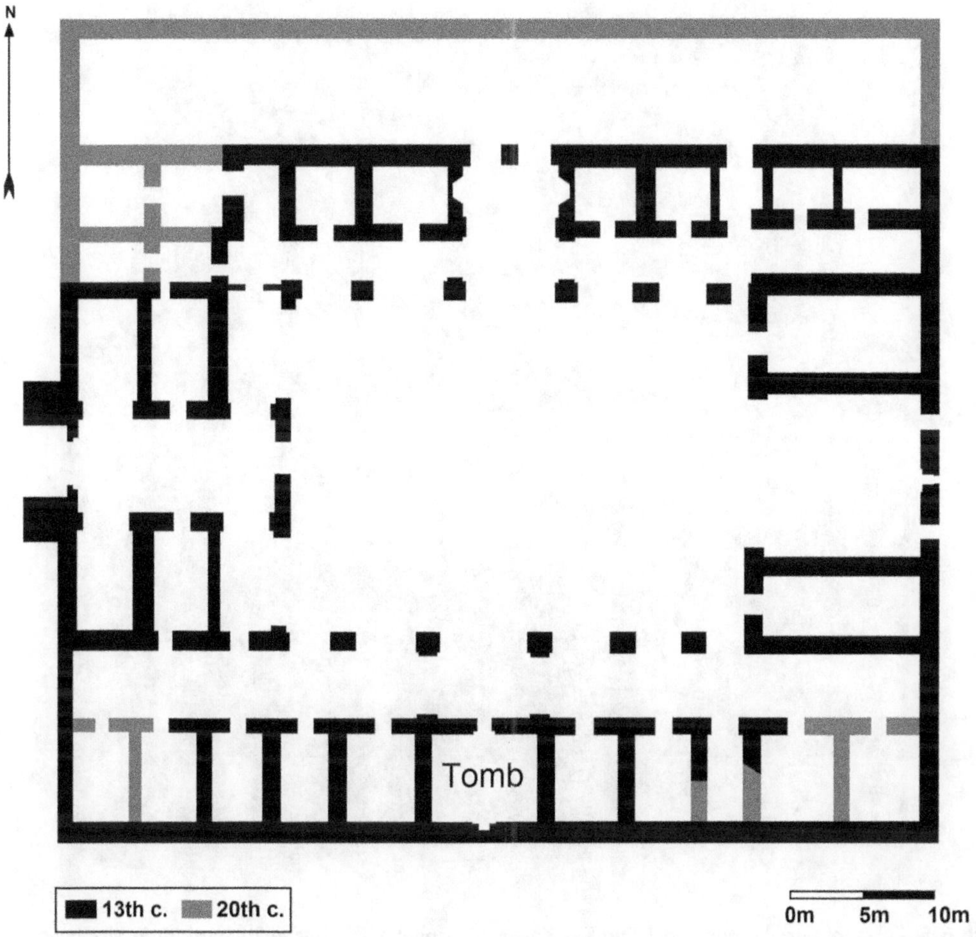

*Dar al-shifa*ʾ or *Bimaristan*?

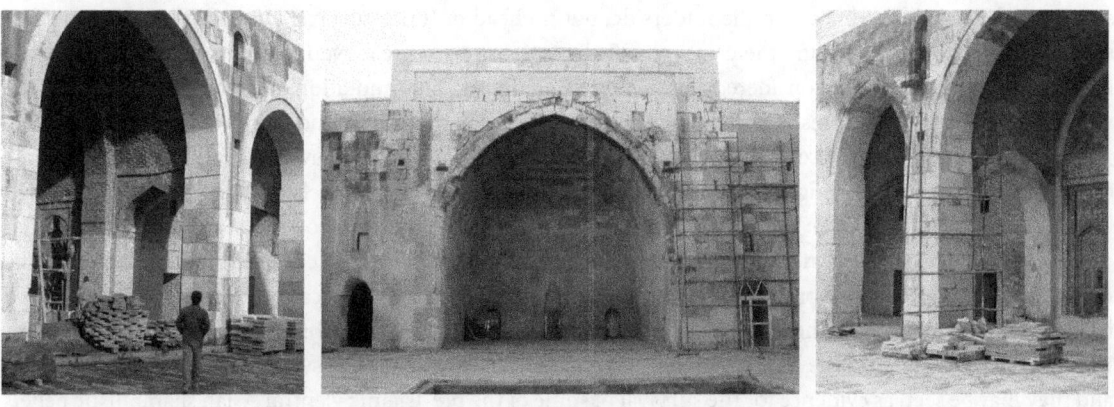

Figure 6.3 Ground plan of the ʿIzz al-Din Kay Kawus I Hospital, Sivas. Image: Richard Piran McClary

Figure 6.4 North, east, and south iwans of the ʿIzz al-Din Kay Kawus I Hospital, Sivas. Image: Richard Piran McClary

105

Health and Architecture

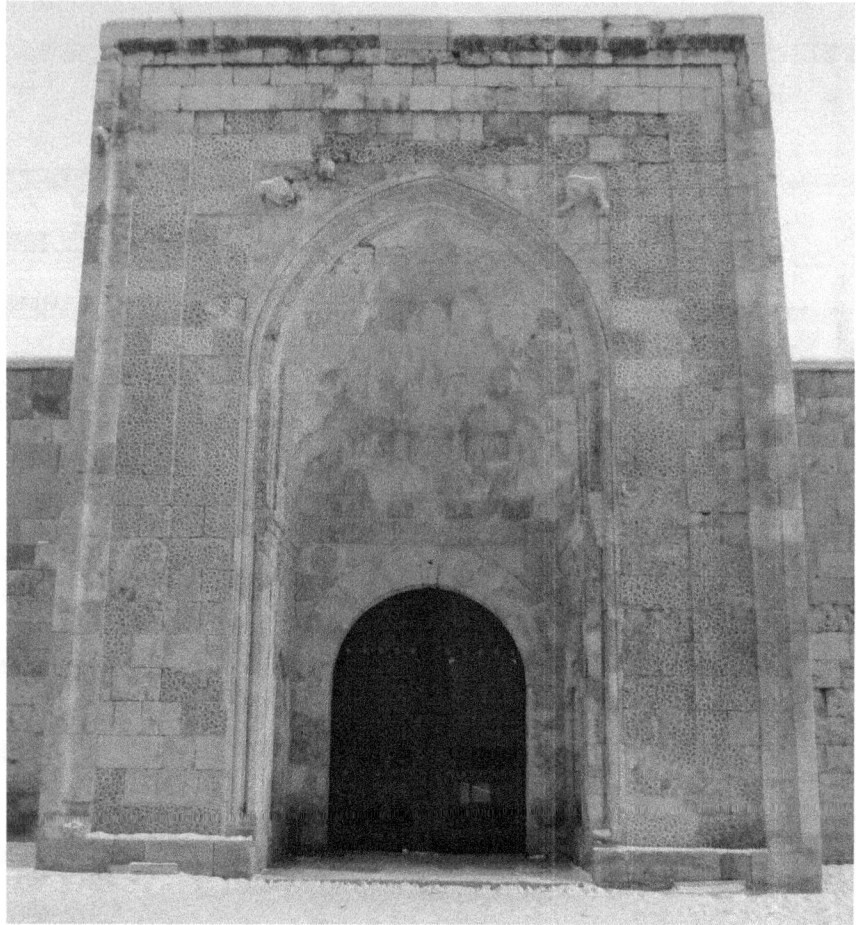

Figure 6.5 Entrance portal of the 'Izz al-Din Kay Kawus I Hospital, Sivas. Image: Richard Piran McClary

leg is missing to reveal a surprisingly pronounced phallus, possibly a symbol of virility that would most likely have been hidden by a leg in its original state. The left-hand sculpture has textile-like decoration on the upper section and lines indicating fur on the underside, but no head or limbs survive. On the upper section there are remains of something riding the creature, but the losses are too great even to speculate as to its original form. The lion has long been considered a protective animal, and the connotation of power associated with the animal helps to explain its presence on the entrance to a hospital that was founded by a sultan.

The courtyard has a large central pool and the large eastern iwan, while heavily restored, features the only other surviving examples of figural sculpture in the complex with two roundels on the spandrels. Although both are damaged, it is clear from the inscriptions and the ray-like form of the surrounding triangular decoration that the north roundel represents the sun, while the south one is a crescent moon. The face in the moon has plaited hair in two braids in the Central Asian manner, and in both cases the heads are surrounded by fragmentary remains of the *shahada* in cursive epigraphy. This integration of what appears to be pre-Islamic solar imagery with the Islamic profession of faith is an example of the syncretic nature of the dynasty, and they may be seen as evidence for the survival of some of the pre-Islamic Central Asian shamanistic beliefs of the Türkmen being blended with Islam.

Like the earlier Damascus hospital, the specific functional role of many of the individual spaces in the complex remains unclear, but the *waqfiyya* does shine some light on the subject. It is worth noting that the *waqfiyya* terms refer to the ideal desires of the patron rather than the actual reality,[56] but they still remain the best source available. The small rooms on either side of the courtyard were intended to be rooms for patients, while the east iwan was a classroom and the large rooms on either side of it were for performing surgery. In addition, the rooms off the entrance corridor were for the treatment of outpatients on one side and the pharmacy (*darukhana*) on the other.[57] The document also makes reference to a cellar for the storage of grain supplies, but no such space has yet come to light during the various excavations and restorations of the site.[58]

Although the earlier Gevher Nesibe Hospital in Kayseri had a hypocaust heating system under the floor of the *hammam*, the Sivas hospital did not have any structurally integrated heating systems, despite the harsh winters experienced in central Anatolia.[59] It must be presumed that, apart from any solar heat gain, the winter heating would have consisted of braziers in individual rooms. Alongside heating, there was a need for hydraulic services for washing patients and filling the large central pool as there was no well on site.[60] It was only during the later Ottoman period that the majority of hospitals had their own well and that most rooms were fitted with a built-in fireplace and chimney. The Ottoman hospital at the Beyazit II complex (1484) in Edirne has a very different plan, with rooms around two courtyards and a large hexagonal structure as the focus of the building. Each room within the building features a fireplace and chimney, allowing for far more effective heating.[61]

The complex, located in the very populous commercial capital of the Rum Seljuq Empire, is the largest foundation dating from the reign of 'Izz al-Din Kay Kawus I, and speaks to the prestige and importance associated with the founding of a hospital. The additional act of including his tomb in the south iwan of the complex, aimed as it was at the poorest and most unwell members of society, adds to the sense of both piety and charity that the patron wished to project. This intention to project piety and humility is supported by the text of one of the glazed Persian inscription plaques on the north side of the courtyard, which refers to the sins of the patron.[62] Although the Sivas complex was based on the plan of the al-Nuri Hospital in Damascus, it was far greater in terms of both scale and ambition. The integration of a royal tomb and a madrasa set the tone for the far larger foundation in Cairo near the end of the century.

The al-Mansur Hospital, Cairo (1284)

Following his treatment for dysentery in the al-Nuri Hospital in Damascus, the Mamluk sultan al-Mansur Qalawun is thought to have been inspired by the social and charitable role of that foundation, and decided to follow the example of Nur al-Din by building a major hospital in Cairo.[63] Prior to the foundation of a hospital in Cairo, he established a small hospital in Hebron in 1281.[64] It was not just the function but also the aesthetic of the al-Nuri Hospital that appealed to him, and it has been claimed that Damascene craftsmen were brought to Cairo to decorate the hospital-tomb-madrasa complex of Qalawun.[65] He bought the site in Bayn al-Qasrayn, in the heart of what had been the Fatimid palace area, in 1283 and construction began the following year, with the whole complex being completed in 1285.[66] The hospital was the first part to be built, with construction taking less than six months.[67] It was intended as the finest medical facility in the Islamic world.[68] There was initially some controversy concerning the speed with which the former residents of the site were removed, as well as the issuance of *fatwas* against praying in the complex due to the use of forced labor by the supervisor of works, 'Alam al-Din Sanjar al-Shuja'i.[69]

The surviving *waqf* document states that the hospital had a capacity of eight hundred beds. The ordinary diet for patients consisted of chicken and mutton in soup and they were to be given food in covered vessels intended for their private use. Such practices, alongside the extensive use of water throughout the complex, demonstrate a clear awareness of the importance of hygiene on the part of the medical staff.[70] An account by the first supervisor of the al-Mansur Hospital, Shihab al-Din al-Nuwayri, shines some light on the specific sources of revenue for the complex, the great majority of which went to the hospital, and which included markets, hotels, shops, bathhouses, trade monopolies, and property in the Levant.[71]

The section of the hospital reserved for the treatment of the mentally ill was one of the few functionally specific areas, and featured cells for the confinement of the most severe cases. The patients were on occasion restrained using iron chains, and a wide array of treatments were employed.[72] The sixteenth-century Ottoman traveler Evliya Çelebi reports that the attendants to the physicians in the hospital would beat the inmates with cherry switches.[73] Throughout the medieval period the treatment of individuals confined to the *maristan* was frequently harsh, and declaring people to be suffering from madness (*junun*) was a tool frequently manipulated by the state to detain people that were seen as a threat to social order.[74]

Although the *waqf* is invaluable for gaining an understanding of the function and funding of the hospital, it does not give a detailed description of the building. The hospital was built on the site of the Fatimid palace of Sayyidat al-Mulk, and the person in charge of the construction, emir 'Alam al-Din al-Shuja'i, appears to have maintained the layout of the palace, with its four iwans and fountains.[75] This is the same pattern as the earlier Tulunid hospital, which was also a converted palace.[76] Such use of the basic layout of an elite home for hospitals makes sense in light of the fact that the primary place of treatment of the sick in the Islamic world until recently was the home, with hospitals primarily serving the poor who, for whatever reason, could not be cared for by their families at home.[77] The tomb and madrasa survive, but the hospital was demolished in 1910, and all that remains are some fragments of carved stucco, wall recesses, two marble basins, and some Fatimid-era wooden beams.[78] Despite such extensive losses, Evliya Çelebi's description of the hospital in the sixteenth century and the plan drawn by the French architect Pascal Coste (1787–1879) in the early nineteenth century, shown in Figure 6.6, allow for a good understanding of the general layout of the building. There is also a drawing of the interior of the courtyard by Coste, that is now in the Bibliothèques de Marseilles (Figure 6.7).[79]

Despite its reported grandeur, the hospital was not visible from the street, but instead accessed via a passageway running between the tomb and madrasa, both of which had a street front facade. The aesthetic of this entrance (Figure 6.8) draws heavily on the style developed in Aleppo and Konya earlier in the thirteenth century, and demonstrates that it was not just the plan that drew on earlier structures from across the region, but aspects of the decoration as well. The passageway ended with a T shape, and if one turned left along the outside of the western end of the madrasa, then right, alongside the north side of the eastern iwan, there was access to the main courtyard. If the visitor turned right instead of left at the T, along the western exterior of the tomb courtyard, they would have accessed the two sections reserved for mental patients, one for the men and the other for the women. These sections were separated from the rest of the complex and could be viewed as a separate hospital.[80]

The hospital had a cruciform plan, with four large halls connected by a series of smaller rooms along the four sides of the courtyard, which measured 21 × 33 meters.[81] There was a polychrome marble portal accessing the hospital, and the inlaid decoration on the two surviving marble columns is in the same style as the decoration of the mausoleum.

Coste depicts two oblong iwans in his plan, each 13 meters deep, facing each other on the east–west axis. Each of these had a fountain at the rear with a channel to carry water to the basin in the center of the courtyard. The northern and southern iwans were both a different size and configuration than the eastern and western ones. Behind the southern iwan was a further cruciform wing with a central basin that served

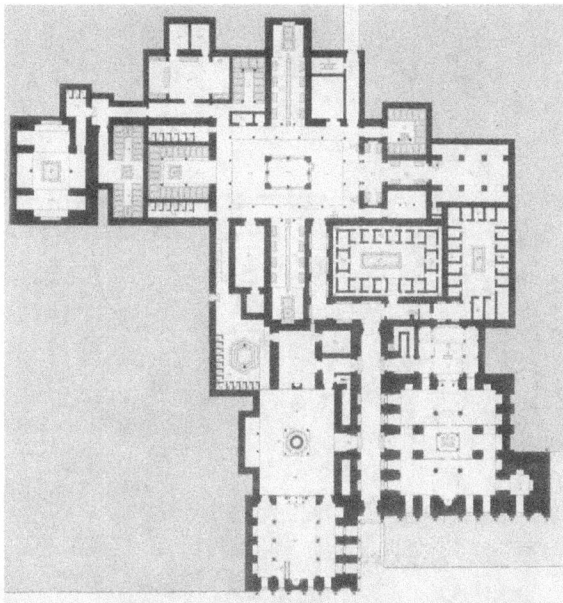

Figure 6.6 Plan of the al-Mansur Hospital, Cairo. Image: After Coste 1839, pl. XV

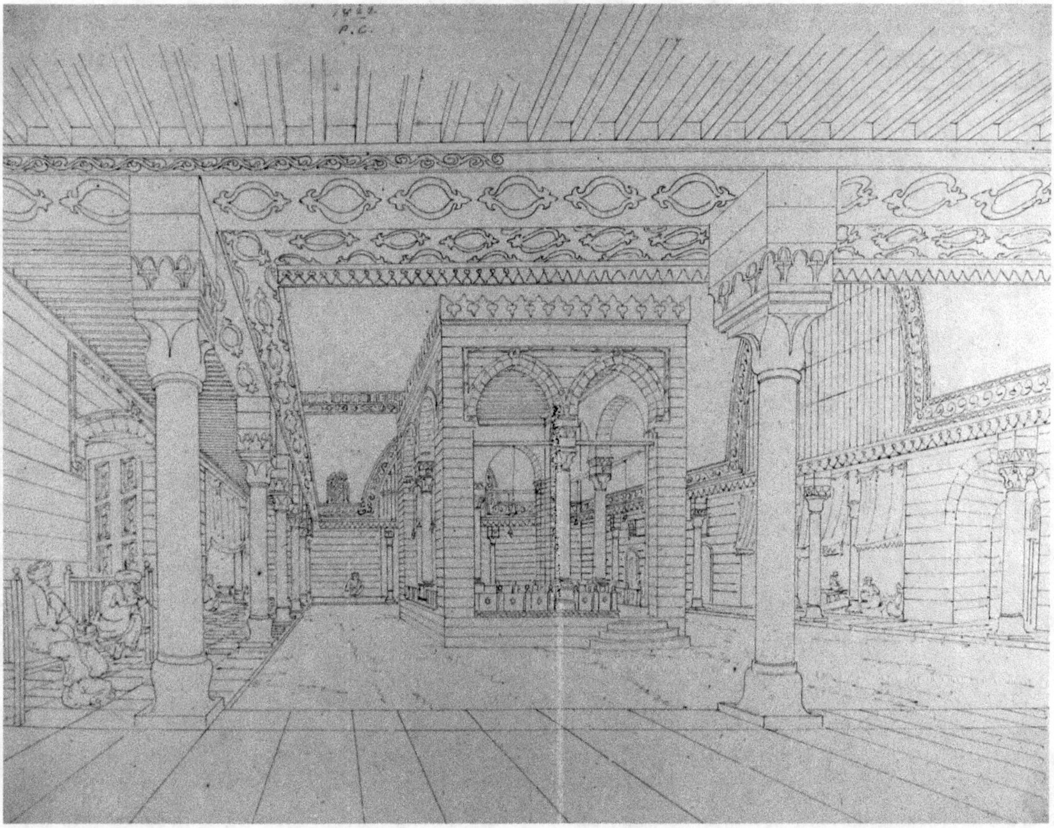

Figure 6.7 Street entrance leading to the al-Mansur Hospital, Cairo. Image: Richard Piran McClary

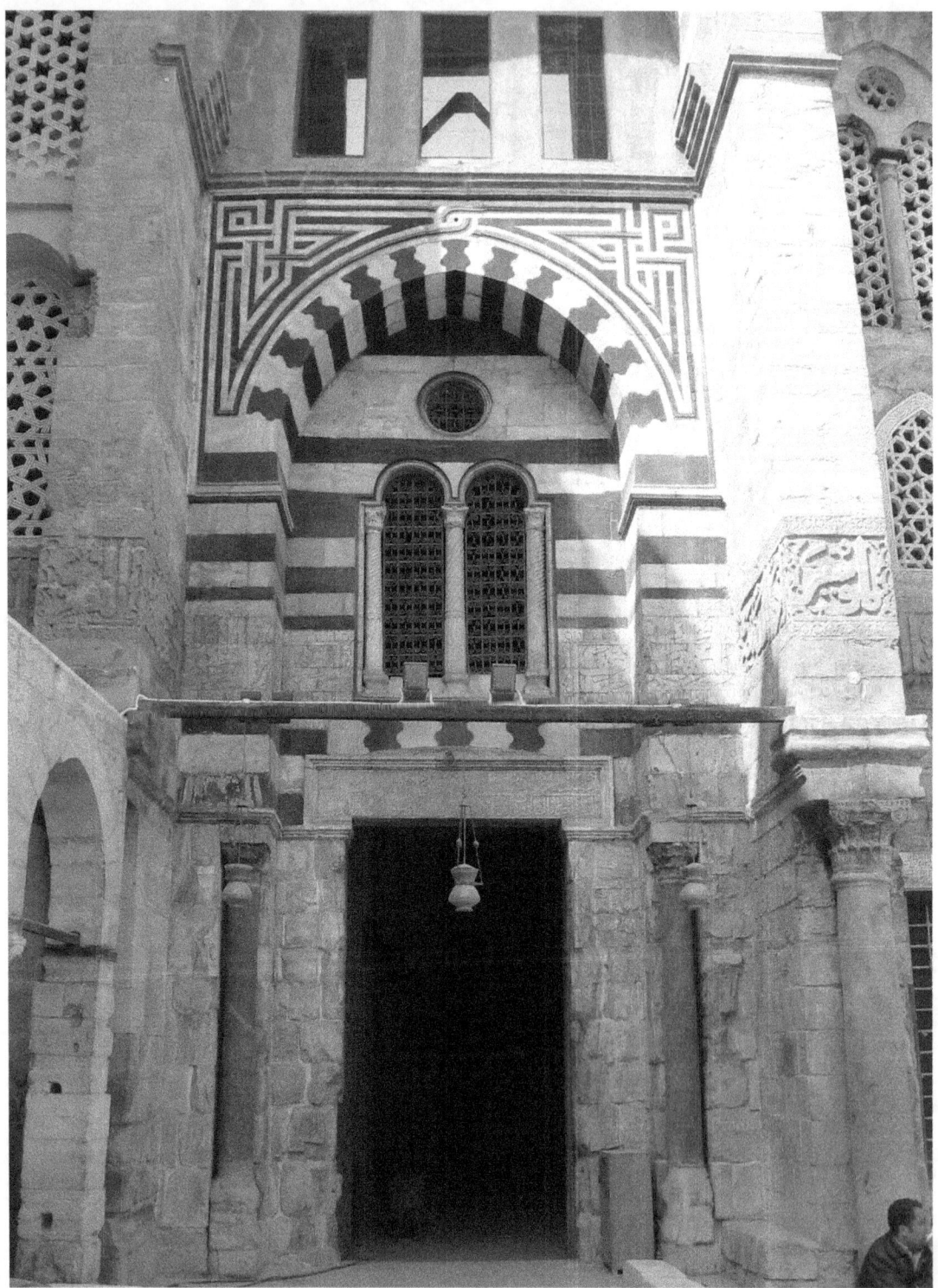

Figure 6.8 The interior of the Qalawun hospital, Cairo. Drawing: Pascal Coste in 1822, Bibliothèques de Marseille

as the women's section. The tripartite space to the south of this wing was a hammam according to the *waqf* document. The northern iwan led to the physician's residence, while the northeast corner of the site was occupied by two further courtyards, each with a central rectangular basin, which were surrounded with cells for male and female mental patients respectively, while the southwestern corner of the site was the location of the kitchens.[82]

A contemporary description of the hospital by Ibn Abi Usaybi'ah states that the hospital was divided into two wings, one for men and the other for women. These were further divided into several smaller halls for ophthalmology[83] and for the types of surgery laid out in the *waqfiyya*. The hall for internal medicine was subdivided into chambers for patients who were suffering from fevers (*al-mahmunin*), depression (*al-mabrudin*), madness (*al-mamrurin*), and diarrhea (*ishal*), with each section having between one and three physicians.[84] Despite these facilities, the *waqfiyya* states that the provision of medicine was the most important function of the hospital, with surgical provision being of secondary importance.[85] Alongside the administration of drugs, musical performances are also known to have been given at the al-Mansur Hospital throughout the medieval period in order to ease the minds of the mentally ill.[86]

The fifteenth-century historian al-Maqrizi provides an accurate description of the building's design and final appearance:

> The king drew the plan of the building including a *bimaristan*, a mausoleum, an orphanage and a madrasa. He invested so much energy in the project that the works were finished within eleven months and few days, having started on the 1st Rabi 683 (1284). As soon as the work was completed, he founded a huge endowment through several *awqaf*, amounting to 1 million dinars per year and he organized the expenses for the *bimaristan*, the mausoleum, the orphanage and the madrasa. He ensured an income for the remedies, the physicians' wages, and everything which was necessary for the sick. He appointed male and female staff to serve the sick, both men and women, set beds and bedding and arranged a special section for each type of disease in four departments (*iwan*), one dedicated to infectious diseases, the second one to ophthalmology, the third one to surgery and the fourth to sick people with diarrhea. Special areas were attributed to women and to those with cold character. Running water was provided throughout the *bimaristan*, a part of which was used for the kitchen and to prepare drugs, drinks, electuaries, and collyrium.[87]

The centrality of water to all the different areas of the hospital can be seen from the plan, with water moving from fountains into channels and thence into basins being a major design element of the complex. While the use of water is central to Islamic palatial architecture,[88] upon which the overall design schema of this hospital was based, the expansion of the network of flowing water into the new elements as well as those based on the earlier Fatimid palace, and its presence in the other two hospitals discussed above, highlights the importance placed on water therapy by the designers of medical establishments across the medieval Islamic world.

The scale and ambition of the hospital, as well as the information provided in the *waqfiyya*, demonstrate the extent of the investment that rulers were willing to make in what were primarily non-religious structures by the end of the thirteenth century. Unlike the earlier hospitals, many of the spaces within the complex were function-specific, and the al-Mansur Hospital marks the beginning of the development of the hospital as the word is understood today, with multiple departments offering a range of different clinical and treatment options.

Conclusion

From at least the eighth century onwards, the Islamic world cultivated a long and continuous tradition of founding hospitals, and the provision of both polyclinical and pharmaceutical services was seen as an important element of a ruler's duty. Despite the large number of foundations across the *dar al-Islam*, the majority of the evidence for understanding both the form and the function of such institutions is to be found primarily in the structural remains and textual accounts of the twelfth- and thirteenth-century foundations built in cities across the Levant and Anatolia.

All of the structures examined above feature the four-iwan plan, and while this is a format that developed in the context of palatial architecture, and was adopted for mosques in Iran under the Seljuqs, it appears to have been ideally suited to the functional requirements of hospitals in the medieval Islamic world from at least the twelfth century onwards, if not before. The prestigious nature of the structures, built by elite patrons and usually at great expense, laid the groundwork for both the scale and the decoration of numerous other buildings with different functions, including madrasas, caravanserais, and mosques, across the region. All the surviving and documented hospitals featured extensive use of water either for pools, fountains, or bathing, and showed a strong emphasis on the treatment, as well as confinement, of patients deemed to be mentally ill, although the basis for establishing such a diagnosis remains far from clear. The construction of hospitals continued into the early modern age, with a large number of foundations built across the region under Ottoman patronage.

In all the cases where travelers' reports or *waqf* documents survive, it can be seen that Islamic hospitals were generous charitable institutions open to all Muslims free of charge.[89] They were political and social structures that served the needs of both the patron and the public at large. Hospitals gave tangible proof of the ruler's involvement in public services, and thus fulfilled a regent's sacred duties of charity and donation, in addition to providing a much-needed service to the Muslim population. They were complex bureaucratic institutions that offered medical treatment on site, distributed food and medicines to the homes of the poor, and served as centers of medical education for surgeons, physicians, and herbalists.

Notes

1. G. Lev and Yaacov Lev, "Politics, Education, and Medicine in Eleventh Century Samarkand. A Waqf Study," *Wiener Zeitschrift für die Kunde des Morgenlandes* 93 (2003): 120.
2. Véronique Pitchon, "Food and Medicine in Medieval Islamic Hospitals: Preparation and Care in accordance with Dietetic Principles," *Food & History* 14, no. 1 (2016): 14.
3. For the best overview of the origins and development of Islamic medical theory and practices in the medieval period, see Peter Pormann and Emily Savage-Smith, *Medieval Islamic Medicine* (Edinburgh: Edinburgh University Press, 2007), 6–143.
4. For the most up-to-date study of the contemporaneous construction of hospitals in Europe, with a focus on the Champagne region, see Adam J. Davis, *The Medieval Economy of Salvation. Charity, Commerce, and the Rise of the Hospital* (Ithaca, NY: Cornell University Press, 2019).
5. Yolande Crowe, "Divriği: Ulu Cami and Hospital" (Ph.D. diss., University of London, 1973), 121.
6. Lev and Lev, "Politics, Education, and Medicine," 139–40. Little is known about the staffing levels of the hospital, but it did have a ward for the mentally ill. Although Ragab suggests that this was the first hospital in Egypt (Ahmed Ragab, *The Medieval Islamic Hospital: Medicine, Religion and Charity* (Cambridge: Cambridge University Press, 2015), 78), Swelim, citing al-Maqrizi, notes the existence of two earlier ones, the *bimaristan* of Zuqaq al-Qandil and the *bimaristan* of Murafir. Tarek Swelim, *Ibn Tulun His Lost City and Great Mosque* (Cairo: American University in Cairo Press, 2015), 45–7.
7. Cyril Elgood, *A Medical History of Persia and the Eastern Caliphate* (Cambridge: Cambridge University Press, 1951), 70–1.

8. Lev and Lev, "Politics, Education, and Medicine," 140. For details of the Baghdad hospital and its staff, see Elgood, *A Medical History of Persia*, 161–71.
9. Elgood, *A Medical History of Persia*, 172, citing Rabbi Benjamin of Tudela's *Itinerary*.
10. Alongside the use of extensive *spolia*, the al-Mansur Qalawun *bimaristan* was set on the foundations of the Fatimid palace of Sitt al-Mulk, retaining the precise layout of the earlier *qaʿah*. Iman R. Abdulfattah, "Theft, Plunder, and Loot: An Examination of the Rich Diversity of Material Reuse in the Complex of Qalāwūn in Cairo," *Mamlūk Studies Review* 20 (2017): 98, citing al-Zahir and al-Maqrizi.
11. In a study on the origins of the Islamic hospital, Dols defined "hospital" as a public charitable institution which provided care to the sick over an extended period of time, see Michael W. Dols, "The Origins of the Islamic Hospital: Myth and Reality," *Bulletin of the History of Medicine* 61 (1987): 370.
12. A *waqf* is an inalienable pious endowment of revenue, usually from either land or shop rents, for the benefit of Muslims. The *waqfiyya* lays out the terms of the *waqf*.
13. The most detailed study of the Sivas hospital is in Richard Piran McClary, *Rum Seljuq Architecture, 1170-1220: The Patronage of Sultans* (Edinburgh: Edinburgh University Press, 2017), 91–178. The earliest major study is Sedat Çetintaş, *Sivas Darüşşifası* (Istanbul: Ibrahim Horoz Basımevi, 1953), although the building is covered in Albert Gabriel, *Monuments turcs d'Anatolie* (Paris: E. de Boccard, 1934), 146–50, including the earliest plan of the site, on 147, fig. 92, as well as in Metin Sözen, *Anadolu Medreseleri: Selçuklular ve Beylikler Devri*, vol. 1 (Istanbul: Istanbul Teknik Üniversitesi Mimarlık Fakültesi, 1970), 94–101. For a Turkish translation of the *waqf*, see M. Cevdet, "Sivas Darüşşifası vakfiyesi ve tercümesi," *Vakıflar Dergisi* 1 (1938): 35–8.
14. Elgood, *A Medical History of Persia*, 174.
15. Doris Behrens-Abouseif, *Islamic Architecture in Cairo: An Introduction* (Leiden: Brill, 1989), 96.
16. For the Arabic text and a Turkish translation, see Hakkı Önkal, *Anadolu Selçuklu Türbeleri* (Ankara: Atatürk Kültür Merkezi, 1996), 381, and McClary, *Rum Seljuq Architecture*, 65, fig. 3.1 for an image of the portal.
17. Ernst Herzfeld, "Damascus: Studies in Architecture: 1," *Ars Islamica* 9 (1942): 2.
18. M. Khadr, "Deux actes de WAQF d'un Qaraḫānide d'Asie centrale," *Journal Asiatique* 255 (1967): 323.
19. Lev and Lev, "Politics, Education, and Medicine," 120. See McClary, *Rum Seljuq Architecture*, 102–3 for the Arabic text and an English translation of the foundation inscription over the doorway of the entrance portal of the Sivas hospital. See Crowe, "Divriği," esp. 75–83 and 120–36 for a study of the hospital in Divriği.
20. Leigh Chipman, "Islamic Pharmacy in the Mamlūk and Mongol Realms: Theory and Practice," *Asian Medicine* 3 (2007): 274.
21. For details of the links between food and drugs with specific reference to Anatolia, see Nicolas Trépanier, *Foodways and Daily Life in Medieval Anatolia* (Austin: University of Texas Press, 2014), 96–8, and for an excellent recent study on the role and importance of food in the wider context of medieval Islamic hospitals, see Pitchon, "Food and Medicine," 13–33. See Chipman, "Islamic Pharmacy," 265–8 for details of the practice of pharmacy and drug production in thirteenth-century Cairo.
22. This theory was based on the idea that the health of the body and the mind was determined by the balance of the four humors: blood, phlegm, yellow bile, and black bile. See Manfred Ulmann, *Islamic Medicine* (Edinburgh: Edinburgh University Press, 1978), 58 for further details of the humors. For details of Galen's theory of qualified experience, and the problems he identified with empiricism, see Kamran I. Karimullah, "Avicenna and Galen, Philosophy and Medicine: Contextualising Discussions of Medical Experience in Medieval Islamic Physicians and Philosophers," *Oriens* 45 (2017): 107–10.
23. Lev and Lev, "Politics, Education, and Medicine," 141–2.
24. An iwan, or eyvan, is a large rectangular-plan vaulted arched space with walls on three sides and open on one, often facing onto a courtyard.
25. Linda S. Northrup, "Qalāwūn's Patronage of the Medical Sciences in Thirteenth-Century Egypt," *Mamluk Studies Review* 5 (2001): 120.
26. In the Süleymaniye, Istanbul, Fatih 5433.
27. Conrad Hirschler, *The Written Word in the Medieval Arabic Lands: A Social and Cultural History of Reading Practices* (Edinburgh: Edinburgh University Press, 2012), 153. See 153–4 of the same work for details of the three-stage classification system used in the inventory.
28. Trépanier, *Foodways and Daily Life*, 99. He adds that while there are numerous references to the preparation of drugs, the description of medical acts such as surgery appears to be largely absent from medieval Islamic sources. However, al-Maqrizi does refer to the presence of a space for ophthalmology and another for surgery in the hospital of Qalawun

in Cairo. Pitchon, "Food and Medicine," 18, translated by Pitchon from al-Maqrizi's *Kitāb al-Mawāʿiẓ wa al-iʿtibār fī dhikr al-khiṭaṭ wa-al-āthār.*

29. Northrup, "Qalāwūn's Patronage," 123. These different roles were all appointed to the hospital founded in Cairo by Qalawun.
30. Herzfeld, "Damascus," 5. Ragab suggests that this small earlier hospital was in fact built by the Seljuq ruler Duqaq ibn Tatash (Ragab, *The Medieval Islamic Hospital*, 52).
31. Yasser Tabbaa, "The Architectural Patronage of Nur al-Din (1146–1174)" (Ph.D. diss., New York University, 1982), 86. See 97–110 and 227–31 of the work for a detailed study of the monument, and 444–75, figs. 150–84 for the most complete visual record of the building and its decoration.
32. Tabbaa, "The Architectural Patronage," 97–8.
33. Northrup, "Qalāwūn's Patronage," 123.
34. Herzfeld, "Damascus," 5.
35. Tabbaa, "The Architectural Patronage," 228.
36. The plan of the hospital in Figure 6.1 is based on elements of both Salaheddine Munajid, *Bimaristan de Nur-ed-Din* (Damascus: n.p., 1946) 19, and Herzfeld, "Damascus," 6, fig. 1.
37. Herzfeld, "Damascus," 5. The inscriptions include Qur'an 10:57 and 26: 78–80.
38. Tabbaa, "The Architectural Patronage," 228–9. Tabbaa adds that the Qur'anic inscriptions were there to remind the doctors that they were merely instruments of Allah, and that it is he, not the doctors, who cures the patients.
39. Ibid., 99. Although Tabbaa credits the Damascus portal as the first, the portal of the Maghak-i Attari Mosque in Bukhara also has stucco muqarnas cells, and, while undated, it is of *c.* mid-twelfth-century vintage.
40. Ibid., 98.
41. Ibid., 98–9.
42. See Pormann and Savage-Smith, *Medieval Islamic Medicine*, 151–3 for details of the inscriptions on the bowls and the role of magic in medical practice in the medieval Islamic world.
43. Tabbaa, "The Architectural Patronage," 102. The earliest was the one at the recently destroyed Imam Dur tomb near Samarra.
44. Ibid., 103.
45. Michael W. Dols, "Insanity and its Treatment in Islamic Society," *Medical History* 31 (1987): 7–8.
46. Also suggested as a possibility by Ragab (Ragab, *The Medieval Islamic Hospital*, 57).
47. For more details, see Tabbaa, "The Architectural Patronage," 107–8.
48. Ibid., 105–7.
49. Ibid., 110.
50. Gülşen Dişli and Zühal Özcan, "An Evaluation of Heating Technology in Anatolian Seljuk Period Hospitals (Darüşşifa)," *METU Journal of the Faculty of Architecture* 33, no. 2 (2016): 184.
51. For an overview of the history and significance of Sivas in the thirteenth century, see McClary, *Rum Seljuq Architecture*, 92–3.
52. The Danişmendid dynasty ruled much of central Anatolia in the twelfth century prior to the rise of the Rum Seljuqs. For details of their rule of Sivas, see McClary, *Rum Seljuq Architecture*, 92. For a list of rulers and brief history of the dynasty, see Clifford Edmund Bosworth, *The New Islamic Dynasties: A Chronological and Genealogical Manual* (Edinburgh: Edinburgh University Press, 1996), 215–16.
53. See McClary, *Rum Seljuq Architecture*, 96, fig. 4.3 for a ground plan of the Çifte Madrasa. For additional details of the structure and its epigraphy, see Önkal, *Anadolu Selçuklu Türbeleri*, 379–82.
54. See Çetintaş, *Sivas Darüşşifası*, 70 and 82–3 for conjectural plans of the lost madrasa, and 88–93 for images of the excavations of the northern section of the complex undertaken in 1937, which have now been built over.
55. See McClary, *Rum Seljuq Architecture*, 100–9 for a detailed study of the portal.
56. Chipman, "Islamic Pharmacy," 271.
57. Betül Bakir and Ibrahim Başağaoğlu, "How Medical Functions Shaped Architecture in Anatolian Seljuk Darüşşifas (Hospitals) and Especially in the Divriği Turan Malik Darüşşifa," *Journal of the International Society for the History of Islamic Medicine* 5, no. 10 (2006): 69.
58. Zühal Özcan and Gülşen Dişli, "Refrigeration Technology in Anatolian Seljuk and Ottoman Period Hospitals," *Gazi University Journal of Science* 27, no. 3 (2014): 1019.
59. There is a single fireplace and chimney in the northwest corner of the complex, but it is a later addition and does not date from the initial period of construction. See Dişli and Özcan, "An Evaluation of Heating Technology," 188, 190, fig. 15.

60. Excavations at the site in 2011 found sectional terracotta pipes along the eastern wall and in the entrance area at the level of the base of the foundations, which would have delivered water to the hospital. See Dişli and Özcan, "An Evaluation of Heating Technology," 185–6 and figs. 3–4.
61. See Doğan Kuban, *Ottoman Architecture* (Woodbridge: Antique Collectors' Club, 2010): 197–200 for details of the functional usage of each space, as well as a plan and images of the hospital.
62. See McClary, *Rum Seljuq Architecture*, 133 for the Persian text and an English translation of the inscription panel, located on the north wall of the courtyard.
63. Ragab, *The Medieval Islamic Hospital*, 94.
64. Ibid., 90–1.
65. Nasser Rabbat, *Mamluk History Through Architecture: Monuments, Culture and Politics in Medieval Egypt and Syria* (London: I.B.Tauris, 2010), 135–6. See Northrup, "Qalāwūn's Patronage," 124–30 and 139 for further details of Qalawun's motives for the building of the hospital.
66. Northrup, "Qalāwūn's Patronage," 122.
67. Doris Behrens-Abouseif, *Cairo of the Mamluks: A History of the Architecture and its Culture* (London: I.B.Tauris, 2007), 134. Work began in Rabi' II 683 (June–July 1284) and was completed by Ramadan (November–December) of the same year.
68. Northrup, "Qalāwūn's Patronage," 120.
69. For details of the controversy, see Ragab, *The Medieval Islamic Hospital*, 98–103.
70. Pitchon, "Food and Medicine," 21.
71. Ragab, *The Medieval Islamic Hospital*, 96–7. See 109–38 of the same work for a detailed study of the *waqfiyya* of the hospital.
72. For a detailed study of the treatment of the insane in the medieval Islamic world, with specific reference to the practices at the al-Mansur Hospital, see Michael W. Dols, "Insanity and its Treatment in Islamic Society," *Medical History* 31 (1987): esp. 6–7 and 10.
73. Boaz Shoshan, "The State and Madness in Medieval Islam," *International Journal of Middle Eastern Studies* 35 (2003): 335.
74. Shoshan, "The State and Madness," 338.
75. Behrens-Abouseif, *Cairo of the Mamluks*, 141.
76. Herzfeld, "Damascus," 2.
77. Dols, "The Origins of the Islamic Hospital," 270.
78. Behrens-Abouseif, *Cairo of the Mamluks*, 141. See Abdulfattah, "Theft, Plunder, and Loot," 118, fig. 5 for a photograph of the surviving stucco window on the north wall of the *bimaristan*'s southeast iwan.
79. Ms. 1309, fol. 28.
80. Ragab, *The Medieval Islamic Hospital*, 193.
81. Behrens-Abouseif, *Cairo of the Mamluks*, 142.
82. The preceding description of the layout of the hospital is largely based on information in Behrens-Abouseif, *Cairo of the Mamluks*, 142.
83. For details concerning the major growth of interest in ophthalmology in the twelfth and thirteenth centuries across Egypt and the Levant, see Pormann and Savage-Smith, *Medieval Islamic Medicine*, 65–7.
84. Chipman, "Islamic Pharmacy," 271–2. See 272 of the same work for details of the different staff and roles provided for in the *waqfiyya*, as well as the types of medicine made available to patients.
85. Chipman, "Islamic Pharmacy," 273.
86. Dols, "Insanity and its Treatment," 8–9. He also notes that the Ottoman traveler Evliya Çelabi reported that in 1648 there were three daily concerts given at the al-Nuri Hospital in Damascus.
87. Pitchon, "Food and Medicine," 18. Translated by Pitchon from al-Maqrizi's *Kitāb al-Mawā'iẓ wa al-i'tibār fī dhikr al-khiṭaṭ wa-al-āthār*.
88. See the presence of pools and water channels in virtually every palace ground plan in Felix Arnold, *Islamic Palace Architecture in the Western Mediterranean: A History* (Oxford: Oxford University Press, 2017).
89. Pitchon, "Food and Medicine," 24.

CHAPTER 7
THE BODY OF THE CITY
MEDICINE AND URBAN RENEWAL IN SIXTUS IV'S ROME
Johanna D. Heinrichs

At a busy corner of Campo de' Fiori in Rome a marble inscription commemorates a project of street repairs ordered by Pope Sixtus IV (Francesco della Rovere, r. 1471–84) in 1483 (Figure 7.1). Sponsored by the *maestri di strada*, municipal officials in charge of Rome's streets, the plaque states that until recently the via Florea (or via Florida) and surrounding streets had been "decaying, squalid, and full of stinking mud." Now, it exhorts passersby to admire "everything in these gleaming places." The text attributes this urban transformation to Pope Sixtus as *salutifero*, the bearer of health.[1]

The Via Florea repairs formed part of Sixtus IV's ambitious program of urban renewal. A woodcut from the 1493 *Liber Chronicarum* portrays the most visible results of his efforts (Figure 7.2). On the left of this bird's-eye view, the Ponte Sisto, founded in 1473, spans the Tiber River. It joins the ancient Ponte Sant'Angelo as the only two bridges selected for depiction. Just inside the Porta del Popolo, in the woodcut's lower right corner, stand the tower and church of Santa Maria del Popolo, whose reconstruction began in 1472. And almost at the center of the composition stands the Hospital of Santo Spirito, with its porticoed infirmary hall facing the river, a short distance from St. Peter's Basilica. From 1473, the pope rebuilt this medieval foundation and endowed its new medical ward with a remarkable fresco cycle. These three Sistine projects, shown to compete with the marvels of the ancient city, encapsulate the pope's program of urban revitalization.[2]

The city of Rome had suffered over a century of neglect, population loss, and diminished prestige during the Avignon papacy (1309–76) and the Papal Schism (1378–1417). Following its definitive reinstatement as the pontifical seat upon Martin V's election in 1417, later fifteenth-century popes sought to restore the city's battered physical fabric—part of a strategy to renew its spiritual and political primacy as the capital of Christendom and to increase pontifical control over civic matters. While Pope Sixtus IV's *renovatio urbis* built on the planning efforts of his predecessors, notably Nicholas V (r. 1447–55), his vision was marked by a new breadth, comprehensiveness, and practicality.[3] In addition to his patronage at the Vatican, Sixtus improved Rome's street system, repaired infrastructure for water supply and waste, and built or restored numerous churches, monasteries, and charitable institutions. His efforts launched the still more ambitious urban programs of the next century—from that of his nephew Pope Julius II (r. 1503–13) to that of his namesake Pope Sixtus V (r. 1585–90). Francesco Albertini's 1510 guidebook, published during Julius's pontificate, stated succinctly: "Sixtus IV began to restore Rome."[4]

In a medal celebrating the foundation of Ponte Sisto in 1473, Sixtus asserted publicly the new duty he had taken upon himself: CURA RERUM PUBLICARUM (care for public things).[5] These Roman capitals span the medal's circular field above a depiction of the arched bridge planted firmly in the swirling Tiber. The image of the bridge makes clear that *cura rerum publicarum* meant care for the urban fabric. Yet Sixtus IV's care for the city should be understood in relation to his self-ascribed role as the "bearer of health": that is, not simply as papal benevolence but explicitly as medical care. This chapter argues that Sixtus IV conceived his urban renewal as the care and healing of the decrepit body of Rome.[6] He crafted a curative vision for the

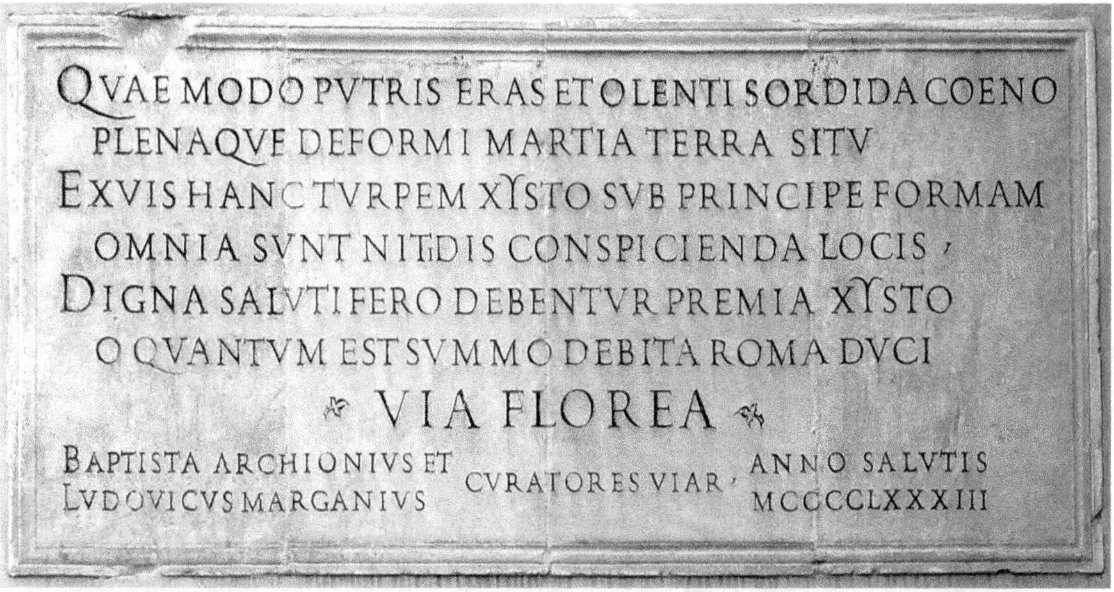

QVAE MODO PVTRIS ERAS ET OLENTI SORDIDA COENO
PLENAQVE DEFORMI MARTIA TERRA SITV
EX VIS HANC TVRPEM XYSTO SVB PRINCIPE FORMAM
OMNIA SVNT NITIDIS CONSPICIENDA LOCIS,
DIGNA SALVTIFERO DEBENTVR PREMIA XYSTO
O QVANTVM EST SVMMO DEBITA ROMA DVCI
VIA FLOREA
BAPTISTA ARCHIONIVS ET   CVRATORES VIAR,   ANNO SALVTIS
LVDOVICVS MARGANIVS   MCCCCLXXXIII

Figure 7.1 Rome, Sistine inscription from Via Florea (Campo de' Fiori), 1483. Photo: Peter1936F, Wikimedia Commons, CC BY-SA 4.0

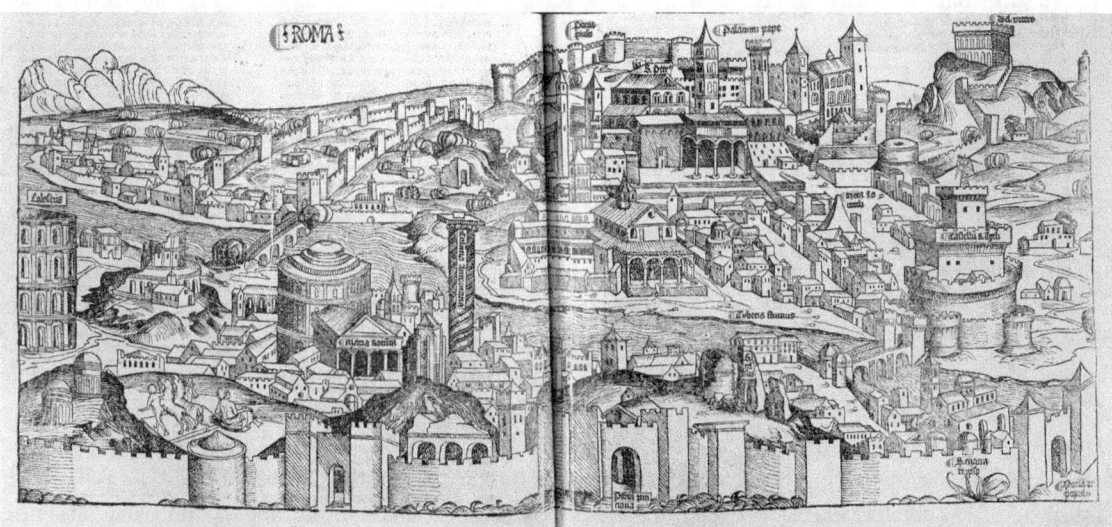

Figure 7.2 View of Rome from Hartmann Schedel, *Liber Chronicarum* (Nuremberg, 1493), woodcut. Source: Chapin Library, Williams College

urban body that invoked principles of ancient and medieval medicine and went so far as to relate parts of the city to bodily organs. This governing corporeal analogy can make sense of the various cultural and urbanistic undertakings of Sixtus's pontificate. It explains the predominantly utilitarian character of his interventions and the prominence he gave to the Hospital of Santo Spirito (Figure 7.3). Indeed, Santo Spirito played a key role in making visible Sixtus's guiding concept. According to Eunice Howe, the hospital's fresco program molded an

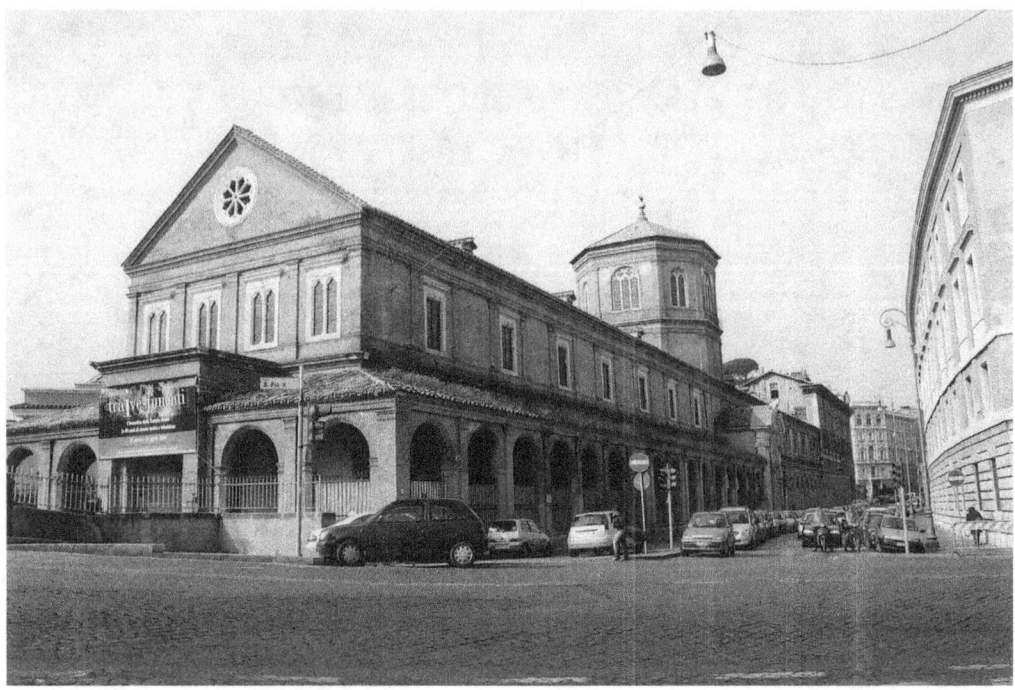

Figure 7.3 Rome, Hospital of Santo Spirito in Sassia, east end and north facade along via Borgo Santo Spirito. Photo: Johanna Heinrichs

image of Sixtus IV as "an imperial authority … but also a figure who represented Christ's charity and healing powers."[7] As an urban presence and an institution dedicated to bodily healing, the hospital communicated and extended this entwined vision of papal care and control across the city.

Sixtus IV's cultural and institutional patronage extended well beyond the Vatican and the Sistine Chapel, for which he is perhaps best known, and encompassed both the sacred and secular realms of the city.[8] In a December 1473 brief regarding the repair of city streets, Sixtus announced that, among his many concerns as pope, he must attend to the cleanliness and beauty of Rome. Adopting the city's traditional epithet, "head of the world" (*caput orbis*), he lamented that its streets and squares had become "foul and deformed" (*sordide et incomposite*).[9] A year later, in January 1475, he issued a papal bull, known as *Etsi universis*, in which he expressed his pragmatic ambitions for the "restoration of the city": "Unhappily, many calamities have befallen [Rome], through which her buildings have fallen into decay, and the number of her citizens has been diminished. We therefore earnestly desire to see her population increased, her houses and palaces rebuilt, and all her other necessities duly provided for."[10] Over the course of Sixtus's pontificate, the humanists and courtiers in his orbit glossed this vision with a rhetoric of renewal and transformation that sought to justify sometimes aggressive urban interventions. Papal briefs, eulogistic texts, and inscriptions such as the one at Via Florea conjured the filth, mud, stench, and squalor of Rome's public spaces.[11] The poet and humanist Aurelio Brandolini (1454–97) declared that Rome before Sixtus was "not a city but a cadaver." But now, "you renew everything, you increase and restore health. Because of you, leader, everything is accessible, everything gleams."[12] The perils of navigating the unpaved, congested streets of the medieval urban center were real.[13] Rhetorical logic, however, dictated that the greater Rome's decrepitude, the more complete and astonishing the transformation realized by the pope.

Sixtus and his unofficial spokesmen also promoted the fundamental practicality of this transformative enterprise, and modern scholars have followed suit. A silver *grosso* coin cast during his reign paired a portrait of the pope as restorer of the city on the obverse, with the phrase UTILITATI PUBLICAE (for the utility of the public) on the reverse.[14] Robert Flemmyng (*c.* 1415–83), an English protonotary at the papal court, claimed that Sixtus did not build obelisks and theaters but "excellent buildings" that "utility, piety, and honesty, not pomp and pride, demand."[15] He cited the construction and renovation of churches and monasteries but could certainly have included Ponte Sisto and the Hospital of Santo Spirito in that category. In the 1475 papal bull cited above, Sixtus posited a direct connection between the health of the physical city and that of its citizens. Santo Spirito stood at the heart of this relationship, representing both healing at an urban scale and the therapeutic care for the individual. Before we look at Sixtus's care and cure of the city and the hospital, we will examine how personal experience and intellectual discourse shaped his corporeal conception of the city.

Health, Medicine, and Theology in Papal Rome

Pope Sixtus IV brought to bear on his program of urban transformation an abiding interest in medical culture and, I will argue, a working knowledge of anatomy and physiology. He also could have drawn on his own experience of bodily affliction. Papal biographies presented illness as a major theme in the early life of Francesco della Rovere, born in 1414 near Savona. The Santo Spirito fresco cycle, which was primarily dedicated to the pope's own life, includes several scenes of the grave illnesses and miraculous recoveries he endured as an infant and child.[16] As a student and later lecturer in philosophy at the University of Padua, the young Franciscan friar came to know some of the physicians in the leading medical faculty in Italy. They may have kindled in him an amateur's interest in medicine. Physical ailments, including debilitating episodes of gout, continued to plague Sixtus throughout his life.[17] In the end pages of a manuscript he acquired while in Padua, he scrawled three medicinal recipes: two concoctions to counteract malarial fever and pleurisy, and a third for herbal pills for the stomach prescribed by his personal physician. Perhaps it is no coincidence that the book contained commentaries on Aristotle's natural philosophy, covering topics such as longevity, youth, and aging.[18]

Health and longevity came to hold greater urgency for Sixtus when his corruptible human body assumed the Petrine office, for the Roman pontiff physically represented Christ on earth.[19] Sixtus and his court, as has been shown, demonstrated a salient concern for "the cure, care, and recreation of the [papal] body."[20] He occasionally sought refuge in the Roman countryside for both leisure and health, and, like his predecessors, escaped the city's pestilential summers by removing his entire curia to the hill towns of Lazio and farther north.[21] New editions of ancient medical literature and modern medical texts were also dedicated to Sixtus. In the opening of the 1475 edition of *Opus ad sanitatis conservationem* by Benedict of Nursia, the publisher Giovanni Filippo Lignamine exhorted the pope to safeguard his health.[22] As we shall see, Sixtus extended his care of the papal body to that of the city.

Sixtus's interest in medicine went beyond personal care and informed his theology. In 1463, the learned Franciscan had been invited by Pope Pius II to participate in a formal debate with Dominican theologians on the controversial subject of the blood of Christ and the status of relics associated with Christ's Crucifixion and Passion. A now damaged fresco from Santo Spirito depicted him making his oration. He later committed his arguments to writing, in a treatise known as *De sanguine Christi*, dedicated to his predecessor Pope Paul II and later published by Lignamine's press in 1472.[23] The Franciscans held that blood was a humoral superfluity extraneous to the essence of Christ's living human nature (*veritas humanae naturae*), meaning that any fallen drops were not reunited with Christ's resurrected body. Instead, blood relics remained potent reminders of his bodily death.[24] The text of *De sanguine Christi* calls upon physiological evidence related to the production of arterial and venal blood to develop this argument. He demonstrates his knowledge of medical literature when he cites the "opinion of skilled physicians," probably textual sources, but he also indicates that he had consulted in person with anatomy experts when he was in Padua.[25]

Sixtus thus knew the essential principles of Galenic thought, which formed the foundation of medieval and early Renaissance medicine. The first-century Greek physician Galen had developed the anatomical and physiological framework suggested by Plato in his description of the tripartite human soul in the *Timaeus*.[26] The widely read *Anatomy* of Mondino de' Liuzzi (c. 1265–1326) followed Galen's basic structure.[27] Three souls—the animal (psychic), vital, and natural (vegetative)—were thought to lodge in the ventricles of the head, thorax, and abdomen and corresponded to three systems of organs and physiological functions. One principal organ ruled each one of these systems and exercised different faculties. Most important was the brain and its psychic faculties. The heart ruled the faculties associated with the vital soul, such as breath and arterial blood flow. Based in the liver, the natural faculties were responsible for the lower-order "operation of the vegetative soul": growth, nutrition, and reproduction.[28] The liver managed the process of sanguification, by converting digested food into *sanguis nutrimentalis*, nutrimental blood, as the future pope explains in his treatise.[29] Galen had described this and other processes in his magisterial *De usu partium* (On the Usefulness of the Parts of the Body) as well as *De facultatibus naturalibus* (On the Natural Faculties), both in use at medical schools in late medieval Italy.

De usu partium was one of Galen's most important works but was not available in a reliable printed translation until 1502, so it is worth assessing whether Sixtus could have read it.[30] He may have encountered it first in Padua, where a corrupt, abridged Latin version of an earlier Arabic translation, known as *De iuvamentis membrorum*, was likely part of the university's medical curriculum.[31] Once in Rome in the 1460s, the future pope could have seen a rare manuscript of the Greek text, dated to the tenth or eleventh century, in the collection of a humanist cardinal in his circle.[32] He also could have studied the Galenic corpus in the Vatican Library.[33] A manuscript of Niccolò da Reggio's authoritative Latin translation of *De usu partium*, entitled *De utilitate particularum libri XVII* (completed 1317), had resided in the papal collection since the time of Eugenius IV (r. 1431–47).[34] It is plausible, then, that Sixtus knew Galen's text in one version or another, and if not, he certainly could have learned the fundamentals of Galenic thought from colleagues in Padua. Both his theological work and his concern for his own bodily health would have informed his interest in Galenic teaching. If he had read Galen or conversed with those who had, he would have discovered that the Greek physician had deployed a host of urbanistic analogies to describe parts and processes of the human body. And Galen's comparison of the human body to the city formed part of a long tradition of thought with which Sixtus most likely was familiar.

Body as City, City as Body

Galen observed in *De usu partium* that the system of veins and other passages in the body made a natural parallel with a system of city streets. For example, food enters by way of the esophagus, "the first and largest street of all" (*maxima et prima omnium via*), while the "narrow streets" (*angustas vias*) of the veins carry blood to individual organs.[35] We use such figurative language today—albeit in reverse—when we refer to a major urban road as an "artery." Galen went on to explain that digested food passes into the liver through a single vein called a gateway or *porta*, "a name which has persisted ever since ... approving the wisdom of the first man who likened the governance of an animal to that of a city."[36] Here Sixtus might have found an echo of Aristotle's comparison of a living organism to that of a "city well-governed by laws" in *De motu animalium*.[37] Whether or not Sixtus studied *De usu partium*, the kinds of analogies the Greek physician had employed were a convenient way to elucidate, in lay terms, complex anatomical structures and physiological processes. One could imagine, for example, Sixtus's colleagues in Padua describing the blood system to him in just this way.

The pope also may have recognized such anthropomorphic imagery from other sources, not least the New Testament, where St. Paul identified the Christian faithful as the body of Christ and as a body of which Christ was the head.[38] By extension, the pope acted in Christ's stead as head of the Church on earth. A rich tradition of political and philosophical thought complemented this theological and ecclesiastical theme. Indeed, the analogy of the state to a living organism was a well-worn trope in medieval political theory and could be traced back to Plato and Aristotle.[39] The philosopher and theologian Nicholas of Cusa (1401–64), who preceded Francesco della Rovere as titular cardinal of the church of San Pietro in Vincoli, used it to analyze the hierarchies of Church and empire, in his *De concordantia catholica* (1433). Calling upon considerable medical knowledge, he developed an elaborate comparison in which he identified the priesthood as the soul that infuses the body of the Christian faithful, with the pope dwelling in the head.[40] Divine laws "circulate" throughout the arteries like vital blood, while canon laws flow through the veins of the ecclesiastical commonwealth. In the secular body-state, the emperor forms the head, and its laws are the nerves that extend from the imperial brain to the rest of the body. Nicholas also compared the emperor to "an expert doctor" who must "keep the body well" with a good humoral balance.[41]

Early Renaissance architects and theorists, following Vitruvius, used the human body as a touchstone as they considered architectural proportions and the relationship of parts in buildings. But, perhaps aware of the political tradition discussed above, they also extended this thinking to the city. In his manuscript treatise of 1461–4, Antonio Averlino, known as Filarete (*c.* 1400–69), noted that "the city ought to be like the human body."[42] Francesco di Giorgio Martini (1439–1501) took up the theme most enthusiastically. In the first version of his architectural treatise, the *Codex Saluzzianus* (before 1486), the human body even generates the form for an ideal fortified city.[43] In his drawing, the city appears as a male figure whose limbs inscribe defensive ramparts, while his belly forms a circular piazza. A round bastion crowns the head, an echo of Galen's comparison of the skull to a ring of walls that protect the brain.[44] As we shall see, Sixtus's conception of Rome as a body shared some of the literalness found in Francesco di Giorgio's graphic interpretation as well as the anatomical specificity of Nicholas of Cusa's political metaphor.

A wide range of discourses of the late medieval and early Renaissance periods made use of the analogy of the human body to conceptualize human institutions, social structures, and inventions, including the city. Medical literature, in turn, went the other way, using the macrocosm of the city to explain the microcosm of the body's interior. Sixtus IV tapped into these mutually reinforcing streams of thought as he envisioned the renewal and restoration of Rome at multiple scales, from the individual to the urbanistic.

Healing the City

If Sixtus, like Nicholas of Cusa's emperor, saw himself as the expert physician, what ills did he diagnose for the city? We can think of his interventions as having focused on three distinct but interrelated aspects of the papal city: infrastructure, including streets, bridges, aqueducts, and sewers; religious sites, including the papal enclave of the Vatican and devotional spaces across the city; and hospitals and charitable institutions. The first step toward reviving the urban corpse was to attend to the city's natural soul—the faculties that enabled its physical well-being and growth. Galen, as we have seen, likened the body's passages for the intake of food and flow of blood to an urban street system. From the beginning of Sixtus's reign, he ordered extensive improvements to Rome's infrastructure, which involved clearing streets of obstructions and widening, straightening, and paving them. Unglamorous but necessary, basic improvements to the systems of communication and circulation formed the foundation of Sistine urbanism, and they enabled the integration of the other two components of his building program.

A healthy body must first be a clean body. According to the regulations of the Order of Santo Spirito, which operated the Hospital of Santo Spirito, the lay sisters were to bathe the infirm on a regular schedule. They washed hair on Tuesdays and feet on Thursdays.[45] In his December 1473 brief, Sixtus first expressed his concern about Rome's "foul and disorderly" public ways, which were muddy, clogged with waste, and constricted by projecting porticoes and balconies from private buildings.[46] An anonymous chronicle attested that impassable, stinking streets were purged of mud, grass, and refuse.[47] In 1480, the papal *camerlengo* (chamberlain) Guillaume d'Estouteville ordered that four of Rome's public squares, the sites of food markets, be cleansed of rubbish on a weekly basis.[48] Sixtus instituted regular street sweeping in some areas and for the first time paved major streets. Finally, he restored part of the Cloaca Maxima, the ancient sewer system in the Foro Boario, perhaps recalling that among the cleansing functions of the body's natural faculties was the elimination of waste by the bladder.[49]

Sixtus articulated his vision for wide, paved streets free of impediments in his 1480 bull *Etsi de cunctarum*, but improvements to the street system had begun early in his reign.[50] By confirming the statutes of the municipal office of the *maestri di strada* and expanding their authority to demolish and expropriate private property, he strengthened the institutional framework for urban hygiene and infrastructure. But to ensure that his vision was realized, Sixtus also subordinated these magistrates to the Apostolic Chamber and the *camerlengo* Cardinal D'Estouteville.[51] Just as veins and arteries provided passage for the blood through the body, the newly cleared and paved streets reduced urban congestion for the easy flow of people and goods. Some of the new and repaired roads sought to facilitate communication within the Vatican Borgo, where St. Peter's Basilica was located. For example, Borgo Santo Spirito was repaired and paved for access to the new hospital and to improve one of the principal routes to the Basilica. Other infrastructure projects eased traffic between the Borgo and the city center lying on the opposite side of the river.[52] At the time the only bridge that connected the Vatican with the city was Ponte Sant'Angelo (see Figure 7.2). The eponymous via Sistina systematized existing streets to create a more direct route between the Borgo (via Ponte Sant'Angelo) and the northernmost city gate, Porta del Popolo, where visitors from many northern locales entered the city. This was also the site of Sixtus's favored church, Santa Maria del Popolo, which he rebuilt from 1472. A marble inscription of 1475 near the Ponte Sant'Angelo celebrated via Sistina's linking of St. Peter's and Santa Maria del Popolo.[53] Sixtus also attended to the three major routes that fanned from the bridge through the dense central zone of the Tiber bend—via Recta; via Papalis, Rome's most important processional way; and via Peregrinorum. These improvements eased the movement of pilgrims among the city's churches, many of them restored by the pope. They also aided access to commercial centers at Campo de' Fiori and Piazza Navona, where Sixtus established a new weekly market.[54] Via Sistina facilitated the delivery of foodstuffs arriving from the north to these sites.[55]

Concerns about commercial traffic as well as food supply prompted Sixtus's construction of the new Tiber bridge, Ponte Sisto (Figure 7.4). The stone bridge, carried on four arches with a classically inspired oculus in the center, was erected over a long-ruined imperial Roman bridge called the pons Aurelius.[56] It was the first new bridge built in papal Rome and connected the city center to the Trastevere neighborhood on the right bank. It encouraged development of this zone and linked it to the central commercial district around Campo de' Fiori.[57] Sigismondo de' Conti, a member of Sixtus's court, marveled that this formerly "dirty and empty district" was now "filled with people and well cared for."[58] The bridge incorporated this peripheral zone into the body of the city.

The Body of the City

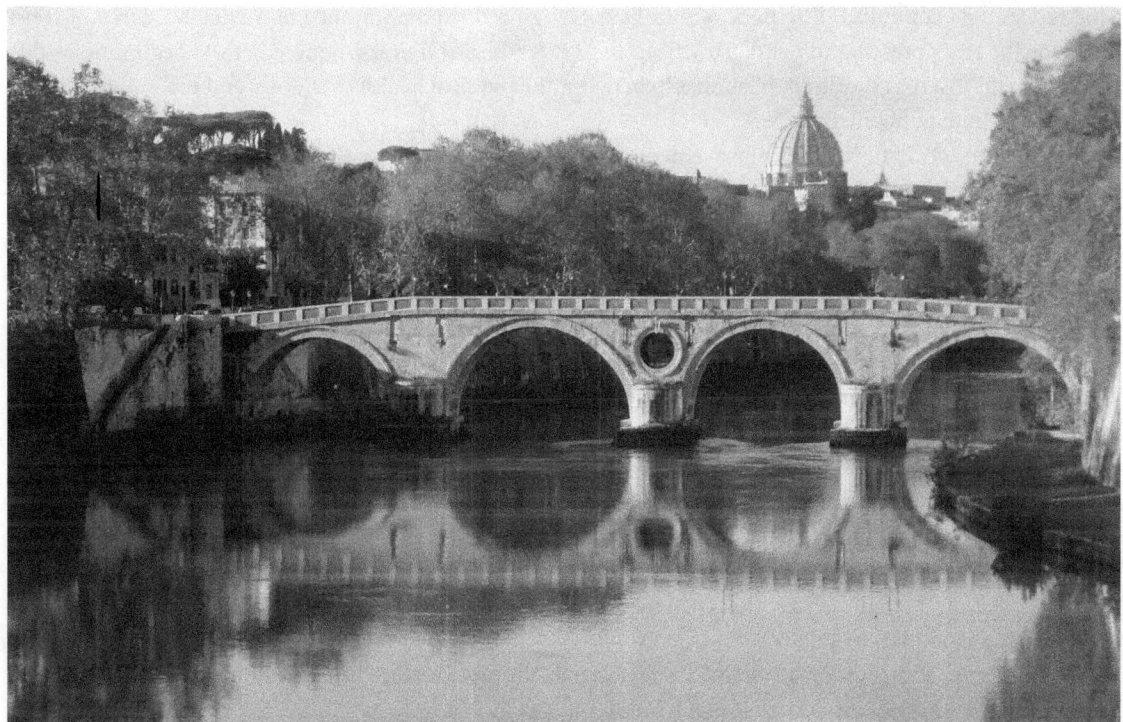

Figure 7.4 Rome, Ponte Sisto. Photo: Scott Moringiello

According to one of the bridge's marble inscriptions, Sixtus erected it for the benefit (*ad utilitatem*) of both the Roman people and pilgrims. His biographer explained that he sought to avoid the tragedy of the 1450 Jubilee, when a stampede on Ponte Sant'Angelo, caused by an obstinate mule, left hundreds of pilgrims dead.[59] Most modern scholars have thus seen the construction of Ponte Sisto as an effort to ease traffic into the Vatican during the 1475 Holy Year.[60] But the location of Sixtus's new bridge at some distance downstream meant that it could do little to alleviate crowding on Ponte Sant'Angelo.[61] The rhetoric of Sistine care for the pilgrim instead masked the pope's intention to gain control of the city's food supply. Nutrition, a precondition for growth, was one of the natural faculties, and thus another facet of Sixtus's care for the urban body. Blood produced by the liver carried essential nutrients to the rest of the body. Galen had compared the stomach to a grain warehouse, from which a vein transports wheat to the "public bakery" of the liver where it is cooked into nutrimental blood.[62] As Carla Keyvanian has recently argued, Sixtus supplanted old supply routes controlled by Roman clans with a new system to bring imported Mediterranean grain into the city. Ponte Sisto forged the crucial link in moving this commodity from the Tiber port of Ripa Grande to the granaries and the market at Campo de' Fiori.[63]

Sixtus also ordered the renovation of the Acqua Vergine, the only ancient aqueduct still functioning and the principal source of fresh water for the densely populated city center. It fed Rome from its outlet at the Trevi Fountain, which had been rebuilt by Pope Nicholas V in 1453. By 1472 the aqueduct required further attention, and bricklayers and masons repaired the above-ground arches, opened clogged channels, and repaired the fountain again.[64] Again Sixtus may have found a precedent in Galen, who invoked Roman engineering ingenuity when he compared the branching structures of veins, arteries, and nerves to an aqueduct and its conduits.⁶⁵ The pope would have recognized the importance of a reliable source of fresh water for the city's preservation and growth. In the 1475 bull *Etsi universis*, quoted at the beginning of this chapter, Sixtus asserted the direct relationship between the physical health of the city and the well-being and growth of its human population.

While many of Sixtus's civic improvements built on those of his predecessors, especially Nicholas V, scholars have emphasized the systematic and comprehensive nature of Sistine renewal.⁶⁶ It embraced the sacred center of the Vatican and the secular city of the Romans, sparsely populated neighborhoods and central market squares. Sixtus's conception of the city as a body provided the framework for this holistic approach. The parallels between the natural faculties, especially the system of veins, on the one hand, and the city's street network and its food and water supply, on the other, offered apt metaphors for the growth of the urban organism and "incorporation" of its disparate parts.

Despite his practically minded emphasis on the urban body's natural faculties, Sixtus did not neglect the other bodily systems—the animal and vital souls. For Galen and his medieval followers like Mondino de' Liuzzi, the natural members belonged in the lowermost cavity of the abdomen because their operations were inferior. The most elevated organ was the brain, with its psychic or animal faculties, such as the nervous system, sensory perception, voluntary motion, and mental activity. It resided in the uppermost cavity of the head, where it could receive abundant sensory impressions, just as "governors of cities do place their watches on high, as in towers and the like, that they may see afar, as Galen doth say."⁶⁷ As we have seen, Galen had compared the skull to a city's defensive ramparts.

Sixtus, as head of the Roman Church, considered the Vatican to be the "head" of Rome's body. The fortified Borgo lay separate from the rest of Rome to which it was linked only by Ponte Sant'Angelo, as the head is distinct from the body, though attached by the neck (Figure 7.2). Sixtus affirmed the primacy of the Vatican and St. Peter's Basilica (rather than the Cathedral of St. John Lateran) as the pontifical seat, a move initiated by Nicholas V.⁶⁸ Sixtus made significant interventions in the Vatican Palace, most notably the expansion of the Vatican Library, which he opened to the public in 1475. His librarian Platina reorganized the precious papal collection of Latin and Greek manuscripts and decorated the reading rooms that housed it, efforts commemorated in the Santo Spirito frescoes.⁶⁹ And, of course, he renovated the great chapel built by Innocent III, now known as the Sistine Chapel, and invited Botticelli, Ghirlandaio, and others to cover its walls with a magnificent cycle of frescoes.⁷⁰ The Borgo under Sixtus became "the definitive headquarters of a triumphant papacy."⁷¹

Nicholas of Cusa, author of *De concordantia catholica*, had likened the pope to the human soul located in the head and placed the inferior ranks of the ecclesiastical hierarchy in progressively lower parts of the body.⁷² For Sixtus, the numerous churches of Rome, run by religious orders, could be seen as the organs and limbs governed by the animal soul in the brain. He built, rebuilt, and renovated dozens of stational churches, and encouraged his cardinals to do the same. His deep devotion to the Virgin Mary expressed itself in his personal patronage of Santa Maria del Popolo (1472–8) and Santa Maria della Pace (1482–4), among others.⁷³ Cardinal d'Estouteville sponsored the church of Sant'Agostino in 1479–83, to which the straightening of via Recta improved access.⁷⁴ We have seen that trade and food supply were an impetus to Sixtus's program of street repairs, but the movement of pilgrims and papal processions through the city further intensified the need for a well-maintained network of streets and public spaces, as Sixtus pointed out in his 1480 bull.⁷⁵ The ritualized itineraries of Christian devotion made visible Rome's nervous system.

Between the animal and the natural lay the vital soul, ensconced in the thoracic cavity and ruled by the heart. Along with the lungs, the heart oversaw respiratory operations and most importantly the dissemination of life-giving *spiritus* (*pneuma* in Greek). The vital blood was thought to be thinner and lighter than nutrimental blood because it transmitted the airy *spiritus*. As Sixtus explained in *De sanguine Christi*, blood from the liver and spirit from the lungs are mixed in the heart and sent coursing through the arteries to all the body's organs.[76] *Spiritus* was also believed to be transmitted by the heart to part of the brain where it was further refined to aid in that organ's functions.[77] If the brain animated the body, the heart enlivened it.

In Sixtus's corporeal framework, the Hospital of Santo Spirito was the heart of the city. As the heart lies between the body's natural and animal members, so the hospital stands between the Vatican and the rest of the city of Rome, near Ponte Sant'Angelo and the intersection of the two networks of streets restored by Sixtus—those in the Borgo and those in the city. The heart's life-giving sustenance combined animating *spiritus* and the liver's nutrimental blood. Likewise, the hospital, with its adjacent church of Santo Spirito, attended to both the physical and spiritual restoration of those who entered its doors. The heart, whose Latin *cor* was thought to be derived from *cura* (care), was understood to be the origin and repository of human charity: "in it resides all solicitude."[78] The heart thus formed the source of solicitous care for others—of charity or *caritas* in the Christian sense of love for God and neighbor. Medieval iconography underscored this correlation: the theological virtue *Caritas* was sometimes represented by a figure with a burning heart.[79] As the principal locus of papal charity, the Hospital of Santo Spirito stood at the head of the Vatican Borgo as a monumental sign of papal munificence marking the approach to St. Peter's (see Figure 7.3).[80]

The Hospital of Santo Spirito

Santo Spirito had been founded by Pope Innocent III around 1204 on the site of the Schola Saxonum, which had served as the quarters of the Anglo-Saxon community in Rome. At the same time he approved the lay Order of Santo Spirito, which was to operate the new institution.[81] Like other medieval foundations the confraternity supported a broad charitable mission of hospitality based on the Corporal Works of Mercy.[82] Members of the order lived out Christ's call from Matthew 25:35–6 as they cared for the ill and indigent, fed the hungry, took in orphans, and sheltered pilgrims. Innocent III's foundation of Santo Spirito and Sixtus's rebuilding nearly three centuries later performed this vocation on an institutional scale. From its beginnings, it was a "beacon of [papal] charity … visible to every Christian pilgrim."[83]

While Italian hospitals began to specialize in medical care over the fifteenth century, under the Franciscan pope Sixtus IV, Santo Spirito continued to serve a diverse population: not only the infirm but also the urban poor and pilgrims, as well as abandoned infants.[84] Sixtus's attention to its finances, income, and administration affirmed its status as the most important charitable foundation in Rome. On March 21, 1478, he re-founded the confraternity with the bull *Illius qui pro dominici* and at the same time inscribed himself personally in its registry of members. Cardinal d'Estouteville, who was closely involved with Sixtus's urban planning initiatives, signed his name immediately below that of the pope.[85] Sixtus also devoted funds and patronage to other hospitals and charitable institutions in Rome.[86]

Through its works of charity and medical care, Santo Spirito was an ideal vehicle through which to make tangible the corporeal underpinnings of Sixtus's program of urban transformation. But by the time of his election it needed a physical fabric that proclaimed its importance. If the city of Rome was a "cadaver" before Sixtus's transformation, the hospital was a "sepulcher," in the words of his librarian and biographer Platina. He related Sixtus's rebuilding to his restoration of the city: the pope "rebuilt it from its foundations as an ornament to the city" and especially "for the comfort of pilgrims and the ill."[87] Sixtus laid the foundation stone in 1473 or 1474, and it was largely complete by 1476, although some work, including decoration of the ward, continued for several more years. The expansion and rebuilding, by an as yet unidentified architect, involved the erection of an immense new medical ward that extended the footprint of Innocent's thirteenth-century hospital building eastward along via Borgo Santo Spirito toward the Tiber.[88] A tall octagonal lantern marked

Health and Architecture

the center of the infirmary hall, and a shallow crossing was formed below it by the main entrance and a slight projection in the opposite south wall, visible in the 1493 view (see Figure 7.2). Santo Spirito's design departed from the influential cruciform plan by Filarete for the Ospedale Maggiore in Milan of the 1450s. The arm that extends southward from the crossing in the 1649 plan by Pierre Saulnier was not part of the original fifteenth-century hospital, and it always remained a distinct space (Figure 7.5).[89]

A group of subsidiary buildings further expanded the hospital complex to the south. Although later construction campaigns and changes of use, some of which are reflected in the 1649 plan, have complicated a reconstruction of the Sistine buildings, it is certain that two large adjacent structures, each defined by a two-story arcaded courtyard at the center, abutted the long hospital ward on its south side. Sixtus's 1478 bull referred to separate accommodations for nobles and for the "women and foundlings."[90] The larger of the two structures, to the west, may have housed the sisters, wet-nurses, and abandoned infants in their care, while the other building, located next to the later cross arm of the hospital ward, seems to have included private rooms for ill, impoverished noblemen on the upper story. It may also have accommodated the *frati*, or confraternity brothers. With round-headed arches carried on ancient spoliated columns, they suggest a monastic typology appropriate to the communal life of the order. Despite uncertainties about the original plan, it is evident that Sixtus's new hospital accommodated a variety of functions and users in distinct spaces according to the occupants' gender, social rank, and status as patient or worker.[91] In 1581 the English priest Gregory Martin described the hospital in urbanistic terms: "as it were a little parish in itself for buildings and distinct roomes."[92]

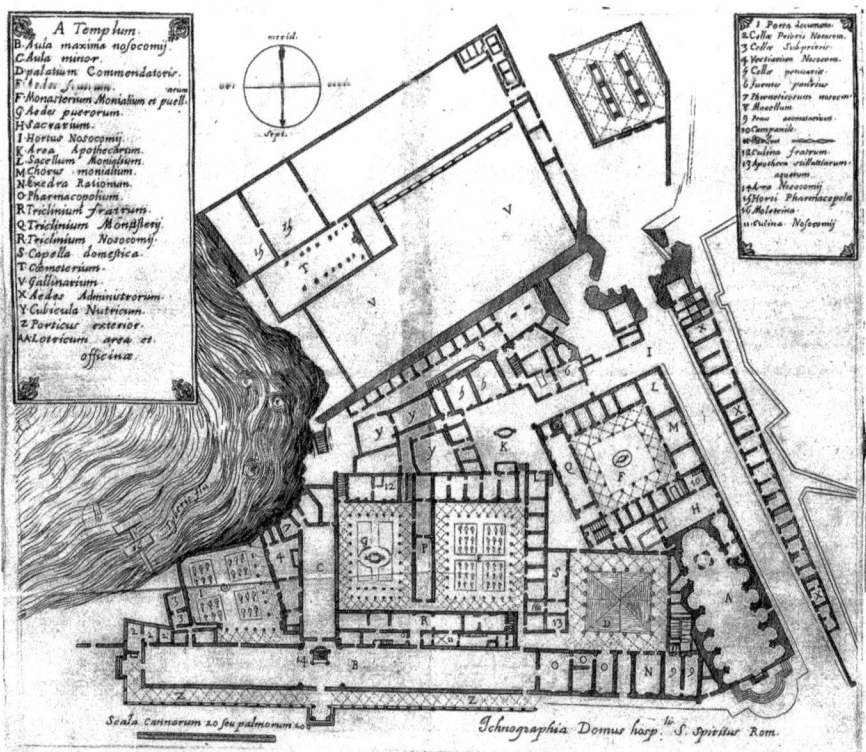

Figure 7.5 Plan of the Hospital of Santo Spirito, from Pierre Saulnier, *De capite sacri ordinis Sancti Spiritus dissertatio* (Lyons, 1649). Source: Wellcome Collection. Attribution 4.0 International CC BY 4.0

These residential courtyards remained hidden from the outside, and it was the hospital's infirmary hall, known today as the Corsia Sistina, that acted as the hospital's public face (see Figure 7.3). The tan brick structure evoked ecclesiastical architecture with its long, nave-like interior, the lantern lit by biforate and triforate windows, and the gabled east side, where a rose window pierced the tympanum.[93] The east end of the hospital stood in a highly visible position facing Castel Sant'Angelo where the three major streets leading through the Borgo to St. Peter's converged. The main facade on the north, with the hospital's entrance portal, extends nearly 130 meters along Borgo Santo Spirito. Tuscan pilasters punctuate this wall's upper register at regular intervals, and between them blank square panels of brick alternate with windows (originally biforate) framed in white marble, which illuminate the ward. Their lintels once bore the words "SIXTUS IIII FUNDAVIT," an inscription that also appears on doorways in the hospital courtyards and proclaimed its papal patronage. At ground level, a spacious portico wraps both the north and east sides of the ward (Figure 7.6). Here the round-headed arches are combined with Tuscan trabeation and pilasters, and they define a liminal area between the street and the ward interior. Unlike the public loggia of Filippo Brunelleschi's Ospedale degli Innocenti in Florence of 1419, however, the Santo Spirito portico was reserved for use by the hospital community. It was shielded from the street by a continuous low wall that connected the socles of the arcade piers. The confraternity sisters and brothers, hospital servants, and, significantly, some patients who were close to recovery could relax, take the air, and even exercise there with some privacy.[94] From this protected shelter, the healing patients and their caregivers would have manifested Sixtus's vision of healing to the broader public.

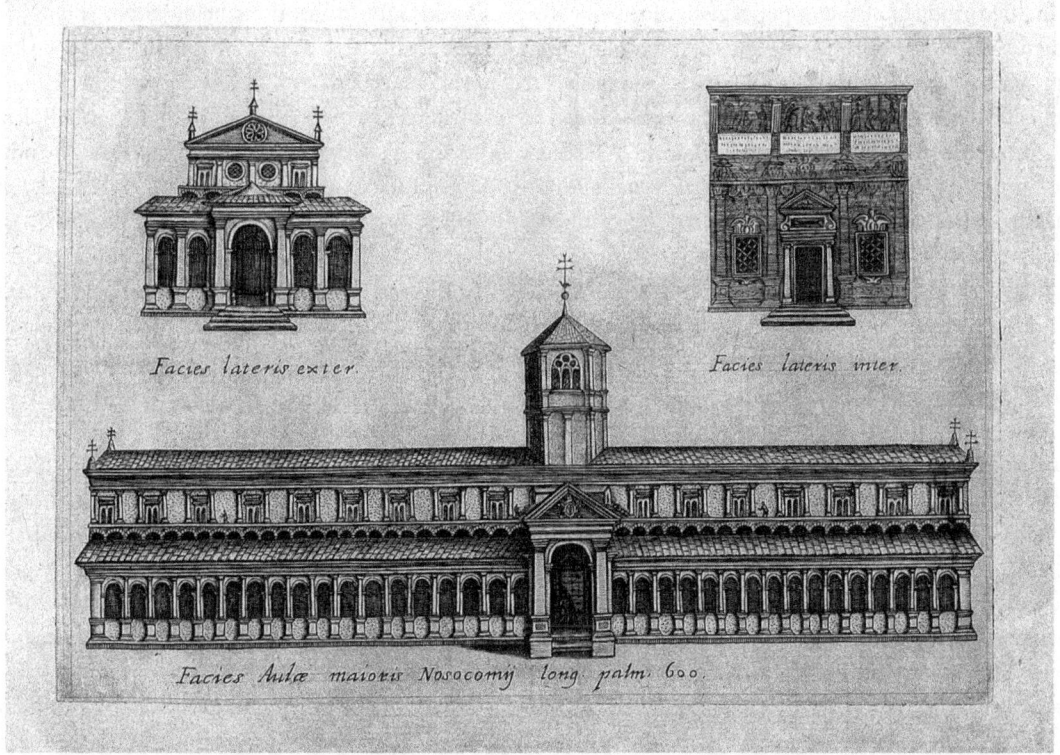

Figure 7.6 Elevations of the east and north facades of the Hospital of Santo Spirito, from Pierre Saulnier, *De capite sacri ordinis Sancti Spiritus dissertatio* (Lyons, 1649). Source: Wellcome Collection. Attribution 4.0 International CC BY 4.0

Health and Architecture

Santo Spirito made its work visible in other ways, namely through daily almsgiving and public processions in which the hospital community participated.⁹⁵ The order's regulations required the sisters and brothers to seek out the indigent and sick in the streets and bring them to the hospital for treatment.⁹⁶ Santo Spirito's urbanistic prominence and the importance of the institution, moreover, gave it an eminent place in the itineraries of pilgrims and visitors to Rome. Hundreds of travelers registered themselves in the confraternity and made donations—and were able to tour the premises.⁹⁷ The ward may even have been used by Sixtus IV for the reception of important dignitaries and royal personages, such as Queen Charlotte of Cyprus in 1478.⁹⁸

Once inside the ward, visitors found themselves in an enormous space whose nave-like character was reinforced by the altar positioned near the south wall under the octagonal lantern (Figure 7.7). Mass was celebrated there daily, and, from the 1550s on, priests used a domed altar ciborium designed by the architect Andrea Palladio.⁹⁹ These sacral associations would have reminded Christian viewers of the relationship between physical and spiritual health.¹⁰⁰ A seventeenth-century English visitor described a scene of impressive order, much like the view in Saulnier's engraving of the ward seen from the crossing: "When you come in, you shall see right out before, on both sides, three hundred beds standing, all hung with very fair curtains, the bedsteads carved, nightgowns, pantables, and other necessaries in order placed by every bed."¹⁰¹ In the print, four rows of cots supplement the permanent, curtained beds, perhaps because of an emergency.¹⁰² While in the ward, the visitor would witness the daily rituals of admission and care for patients. These were identified by Gregory Martin in 1581 as "the common sorte of sicke persons"—that is, pilgrims and the poor without noble rank.¹⁰³

The cavernous height of the Corsia Sistina was believed to encourage the rise and dispersal of noxious air exhaled by the ill patients.¹⁰⁴ The high walls also provided a field for fresco decoration that could be enjoyed by the bed-ridden. In the upper register, forty-six frescoes with Latin inscriptions below them spoke to an audience that included not only those patients and their caregivers but also physicians and surgeons, visitors, pilgrims, and clergy.¹⁰⁵ Devised by Sixtus's humanist advisors and executed by a largely anonymous *équipe* of painters between 1476 and 1478, the cycle mixed legend and fact as it presented events in both Santo Spirito's institutional history and the life of its patron.¹⁰⁶ The first seven scenes, which begin on the east wall, introduce Pope Innocent III's foundation of the Hospital and Order of Santo Spirito, casting it as a merciful response to the pressing social problem of infanticide, graphically invoked by multiple images of dead babies.¹⁰⁷ After the hospital's early history, the cycle turns to focus in the remaining thirty-nine scenes on the life of Sixtus IV, including his childhood illnesses and precocious entry into the Franciscan order. A survey of his career includes university lectureships, the dispute over the Blood of Christ, and his rise through the ecclesiastical hierarchy. The cycle thus highlights Sixtus's own experience of bodily illness and harm, as well as his theological training and medical knowledge.

Toward the end of the south wall, the newly elected pope's procession through the city to the Lateran introduces a sequence dedicated to his rebuilding of Santo Spirito and other urban projects. He first inspects the decrepit old hospital and, in the next scene, greets a kneeling crowd of confraternity members and female orphans, or *zitelle*. Like Pope Innocent before him, he is moved to pity for the young girls and resolves to rebuild the hospital. The two scenes demonstrate the pope's dual concern for the building and the people it housed. A depiction of the Ponte Sisto then unexpectedly interrupts the sequence. On the left, Sixtus extends a benedictory hand toward the industrious laborers on the bridge, who meet his gesture with raised hammers. Then follow two more events related to Santo Spirito: the old hospital's demolition (now damaged) and its reconstruction. In the latter, the pope again appears to bless and supervise the building works as masons labor on the roof. The adjacent west wall then returns to the hospital, where the pope dedicates the wards for women and foundlings and for nobles, again with a focus on the hospital's inhabitants gathered in the newly constructed courtyards. Finally, his rebuilding of the church of Santa Maria del Popolo concludes this sequence.

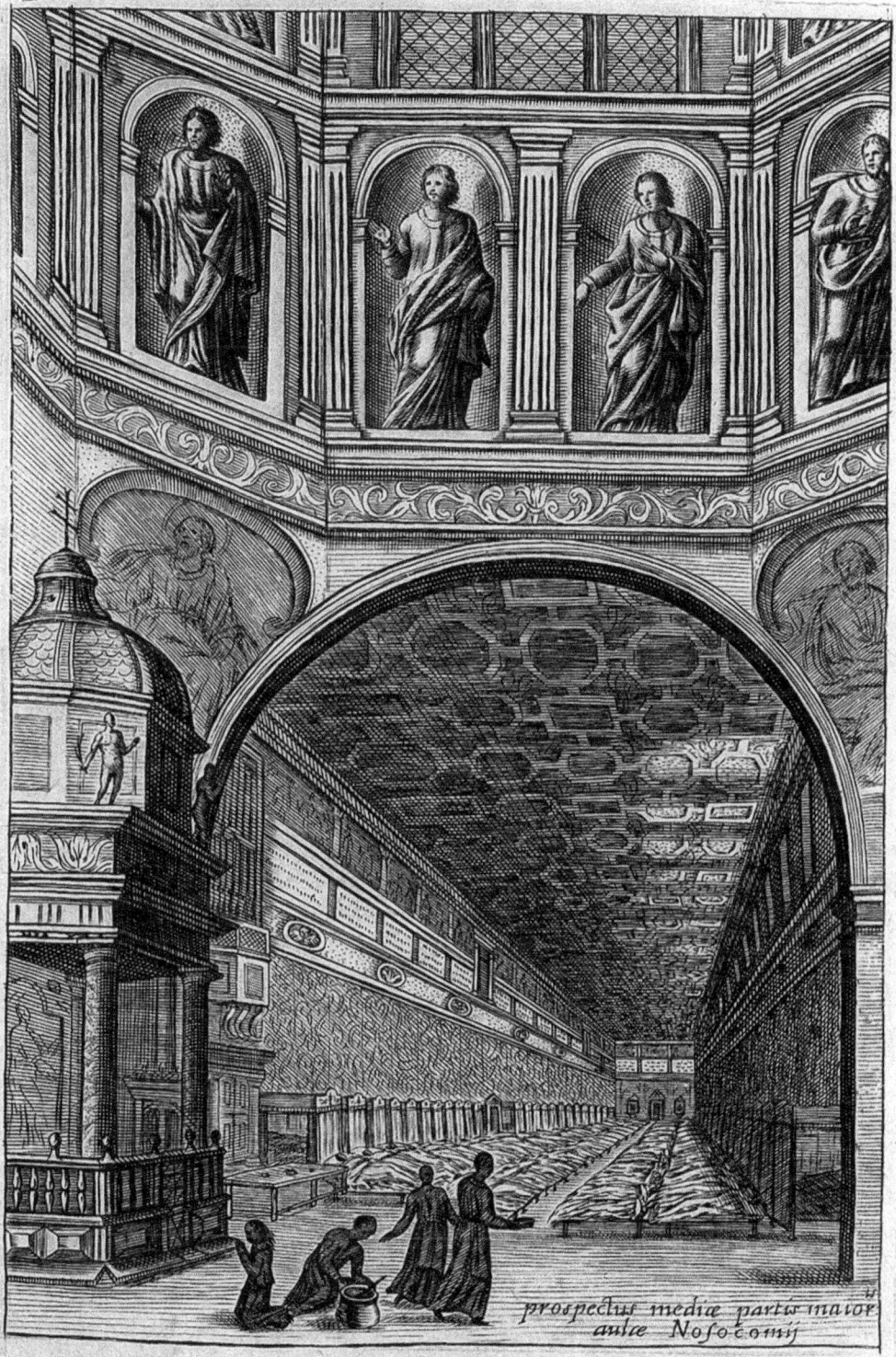

Figure 7.7 View of the interior of the Corsia Sistina, from Pierre Saulnier, *De capite sacri ordinis Sancti Spiritus dissertatio* (Lyons, 1649). Source: Wellcome Collection. Attribution 4.0 International CC BY 4.0

Health and Architecture

It is worth noting that the original Latin texts of the inscriptions cast the Santo Spirito and Ponte Sisto projects explicitly as *rebuildings*, not as ex novo foundations. Sixtus "restored" them "from the foundations," a theme that surfaces elsewhere in Sistine rhetoric.[108] Such an emphasis not only posited a salient historical continuity with earlier foundations—the ancient bridge, the Innocentine hospital—but it also resonated with the therapeutic context of the hospital. The architect Filarete had observed that buildings, like people, sicken and die. But "if it has a doctor when it becomes ill, that is, the master who mends and cures it, it [will] stand a long time in good state."[109] Of course, he envisioned the architect as the physician, but so too could a patron play that role—just as they often took credit for the authorship of buildings in this period.[110] We find such a claim made for Pope Sixtus IV in the fresco cycle at Santo Spirito. The inscriptions for the hospital demolition and rebuilding scenes ascribe these acts to the pontiff, not the laborers: "He demolished this antiquated and dirty hospital right down to the foundations in order to rebuild a larger and more commodious one." Then, "having called the best architects and a great number of workmen from all over, he constructed the hospital itself with much care."[111] The new hospital's designer may be the figure who kneels in front of the pontiff, but his subservience highlights the pope's dominant role as the skilled physician who brought the decrepit institution back to life.

Conclusion

The fresco cycle positions the restoration of Santo Spirito within Sixtus's larger program of urban renewal. As others have noted, the prominent Latin "captions" below each painting evoke numerous marble plaques installed throughout the city to commemorate Sixtus's improvements—such as those at Via Florea and Ponte Sisto (see Figure 7.1). Text and image together invite the audience on a virtual tour of major Sistine sites, guided by the pope himself. Accompanied by his red-hatted cardinals, he appears in each scene in profile, garbed in full papal regalia, with a gesture of blessing; his figure provides visual continuity across the sequence.[112] The physician who revived the hospital is also the healer of the city, the *urbis renovator*, as he claimed on inscriptions, coins, and medals. The hospital, bridge, and church featured in the thematic sequence of his civic works exemplify his three main targets of intervention in Rome: charitable institutions, infrastructure, and religious sites. These exempla reappear in the cycle's penultimate episode, where we have fast-forwarded to the end of Sixtus's life. In the left foreground, the pope kneels on the ground between the Virgin Mary and St. Francis, who present him to God the Father, at the upper right. A group of angels precede them, bearing evidence of the pope's good works: models of two churches, of the Ponte Sisto and, the largest, of the Hospital of Santo Spirito. These models stand as a visual shorthand for Sixtus's *renovatio urbis*.[113] They are the organs of the urban body of Rome and govern its corporeal faculties.

If the frescoes show Santo Spirito as an integral part of this urban renewal, conversely, they also present Sixtus's civic works as embedded in a narrative of Christian charity initiated by Innocent III. Both popes are shown to assume personal responsibility for the care of the city, both its people and its physical fabric. Sixtus has restored the city to wholeness—just as the hospital patients are nursed to health by members of the Order of Santo Spirito. As a charitable institution, a physical presence in the city, and most explicitly in its decoration, the Hospital of Santo Spirito manifested Sixtus's project for healing the broken body of Rome. Viewing the fresco narrative as he stood within a living scene of medical care, the viewer was urged to see the relationship of the individual healing bodies in the beds to the *corpus* of the physical city, and also to the corporate body of Roman citizens and the entire Christian faithful. For Sixtus, the stakes of *renovatio urbis* in Rome went beyond the city's well-being, and even beyond the desire to expand the papacy's temporal authority. Bodily restoration was preparation for spiritual transformation. In Latin the word for health—*salus*—also signified salvation; as *salutifero*, Pope Sixtus saw himself as the bearer of not only physical health but also the possibility of salvation. The healing of the city of Rome thus augured the eschatological union of the city of God on earth with that in heaven.

Acknowledgments: This chapter stems from research completed for my 2004 M.Phil. dissertation, supervised by Deborah Howard of the University of Cambridge, to whom I offer my heartfelt gratitude. My thanks also go to Williams College and the Herchel Smith Fellowship and the staff of the Wellcome Library, Warburg Institute Library, British Library Rare Books Room, and Cambridge University Library. For help at various stages of this project, I would like to thank Scott Moringiello, Eugene J. Johnson, John Pinto, Marion Riggs, Diana Bullen Presciutti, and our editor Mohammad Gharipour, and the other members of the panel, "A Matter of Life and Death," at the 2018 Society of Architectural Historians Annual Conference in St. Paul, Minnesota.

Notes

1. Paola Guerrini, "L'epigrafia sistina come momento della 'restauratio Urbis,'" in *Un pontificato ed una città: Sisto IV (1471–1484)*, ed. Massimo Miglio et al. (Vatican City: Associazione Roma nel Rinascimento, 1986), 472–3; Iiro Kajanto, *Papal Epigraphy in Renaissance Rome* (Helsinki: Suomalainen Tiedeakatemia, 1982), 83; J. Brian Horrigan, "Imperial and Urban Ideology in a Renaissance Inscription," *Comitatus* 9 (1978): 75–6.
2. On the bridge and the hospital as complementary and highly public undertakings, see Eunice D. Howe, *The Hospital of Santo Spirito and Pope Sixtus IV* (New York: Garland, 1978), 32–7; Flavia Cantatore, "Sisto IV committente di architettura a Roma tra magnificenza e conflitto," in *Congiure e conflitti. L'affermazione della signoria pontificia su Roma nel Rinascimento: politica, economia e cultura*, ed. Myriam Chiabò et al. (Rome: Roma nel Rinascimento, 2014), 316.
3. For an introduction to fifteenth-century Rome and its urban form, see Torgil Magnuson, *Studies in Roman Quattrocento Architecture* (Stockholm: Almquist & Wiksell, 1958); James S. Ackerman, "The Planning of Renaissance Rome, 1450–1580," in *Rome in the Renaissance: The City and the Myth*, ed. P. A. Ramsey (Binghamton, NY: Center for Medieval & Early Renaissance Studies, 1982), 3–17; Linda Pellecchia, "The Contested City: Urban Form in Early Sixteenth-Century Rome," in *Cambridge Companion to Raphael*, ed. Marcia Hall (Cambridge: Cambridge University Press, 2005), 59–61. On Nicholas V, see Carroll William Westfall, *In this Most Perfect Paradise: Alberti, Nicholas V, and the Invention of Conscious Urban Planning in Rome, 1447–55* (University Park, PA: Pennsylvania State University Press, 1974); Charles Burroughs, *From Signs to Design: Environmental Process and Reform in Early Renaissance Rome* (Cambridge, MA: MIT Press, 1990).
4. "Sixtus Quartus … cepit urbe[m] instaurare." Francesco Albertini, *Opusculum de mirabilibus novae et veteris urbis Romae* [1510] (Basel: [n.p.], 1519), fol. 75v, accessed May 30, 2018. https://books.google.com/books?id=bsJbAAAAQAAJ. See also Allan Ceen, "The Quartiere de' Banchi and Urban Planning in Rome in the First Half of the Cinquecento" (Ph.D. diss., University of Pennsylvania, 1977), 37.
5. Fabio Benzi, *Sisto IV Renovator Urbis: Architettura a Roma 1471–1484* (Rome: Officina, 1990), 27; Jill E. Blondin, "Power Made Visible: Pope Sixtus IV as 'Urbis Restaurator' in Quattrocento Rome," *The Catholic Historical Review* 91, no. 1 (January 2005): 1. On the medal, see Roberto Weiss, *The Medals of Pope Sixtus IV (1471–1484)* (Rome: Edizioni di Storia e Letteratura, 1961), 18; Antonio Bertino, "Arte e storia nelle medaglie di Sisto IV e di Giulio II," in *Sisto IV e Giulio II mecenati e promotori di cultura*, ed. Silvia Bottaro, Anna Dagnino, and Giovanna Rotondi Terminiello (Savona: Coop Tipograf, 1985), 127–35.
6. On the Augustinian roots of Sixtus's "corporate" conception, see Benzi, *Renovator Urbis*, 9, 30. On urban renewal in relation to Sixtus's care of the papal body, Starleen Kay Meyer, "The Papal Series in the Sistine Chapel: The Embodiment, Vesting and Framing of Papal Power" (Ph.D. diss., University of Southern California, 1998), 319. For a transhistorical consideration of the theme of city and body, see Richard Sennett, *Flesh and Stone: The Body and the City in Western Civilization* (New York and London: W. W. Norton, 1994).
7. Eunice D. Howe, *Art and Culture at the Sistine Court: Platina's "Life of Sixtus IV" and the Frescoes of the Hospital of Santo Spirito* (Vatican City: Biblioteca Apostolica Vaticana, 2005), 139.

8. Giorgio Simoncini, *Roma: Le trasformazioni urbane nel Quattrocento*, vol. 1, *Topografia e urbanistica da Bonifacio IX ad Alessandro VI* (Rome: Leo S. Olschki, 2014), 202–3.
9. Brief of December 7, 1473, authorizing Girolamo de' Gigantis to oversee street repairs, in Eugène Müntz, *Les Arts à la cour des papes pendant le XVe et le XVIe siècle. Troisième partie: Sixte IV–Léon X* (Paris: E. Thorin, 1882), 179, citing Archivio Segreto Vaticano, Divers. Cam., 1471-8, fols. 210v–211r. See also Egmont Lee, *Sixtus IV and Men of Letters* (Rome: Edizioni di Storia e Letteratura, 1978), 131, 135; Blondin, "Power Made Visible," 10.
10. The bull, dated January 1, 1475, regulated ownership of property and buildings in Rome. "Cupientes igitur pro instauratione dictae Urbis, quae causantibus sinistris eventibus in civibus, incolis et aedificiis plurimum diminuta est, ut annuente Altissimo virorum copia instauretur, et quantoties ipsius structurae et aedificia refectionem et reparationem pro ejus venustate et decore consequantur, suisque statui et necessitati opportunis remediis consulatur." Translation from Ludwig Pastor, *The History of the Popes from the Close of the Middle Ages* (St. Louis, MO: B. Herder, 1923), 4:277. Full Latin text in Müntz, *Les Arts*, 180; see also Giorgio Simoncini, ed., *Roma: Le trasformazioni urbane nel Quattrocento*, vol. 2, *Funzioni urbane e tipologie edilizie* (Rome: Leo S. Olschki, 2014), 264–5. On the bull, Lee, *Sixtus IV*, 130; Simoncini, *Topografia*, 185–6.
11. On the Via Sistina project: "Publica quum nuper via ad alta palacia ducens abs tumulo, o Adriane, tuo, rupta, horrida, turpis plenaque deformi coenoque lutoque fuisset, nec lapis haereret lapidi, nec tempore quisquam hiberno posset pedes illac aut eques ire." Robert Flemmyng, *Lucubraciuncolae tiburtinae* (c. 1477), published in Vincenzo Pacifici, *Un carme biografico di Sisto IV del 1477* (Tivoli: Società Tibertina di Storia e Arte, [1923]), 24 (ll. 595–9), accessed May 30, 2018. https://hdl.handle.net/2027/njp.32101073446377. For the attribution to Flemmyng: Howe, *Hospital*, 246–7. On Via Papalis: "Sordibus et coeno immundae vix pervia plebi/Haec via dicta tamen Pontificalis erat." Aurelio Brandolini, *Ad Sixtum IV pontificem maximum de urbe ab eo instaurata epigrammata et aliis eius laudibus*, epigram 24 (Biblioteca Apostolica Vaticana [hereafter BAV], Ms. Urb. lat. 739, fol. 85v, accessed May 30, 2018. https://digi.vatlib.it/view/MSS_Urb.lat.739); also quoted in Blondin, "Power Made Visible," 14 n. 38.
12. Brandolini, *Ad Sixtum IV*, epigram 18: "Non urbs, iam Roma cadaver erat." From epigram 17: "Tu totam instauras, auges reddisque salubrem,/Pervia te tota est principe, tota nitet." BAV, Ms. Urb. lat. 739, fols. 82v, 81v, accessed May 30, 2018. https://digi.vatlib.it/view/MSS_Urb.lat.739. Excerpted in Tillman Buddensieg, "Die Statuenstiftung Sixtus' IV. im Jahre 1471," *Römisches Jahrbuch für Kunstgeschichte* 20 (1983): 63. See also Blondin, "Power Made Visible," 14.
13. Piero Tomei, "Le strade di Roma e l'opera di Sisto IV," *L'Urbe* 2 (1937). 15, Blondin, "Power Made Visible," 10.
14. Giancarlo Alteri, "Il Giubileo di Sisto IV attraverso alcune testimonianze numismatiche dirette e indirette," in *Sisto IV: Le Arti a Roma nel Primo Rinascimento*, ed. Fabio Benzi (Rome: Edizioni dell'Associazione Culturale Shakespeare and Company, 2000), 152; Benzi, *Renovator Urbis*, 27.
15. "praestantibus aedibus … iis quas utilitas, pietas vel honestas denique poscit, non pompa aut fastus." Flemmyng, *Lucubraciuncolae tiburtinae*, in Pacifici, *Un carme*, 30, also 22. See also Platina, "Life of Sixtus IV," in Howe, *Art and Culture*, 193. Modern assessments in Blondin, "Power Made Visible," 16 n. 44; Marcello Fagiolo and Maria Luisa Madonna, *Roma 1300-1875. La città degli anni santi: Atlante* (Milan: A. Mondadori, 1985), 104; Benzi, *Renovator Urbis*, 26, 28.
16. For the frescoes' subjects, inscriptions, and their written sources, Howe, *Hospital*, 345–52. On the theme of childhood illness, ibid., *Art and Culture*, 159.
17. Lee, *Sixtus IV*, 20; Meyer, "Papal Series," 315; Pastor, *History of the Popes*, 4:384–5.
18. Joannes Buridanus (Jean Buridan), *Expositiones in Aristotelis libros naturales*, BAV, Ms. Vat. lat. 2162, fol. 168r, accessed May 14, 2018. https://digi.vatlib.it/view/MSS_Vat.lat.2162. See Anneliese Maier, "Alcuni autografi di Sisto IV," in *Ausgehendes Mittelalter: Gesammelte Aufsätze zur Geistesgeschichte des. 14. Jahrhunderts* (Rome: Edizioni di storie e letteratura, 1967), 2:138–9; Paola Scarcia Piacentini, "Ricerche sugli antichi inventari della Biblioteca Vaticana: I codici di lavoro di Sisto IV," in Miglio et al., *Un pontificato*, 160. See also Lee, *Sixtus IV*, 20 n. 46; Meyer, *Papal Series*, 316, 470. Buridan's manuscript included commentaries on *De iuventute et senectute*, *De longitudine et brevitate vitae*, and *De motu animalium*.
19. Agostino Paravicini-Bagliani, *The Pope's Body*, trans. David S. Peterson (Chicago and London: University of Chicago Press, 2000), 59.
20. Meyer, *Papal Series*, 278, 313–20. On the "papal body," see Paravicini-Bagliani, *Pope's Body*.
21. Pastor, *History of the Popes*, 4:288–9; Howe, *Art and Culture*, 83–5; Meyer, *Papal Series*, 318.
22. Lee, *Sixtus IV*, 101, citing Benedict of Nursia (Benedetto Reguardati), *Opus ad sanitatis conservationem* (Rome: Giovanni Filippo Lignamine, 1475). Around 1475-8 Jacopo Ravaldi, a French miniaturist in the papal circle, produced a copy of Guy de Chauliac's *De chirurgia et de medicina* for Sixtus (BAV, Ms. Vat. lat. 4804). See Gennaro Toscano, "La

miniatura '*all'antica*' tra Roma e Napoli all'epoca di Sisto IV," in Benzi, *Sixtus IV: Le arti a Roma*, 265. For editions of Hippocrates dedicated to Sixtus by Andrea Brenta, see Meyer, *Papal Series*, 320.

23. Francesco della Rovere, *De sanguine Christi*, BAV, Ms. Vat. lat. 1051, accessed May 9, 2018. https://digi.vatlib.it/view/MSS_Vat.lat.1051; ibid., *Tractatus de sanguine Christi* (Rome: Giovanni Filippo Lignamine, 1472). On the debate, see Lee, *Sixtus IV*, 19–20; Lorenzo Di Fonzo, "Sisto IV. Carriera scolastica e integrazioni biografiche (1414–84)," *Miscellanea Francescana* 86, nos. 2–4 (1986): 278–85; Concetta Bianca, "Francesco della Rovere: un Francescano tra teologia e potere," in Miglio et al., *Un pontificato*, 26–40.

24. Caroline Walker Bynum, *Wonderful Blood: Theology and Practice in Late Medieval Northern Germany and Beyond* (Philadelphia: University of Pennsylvania Press, 2007), 120–5, 127–30. On the connection to Botticelli's *Temptation of Christ / Cleansing of the Leper* in the Sistine Chapel, see Leopold Ettlinger, *The Sistine Chapel before Michelangelo: Religious Imagery and Papal Primacy* (Oxford: Clarendon Press, 1965), 83–4. (Bynum notes his misreading of the Dominican position.) The building in the fresco's background resembles the Hospital of Santo Spirito, on which see Carla Keyvanian, *Hospitals and Urbanism in Rome, 1200–1500* (Leiden and Boston: Brill, 2015), 345–51; cf. Eunice D. Howe, "A Temple Facade Reconsidered: Botticelli's *Temptation of Christ*," in Ramsey, *Rome in the Renaissance*, 209–21.

25. "Quibus sic stantibus arguimus sic: tempore passionis sacratissime nostri salvatoris dulcissimi Iesu Christi in corpore eius non solum fuit sanguis arterialis, sed etiam venalis; quod declaro ex sententia peritorum medicorum; que etiam satis clara est apud eos qui anothomiam viderunt, quam et ipse, dum Padue legerem, propriis luminibus sum intuitus." Della Rovere, *De sanguine Christi*, fols. 96v–97r. See also Bianca, "Francesco della Rovere," 37; Benzi, *Renovator Urbis*, 21.

26. For an overview of the Platonic-Galenic framework, see May, "Introduction," in Galen, *On the Usefulness of the Parts of the Body*, trans. Margaret Tallmadge May, 2 vols. (Ithaca, NY: Cornell University Press, 1968), 1:45–50; Nancy G. Siraisi, *Medieval & Early Renaissance Medicine: An Introduction to Knowledge and Practice* (Chicago and London: University of Chicago Press, 1990), 107–9; Andrew Cunningham, *The Anatomical Renaissance: The Resurrection of the Anatomical Projects of the Ancients* (Aldershot: Scolar, 1997), 10–13, 28–9.

27. Mondino de' Liuzzi, *Anatomia* (Venice, 1494), in *Medicina medievale: Testi dell'Alto Medioevo*, ed. Luigi Firpo (Turin: L'Unione Tipografico-Editrice Torinese, 1972), 165–204. See also Edward Grant, ed., *A Source Book in Medieval Science* (Cambridge, MA: Harvard University Press, 1974), 729–39.

28. Della Rovere, *De sanguine Christi*, fol. 95r; see Galen, *On the Natural Faculties*, trans. Arthur John Brock (Cambridge, MA: Harvard University Press, 1963), 19 (Book 1, ch. 5).

29. Della Rovere, *De sanguine Christi*, fols. 96v–97r.

30. Niccolò da Reggio's Latin translation of *De usu partium* first appeared in print in Venice in 1502, as part of Galen's *Opera omnia*, and in Paris in 1528 on its own. See Richard J. Durling, "A Chronological Census of Renaissance Editions and Translations of Galen," *Journal of the Warburg and Courtauld Institutes* 24, no. 3–4 (1961): 255; Stefania Fortuna, "The Latin Editions of Galen's *Opera omnia* (1490–1625) and Their Prefaces," *Early Science and Medicine* 17, no. 4 (2012): 395. On *De usu partium*'s Renaissance reception, see Nancy G. Siraisi, "Life Sciences and Medicine in the Renaissance World," in *Rome Reborn: The Vatican Library and Renaissance Culture*, ed. Anthony Grafton (Washington, DC: Library of Congress, 1993), 180; Donald F. Jackson, "Greek Medicine in the Fifteenth Century," *Early Science and Medicine* 17, no. 4 (2012): 378–90.

31. It is listed in Bologna's surviving curricular statutes. See Tiziana Pesenti, "The Libri Galieni in Italian Universities in the Fourteenth Century," *Italia medioevale e umanistica* 42 (2001): 120. On this text, see R. K. French, "*De iuvamentis membrorum* and the Reception of Galenic Physiological Anatomy," *Isis* 70, no. 1 (March 1979): 96–109.

32. BAV, Ms. Urb. gr. 69; Siraisi, "Life Sciences," 180–1. For its ownership by Cardinal Jacopo Ammannati, see Montserrat Moli Frigola, "Iakobo," in *Scrittura, biblioteche e stampa nel Quattrocento: Aspetti e problemi*, ed. Concetta Bianca et al. (Vatican City: Scuola Vaticana di Paleografia, Diplomatica e Archivistica, 1980), 198. On Ammannati and Sixtus IV, see Lee, *Sixtus IV*, 17–19.

33. The 1474 inventory by Sixtus's librarian Platina lists eleven Galen manuscripts in the Latin collection and three Greek texts. Among the Latin translations are several described in generic terms such as "various" works of Galen, which may have contained *De iuvamentis membrorum*. See Eugène Müntz and Paul Fabre, *La Bibliothèque du Vatican au XVe siècle d'après des documents inédits* (Paris: Ernest Thorin, 1887), 214–16, 234–5.

34. Galen, *De utilitate particularum libri XVII*, trans. Niccolò da Reggio, BAV, Ms. Vat. lat. 2380, accessed May 16, 2018. https://digi.vatlib.it/view/MSS_Vat.lat.2380, on which see Pesenti, "Libri Galieni," 121. It is identifiable by its *incipit* in the 1443 inventory of Pope Eugenius IV's collection; see Müntz and Fabre, *La Bibliothèque*, 23–4. It is not, however, listed by this title nor the *incipit* in Platina's 1474 inventory. For Niccolò's translation, see Durling, "Chronological

Census," 233; Stéphane Berlier, "Niccolò da Reggio traducteur du *De usu partium* de Galien. Place de la traduction latine dans l'histoire du texte," *Medicina nei secoli* 25, no. 3 (2013): 957–78.

35. See Galen, *De utilitate*, fol. 49; Galen, *Usefulness of the Parts*, 1:204 (Book 4, ch. 1). I have also consulted the 1528 print edition: Claudius Galenus, *De usu partium* (Paris: Simonis Colinaei, 1528), 101, accessed June 1, 2018. https://hdl.handle.net/2027/uc1.31378008366729.

36. See Galen, *Usefulness of the Parts*, 1:205 (Book 4, ch. 2); Galen, *De utilitate*, fol. 49–50. See also Galen, *On the Natural Faculties*, 37 (Book 1, ch. 10).

37. Aristotle, *De motu animalium*, 703a29–30; Martha Craven Nussbaum, *Aristotle's De Motu Animalium: Text with Translation, Commentary and Interpretive Essays* (Princeton: Princeton University Press, 1978), 52. Sixtus's copy of Buridan's commentary on this Aristotle text (see above, n. 18) inexplicably cuts off before chapter 5, which addresses the relevant passage. It nonetheless suggests that he knew the Aristotelian text. Peter of Auvergne's commentary on the same text is listed in Platina's 1474 Vatican Library inventory; see Petrus de Alvernia, *Expositio sup. Lib. Arist. de motu animalium* BAV, Ms. Vat. lat. 2181, fols. 1r–7v, accessed May 18, 2018. https://digi.vatlib.it/view/MSS_Vat.lat.2181; Müntz and Fabre, *La Bibliothèque*, 211.

38. Romans 12:4–5; 1 Corinthians 12: 12–27; Ephesians 5:23; Colossians 1:18. See Leonard Barkan, *Nature's Work of Art: The Human Body as Image of the World* (New Haven and London: Yale University Press, 1975), 69.

39. Paul Archambault, "The Analogy of the 'Body' in Renaissance Political Literature," *Bibliothèque d'Humanisme et Renaissance* 29, no. 1 (1967): 22–35.

40. Nicholas of Cusa, *The Catholic Concordance*, trans. Paul E. Sigmund (Cambridge and New York: Cambridge University Press, 1995), 215 (Book 3, ch. 1). See also Morimichi Watanabe, *The Political Ideas of Nicholas of Cusa with Special Reference to his* De concordantia catholica (Geneva: Librairie Droz, 1963), 180–3; Barkan, *Nature's Work of Art*, 73–4. On Cusano's and Sixtus's shared patterns of philosophical thought, see Benzi, *Renovator Urbis*, 20–1.

41. Nicholas of Cusa, *The Catholic Concordance*, 318–21 (Book 3, ch. 41).

42. "Una citta debba essere quasi come uno chorpo humano." See Antonio Averlino (Filarete), *Treatise on Architecture*, trans. John R. Spencer (New Haven and London: Yale University Press, 1965), 1:45; 2:25v for the original. See also Leon Battista Alberti, *On the Art of Building in Ten Books*, trans. Joseph Rykwert, Neil Leach, and Robert Tavernor (Cambridge, MA: MIT Press, 1988), 23 (Book 1, ch. 9).

43. Francesco di Giorgio Martini, *Trattati di architettura ingegneria e arte militare*, ed. Corrado Maltese (Milan: Il Polifilo, 1967), 1:3–4, 20. On the influence of political thought on Martini, see Lawrence Lowic, "The Meaning and Significance of the Human Analogy in Francesco di Giorgio's Trattato," *Journal of the Society of Architectural Historians* 42, no. 4 (December 1983): 362–3. See also Angeliki Pollali, "Human analogy in *Trattati I*: The *Ragione* of Modern Architecture," in *Reconstructing Francesco di Giorgio Architect*, ed. Berthold Hub and Angeliki Pollali (Frankfurt am Main: Peter Lang, 2011), 59–84.

44. On this image, see Simon Pepper, "Body, Diagram, and Geometry in the Renaissance Fortress," in *Body and Building: Essays on the Changing Relation of Body and Architecture*, ed. George Dodds and Robert Tavernor (Cambridge, MA and London: MIT Press, 2002), 115–16. Galen, *Usefulness of the Parts*, 1: 379 (Book 7, ch. 21).

45. *Regula Hospitalis S. Spiritus*, BAV, Ms. Borgh.242, fol. 3r, ch. 37, accessed May 15, 2018. https://digi.vatlib.it/view/MSS_Borgh.242; Pietro de Angelis, *L'Ospedale di Santo Spirito in Saxia* (Rome: [n.p.], 1962), 1:259. See also Anna Esposito, "Assistenza e organizzazione sanitaria nell'Ospedale di Santo Spirito," *Il Veltro* 45, no. 5-6 (September-December 2001): 203; Flavia Colonna, *L'ospedale di Santo Spirito in Sassia: Lo sviluppo dell'assistenza e le trasformazioni architettonico-funzionali* (Rome: Edizioni Quasar, 2009), 50, 54; John Henderson, *The Renaissance Hospital: Healing the Body and Healing the Soul* (New Haven and London: Yale University Press, 2006), 163.

46. Text in Müntz, *Les arts*, 179–80. See also Simoncini, *Topografia*, 172–3.

47. "Vi spese una buona somma d'oro, essendo le strade di Roma in alcune parti impraticabili, dove vi nasceva financo l'erba, et che rendevano puzzore, et altre strade che erano piene di fango, e di immonditie." *Diario di Sisto IV*, in BAV, Ms. Urb. lat. 1641, fols. 33v–34r, accessed July 2, 2018. https://digi.vatlib.it/view/MSS_Urb.lat.1641. See also Simoncini, *Topografia*, 172.

48. The decree of January 8, 1480 is in Camillo Scaccia Scarafoni, "L'antico statuto dei 'Magistri Stratarum' e altri documenti relativi a quella magistratura," *Archivio della Società Romana di Storia Patria* 50 (1927): 283. See Anna Modigliani, "L'approvigionamento annonario e i luoghi del commercio alimentare," in Simoncini, *Funzioni urbane*, 43–4.

49. For street sweeping and the Cloaca Maxima, see Lee, *Sixtus IV*, 135. On paving, Ceen, "Quartiere de' Banchi," 30. See also Galen, *Usefulness of the Parts*, 1:205 (Book 4, ch. 3), 206 (ch. 4), 207 (ch. 6), 240 (ch. 18).

50. Müntz, *Les arts*, 182–7; Simoncini, *Funzioni urbane*, 272–7.
51. On the *maestri*, see Scaccia Scarafoni, "L'antico statuto"; Magnuson, *Roman Quattrocento Architecture*, 35–41; Orietta Verdi, "Da ufficiali capitolini a commissari apostolici: I maestri delle strade e delle edifici di Roma tra XIII e XVI secoli," in *Il Campidoglio e Sisto V*, ed. Luigi Spezzaferro and Maria Elisa Tittoni (Rome: Edizioi Carte Segrete, 1991), 57. See also Jill Elizabeth Blondin, "Constructing History: The Visual Legacy of Pope Sixtus IV" (Ph.D. diss., University of Illinois, Urbana-Champaign, 2002), 105–7; Simoncini, *Topografia*, 184–5. On d'Estouteville, Pastor, *History of the Popes*, 4:455.
52. The following is based on: Tomei, "Le strade," 13–14; Ceen, "Quartiere de' Banchi," 29–37; Lee, *Sixtus IV*, 127–9; Fagiolo and Madonna, *Roma 1300–1875*, 107–10; Blondin, "Power Made Visible," 11–14; Simoncini, *Topografia*, 172–84, catalog of street improvements, 269–84.
53. Blondin, "Power Made Visible," 12 n. 32; Kajanto, *Papal Epigraphy*, 83. See also Ceen, "Quartiere de' Banchi," 34–5; Fagiolo and Madonna, *Roma 1300–1875*, 107.
54. Blondin, "Power Made Visible," 11–12; Cantatore, "Sisto IV committente," 319; Keyvanian, *Hospitals and Urbanism*, 376–7.
55. Simoncini, *Topografia*, 176–7; Cantatore, "Sisto IV committente," 319.
56. Luigi Spezzaferro, "Ponte Sisto," in *Via Giulia: una utopia urbanistica del '500*, ed. Luigi Salerno, Luigi Spezzaferro, and Manfredo Tafuri (Rome: A. Staderini, 1975), 521–6; Gaetano Miarelli Mariani et al., eds., *Ponte Sisto (1475–1975; 1877–1977): Ricerche e proposte* (Rome: Multigrafica Editrice, 1977); Maurizio Gargano, "Ponte Sisto a Roma, nuove acquisizioni (1473–1475)," *Quaderni dell'Istituto di storia dell'architettura* 21 (1994): 29–38; Minou Schraven, "Founding Rome Anew: Pope Sixtus IV and the Foundation of Ponte Sisto, 1473," in *Foundation, Dedication and Consecration in Early Modern Europe*, ed. Minou Schraven and Maarten Delbeke (Leiden: Brill, 2012), 129–50.
57. Lee, *Sixtus IV*, 126–7, 242; Fagiolo and Madonna, *Roma 1300–1875*, 106; Spezzaferro, "Ponte Sisto," 523–4; Simoncini, *Topografia*, 171–2.
58. "Pontem etiam media Urbis regione Tyberis … instauravit … cuius pontis opportunitate tota regio illa transtyberina, quae inanissima, et immundissima erat, frequentissima et cultissima reddita est." Sigismondo dei Conti, *Le storie de' suoi tempi dal 1475 al 1510*, 2 vols. (Florence: G. Barbèra, 1883–5), 1:205–6, accessed July 2, 2018. https://books.google.com/books?id=R1YhHQAACAAJ.
59. Epigraph text in Guerrini, "L'epigrafia," 471. Platina, "Life of Sixtus IV," in Howe, *Art and Culture*, 193.
60. Ceen, "Quartiere de' Banchi," 33; Lee, *Sixtus IV*, 129–30; Howe, *Hospital*, 34–5; Fagiolo and Madonna, *Roma 1300–1875*, 102–7; Simoncini, *Topografia*, 161–2; Cantatore, "Sisto IV committente," 315–16.
61. Keyvanian, *Hospitals and Urbanism*, 368.
62. Galen, *Usefulness of the Parts*, 1:204 (Book 4, ch. 2).
63. Keyvanian, *Hospitals and Urbanism*, 370–83. On the commercial importance of Ponte Sisto, see also Modigliani, "L'approvigionamento annonario," 60–1; Spezzaferro, "Ponte Sisto," 524.
64. On the Acqua Vergine and Nicholas V., Cesare D'Onofrio, *Acque e fontane di Roma* (Rome: Staderini, 1977), 15–42; John Pinto, *The Trevi Fountain* (New Haven and London: Yale University Press, 1986), 28–31; David Karmon, "Restoring the Ancient Water Supply System in Renaissance Rome: The Popes, the Civic Administration, and the Acqua Vergine," *The Waters of Rome* 3 (2005): 6–7; Simoncini, *Topografia*, 133. For Sixtus's interventions, see Pastor, *History of the Popes*, 4:274; D'Onofrio, *Acque e fontane*, 22; Lee, *Sixtus IV*, 142–3, 247–8; Simoncini, *Topografia*, 190. Archival documents for the repairs in Müntz, *Les arts*, 174–6.
65. Galen, *Usefulness of the Parts*, 2:682 (Book 16, ch. 1); also 1:207 (Book 4, ch. 5).
66. Ceen, "Quartiere de' Banchi," 36; Lee, *Sixtus IV*, 134; Blondin, "Power Made Visible," 1; Simoncini, *Topografia*, 203; Cantatore, "Sisto IV committente," 315, 322–3.
67. De' Liuzzi, *Anatomia*, 167; translation from Grant, *Source Book*, 730–1. See also Galen, *Usefulness of the Parts*, 1:396 (Book 8, ch. 5).
68. Westfall, *In this Most Perfect Paradise*, 130.
69. Leonard E. Boyle, O.P., "Sixtus IV and the Vatican Library," in *Rome: Tradition, Innovation and Renewal*, ed. C. Brown, J. Osborne, and C. Kirwin ([Victoria, BC]: [University of Victoria], 1991), 65–73; Anthony Grafton, "The Vatican and Its Library," in Grafton, *Rome Reborn*, 34; Antonio Manfredi, "La nascita della Vaticana in età umanistica da Niccolò V a Sisto IV," in *Storia della Biblioteca Vaticana I: Le origini della Biblioteca Vaticana tra umanesimo e rinascimento (1447–1534)*, ed. Antonio Manfredi (Vatican City: Biblioteca Apostolica Vaticana, 2010), esp. 149, 198, 212; Blondin, "Constructing History," 121–8. On the library's architecture, see Flavia Cantatore, "La Biblioteca Vaticana nel palazzo di Niccolò V," in Manfredi, *Storia della Biblioteca Vaticana I*, 383–412.

70. Ettlinger, *Sistine Chapel*; Keyvanian, *Hospitals and Urbanism*, 342–3.
71. Keyvanian, *Hospitals and Urbanism*, 361.
72. Nicholas of Cusa, *The Catholic Concordance*, 318 (Book 3, ch. 41).
73. A list of churches is in Cantatore, "Sisto IV committente," 328–9. See also Pastor, *History of the Popes*, 4:275, 456; Lee, *Sixtus IV*, 143–5; Fagiolo and Madonna, *Roma 1300–1875*, 103–04. For the Marian churches, Benzi, *Renovator Urbis*, 99–107, 114–19.
74. Benzi, *Renovator Urbis*, 108–13, 120–3. For d'Estouteville, see also Simoncini, *Topografia*, 177–8.
75. For the text of the bull, see Müntz, *Les arts*, 182; Simoncini, *Funzioni urbane*, 273.
76. Della Rovere, *De sanguine Christi*, fol. 97r. On the heart, see Galen, *Usefulness of the Parts*, 278–334 (Book 6).
77. Siraisi, *Medieval & Early Renaissance Medicine*, 108.
78. Isidore of Seville, *The Etymologies of Isidore of Seville*, trans. Stephen A. Barney et al. (Cambridge and New York: Cambridge University Press, 2006), 238. This text was in Sixtus's Vatican Library; see Müntz and Fabre, *La Bibliothèque*, 187–8.
79. See, for example, Ambrogio Lorenzetti's depiction of *Caritas* in his *Allegory of Good Government* (*c.* 1339) in the Palazzo Pubblico of Siena.
80. Howe, *Hospital*, 57–8; Blondin, "Constructing History," 36; Keyvanian, *Hospitals and Urbanism*, 361.
81. On the early history of the hospital: De Angelis, *L'Ospedale*, 1:205–24; Howe, *Hospital*, 3–27; Colonna, *L'Ospedale*, 7–9; Keyvanian, *Hospitals and Urbanism*, 79–85.
82. As reflected in the *Liber regulae* of the order of Santo Spirito and Innocent's bull founding the hospital, in De Angelis, *L'Ospedale*, 1:241, 381–4. Also, Anna Esposito, "Gli ospedali romani tra iniziative laicali e politica pontificia (secc. XIII–XV)," in *Ospedali e città. L'Italia del Centro-Nord, XIII–XVI secolo*, ed. Allen J. Grieco and Lucia Sandri (Florence: Casa Editrice Le Lettere, 1997), 234–5.
83. Eunice D. Howe, "Appropriating Space: Women's Place in Confraternal Life at Santo Spirito in Sassia, Rome," in *Confraternities and the Visual Arts in Renaissance Italy: Ritual, Spectacle, Image*, ed. Barbara Wisch and Diane Cole Ahl (Cambridge: Cambridge University Press, 2000), 235. On the theme of charity at Santo Spirito, see also Howe, *Art and Culture*, 146–57, 163–4.
84. Howe, *Hospital*, 43; Giorgio Cosmacini, *Storia della medicina e della sanità in Italia dalla peste europea alla Guerra Mondiale, 1348–1918* (Rome and Bari. Laterza, 1987), 57; Esposito, "Gli ospedali romani," 235. On the importance of abandoned infants at Santo Spirito, see Diana Bullen Presciutti, "Dead Infants, Cruel Mothers, and Heroic Popes: The Visual Rhetoric of Foundling Care at the Hospital of Santo Spirito, Rome," *Renaissance Quarterly* 64, no. 3 (2011): 752–99. On hospital specialization, see Cosmacini, *Storia della medicina*, 43–68; Henderson, *Renaissance Hospital*, 25–8.
85. For the bull and registry of names, see De Angelis, *L'Ospedale*, 2:104–10, 648–54. See Lee, *Sixtus IV*, 139–41; Howe, *Hospital*, 38–47, on Sixtus's attention to the hospital finances and the order from 1472–84.
86. Flavia Colonna, "Distribuzione urbana e tipologie degli edifici assistenziali," in Simoncini, *Funzioni urbane*, 166–7; Cantatore, "Sisto IV committente," 328.
87. "Hospitale item Sancti Spiritus sepulchrum potius ob situm et incommoditatem loci, quam pauperum et aegrotantium hospitium, restituere adorsus, magna iecit fundamenta, cum ad ornatum Urbis, tum vel maxime ad perigrinoram et aegrotantium commoditatem." Platina, "Life of Sixtus IV," in Howe, *Art and Culture*, 193.
88. For the building chronology, see Howe, *Hospital*, 32–3, 39–41. Colonna argues that the new ward was in fact a completion of an unfinished project by Paul II, to which Sixtus added the exterior portico and the hospital cloisters. See Colonna, *L'Ospedale*, IX–XX, 25–39; ibid., "Paolo II Barbo e un suo possibile intervento nel quattrocentesco ospedale di S. Spirito," *Il Veltro* 45, no. 5–6 (2001): 331–9. Cf. Keyvanian, *Hospitals and Urbanism*, 352 n. 21. On the extension of the Innocentine structure, see ibid., 350–1. On the various attributions, see Colonna, *L'Ospedale*, 39–41.
89. This wing is known from the 1530s as the "Ospedaletto" and described as a separate space. It does not appear in Schedel's 1493 view in Figure 7.2. See Howe, *Hospital*, 65–8; ibid., "L'ospedale di Santo Spirito come città ideale," *Il Veltro* 45, no. 5–6 (2001): 347. But cf. Colonna, *L'Ospedale*, 86 n. 20. On the Ospedale Maggiore, see Philip Foster, "Per il disegno dell'Ospedale di Milano," *Arte lombarda* 18, no. 38–9 (1973): 1–22.
90. De Angelis, *L'Ospedale*, 2:649. My description of the layout is based on Howe, "Appropriating Space," 246–7; Howe, "Città ideale," 347–9. These adapt her earlier analysis: Howe, *Hospital*, 56, 62–5. Later, the nobles' quarters instead may have occupied two wings on the east side of the cross arm. See Colonna, *L'Ospedale*, 33 n. 32; Howe, *Hospital*, 65.
91. See also Colonna, *L'Ospedale*, 33, 44; Howe, "Città ideale," 349.

92. Gregory Martin, *Roma Sancta*, ed. George Bruner Parks (Rome: Edizioni di Storia e Letteratura, 1969), 185. On the hospital as an "ideal city," see Howe, "Città ideale," 349, 351.
93. The east end we see today is a result of a restoration campaign in the 1940s, following the demolition of an eighteenth-century extension. The four windows below the gable were added at that time; the original façade contained two oculi in place of the middle pair. See Howe, "Temple Façade"; Colonna, *L'Ospedale*, 97–104, 122–3.
94. Gasparo Alveri, *Roma in ogni stato*, 2 vols. (Rome: Fabio Falco, 1664), 2:255–6, accessed July 5, 2018. https://books.google.com/books?id=s0kokCu_dugC. See Howe, *Hospital*, 59; ibid., "Città ideale," 347.
95. On processions, see Howe, "Appropriating Space," 248–9. For almsgiving, Edward P. de G. Chaney, "Giudizi inglesi su ospedali italiani, 1545–1789," in *Timore e carità: i poveri nell'Italia moderna*, ed. Giorgio Politi, Mario Rosa, and Franco della Peruta (Cremona: Biblioteca Statale, 1982), 92.
96. Anna Esposito, "Assistenza," 203; De Angelis, *L'Ospedale*, 1:259 (ch. 35 of the *Regula*).
97. For the registers, De Angelis, *L'Ospedale*, 2:111–302.
98. Howe, *Hospital*, 162, 177–8 n. 3; Keyvanian, *Hospitals and Urbanism*, 354. On the reception of Queen Charlotte, see Albertini, *Opusculum*, fol. 84v. This source is, however, much later than the queen's visit on March 27, 1478. See Pietro de Angelis, *L'architetto e gli affreschi di Santo Spirito in Saxia* (Rome: Nuova Tecnica Grafica, 1961), 244–5. The fresco in the Corsia Sistina places the event in a generic outdoor setting, like the other scenes of reception on the same wall.
99. Colonna, *L'Ospedale*, 67–8.
100. On the Corsia's church-like character, Howe, *Hospital*, 186–7. On care for soul and body, see Henderson, *Renaissance Hospital*.
101. Anonymous seventeenth-century description cited in Chaney, "Giudizi inglesi," 94.
102. Henderson, *Renaissance Hospital*, 165.
103. Martin, *Roma Sancta*, 185.
104. Henderson, *Renaissance Hospital*, 158–9.
105. On this broad audience, see Howe, *Art and Culture*, 163; Presciutti, "Dead Infants," 757, 767.
106. Five of the scenes, at the east side of the north wall, were painted in 1599. The most extensive treatment of the fresco cycle, including the dating, is Howe, *Hospital*, 93–304; Howe, *Art and Culture*. Howe assigns the lead role to Antoniazzo Romano, and the program to Sixtus's librarian Platina. See also Maria Alessandra Cassiani, "L'Ospedale di Santo Spirito in Sassia: cultura francescana e devozione nel ciclo pittorico della corsia sistina," in Benzi, *Sisto IV*, 167–73; Massimo Miglio, "Una biografia pontificia per immagini: Sisto IV e l'Ospedale di Santo Spirito," *Il Veltro* 45, no. 5–6 (2001): 111–24. The frescoes are illustrated in full in Howe, *Hospital*, and de Angelis, *L'architetto*.
107. On this part of the cycle, see Presciutti, "Dead Infants," 760–83.
108. Translation and original text in Howe, *Hospital*, 359, 361. On the theme of rebuilding vs. new construction, see Fagiolo and Madonna, *Roma 1300–1875*, 105; Kajanto, *Papal Epigraphy*, 83; Simoncini, *Topografia*, 203.
109. Averlino, *Treatise on Architecture*, 1:12 (Book 1); original text in 2:6r. See also Alberti, *Art of Building*, 320 (Book 10, ch. 1).
110. Dale Kent, *Cosimo de' Medici and the Florentine Renaissance: The Patron's Oeuvre* (New Haven and London: Yale University Press, 2000), 5–6.
111. Translation and original text in Howe, *Hospital*, 363.
112. Howe, *Hospital*, 305; Blondin, "Constructing History," 40–1; ibid., "Power Made Visible," 24.
113. See also Benzi, *Renovator Urbis*, 26–7; Blondin, "Constructing History," 127.

CHAPTER 8
SPACES OF HEALING IN EARLY MODERN PORTUGUESE EMPIRE
CHANGING PUBLIC HEALTH AND HOSPITAL BUILDINGS ON MOZAMBIQUE ISLAND
Eugénia Rodrigues

Research on hospital buildings and sites in the Western world has shown how, throughout the early modern period, the typology of edifices, architectural styles, and their location changed according to various historical contexts. From the eighteenth century onward, the shift in care for patients from being a religious charitable act to active medicalization as well as the resurgence of environmental perspectives on disease and health changed the characteristics of hospital buildings and the organization of their internal spaces. The rise of public policies for healthcare and the emphasis on preventive medicine increased the number of hospitals and resulted in their reorganization according to new medical models, as well as a mechanism to better monitor patients and medical staff.[1] Hospital architecture is also discussed as part of spatial practices in the context of European urbanization, with a focus on the landscape in which hospitals were built, which articulates internal and external changes.[2] European powers tended to transfer domestic models to their empires. However, as David Arnold, a historian of medicine in India, highlights in relation to medicine in the tropics, it is necessary to also consider the impact of local factors. Thus, these transpositions from Europe to overseas domains were not mimetic and entailed their own cultural configurations.[3]

In the case of Portugal and its overseas empire, scholarly literature has paid scant attention to the architecture of hospitals and how it was incorporated into the urban landscape, generally mentioning it only in the context of broader research. For example, this is the case with studies on All Saints Royal Hospital in Lisbon, which was established in 1492 by the Portuguese Crown in the framework of reforms providing for poor relief and healthcare. These studies demonstrate that the regulation of the hospital in Lisbon followed the model of organization and functioning of Italian hospitals, especially Santa Maria Nuova hospital in Florence, and that it was inspired by the architectural layout of the Lombard hospitals. Set out as a Greek cross, the large All Saints Royal Hospital consisted of three-story buildings in a symmetrical structure. As Santa Maria Nuova hospital it was organized into several gendered infirmaries, a church, administrative rooms, and spaces for daily life. Occupying a central location in the Portuguese capital, which was enjoying a spurt of urban growth due to its standing as a leading maritime Atlantic port, the new hospital also served as an affirmation of royal power.[4] Pointing to the same kind of legitimation, the Queen's House established a thermal hospital at Caldas da Rainha, approximately 100 kilometers north of Lisbon, whose regimen was similar to that of All Saints Royal Hospital.[5] However, most of the hospitals in Portugal were small institutions scattered across the countryside, such as those maintained by the Holy Houses of Mercy (Santas Casas da Misericórdia), which deserves some scrutiny from scholars.[6] The architecture of the military hospitals that were established in Portugal during the seventeenth century—some in buildings that were adapted while others were specifically built for that purpose—has also been studied.[7] In turn, the growing literature on hospitals in the Portuguese Empire, mainly in Brazil and India, explores some physical characteristics of the edifices.[8]

In relation to Mozambique Island, in modern-day Mozambique, the subject of this chapter, some studies have analyzed health policies and the administration of hospitals, but shed little light on the buildings themselves.[9] This chapter addresses the progressive transformation of the hospital established by the Portuguese Crown on Mozambique Island in the early sixteenth century, as well as the role played by the hospital run by the Santa Casa da Misericórdia that was settled during the eighteenth century. Instituted by the Portuguese Crown as a mechanism to build its empire in the Indian Ocean, the royal hospital underwent changes in the location and structure of the edifices in response to prevailing medical perspectives. Notions about health and disease and public policies that supported changes in hospitals in Europe also shaped the configuration of hospital buildings on Mozambique Island, although they had to take local contexts into account. Over time, concerns about the building's role varied, reflecting different medical, social, and urban contexts. Changes in hospital architecture were particularly noticeable during the eighteenth century, when the former structure was progressively expanded and redesigned in attempts, often deemed unfruitful, to provide suitable conditions for healing patients. While outlining the evolution of health politics and the royal hospital on Mozambique Island, this chapter discusses how European models of architecture were transposed to imperial territories and interacted with local cultures.

Empire and Health: The Royal Hospital on Mozambique Island

To a great extent, the Portuguese Empire in the Indian Ocean was a Crown-run enterprise, and this conditioned health services policies. From the sixteenth century onward, the Portuguese Crown assumed responsibility for maintaining hospital facilities in the Indian Ocean, just as it did in Lisbon at the Real Hospital de Todos os Santos.[10]

In the early sixteenth century, the Portuguese established factories in various cities along the East African coast, including Sofala and Mozambique Island, in present-day Mozambique, as part of their strategy to build an empire in the Indian Ocean. As was the case with other Swahili port cities, Mozambique Island, situated in the bay of Mossuril, north of Mozambique, was governed by a Muslim elite, represented by a sheik, and had close ties with Kilwa in what is now Kenya. Measuring almost 3 kilometers in length and with a maximum width of 500 meters, the island was a narrow, sandy area that depended on supplies of food and water from the neighboring mainland. Even though it was not a well-known trading station at the time, it played a crucial function in supporting the route linking Kilwa and Sofala—the main port for trading gold procured from the Karanga plateau south of the Zambezi River. Vessels stopped there for repairs and supplies.[11]

The role it played in providing assistance for navigation also attracted the Portuguese to Mozambique Island. In 1507, they built a small fortification, the Tower of São Gabriel, with warehouses to complement their factory in Sofala (1505) in central Mozambique. While the shallow waters along the Sofala coast were an obstacle for Portuguese carracks, Mozambique Island offered a sheltered deep-water port, and thus increasingly became the main port of call on the India route. The carracks that set out every year from Lisbon for India, and some on the return voyage, would stop there to replenish their supplies of fresh food and water, while soldiers, crewmates, and passengers could recover after a long voyage. The vessels often had to winter on the island, staying there for several months for repairs or awaiting favorable monsoon winds.[12]

By the 1530s, Mozambique Island had become the political seat of Portuguese establishments in Southeast Africa, integrated into the Estado da Índia (State of India) and governed from Goa, India. Simultaneously, its port acquired an increasingly important role in African trade as the Portuguese expanded their networks along the coast and the Zambezi River Valley. It became a military base from the 1540s onward due to the island's relevance as a way station on the India route and hub for African trade. The São Sebastião fortress was constructed on the northeastern tip to contain Ottoman expansionism and, subsequently, the rise of other

European powers. The fortress was intended to house three hundred soldiers, although that figure was rarely achieved. Military expeditions sent to the Zambezi Valley to conquer the famed Monomotapa, from the 1570s onward, also increased the total number of soldiers on the island.[13]

The political, military, and economic importance of Mozambique Island resulted in its urban growth, which, however, was not very significant. The Portuguese town was located in the central part of the island on the western side, next to the port and facing the continent. As the Portuguese progressively dominated the territory, the Swahili sheik was obliged to shift his settlement to the mainland, although part of the population remained on the island. Just like the Swahili, the Portuguese depended on supplies of water and produce from the neighboring mainland, but that practice proved to be insufficient to meet the needs of a burgeoning population and the many carracks that docked at the island. Foodstuffs were imported from more distant places, including the Zambezi Valley, Madagascar, and India.[14]

Keeping an important position in the Indian Ocean mercantile networks while later extending its influence to the Atlantic through its participation in slave trading, Mozambique Island developed multidirectional connections with other cultures. Although the island was under colonial rule, these specific historical conditions led to the emergence of a multicultural society in which diverse groups interacted, including in terms of medical practices. Indeed, throughout the early modern period, the medicine of the colonizers incorporated practices of other social actors who inhabited the island and the mainland, as well as those who stayed there for long periods for commercial reasons.[15] Health services for the colony's population as well as for the individuals arriving aboard the carracks integrated the policy of building the empire. In 1507, hospital facilities were installed at the island in a wooden building, located outside the walls of the first fortress that the Portuguese erected next to the port. This edifice, constructed by soldiers who stayed on the island, was described as a large house with a rear veranda, with separate houses for the nurse, the attending medic, and the pharmacy.[16] In 1538, it was replaced by a stone structure, with a rectangular shape and an inner courtyard according to its appearance on a map of Mozambique Island.[17] Similar to hospitals in Europe, it had religious facilities, the small church of Holy Spirit, and most likely a single hall.[18] Thus, along with the movement of people, European hospital patterns circulated across the territories of the empire as well.

The edifice was probably erected in keeping with the architecture of Portuguese hospitals and used both rocks found on the island as well as stones carried as ballast on ships sailing from Lisbon to Goa. The same combination of local and imported materials is found in the construction of the Sofala in the same period. This hospital was certainly spacious. In 1563, for example, a Jesuit father mentioned that there were more than 370 patients at the hospital, a number that was equivalent to those found in leading military hospitals in Europe during this period.[19] Despite its relatively large size, the hospital was located amid narrow streets that shaped the settlement.

However, little is known about the hospital operation during the sixteenth and seventeenth centuries. It was managed by local institutions, including the charitable institution Holy House of Mercy (Santa Casa da Misericórdia), a brotherhood commissioned by the Crown in 1564 to administer civil hospitals in Portugal.[20] The hospital was not designed to assist Africans but the soldiers and settlers as well as all those who arrived there aboard ships from Lisbon and from Indian Ocean ports.[21] Because local residents or *moradores*—Portuguese, Indian, and mixed-race people—received treatment primarily at home, most of the patients at the hospital were resident soldiers or sailors. The number of patients rose seasonally as the carracks arrived and increased even further when the ships were obliged to winter there. Without adequate food and water, the lengthy journey from Portugal would result in several diseases such as scurvy.[22] Sometimes the number of these mobile patients exceeded the hospital's capacity and it was necessary to build temporary shelters for them.[23]

As historian of European medicine Mary Lindemann argues, most scholars are of the view that early modern hospitals "offered little medical care, or at the very least, that was not their primary function."[24] It is not known exactly what care was provided in Mozambique since there were often no surgeons or bleeders. Individuals sailing aboard the carracks frequently provided therapeutic care since it was common for missionaries to spend their time on land caring for the sick.[25] However, in the sixteenth century, just as in the royal hospital in Goa, the hospital in Mozambique had a reputation for providing good accommodation, food, and medicines to patients.[26] In fact, the hospital was intended not only to house and feed the sick but also to provide medical care, following the pattern of royal hospitals in Lisbon.[27] For example, a royal letter dating from 1562 emphasizes "curing and healing the sick," ordering that the hospital should be consistently well supplied with "remedies and pharmacy drugs."[28]

In an age when the concept of illness was rooted in humors, as per the Hippocratic-Galenic tradition, health was understood to be derived from a balance of these fluids in the human body and disease was viewed as the outcome of imbalanced humors, influenced by environmental factors, including food and beverages. Medical therapies sought to readjust the proportion of fluids in each individual by means of bleeding, purges, sweating, vomiting, and drugs. The "pharmacy drugs" mentioned in the letter penned by the Portuguese king were also used to correct such imbalances. Moreover, for Christians, as for the Portuguese, the natural causes of illnesses, as explained by Hippocratic-Galenic medicine, mingled with religious convictions that attributed some ailments to divine entities and endorsed the role of prayer to obtain God's intervention in the healing process. The strong presence in the hospital of missionaries who arrived aboard the carracks and provided spiritual cures in addition to physical healing thus also helped ensure the hospital's good reputation.[29]

The standing of the hospital in Mozambique worsened considerably during the seventeenth century. The hospital building was destroyed during the Dutch sieges on Mozambique Island (1607–8) and the government installed it in some rented houses. The Portuguese administration was not able to erect a new building until in the 1630s. Since the ground on which the former hospitals were built had been leased to a private individual, the new structure was constructed at another site within the urban center, but its exact location is not clear. As had been the case in Goa, the hospital's administration was entrusted to the Jesuits in 1629, even before the construction was concluded.[30] Thus, unlike in Europe, where during the early modern period hospitals tended to be transferred from religious to civil authorities, the opposite happened in Mozambique and continued until the mid-eighteenth century.[31] As before, the hospital functioned under a contractual system in which the Crown paid the religious a certain amount annually in exchange for assistance provided to the sick. The hospital also benefited from pious endowments and testamentary legacies that allowed it to increase its budget. However, facing continuous complaints about the quality of care, in 1680 the Jesuits refused to continue with the responsibility of the hospital's administration.[32]

From the late 1670s, proposals were circulated to hand over the hospitals in the Estado da Índia to the Brothers Hospitallers of Saint John of God. This order was created by the disciples of the Portuguese soldier João de Deus (1495–1550), who was renowned for his care of the sick in Granada, Spain. Recognized as an order by Pope Pius V in 1572, the Brothers Hospitallers ensured the operation of military hospitals in Portugal from the early seventeenth century. Thus the Hospitallers were commissioned to run the hospital in Mozambique, as well as those in Goa, Bassein, Daman, and Diu, in the Portuguese State of India.[33] Preparations for this transition began in 1680, and in the following year a warrant issued by the regent, Dom Pedro, entrusted the Order of Hospitallers with the task of establishing a hospital on Mozambique Island, "not only to heal the soldiers at the fortress and the local residents but all the soldiers who arrive there, including those traveling aboard the carracks, to convalesce or to continue on their voyage."[34] The Crown maintained with the Hospitallers the former system of contract in which the budget was managed by the prior of the convent and administrator of the hospital. The Brothers were the main caregivers for the patients, along with a chief-surgeon, since the chief physician who had been appointed at the time had died and was not replaced. Just as in many European hospitals, missionaries served as nurses.[35] Although most of the patients were soldiers, they included individuals of Portuguese, Goan, and mixed-race origin that composed the regiment of infantry. The African slaves pertaining to the Portuguese government, the so-called king's slaves, were also healed in the hospital.

The transfer of the hospital's administration to the Hospitallers was accompanied by the decision to change its location. The site chosen for the new royal hospital was outside the town on an open field south of the settlement. Instead of building a new structure, the Portuguese Crown decided to purchase two houses that had been the residence of a deceased merchant, Vicente Dourado, "as they are suitable and there are no other buildings in the said settlement that could serve the said purpose."[36] The hospital was also located opposite the fortress of São Sebastião, in the north of the island, the area from which most of the patients came. The property had a brackish water well and a cistern, which were invaluable assets considering that water was an extremely scarce resource. The houses were surrounded by a fence that extended up to the island's west coast toward the bay. The estate offered space for cultivation where innumerable palms were planted, along with a garden in which the plants habitually used to cure patients were grown (Figure 8.1).[37] Such features were also common in European hospitals—specifically in the military hospitals administered by the Brothers Hospitallers in Portugal.[38]

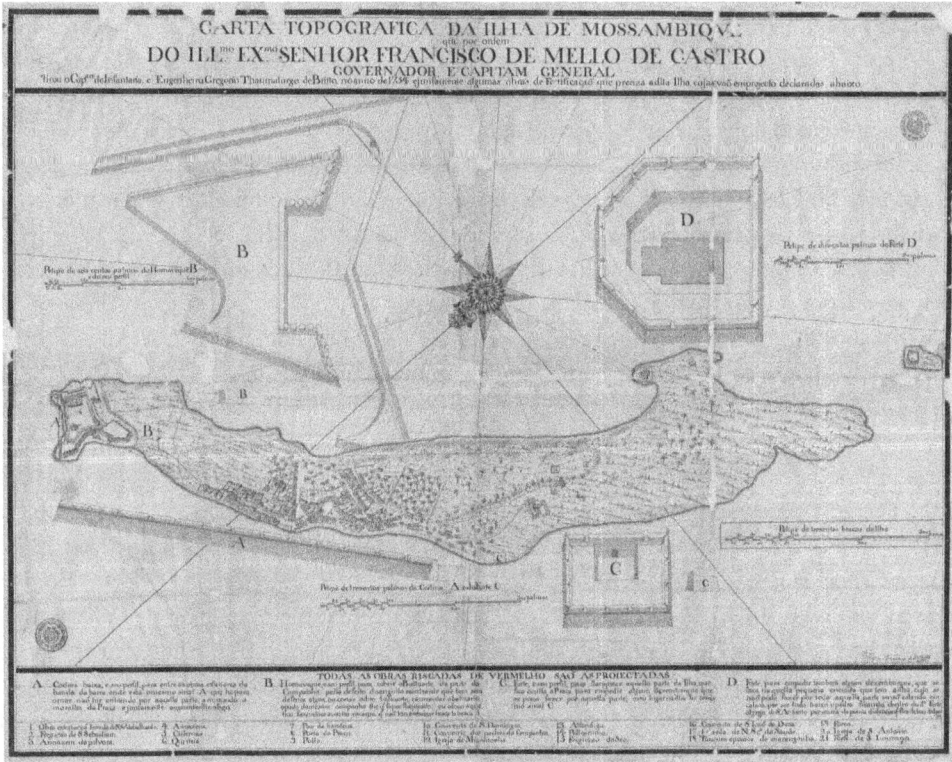

Figure 8.1 Map of Mozambique Island that shows the stone quarter to the west and the *macuti* palm huts scattered to the east and south of the stone town. The hospital appears in an isolated location south of the town. "Carta topografica da ilha de Mossambique," 1754, by Capitão de infantaria e engenheiro Gregório Taumaturgo de Brito. Arquivo Histórico Ultramarino, Lisbon. Courtesy of AHU

The houses that had been built as a private residence were adapted by means of small-scale works. The hospital began operating there in 1682. The architecture of these houses as well as of the structures that were later added to the hospital would undoubtedly have followed the building models and techniques that were already prevalent on Mozambique Island at this time. In the colonies the Portuguese had to adapt their architectural style to the existing materials and local expertise. When transferring European models to Mozambique, the Portuguese faced a continuum of cultural influences that interacted with their homeland styles on Mozambique Island. These influences came not only from mainland Africa, but were also related to the broader context of human mobility and trading networks in the Indian Ocean. The island received myriad influences from flows of people arriving from diverse continental regions and Indian Ocean islands—mainly from Swahili port cities, Arabia, Persia, and India— importing these peoples' own architectural culture and knowledge. The mainland Africans, who made up most of the labor force of slaves that worked on the construction of the buildings, undoubtedly contributed their knowledge of materials.

In the island's edifices, known as "stone and lime" construction, the walls were built with large blocks of coralline rocks extracted from the island's soil, which was the coral architecture found in other Swahili port cities.[39] These blocks were bound together with a lime mortar made from coral or marine shells. Instead of European-style roofs, the buildings were thatched with palm leaves, which were progressively substituted by terraces to gather rainwater that was then channeled into cisterns. This was similar to houses in southern Portugal, a dry region that evidenced a strong Islamic influence, as well as in the Swahili port cities, with which the island maintained close ties (Figure 8.2).

These terraces were constructed with very large girders of *mecrusse* wood (Lebombo ironwood, *Androstachys Johnsonii Prain*).[40] Narrower beams, generally of mangrove wood, were arrayed transversally over this visible wooden structure. Various layers of a mortar made of sand, crushed coral, and lime fabricated from marine shells covered this entire structure. Finally, everything was covered with a better-quality limestone plaster that incorporated sesame oil and *murrapa* oil extracted from a small shrub, producing a durable, elastic, and waterproof material. The same limestone plaster was used on the floor, due to the scarcity of wood. This construction technique ensured that the buildings maintained a comfortable temperature. These structures had a rectangular plan with many rooms, and large patios at the rear that housed the kitchen and living quarters for the domestic slaves. The patios, which sometimes had verandas, also provided spaces for social and leisure activities due to the cool shade from innumerable fruit trees, such as coconut palms, and orange and lemon trees.[41]

The type of materials that were available also influenced the aesthetics of the buildings. Since limestone that is easily worn away by rain could not be used to build European-style stonework, constructions used a stripped architecture with simple lines and plain surfaces. In contrast, facades had decorative elements made from lime mortar and doors were ornamented, becoming symbols of the wealth and social status of the owners (Figure 8.3). The product of cross-cultural encounters, the decorative elements had Indo-Portuguese origins and combined Portuguese and Indian motifs, derived particularly from Gujarat in northwest India from where most of the artisans were recruited, as well as Swahili roots. Seeking similarities between Mozambique Island and European towns, several visitors noted the grandeur of noble residences, the monumental scale of public buildings, and the combination of architectural styles. For example, the British traveler Henry Salt considered that the town, as did its people, presented "a strange mixture of Indian, Arabian and European costume, not blending very harmoniously together, and of which it is difficult to convey and adequate idea to any one unacquainted with three countries."[42] Conversely, a group of Danish architects, who conducted a study on Mozambique Island between 1982 and 1985, concluded that "architectural character of the 'stone built town', created through 400 years, is remarkable for its homogeneity."[43] More than a hybrid architecture, it was a new architecture. Indeed, the architecture promoted mainly by merchants and landlords on Mozambique

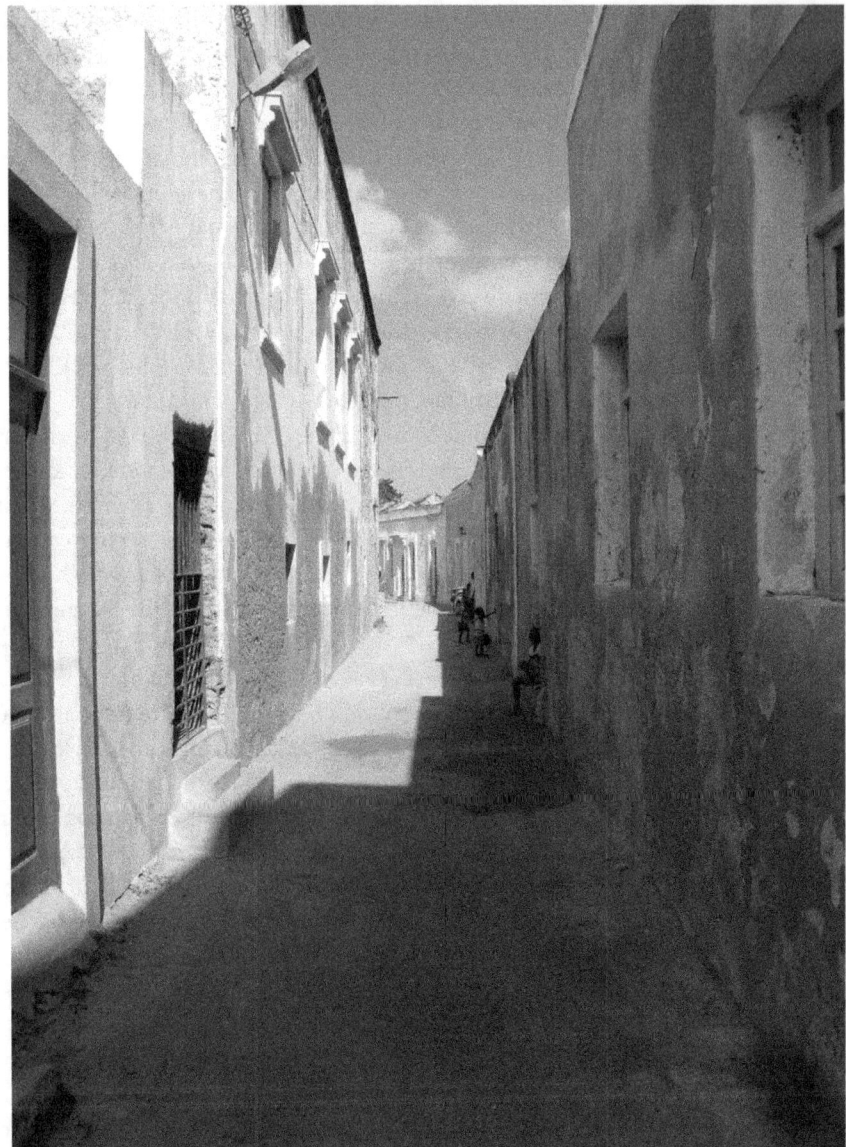

Figure 8.2 A view of a street in the stone town. Photo: Eugénia Rodrigues

Island, including the hospital edifices, mingled together in a unique way the use of materials, techniques, and aesthetics rooted in diverse worlds. The use of the same materials and techniques for centuries has given the island's buildings a stylistic homogeneity.

Nonetheless, nothing is known about the actual features of the two houses where the hospital was established in 1682. It would undoubtedly have had various rooms and could ostensibly house four hundred patients, but it only had a hundred beds.[44] Even if two patients could be housed in each bed, as was often the case in Europe at the time, the hospital would be able to accommodate a maximum of two hundred patients. Conceived along the lines of European institutions, the hospital depended on the dynamics of trade in the Indian Ocean that gave it a local touch: beds, linen, cushions, utensils, pharmaceuticals, and other paraphernalia were imported

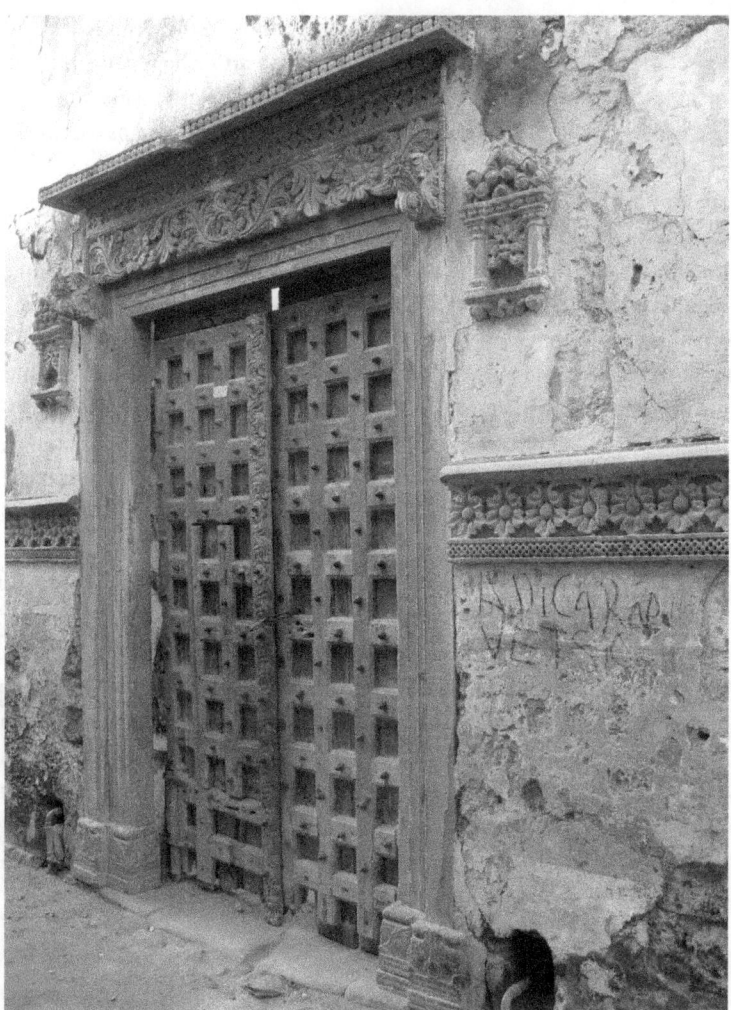

Figure 8.3 Carved entrance door. Photo: Eugénia Rodrigues

from Chaul, India.⁴⁵ According to subsequent criticism, the building only housed patients. Medicines, for example, were acquired from a private pharmacy; there was no room in which they could be prepared.⁴⁶

The hospital's history was inextricably intertwined with that of two other buildings that were indispensable to its functioning, the church and convent of St. John, and the pre-existent church of Good Health. Construction of the convent and church began in 1682, thanks to the generosity of a rich merchant, João Dias Ribeiro, and, after his demise in 1690, to the alms contributed by the island's residents.⁴⁷ As in the previous hospital edifices, the construction of a church adjacent to the hospital buildings was part of the European tradition of "mending the bodies, saving souls."⁴⁸

Indeed, during an age when, for European friars, curing the body was inseparable from curing the soul, the location of the church alongside the infirmary allowed patients direct access to religious ceremonies. This church had three altars, one of which was certainly dedicated to St. John, as was habitual in the hospitals run by the Brothers Hospitallers in Portugal.⁴⁹ References to the convent portray it as a building that was never completed due to a shortage of funds. The ground floor had two cloisters, while the upper floor, built over one of the cloisters, was limited to eight cells, to house the Brothers who had arrived on the island.⁵⁰ The spatial articulation among these constructions is not known precisely, though the complex is often referred to as the convent-hospital. The set of houses would probably have formed an L shape with the church and one of the cloisters adjoining the hospital buildings and the second cloister on the other side. The church of Good Health situated nearby was given over to the Hospitallers, who used the churchyard as a cemetery for patients who died at the hospital.[51]

Alongside these buildings, but within the surrounding fence, houses were built for African slaves who worked in the hospital and convent.[52] While the hospital, convent, and church were built from the limestone used on the island, the houses of the slaves were described as huts, and were probably made of adobe or were wooden and thatched with *macuti* palm leaves, as most African houses on the island were. The set of buildings that formed the hospital complex thus constituted a dialogue between stone structures and palm-thatched houses, which characterized the settlement until the nineteenth century, when the municipal authorities segregated the thatched housing, limiting it to the southern part of the island (Figure 8.4).[53]

The private residence of a rich merchant soon proved to be insufficient to house the patients. In 1692, for example, one of the officials on the island had to transform his home into "a second hospital."[54] In 1701, due to the "limited accommodation" and ruined walls of the hospital houses, the administrator Friar Francisco de São Tomás began to construct "a suitably large and enduring building."[55] When he left the island in 1704, it was almost completed and it was probably concluded in 1708, according to an inscription above the door.[56] The new infirmary was funded by the Royal Treasury, which stipulated the payment of a given sum for every section of the building that the missionaries were able to erect.[57] References to continuous construction, amid innumerable disputes with the administration in Mozambique, suggest that the construction work extended over several years. In addition to this building, one of the cloisters was transformed into a new infirmary, or "corridor," as it was also called, by enclosing the arches. Due to a lack of funding, the original houses were not rebuilt.[58] A 1754 map of the island shows that, with the new construction, the set of buildings were arrayed almost in the shape of a U around a large inner courtyard, delimited on the other side by a wall (Figure 8.5).[59] The hospital's architecture thus reflected monastic structures, and hence, as Mary Lindemann argues regarding many European hospitals, it is "artificial to separate monasteries from hospitals."[60]

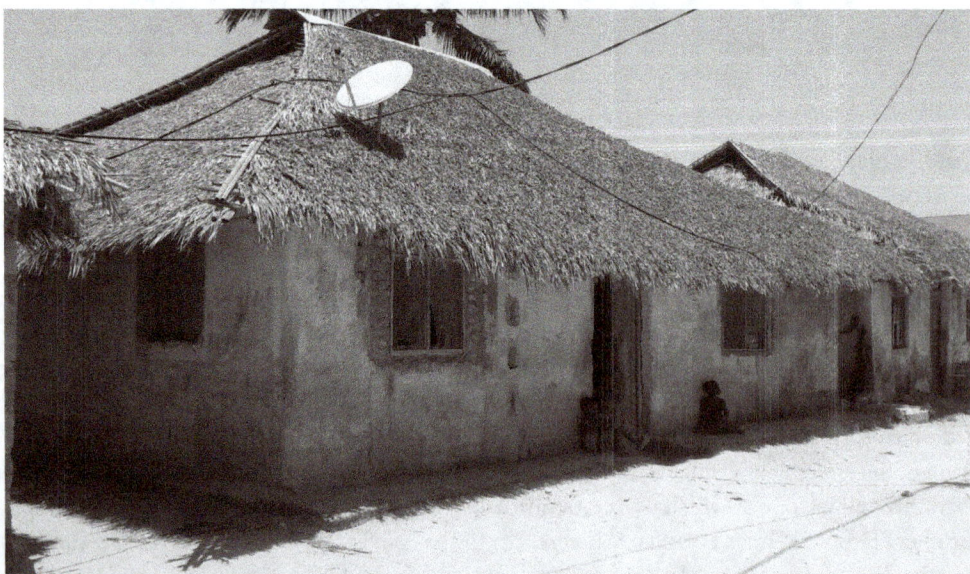

Figure 8.4 Present-day *macuti* houses in the southern part of Mozambique Island. Photo: Eugénia Rodrigues

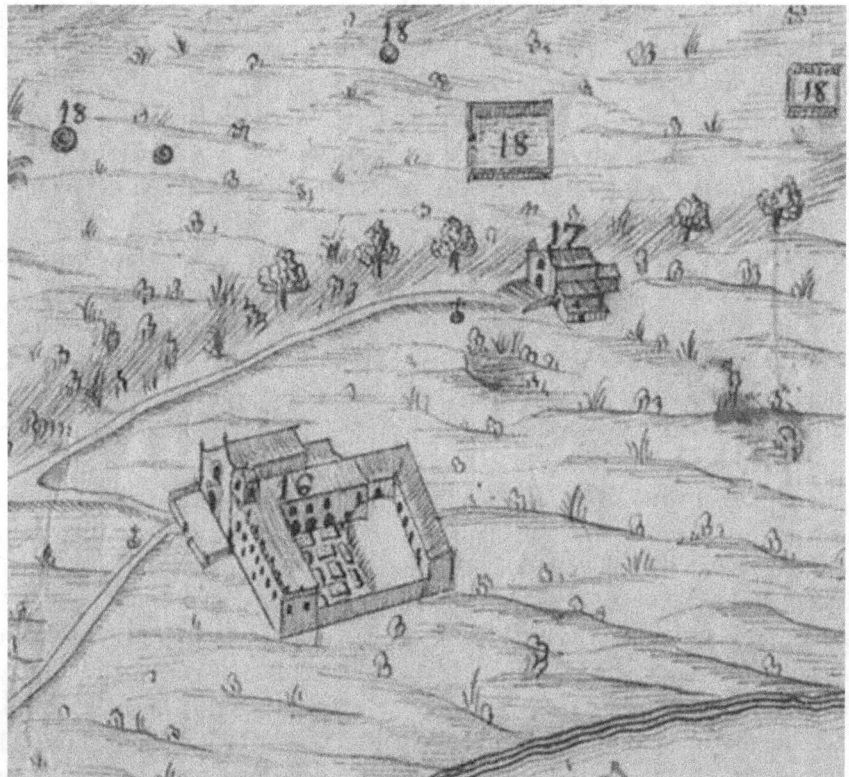

Figure 8.5 Detail from the 1754 map of Mozambique Island showing the hospital, convent, and church of St. John (16) and further away the church of Good Health (17). "Carta topografica da ilha de Mossambique," 1754, by Capitão de infantaria e engenheiro Gregório Taumaturgo de Brito. Arquivo Histórico Ultramarino, Lisbon. Courtesy of AHU

By the mid-eighteenth century, complaints about the limited space in the hospital increased, while the Hospitallers highlighted the need to carry out new construction work at the building. The hospital always incurred high expenditure and, according to the Brothers, its costs exceeded the royal funding, resulting in constant tension with the royal administration. When the number of patients increased, they were accommodated on mats distributed throughout the second cloister situated below the cells of the friars and the entrance to the convent, and were thus exposed to the vagaries of the weather. They sometimes had to be taken to the fortress at the other end of the island or to private homes.[61] There was thus some fluidity between the hospital buildings and other spaces that made the hospital an open institution. With the changes that occurred in medical theories in Europe and new views on the role of the state in looking after the health of subjects, the Hospitallers and the healthcare they provided were increasingly criticized.

Enlightening the Royal Hospital

In the context of the affirmation of European absolutist states, a state's power and wealth were associated with the existence of a numerous and physically robust population. These ideas were particularly expressed in the concept of medical policing, in which the government was to establish a set of policies in the health sector, such as the creation and overhauling of hospitals to promote broader medical facilities, to ensure a healthy population. Although its roots can be traced back to the seventeenth century, the concept of medical policing gained ground during the second half of the eighteenth century.[62] Ideas advocating state intervention to safeguard the health of subjects emerged in Portugal as well.[63]

The evolution of medical theories, namely reinforcing the notion of prevention, required changes in the structure and location of hospitals. The resurgence of environmentalism, which had already been an integral part of medical knowledge in Europe from the time of Hippocrates, reinforced the belief in the noxious effects that the environment could have on the human body and hence on health. In particular, environmentalism claimed that the earth exuded miasmas, i.e., fetid elements dissolved in the atmosphere and in stagnant waters, derived from decomposing organic matter.[64] In the case of imperial territories, the influence of environmental factors was accentuated by the portrayal of the tropics as a different and threatening world for Europeans. As David Arnold argues, "'the tropics' became a way of defining something culturally alien to, as well as environmentally distinct from, Europe and other parts of the temperate World."[65] According to this representation, Europeans were vulnerable to diseases in hot and humid tropical regions, as opposed to the pleasant climate of temperate zones.[66]

From the mid-eighteenth century onward, the ideas that emerged in Europe also circulated throughout the European empires, giving rise to harsh disapproval of the healthcare that was available in Mozambique.[67] This period coincided with a time when Mozambique became autonomous from the Estado da Índia, now being administered directly from Lisbon (1752). Several contingents of soldiers were sent to Mozambique, which increased the pressure on the hospital. Criticism of the healthcare available in Mozambique was aimed, first and foremost, at the actions of the Hospitallers, who were accused of a lack of "charity" while treating patients, among a vast range of issues, such as nutrition, clothing, drugs, bed linens, and the cleanliness of the facilities. Second, the disapproval addressed the hospital facilities. In addition to underlining the small scale of the infrastructure, censure focused on the location and structure of the building as factors promoting diseases.

In effect, the previous assessment of the hospital in Mozambique ended up being combined with Enlightenment perspectives that viewed old hospitals as "gateways to death."[68] The governor-general, Francisco de Melo e Castro (1750–8), expressed the need for improvements, stating that the hospital was a "pigsty which had been given another name." The two infirmaries only had fifty or sixty beds and patients were thus distributed throughout the cloisters on African *quitandas*, i.e., bed frames strung with coir, with mats for mattresses. The luxurious beds imported from India had been replaced by the more Spartan, locally made beds, contributing to the hospital's broader image of decline. Moreover, the infirmaries were very damp and dark even during the summer, which threatened the health of patients. The governor also questioned the fact that there was no infirmary for officers, a social distinction in terms of healthcare that was gaining ground in Europe. Finally, he asked the Portuguese Crown to construct a new building that could house 250 to 300 beds, which was the usual number of patients.[69]

While refuting the criticism leveled at the Hospitallers, the hospital's administrator, Friar Vicente da Encarnação, highlighted that the location of the infirmaries and the building itself contributed to patient deaths. He argued that since it was in the middle of the island the hospital was not "bathed by purifying air … that would cleanse away so many diverse ailments." Moreover, the cloister transformed into an infirmary had to be closed completely, because it faced west, "which faces the brunt of harsh weather in this land," while the second cloister, located below the cells, was "underground" and susceptible to "evil vapors" that even killed the friars. These conditions were aggravated by the region's climate, which was "the most hostile for Europeans … this side of the Cape of Good Hope." He contended that patients sent to convalesce in the "pestilent" fortress returned to the hospital to die from the "contagion this climate produces." In addition, Friar Encarnação felt that the former residences that had been acquired by the Royal Treasury were not suited for infirmaries because they were located in the middle of the island and adjoined the cemetery. He asked the king to build a new hospital "near the sea for better comfort and cleanliness."[70] The surgeon himself, José Alvares, declared that the site of the infirmary was unsuitable.[71] In short, as in Europe, debates in Mozambique also insisted that the hospital caused ailments.[72] Concepts relating to disease thus had an impact on assessing the architecture and location of hospitals, and demanded that healthier environments be created for patients. The criticism in Mozambique also coincided with the renovation of the hospital in Lisbon after the 1755 earthquake, which seemed to sustain similar arguments throughout the empire.[73]

In the context of complaints from Mozambique, the Portuguese Crown adopted two kinds of measures in keeping with the idea of state intervention to safeguard the health and lives of subjects. First, the Crown ordered a new hospital be constructed. In 1754, the Overseas Council in Lisbon agreed that it was crucial for the king to look after the "comfort and health of his vassals as well as his domains." As requested by the governor of Mozambique, the new hospital was to have a capacity of 250 to 300 patients and include houses for staff and other necessary facilities. A part of the customs revenues for ten years was allocated to build the hospital.[74] However, the construction never commenced due to a lack of funding. Second, in the 1761 *Instructions* for the captaincy's government, the more important regulations after Mozambique began to be administered directly from Lisbon, the Crown ordered that the hospital's management was to be transferred to the Royal Treasury so as to safeguard the health of Portuguese vassals. The Hospitallers were to continue as nurses and chaplains.[75]

These measures were implemented progressively. In 1763, the government of Mozambique appointed a storekeeper and a clerk to administer the hospital, subsequently designating other staff.[76] Nevertheless, considering the shortage of funds, the political choices made in Mozambique favored a gradual improvement and upgrade of the existing hospital instead of constructing a new edifice. Changes to the building's structure aimed to expand and specialize spaces, pursuant to medical trends that were gaining ground in Europe. As Dana Arnold argues, "improvements in medical knowledge impacted on the design and layout of hospitals, with distinctive designs to create healthier environments for patients and staff."[77]

In 1765, Governor Baltazar Pereira do Lago (1765–77) began work to "ensure these men live, so our state does not die."[78] Clearly inspired by theories claiming that a strong state depended on the number of subjects, and by the reorganization of hospitals then underway in Portugal, the governor built a new infirmary with thirty or forty beds to house patients with contagious diseases. One of his censures of the hospital was that "in one small infirmary remedies and cures were administered amidst utter confusion and tumult to all types of patients," as well as the existence of "a mix [at the same infirmary] of all kinds of fevers, different ailments and contagious diseases" which often led to the death of patients.[79] In the European hospital model, spaces began to be specialized according to ailment, creating specific hospitals or infirmaries. As the historian of architecture Harriet Richardson stresses, "Specialism was the key of the development of hospital architecture."[80] In Mozambique, it was imperative to introduce some rationality in the infirmaries, organizing spaces according to diverse diseases. Moreover, the governor built a house for convalescents who, after being sent to the fortress at the "first sign of recovery," soon returned to the hospital after relapsing.[81] As Guenter Risse, the historian of medicine, emphasizes, in a "more medicalized context, the issue of physical recovery began to loom larger after the Renaissance, based on more optimistic notions of health and illness."[82] This new infirmary was probably built by joining the ends of the U that formed the hospital's layout.

The governor also ordered the restoration of the old cistern because it was choked with debris and patients were "at the mercy of those who gave them putrid water to drink, and the tanks next to the said hospital are

Health and Architecture

even filthier."[83] Indeed, European medicine viewed beverages as a factor for health or illness. Furthermore, the governor implemented projects to streamline the hospital's functioning. He rebuilt the ruined houses in which the hospital had initially been installed to store food, medicines, beds, and other equipment. These goods had been kept in the storekeeper's house and transported daily to the hospital by slaves.[84] Thus, medicalization was reflected in the hospital's architecture: the infirmaries became differentiated while the increasingly complex tasks within the hospital resulted in the creation of new spaces.

The ruler established simultaneously a new hospital for twelve patients at the Holy House of Mercy (Santa Casa da Misericórdia), in the heart of the stone quarter, close to the port and the new government palace of Saint Paul, the former residence of the Jesuit fathers (Figure 8.6).[85] Although designated to assist

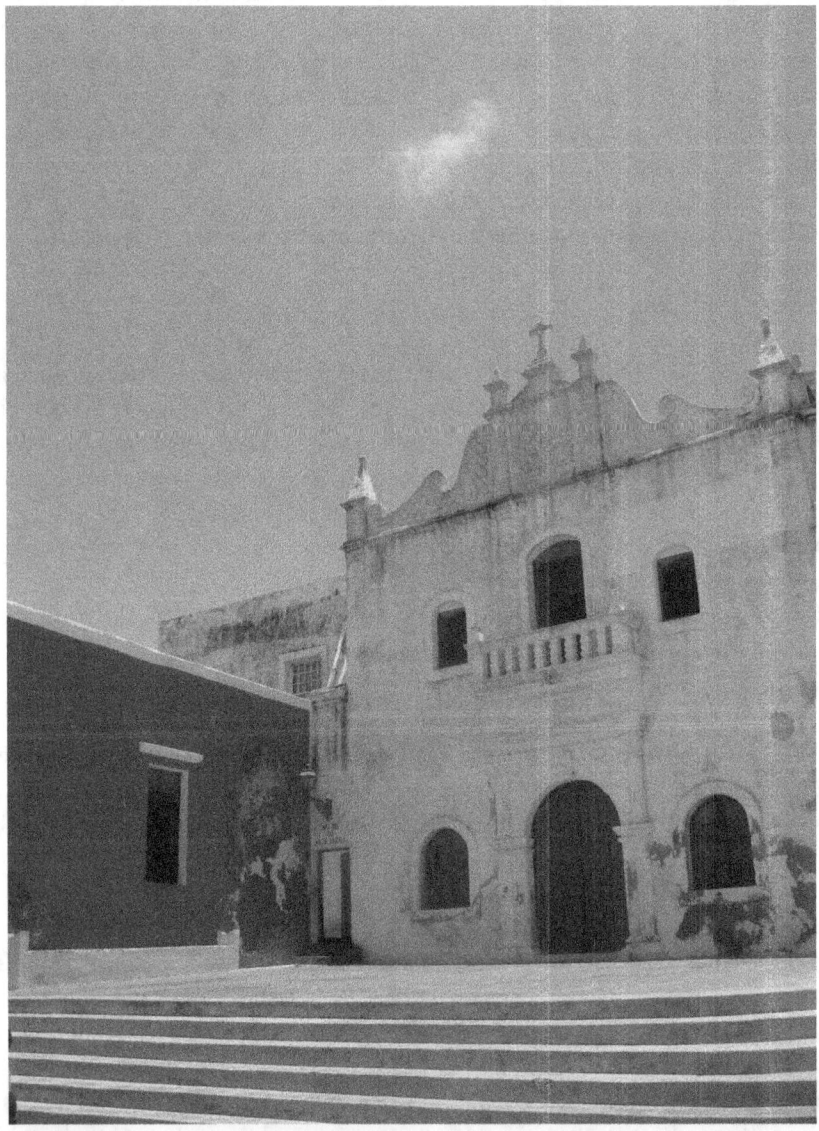

Figure 8.6 The Misericórdia church with a building attached to the left, where the charitable hospital for the poor was located on the ground floor. Photo: Eugénia Rodrigues

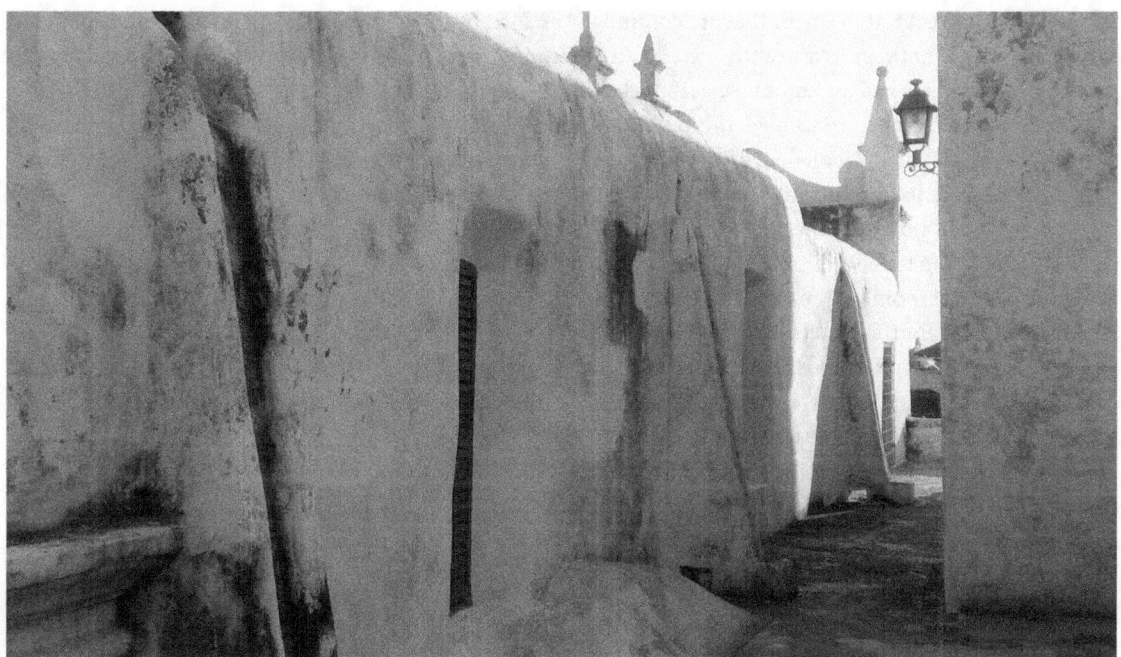

Figure 8.7 A pipe system on the Misericórdia terrace to conduct water to the cistern. Photo: Eugénia Rodrigues

the poor, the Holy House hospital also treated private patients, mainly crew from private vessels, at a time when the slave trade was expanding.[86] This small hospital was installed on the ground floor of the building adjoining the Misericórdia church and had specialized compartments and a chapel.[87] The system of terraces and pipes to use rainwater, which is still visible, likewise indicates the existence of a cistern (Figure 8.7). This initiative appears to have been part of the governor's policy of promoting the Holy House since he was also the trustee of the brotherhood, and not just due to the notions of medical exclusivity circulating in Europe that affirmed that hospitals should be free from the task of looking after the poor.[88] The Misericórdia hospital operated for a few years since, in 1789, the brotherhood and a new governor felt there was a shortage of medical staff to regularly tend to the sick and hence the institution was "a pitiful depository, where many of those miserable patients died in a few days." An agreement was then established with the Royal Treasury by which patients entrusted to the Misericórdia began to be treated at the royal hospital in exchange for payment.[89]

These reforms did not silence critics. In 1780, Governor José Vasconcelos e Almeida (1779–81) stated that the "hospital was so horrible, that it seemed more suitable to bury the dead than for patients to recover their health there." Considering the building to be limited and the infirmaries "damp and unsuitable, located at ground level," he began to renovate existing spaces and to build two new halls on the upper floor.[90] The theory that "corrupt" air was a contributing factor of disease made the provision of proper air circulation and adequate ventilation through window slits imperative, which could not be achieved in ground-floor infirmaries. In addition to intervening in the building, hospital rules adopted measures to eliminate the causes of the diseases that ran rife there, believing that it was impossible to heal patients where the "atmosphere was putrid or impregnated with rotten and contagious particles." Thus, the chief physician was to pay special attention to "ventilation and circulating" the air, "issuing orders to always keep a suitable number of windows open pursuant to the weather and the diseases." Air circulation was complemented by the daily burning of aromatics "to correct rotten smells that are continually exuded by the bodies and excrement of many patients, so as to always keep them in a healthy state."[91] As in Europe, ventilation and perfuming became mandatory practices to eliminate bad air and make edifices healthy.[92]

Subsequent governors continued the building's refurbishment even though the structure was deemed unsuitable. For instance, Lieutenant-Colonel Vicente da Maia e Vasconcelos, the commander of the infantry regiment of Mozambique and interim governor (1781–2), concluded that the works had been "designed by someone who had no experience of troops or hospitals." He highlighted the absence of a prison for criminal patients, who at the time were treated at the fortress, as well as the lack of halls to cure syphilis, a dispensary, and other essential rooms.[93] The work extended through the 1780s, with slow progress due to limited funding.[94] Small works to adapt the structure were carried out later, such as to the installation of a pharmacy in 1795.[95] Thus, the small hospital of the late seventeenth century was transformed into a complex of larger buildings, especially when considering the scale of buildings on the island, and had acquired specialized spaces, in keeping with changes in medical practices

These architectural alterations were accompanied by the preparation of successive highly detailed regulations (1779, 1783, and 1788), aimed at political control of the hospital and its medicalization in keeping with trends at European hospitals.[96] For example, the 1788 regulations were prepared with the involvement of the chief physician João Domingos Toscano (1788–93), a native of Piedmont, Italy, where public control of healthcare was well established. This set of norms—designed to adapt the patients' treatment to the "lights of medicine"—established greater differentiation and specialization of spaces aimed at medical efficiency. While convalescents were kept in their own hall, patients were now organized into two infirmaries, one for medicinal treatment and the other for surgery. Within each infirmary they were distributed according to illnesses to avoid epidemics and to facilitate the work of the doctors.[97] Grouping patients according to diseases provided a spatial structure that contributed toward changing the medical focus, which instead of highlighting the individual patient now focused on the disease.[98] However, it is important to note that these changes were not linear and were often not institutionalized. Their application depended considerably on the incumbent governor and the chief physician, who was now responsible for managing the hospital, and hence criticism and disputes relating to the hospital continued throughout the early modern period.[99]

Available sources suggest that no major changes were made to the structure of the hospital building until the early decades of the nineteenth century. In 1821, the governor reorganized the space to promote greater specialization and patient monitoring. Soldiers, who comprised about 82 percent of the patients, now occupied the upper floor, known as the military hospital, while civilians were relegated to the ground floor—perceived as being more "damp" and "dark"—which began to be called the Misericórdia hospital. According to the governor, the hospital had 80 beds that were each 7.5 spans (1.65 meters) away from each other. This arrangement of the beds sought to reduce contagion among patients, which was in keeping with the organization of European hospitals, where clinics required space to conduct medical examinations on patients.[100] The governor simultaneously made it compulsory for nurses, the pharmacist, and his assistant to reside at the hospital.[101]

A plan of the hospital dating from 1821 reveals that the building continued to be organized around the large quadrangle courtyard. Another external courtyard expanded the space for patients to recuperate. These outdoor areas with gardens were understood to have a benign influence on health. Two wings on the ground floor were allocated for the Misericórdia hospital. The pharmaceutical services were distributed over the third wing: the pharmacy and its affiliated spaces (the kitchen or laboratory and the storehouse), along with the lodgings for the incumbent pharmacist and his assistant. Accommodations for the nurse and his assistant were located in the last wing that adjoined the church, as was the pantry, a guardhouse, and the cistern. This wing was connected to the kitchen located outside behind the infirmary by means of a doorway. On the upper floor, four halls accommodated military patients, with a small room that was reserved for the nurse. The cells of the Hospitallers were placed in the other two wings.[102] The hospital did not limit itself only to healing patients. For example, the Genoese doctor Luís Vicente de Simoni, another native from the Italian Peninsula who served as chief physician between 1819 and 1821, mentioned that he researched diseases by carrying out autopsies on cadavers, probably in a small room.[103] Moreover, new medical professionals were also occasionally given training at the hospital.[104]

Shortly thereafter, in 1826, Governor Sebastião Xavier Botelho (1825–9) carried out new works on the building—to all appearances, mere repairs—and he reorganized medical services in Mozambique. First, he reopened the erstwhile hospital at the Holy House of Mercy where poor patients were transferred, freeing up space at the royal hospital. Secondly, since the number of Hospitallers had diminished significantly, he transformed a part of the upper floor into an infantry barracks. He separated the hospital infirmaries between high-ranking officers and lower ranks, accentuating the aforementioned social distinction. At this time there were "two airy halls for convalescents." The number of beds in the infirmaries rose to two hundred, probably achieved by reducing the space between them. The hospital retained its military features. No ward was set up to accommodate women; it was only in the 1830s that they were admitted to the infirmaries.[105] Thus, throughout the early modern period the gendered differentiation prevailing in European hospitals was not replicated on Mozambique Island. According to the governor, after these changes, the hospital was a good building with a beautiful front.[106] While rooted in local architecture styles, the hospital's shape resulted from the successive plans of several social actors, such as governors, religious, military officials, and doctors, whose ideas about healthcare were based mainly on European culture.

Urban improvements were also carried out to ensure that patients had healthy surroundings, as practiced in Europe. In the eastern area of the hospital African people built *macuti* houses, giving rise to the new neighborhood of Marangonha. In this space wells providing brackish water and some tanks were built; African people would wash their clothes in these tanks. However, the dirty water would then run off directly into the ground "and with no outlet would stagnate, become putrid, infest the air and cause serious ailments, despite the strong winds that blew over the island every evening." In 1825, the governor ordered channels to be dug that would divert the water into a drain that led to the sea, making this site "usable and healthy."[107] According to the ideas about the environment and its effects on human health, the well-drained ground would reduce the presence of miasma at the hospital site. This measure was part of the politics to control the urban space that was "perhaps the most dangerous environment for the population."[108] In fact, the government's interventions in the hospital buildings and surroundings were part of a broader operation to reshape the urban arrangement.

These changes occurred at a time of well-known urban growth that extended the southern limit of the stone quarter up to the hospital. The new stone and lime neighborhood of São João, established in the 1770s, now occupied all the space up to the hospital, while *macuti* houses spread out to the east at the Missanga quarter (Figure 8.8). What had once been an open field had become a square located east of the hospital. During the early decades of the nineteenth century, the hospital was the most impressive building on Mozambique Island, as noted by British surgeon James Prior in 1812: "At the western extremity is a capacious hospital for the sick, which, at certain seasons, are sometimes numerous."[109] In short, the successive expansions and restructuring of the hospital had transformed it into a landmark in the city. In a period when the growth of commerce, especially slave trading, drew many people to the island, the large hospital demonstrated the power of the Portuguese Crown to the local inhabitants and foreign visitors.

Health and Architecture

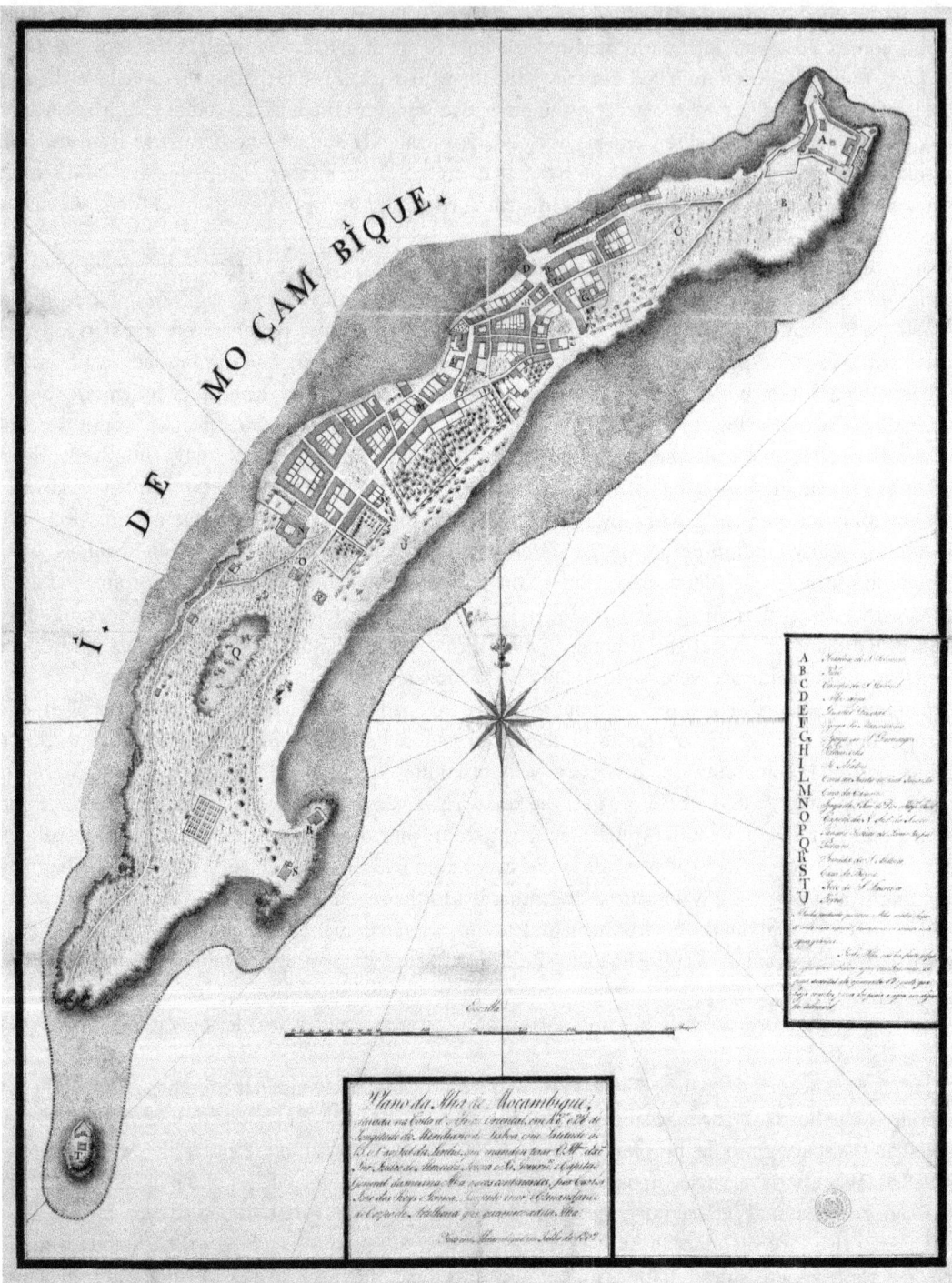

Figure 8.8 An early nineteenth-century map of Mozambique Island that shows how the stone quarter extended up to the hospital buildings (N) as well as the *macuti* houses to the east. "Plano da ilha de Moçambique," Sargento-mor e comandante do corpo de artilharia, Carlos José dos Reis e Gama. 1802. Arquivo Histórico Ultramarino, Lisbon. Courtesy of AHU

Conclusion

The Portuguese Crown established a royal hospital on Mozambique Island in the early sixteenth century to serve the commercial and military interests of its empire in the Indian Ocean. As the island became the main port of the Portuguese in Southeast Africa and the capital of their colony, the hospital achieved increasing importance. The Portuguese hospitals provided the template for the construction of other hospitals in the empire and on Mozambique Island. The hospital was crucial in offering European models of assistance to residents and soldiers in the Portuguese colony, as well as to those who called in at the island on voyages between Europe and India. In this context, the patients were mainly soldiers, including those residents on the island as well as those in transit. However, it is important to stress that the initial European army changed over time to include individuals of Goan, African, and mixed-race origin. Thus, the hospital was not an enclave for Europeans even though they constituted most of the patients, and there were asymmetrical relations of power between these groups. The interaction between these cultures influenced the hospital's daily life and medical practices. The royal hospital was always funded by the Portuguese Crown even though it underwent diverse forms of administration. In the 1760s it was supplemented by the hospital run by the Holy House, sponsored by this lay brotherhood. From the time the royal hospital was established, Renaissance European models of healthcare for patients based on charity and religious support seem to have dominated in Mozambique, even though the provision of medicines was a Crown concern. In 1682, the transfer of the hospital's administration to the Brothers Hospitallers strengthened the association between healthcare and religious institutions, in contrast to what occurred in Europe. With the emergence of medicalization in the eighteenth century, the hospital was harshly criticized, and its management was transferred from the religious to the Royal Treasury. Nevertheless, healthcare continued to be shaped by funding constraints, as most political decision-makers sought to keep expenditure low.

While continuing to act as a symbol of colonial power, throughout the early modern period the royal hospital was located in diverse sites, establishing different relationships with the town. It was initially placed at the heart of the urban matrix, being closely linked to the everyday activities of residents and to the port that connected Mozambique Island to other worlds. It was constructed alongside the first small fortress the Portuguese built on the island, outside the surrounding walls, and was associated with the port and military facilities from which most patients arrived. When its location was changed to a field south of the settlement in 1682 the hospital lost this close link with the town, which only resumed when it expanded southward from the final decades of the eighteenth century onward. At this time the hospital marked the southern edge of the stone and lime quarters. Conversely, the Holy House hospital, which operated intermittently, kept its facilities in the stone and lime building next to the brotherhood church in the center of the city.

As has been stated in this chapter, little is known about the features of the buildings of the former hospitals located at the heart of the settlement. In the initial organization of their colonial settlement on Mozambique Island, the Portuguese privileged their homeland paradigms of architecture and urban landscapes. Yet sources suggest that European models evolved toward a local architecture, adapted to the materials and techniques available in the region, and utilized aesthetics that reflected mainly Swahili and Indo-Portuguese influences. In fact, the transfer of the European paradigms to the colonial settings carried important differences between the diverse regions to which they were transported. It is important to consider the agency of local actors along with the movement of architectural cultures between different worlds. Due to its role as a seaport that was related to the ports of the broader Indian Ocean and its capacity to attract different peoples, locality on Mozambique Island was produced through the lasting interconnection with other worlds.

The first of these hospital edifices was a precarious wooden structure that was replaced by a rectangular stone building with a church. This latter structure was of considerable size to accommodate a number of patients comparable to those housed in military hospitals in Renaissance Europe. There is scarce information about the features of the hospital that replaced this building after it fell into disrepair. The new edifice was erected during the 1630s in the center of the town, albeit at an unknown location. The building, if not its antecessor, was certainly based on local construction techniques, adapted to the use of coral limestone blocks and cemented with a mortar made of sand, coral, and lime.

Unlike the earlier constructions, designed specifically to host patients, the last royal hospital of the early modern period was established in 1682 in existing residential houses, which were augmented by a church and a residence for the friars. These buildings were undoubtedly built in the same manner as the "stone and lime" houses in the city, as were the wings that were added later. The changes that took place over the course of the eighteenth century occurred in response, first, to the need to expand the space for housing patients and, subsequently, to adapt the hospital's structure to the evolution of medical theories. Grappling with the challenges of the medicalization of healthcare, the dissemination of environmental perspectives on disease and the adoption of theories associating strong states with healthy subjects, by the mid-eighteenth century political decisions on whether to construct a new hospital in an environment considered to be healthier or to enlarge the existing building also depended on available funding. This interplay resulted in the decision to expand the old edifice with the sequential construction of new infirmaries and specialized halls. As this chapter has shown, medical specialization entailed a fragmentation of the space and the creation of differentiated rooms for patients, medical procedures, and lodging for hospital staff in a manner similar to the ongoing contemporaneous process in Europe. The enlargement of the hospital changed the building's layout, altering its formerly L-shaped plan, including the church, to a square edifice set around a courtyard, with the addition of an upper floor. Due to these changes, the royal hospital became a key visual landmark on the island, for its facade and its dimensions.

Despite the scant information available on the specific features of the buildings, a study of the hospitals on Mozambique Island reveals how multiple cultural influences—Portuguese, mainland African, Swahili, and Indian—mingled together in the town, creating a singular architecture. It also paves the way for researching comparative perspectives on the ways in which European models were transposed to imperial territories and articulated with local models of construction, giving rise to buildings with unique characteristics. The study of hospitals on Mozambique Island unveils how circulation of European models of hospital architecture has been interpreted and localized in non-European worlds.

Notes

1. For more about changes in medicine and hospitals, see, for example, Guenter B. Risse, *Mending Bodies, Saving Souls. A History of Hospitals* (New York: Oxford University Press, 1999); Mary Lindemann, *Medicine and Society in Early Modern Europe* (Cambridge: Cambridge University Press, 2010); Laurence I. Conrad et al., eds., *The Western Medical Tradition: 800 BC–1800 AD* (Cambridge: Cambridge University Press, 1995); John Henderson, *The Renaissance Hospital: Healing the Body and Healing the Soul* (New Haven: Yale University Press, 2006); *The Impact of Hospitals, 300–2000*, ed. John Henderson, Peregrine Horden, and Alessandro Pastore (Oxford: Peter Lang, 2007); Michel Foucault, "The Politics of Health in the Eighteenth Century," in Michel Foucault, *Power/Knowledge*, ed. Colin Gordon (New York: Pantheon Books, 1980), 166–82; Michel Foucault, *The Birth of the Clinic* (London: Routledge, 2003). On architectural changes in Western World hospitals, see Harriet Richardson, ed., *English Hospitals, 1660–1948: A Survey of Their Architecture and Design* (Swindon: Royal Commission on the Historical Monuments of England, 1998); Jeanne Kisacky, *Rise of the Modern Hospital: An Architectural History of Health and Healing, 1870–1940* (Pittsburgh: University of Pittsburgh Press, 2017); Christine Stevenson, *Medicine and Magnificence: British Hospital and Asylum Architecture, 1660–1815* (New Haven: Yale University Press, 2000).
2. See, for example, Dana Arnold, *The Spaces of the Hospital: Spatiality and Urban Change in London 1680–1820* (New York: Routledge, 2013).

3. David Arnold, "The Place of 'the tropics' in Western Medical Edeas since 1750," *Tropical Medicine and International Health* 2, no. 4 (1997): 303–13.
4. Luís A. de Oliveira Ramos, "Do Hospital Real de Todos os Santos. A história hospitalar portuguesa," *Revista da Faculdade de Letras* 10 (1993): 333–50; Paulo Pereira, ed., *O Hospital Real de Todos os Santos: 500 Anos. Catálogo* (Lisbon: Câmara Municipal de Lisboa, 1993); António Fernando Bento Pacheco, "De Todos-Os-Santos a São José: Textos e Contextos do 'esprital grande de Lixboa'" (MA diss., New University of Lisbon, 2008); Jon Arrizabalaga, "Medical Theory and Surgical Practice: Coping with the French Disease in Early Renaissance Portugal and Spain," in *Hospital Life: Theory and Practice from the Medieval to the Modern*, ed. Laurinda Abreu and Sally Sheard (Bern: Peter Lang, 2013), 93–117; Laurinda Abreu, "Training Health Professionals at the Hospital de Todos os Santos (Lisbon) 1500–1800," in *Hospital Life*, 119–37. On Italian hospitals, see Henderson, *The Renaissance Hospital*; Philip Foster, "Per il disegno dell'Ospedale di Milano," *Arte Lombarda* 38, no. 39 (1973): 1–22; Renzo Baldasso, "Function and Epidemiology in Filarete's Ospedale Maggiore," in *Medieval Hospital and Medical Practice*, ed. Barbara S. Bowers (Aldershot: Ashgate, 2007), 107–22.
5. Lisbeth de Oliveira Rodrigues, "Os hospitais portugueses no Renascimento (1480–1580): o caso de Nossa Senhora do Pópulo das Caldas da Rainha" (Ph.D. diss., University of Minho, 2013); André Costa Aciole da Silva, "'Queremos e mandamos … que o dito hospital … cure os enfermos …': poder e medicina no hospital de Nossa Senhora do Pópulo (séc. XVI–XVII)" (Ph.D. diss., Federal University of Goiás, 2015).
6. Joana Maria Balsa Carvalho de Pinho, "As Casas da Misericórdia: confrarias da Misericórdia e a arquitectura quinhentista portuguesa" (Ph.D. diss., University of Lisbon, 2012).
7. Augusto Moutinho Borges, *Reais Hospitais Militares em Portugal (1640–1834)* (Coimbra: Imprensa da Universidade de Coimbra, 2009).
8. For some studies, see Ermelinda Pataca, "Entre a engenharia militar e a arquitetura médica: representações de Alexandre Rodrigues Ferreira sobre a cidade de Belém no final do século XVIII," *História, Ciências, Saúde. Manguinhos* 25, no. 1 (2018): 89–113; Artur Teodoro de Matos, "A Glimpse of the Hospitallers of Diu in the late 18th Century," in *Goa and Portugal: History and Development*, ed. Charles J. Borges, Oscar Guilherme Pereira, and Hannes Stubbe (New Delhi: Concept Publishing, 2000), 231–7; Fátima da Silva Gracias, *Health and Hygiene in Colonial Goa, 1510–1961* (New Delhi: Concept Publishing, 1994); Cristiana Bastos, "Hospitais e sociedade colonial. Esplendor, ruína, memória e mudança em Goa," *Ler História* 58 (2010): 61–80; Cristiana Bastos, "Together and Apart: Catholic Hospitals in Plural Goa," in *Hospitals in Iran and India, 1500–1950*, ed. Fabrizio Speziale (Leiden: Brill, 2012), 133–57.
9. Banha de Andrade, "O hospital de Moçambique durante a administração dos Almoxarifes," *Portugal em África* 13, no. 78 (1956): 357–70; Banha de Andrade, "O Hospital de Moçambique durante a administração dos religiosos de S. João de Deus," *Portugal em África* 13, no. 77 (1956): 261–2; Banha de Andrade, "Os Hospitaleiros de S. João de Deus na Índia," *Portugal em África* 14, no. 80 (1957): 107–19; Banha de Andrade, "Fundação do Hospital Militar de S. João de Deus, em Moçambique," *Stvdia* 1 (1958): 77–89. For studies focusing on hospital buildings, see Pedro Quirino da Fonseca, "Algumas descobertas de interesse histórico-arqueológico na ilha de Moçambique," *Monumenta* 8 (1972): 55–71; Pedro Dias, "Algumas Misericórdias no Estado da Índia. Apontamentos para a história da construção dos seus edifícios," in *A Misericórdia de Vila Real e as Misericórdias no Mundo de Expressão Portuguesa*, ed. Natália Marinho Ferreira-Alves (Porto: CEPESE, 2011), 555–62.
10. For more on hospitals in the Portuguese Indian Ocean Empire, see Germano de Sousa, *História da Medicina Portuguesa durante a Expansão* (Lisbon: Temas e Debates, 2013), 149–95; Gracias, *Health and Hygiene*; Bastos, "Hospitais e sociedade"; Bastos, "Together and Apart."
11. Michael N. Pearson, *Port Cities and Intruders. The Swahili Coast, India, and Portugal in the Early Modern Era* (Baltimore: Johns Hopkins University Press, 1998); Malyn Newitt, "Mozambique Island: The Rise and Decline of a Colonial Port City," in *Portuguese Colonial Cities in the Early Modern World*, ed. Liam Matthew Brockey (Farnham: Ashgate, 2008), 105–27.
12. C. R. Boxer, "Moçambique Island and the 'carreira da Índia,'" *Stvdia* 8 (1961): 95–132; Malyn Newitt, *A History of Mozambique* (London: Hurst & Company, 1995), 1–30; Newitt, "Mozambique Island."
13. Eric Axelson, *Portuguese in South-East Africa 1600–1700* (Johannesburg: Witwatersrand University Press, 1969), 15–29; Newitt, *A History*, 157–72; Newitt, "Mozambique Island"; Eugénia Rodrigues, *Portugueses e Africanos nos Rios de Sena. Os Prazos da Coroa em Moçambique nos Séculos XVII e XVIII* (Lisbon: Imprensa Nacional-Casa da Moeda, 2013), 123–5.
14. Alexandre Lobato, "Ilha de Moçambique: Notícia Histórica," *Arquivo* 4 (1988): 79–83; Newitt, "Mozambique Island."

15. Eugénia Rodrigues, "Moçambique e o Índico: a circulação de saberes e práticas de cura," *Métis: História & Cultura* 19 (2011): 15–42; Eugénia Rodrigues, "Crossing the Indian Ocean: African Slaves and Medical Knowledge in Goa," in *Learning from Empire: Medicine, Knowledge and Transfers under Portuguese Rule*, ed. Poonam Bala (Newcastle upon Tyne: Cambridge Scholars Publishers, 2018), 74–96.
16. Gaspar Correia, *Lendas da Índia* (Coimbra: Imprensa da Universidade de Coimbra, 1921), 785; Boxer, "Moçambique Island," 105.
17. Manuel Godinho de Herédia, *O lyvro de plantaforma das fortalezas da India* (Lisbon: Ministério da Defesa, 1999).
18. João dos Santos, *Etiópia Oriental e Vária História de Cousas Notáveis do Oriente* (Lisbon: CNPCDP, 1999), 256–7.
19. "Carta do Irmão Jácome de Braga S.J., Goa, 2 de Dezembro de 1563," in *Documentação para a história do padroado português do Oriente. India*, vol. 9, ed. A. da Silva Rego (Lisbon: AGU, 1953), 214. On European military hospitals, see Lindemann, *Medicine and Society*, 186.
20. Eugénia Rodrigues, "As Misericórdias de Moçambique e a administração local, c. 1606–1763," in *O reino, as ilhas e o mar oceano. Estudos em homenagem a Artur Teodoro de Matos*, vol. 2, ed. Avelino de Freitas de Menezes and João Paulo Oliveira e Costa (Lisbon: CHAM, 2007), 709–29. On the role of Misericórdias in the administration of hospitals in Portugal, see Abreu, "Training Health Professionals," 125–9. For more about Misericórdias, see Isabel dos Guimarães Sá, *Quando o rico se faz pobre: Misericórdias, caridade e poder no império português 1500–1800* (Lisbon: CNCDP, 1997).
21. Boxer, "Moçambique Island," 106–7.
22. Ibid., 100–5.
23. Sousa, *História da Medicina*, 112.
24. Lindemann, *Medicine and Society*, 159–60.
25. Boxer, "Moçambique Island"; Sousa, *História da Medicina*, 111–14.
26. For some testimonies, see Boxer, "Moçambique Island." On hospitals in Goa, see Bastos, "Hospitais e sociedade"; Bastos, "Together and Apart"; Gracias, *Health and Hygiene*.
27. On All Saints Hospital in Lisbon, see Pacheco, "De Todos-Os-Santos a São José."
28. "Carta régia,13 Março de 1562," *Arquivo Português Oriental* 5, no. 2 (1865): 501.
29. J. Worth Estes, "Food as Medicine," in *The Cambridge World History of Food*, vol. 2, ed. Kenneth F. Kiple and Kriemhild Conèe Ornelas (Cambridge: University of Cambridge Press, 2000), 1534–53; Jean-Louis Flandrin and Massimo Montanari, eds., *Histoire de l'Alimentation* (Paris: Fayard, 1996); Lindemann, *Medicine and Society*, 12–17.
30. Boxer, "Moçambique Island," 107; Andrade, "Fundação do Hospital"; Rodrigues, "Misericórdias de Moçambique."
31. Risse, *Mending Bodies*, 218.
32. Axelson, *Portuguese*, 117–19.
33. The Brothers Hospitallers of Saint John of God also run hospitals in Spain and Italy. Borges, *Reais Hospitais*; Andrade, "Os Hospitaleiros de S. João de Deus."
34. "Alvará do príncipe regente D. Pedro," March 24, 1681, Arquivo Histórico Ultramarino (Overseas Historical Archive, Lisbon; hereafter AHU), Conselho Ultramarino, cod. 1545, fol. 2–2v.
35. On European hospitals, see Lindemann, *Medicine and Society*, 163.
36. "Provisão do vice-rei do Estado da India," January 3, 1682, AHU, Conselho Ultramarino, cod. 1545, fols. 2v–3.
37. "Carta do príncipe regente D. Pedro para o vice-rei D. Pedro de Almeida," March 20, 1680, AHU, Índia, cx. 56; Frei Bartolomeu dos Mártires, "Memoria Chorografica da Provincia ou Capitania de Mossambique na Costa d'Africa Oriental conforme o estado em que se encontrava no anno de 1822," 1823, Arquivo Histórico de Moçambique (Mozambique Historical Archive, Maputo; hereafter AHM), SE aIII P 9, no. 216a.
38. Borges, *Reais Hospitais*.
39. The Swahili stone domestic architecture developed from the fifteenth century onward. However, it was only in the eighteenth century that stone houses became common in Swahili cities. Andrew Petersen, *Dictionary of Islamic Architecture* (London and New York: Routledge, 2002), 75–6.
40. *Mecrusse* is a very hard wood, which was durable and resistant to the lime used to build houses and the termites that abounded in the region.
41. For more about techniques of construction on Mozambique Island, see Pedro Quirino da Fonseca, "Breves notas sobre a evolução da habitação e construção em Moçambique," *Monumenta* 4 (1968): 45–8; *Ilha de Moçambique. Relatório–Report 1982–85* (Maputo: Secretaria de Estado da Cultura—Moçambique & Arkitektskolen i Aarhus—Danmark, n.d). On Swahili towns, see Prita Meier, *Swahili Port Cities: The Architecture of Elsewhere* (Bloomington, IN: Indiana University Press, 2016).

42. Henry Salt, *A voyage to Abyssinia, and Travels Into the Interior of that Country, Executed Under the Orders of the British Government, in the Years 1809 and 1810* (Philadelphia: M. Carey; Boston: Wells & Lilly, 1816), 29.
43. *Ilha de Moçambique*, 59. See also Alexandre Lobato, *Ilha de Moçambique. Panorama Histórico* (Lisbon: AGU, 1967).
44. "Carta do príncipe regente D. Pedro para o vice-rei," March 20, 1680, AHU, Índia, cx. 56; Andrade, "Fundação do Hospital."
45. "Cópia do assento para o vedor da fazenda geral mandar uma botica de medicina e camas para a enfermaria e mais fabricas necessárias para o hospital novo de Mossambique," November 26, 1681, AHU, Conselho Ultramarino, cod. 1545, fol. 6–6v; "Lista das cousas enviadas de Goa para o novo hospital de Moçambique," AHU, India, cx. 56.
46. For more on the pharmacy, see Andrade, "Fundação do Hospital."
47. "Carta de Frei Vicente da Encarnação para o rei," December 23, 1758, AHU, Moçambique, cx. 15, doc. 39. See also Andrade, "Fundação do Hospital."
48. Risse, *Mending Bodies*.
49. On hospitals in Portugal, see Borges, *Reais Hospitais*.
50. "Carta de Frei Vicente da Encarnação para o rei," December 23, 1758, AHU, Moçambique, cx. 15, doc. 39.
51. "Provisão da Igreja da Saúde," August 7, 1711, AHU, Conselho Ultramarino, cod. 1545, fols. 20v–21.
52. The Portuguese Crown initially bought ten slaves to work in the hospital, but this number varied over time. "Provisão do conde vice-rei," January 3, 1682, AHU, Conselho Ultramarino, cod. 1545, fols. 4v–6.
53. For more on houses built in lime and stone and *macuti*, see *Ilha de Moçambique*.
54. Quoted by Boxer, "Moçambique Island," 109. See also Andrade, "O Hospital de Moçambique durante a administração dos religiosos de S. João de Deus," 261–2.
55. Quoted by Andrade, "O Hospital de Moçambique durante a administração dos religiosos de S. João de Deus," 261–2.
56. The date above the door appears on a hospital plan from 1847. "Plano do Hospital Militar de Moçambique," October 9, 1847, AHU, Secretaria de Estado da Marinha e do Ultramar, Direcção Geral do Ultramar, cx. 1507.
57. "Cópia do assento para o feitor de Mossambique do dinheiro da sua receita dar aos religiosos de São João de Deos quinhentos cruzados de ajuda de custo por cada lanço da caza da infirmeria que levantarem," January 14, 1703, AHU, Conselho Ultramarino, cod. 1545, fol. 13.
58. "Carta do governador Francisco de Melo e Castro para o secretário de estado," July 28, 1753, AHU, Conselho Ultramarino, cod. 1310, fol. 11v; "Carta do governador Francisco de Melo e Castro para o secretário de estado," December 30, 1753, AHU, Moçambique, cx. 9, doc. 32; "Carta de Frei Vicente da Encarnação para o rei," December 23, 1758, AHU, Moçambique, cx. 15, doc. 39.
59. "Carta topográfica da ilha de Mossambique," 1754, Capitão de infantaria e engenheiro Gregório Taumaturgo de Brito, AHU, Cartografia Manuscrita, D.518.
60. Lindemann, *Medicine and Society*, 166–7.
61. Andrade, "O hospital de Moçambique durante a administração dos Almoxarifes."
62. George Rosen, *From Medical Police to Social Medicine: Essays on the History of Health Care* (New York: Science History Publications, 1974); Roy Porter, "The Eighteenth Century," in *The Western Medical Tradition*, 465–6; Risse, *Mending Bodies*, 236–43.
63. Laurinda Abreu, *Pina Manique. Um reformador no Portugal das Luzes* (Lisbon: Gradiva, 2013).
64. Ludmilla Jordanova, "Earth Science and Environmental Medicine: The Synthesis of the Late Enlightenment," in *Images of the Earth: Eessay in the History of the Environmental Sciences*, ed. Ludmilla Jordanova and Roy Porter (Chalfont St. Giles: British Society for the History of Science, 1979), 119–46; Anthony Kessel, *Air, the Environment and Public Health* (Cambridge: Cambridge University Press, 2010); Lindemann, *Medicine and Society*, 109–12.
65. Arnold, "The Place of 'the tropics.'"
66. See, for example, David Arnold, "Introduction. Tropical Medicine before Manson," in *Warm Climates and Western Medicine: The Emergence of Tropical Medicine, 1500–1900*, ed. David Arnold (Amsterdam and Atlanta: Rodopi 1996), 1–19; David Arnold, *Science, Technology and Medicine in Colonial India* (Cambridge: Cambridge University Press, 2004), 50–76; Mark Harrison, *Climates and Constitutions: Health, Race, Environment and British Imperialism in India, 1600–1850* (New Delhi: Oxford University Press, 1999).
67. For similar topics in the British Empire see, for example, Pratik Chakrabarti, "'Neither of meate nor drink, but what the Doctor alloweth': Medicine amidst War and Commerce in Eighteenth-Century Madras," *Bulletin of the History of Medicine* 80, no. 1 (2006): 1–38.
68. Lindemann, *Medicine and Society*, 160; Risse, *Mending Bodies*, 5.

Health and Architecture

69. "Carta do governador Francisco de Melo e Castro para o secretário de estado," December 20, 1753, AHU, Moçambique, cx. 9, doc. 4. See also, "Carta do governador Francisco de Melo e Castro para o secretário de estado," July 28, 1753, AHU, Conselho Ultramarino, cod. 1310, fol. 11v.
70. "Carta de Frei Vicente da Encarnação para o rei," December 23, 1758, AHU, Moçambique, cx. 15, doc. 39. See also Andrade, "O hospital de Moçambique durante a administração dos Almoxarifes."
71. "Carta do cirurgião José Álvares," December 22, 1758, AHU, Moçambique, cx. 15, doc. 39.
72. On Europe, see, for example, Lindemann, *Medicine and Society*, 161; Foucault, "The Politics of Health," 180.
73. On hospital in Lisbon, see Abreu, "Training Health Professionals."
74. "Consulta do Conselho Ultramarino," October 14, 1754, AHU, Moçambique, cx. 10, doc. 14. See also "Carta régia," April 14, 1755, AHU, Conselho Ultramarino, cod. 1327, fol. 155.
75. "Instrução ao governador de Moçambique Calixto Rangel Pereira de Sá," May 7, 1761, AHU, Moçambique, cx. 19, doc. 63-A.
76. Rodrigues, "Moçambique e o Índico."
77. Arnold, *Spaces of the Hospital*, 7. See also Lindemann, *Medicine and Society*, 161
78. "Carta do governador Baltazar Pereira do Lago para o secretário de estado," August 24, 1766, AHU, Moçambique, cx. 25, doc. 69.
79. "Instrução do governador Baltazar Manuel Pereira do Lago ao seu sucessor," AHU, Conselho Ultramarino, cod. 1325, fols. 176-9. On hospitals in Portugal, see Abreu, "Training Health Professionals."
80. Richardson, *English Hospitals, 1660-1948*, 15.
81. "Instrução do governador Baltazar Manuel Pereira do Lago ao seu sucessor," AHU, Conselho Ultramarino, cod. 1325, fols. 176-9.
82. Risse, *Mending Bodies*, 7.
83. "Instrução do governador Baltazar Manuel Pereira do Lago ao seu sucessor," AHU, Conselho Ultramarino, cod. 1325, fols. 176-9. See also "Carta do governador Moçambique Baltazar Pereira do Lago para o secretário de estado," August 20, 1766, AHU, Moçambique, cx. 26, doc. 83
84. Ibid.
85. The Jesuits had been expelled from Portugal and its empire in 1759.
86. "Bando do governador António de Melo e Castro," June 8, 1789, AHU, Moçambique, cx. 58, doc. 16. For more about the slave trade, see José Capela, *O tráfico de escravos nos portos de Moçambique, 1733-1904* (Porto: Afrontamento, 2002).
87. "Certidão passada por Frei Bernardo da Anunciação," June 20, 1773, AHU, Conselho Ultramarino, cod. 1332, fols. 111v-12.
88. On Europe, see Lindemann, *Medicine and Society*, 161.
89. "Alvará do governador António de Melo e Castro," June 5, 1789, AHU, Moçambique, cx. 58, doc. 14.
90. "Carta do governador José Vasconcelos e Almeida para o Marquês de Angeja," August 26, 1780, AHU, Moçambique, cx. 34, doc. 53. See also "Carta do governador José Vasconcelos e Almeida," February 21, 1780, AHU, Conselho Ultramarino, cod. 1339, fol. 236.
91. "Regimento do Hospital," December 30, 1788, AHU, Moçambique, cx. 56, doc. 72. See also "Regimento do Hospital," August 1, 1783, AHU, Moçambique, cx. 43, doc. 12.
92. See, for example, Christian Cheminade, "Architecture and Medecine in the Late 18th Century: Ventilation in Hospitals, from the Encyclopédie to the Debate on the Hôtel-Dieu in Paris," *Recherches sur Diderot et sur l'Encyclopédie* 14 (1993): 85-109; Risse, *Mending Bodies*, 151, 242-3.
93. "Carta do governador interino Vicente Caetano de Maia e Vasconcelos para o secretário de estado," August 18, 1781, AHU, Conselho Ultramarino, cod. 1345, fols. 96v-100v. Syphilis treatments required a mercury pomade to be applied all over the patient's body in a heated room in order to induce sweating and thus expel noxious humors. Jon Arrizabalaga, John Henderson, and Roger French, *The Great Pox. The French Disease in Renaissance Europe* (New Haven and London: Yale University Press, 1997). All Saints Hospital in Lisbon also had a pox house from the early sixteenth century. Arrizabalaga, "Medical Theory," 94. The same kind of medicine was used in hospitals in colonial India. Erica Wald, *Vice in the Barracks: Medicine, the Military and the Making of Colonial India, 1780-1868* (Basingstoke: Palgrave Macmillan, 2014).
94. "Representação do governador interino Vicente da Maia Caetano de Vasconcelos aos outros governadores," January 17, 1784, AHU, Conselho Ultramarino, cod. 1352, fols. 6v-8v; "Regimento do Hospital," December 30, 1788, AHU, Moçambique, cx. 56, doc. 72.

95. "Carta do governador D. Diogo de Sousa para o secretário de estado," August 22, 1794, AHU, Moçambique, cx. 68, doc. 60.
96. Lindemann, *Medicine and Society*, 159–61.
97. "Regimento do Hospital," December 30, 1788, AHU, Moçambique, cx. 56, doc. 72.
98. Foucault, *The Birth*; Kisacky, *Rise of the Modern Hospital*, 18.
99. For more about the profile of the medical staff, see Rodrigues, "Moçambique e o Índico"; Eugénia Rodrigues, "Eating and Drinking at the Royal Hospital of Mozambique Island: Medicine and Diet Change between the End of the 18th and the Early 19th Century," *Afriques. Débats, méthodes et terrains d'histoire* 5 (2014), accessed January 30, 2015. http://afriques.revues.org/1553.
100. Foucault, *The Birth*, 139–87. However, the pattern of separate beds had already been adopted in All Saints Hospital in Lisbon during the sixteenth century. Pacheco, "De Todos-Os-Santos a São José," 50.
101. "Carta do governador João Manuel da Silva para o secretário de estado," November 27, 1821, AHU, Moçambique, cx. 181, doc. 121. On the number of the military patients, see Rodrigues, "Eating and Drinking."
102. "Planta do Hospital Militar da Cidade de Mossambique," n.a. [Xavier Shmid von Belliken], n.d. [1821], Ministério da Defesa, Direcção de Infra-estruturas do Exército (Ministry of Defense, Directorate of Infrastructures of the Army, Lisbon), GEAM/DIE, 1218–2A-24A-111.
103. Luís Vicente de Simoni, "Tratado Medico sobre o Clima e Enfermidades de Moçambique," 1821, Biblioteca Nacional (National Library, Rio de Janeiro), Secção de Manuscritos, cod. I–47, 23, 17, fol. 12.
104. Rodrigues, "Moçambique e o Índico."
105. "Carta do governo interino para o administrador do hospital Matias Antunes de Sousa," May 3, 1838, AHM, Fundo Século XIX, cod. 11–6 Da6, fol. 67.
106. Sebastião Xavier Botelho, *Memória estatística sobre os domínios portugueses na África Oriental* (Lisbon: Tipografia José Baptista Morando, 1835), 330–2.
107. Ibid., 334.
108. Foucault, "The Politics of Health," 175.
109. James Prior, *Voyage Along the Eastern Coast of Africa, to Mosambique, Johanna and Quilloa; St. Helena; to Rio de Janeiro, Bahia, and Pernambuco in Brazil in the Nisus Frigate* (London: Printed for Sir Richard Phillips and Co, 1819), 34.

CHAPTER 9
FROM EXIGENCY TO CIVIC PRIDE
THE DEVELOPMENT OF EARLY AUSTRALIAN HOSPITALS
Julie Willis

The idea of the hospital as a dedicated place for the care of the sick has a long history in Western civilization, stretching back thousands of years. The military hospitals of the Romans and the monastic hospitals across Europe formed the basis of a tradition of spaces that provided succor to the sick, the indigent, and the insane. The Renaissance saw the further development of the hospital, with large-scale secular institutions built to dispense benevolent care within grand edifices. In Britain, at least, this was supplemented by the creation of cottage hospitals that appeared in smaller towns. The hospital was thus a permanent and public building that was a cornerstone of social welfare, if not yet a social welfare state. Importantly, it wasn't just hospitals in Britain and Europe that provided healthcare; they were supplemented by a surrounding infrastructure of doctors, barber-surgeons, apothecaries, and midwives. Most people thus had a reasonable chance of accessing some kind of healthcare, whether through charitable or private means.

The colonial settlement of Australia in 1788 cannot be dated to the pre-modern period, but its isolation and privation in its early years, and the way its hospitals were provided, speaks to the difficulties of establishing a functioning medical infrastructure *de novo*. In the early years of colonial settlements, when only a handful of doctors would struggle against widespread outbreaks of disease without permanent buildings or medical supplies, the surgeons and their superiors must have believed they had returned to pre-modern times, where death, despair, and dire needs were the order of the day and salvation a distant hope. There was not the luxury of designing hospitals as places of healing or repose, instead they were structures built of necessity, shelters in which, at best, very basic medical care could be dispensed.

Australian colonial hospitals stood in stark contrast to the grand edifices of charity and small cottage hospitals that underpinned the contemporaneous British hospital system. The designs of colonial hospitals drew on the military field hospital and, more often, military barracks: they were simple structures designed to accommodate the bed-ridden. Within the newly settled colonies, the hospital was believed to be an important facility—so important that, in several instances, prefabricated structures were transported with settlers, their construction prioritized above all else—yet for decades these societies lacked a functioning medical community beyond the colonial surgeon and his barebones hospital. These first hospitals were scarcely more than huts or tents to shelter the injured, sick, and dying, and to dispense what little medicine might be available. Little thought was expended on making the hospitals places of healing, and their designs generally bore scant recognition of the need for proper ventilation and sanitation. The more permanent hospitals that replaced the first incarnations were an improvement: wards were usually placed so that they could have windows on at least two walls, but generally these were arranged to arrive at a plan that was aesthetically pleasing rather than highly functional. More often than not, no provision was made at all for spaces of ablution or supervision. The architectural embellishment evident in early Australian hospitals, through the use of styles that indicated their status, showed them to be important public buildings in the colonies and just as much part of civic infrastructure as the courthouse or custom house.

This chapter examines the establishment and development of colonial hospitals in the Australian colonies from 1788 to 1850. It focuses on the conundrum that, while these hospitals were evidently valued highly in these settlements, they suffered from manifestly inadequate provisioning, as if the availability of a hospital was more important than its capacity to function. In contrast to Britain, from the outset the primary provider of hospitals and healthcare in the Australian colonies was the state rather than private citizens through subscription and charitable efforts. While this was understandable in the penal colonies, such as New South Wales, where nearly the entire population was dependent on the Crown for their support, it was perhaps less so in the free Australian colonies where the state would also be an important catalyst in the provision of hospitals.

Colonial Settlement in Australia

The history of hospitals in Australia is intimately tied to its history as a collection of penal and settler colonies from England in the late eighteenth and early nineteenth centuries. The Australian continent's history of human settlement stretches back at least 50,000 years. Connections to Western civilization were evident through trade as early as the thirteenth century,[1] and European sightings of the land from 1606, but it was the voyage of Captain James Cook up its east coast in 1770 that ultimately prompted its annexation by the British Empire.[2] British settlement commenced with the arrival of the First Fleet in the early weeks of January 1788, after an eight-month journey that left Portsmouth, England in May 1787. The fleet—eleven ships in total, carrying just over 1,000 people, 750 of whom were convicts—was to establish a penal colony on the east coast of Australia. The only shelter available to them was what they brought themselves, as the arrangements for the advance party had failed[3] and the local Indigenous inhabitants built structures and shelters that could not be immediately appropriated or commandeered.[4]

The colonization of Australia began with the Sydney settlement of 1788. Over a period of some seventy years, six independent colonies, all founded by the British, were created on the Australian mainland and its immediate surrounding islands. These colonies federated in 1901 to create the nation of Australia, comprising (in order of legal establishment): New South Wales (1787); Tasmania (1825, known then as Van Dieman's Land); Western Australia (1829); South Australia (1836); Victoria (1851); and Queensland (1859). In its earliest incarnation, New South Wales was declared as the entire eastern part of the continent, from which both Victoria and Queensland were then formally excised. Both Western Australia and South Australia were created through directives of the British government and promoted as settler idylls, but their harsh reality bore little relation to the paradise promised. Each colony's primary towns, later state capitals, were founded near the coast, for the vast distances between them and any other developed ports meant the only viable transportation route was by sea. All the colonies were highly dependent on government auspices, whether it be the British Parliament of Westminster or, later, their own colonial administrations: in those places where transported convicts made up a significant portion of the population (including New South Wales, Tasmania, and later Western Australia), the state was responsible for their care and shelter; elsewhere, the state held less social responsibility.

The Sydney Hospital: The First Public Building

The civil and military contingent that arrived in Sydney in the early days of 1788 had included medical staff consisting of a principal surgeon, three assistant surgeons, and one junior surgeon who, upon disembarking, immediately set about creating accommodation for a hospital. The entire community in its first days ashore was housed under canvas, and the hospital thus consisted of a series of tents, several reserved for the sick and one as a dispensary and consulting room.[5] Despite the multiple pressing needs for more permanent accommodation, Governor Phillip prioritized the building of a hospital and a stores building, directing all his convict carpenters to the effort in mid-February 1788.[6] The hospital was thus the first public building erected in the colony and its third permanent structure, after the Governor's house (brought prefabricated in the fleet's cargo) and the stores.

The hospital that was built, adjacent to the tent hospital on the western side of Sydney Cove (in the area now known as the Rocks), was a timber-framed structure clad in pine shingles that were attached by pegs made by the female convicts.[7] The lack of available lime deposits in the Sydney area meant that there was no mortar for bricks or the plastering of walls, so the single-skin shingle roof, walls built on the ground, and the dirt floor barely gave protection from the weather, let alone appropriate accommodation for the sick. The building, measuring 23 × 84 feet (7 × 25.6 m) was designed to hold up to eighty patients, with separate sections for the dispensary, the convict patients, and the military patients.[8] This initial separation of the military from the convict contingent was not surprising, but would become clearer in the later provision of hospitals. The hospital was unable to provide much more than shelter: there had been provision of medicines and surgical instruments in the fleet's cargo, but no blankets or sheets, and many of the medical stores were found to have perished on the long journey.[9] With new supplies years away (the medical staff were obliged to seek out substitute compounds, presumably with the help of the local Aboriginal people), the colony remained in a parlous situation with regards to proper medical care for some time.

Underscoring the importance of the hospital to the New South Wales colony, a prefabricated hospital building (Figure 9.1) was carried in the cargo of the Second Fleet, which arrived at Sydney in June 1790, nearly two-and-a-half years after the arrival of the first. Designed by architect Samuel Wyatt in London, the

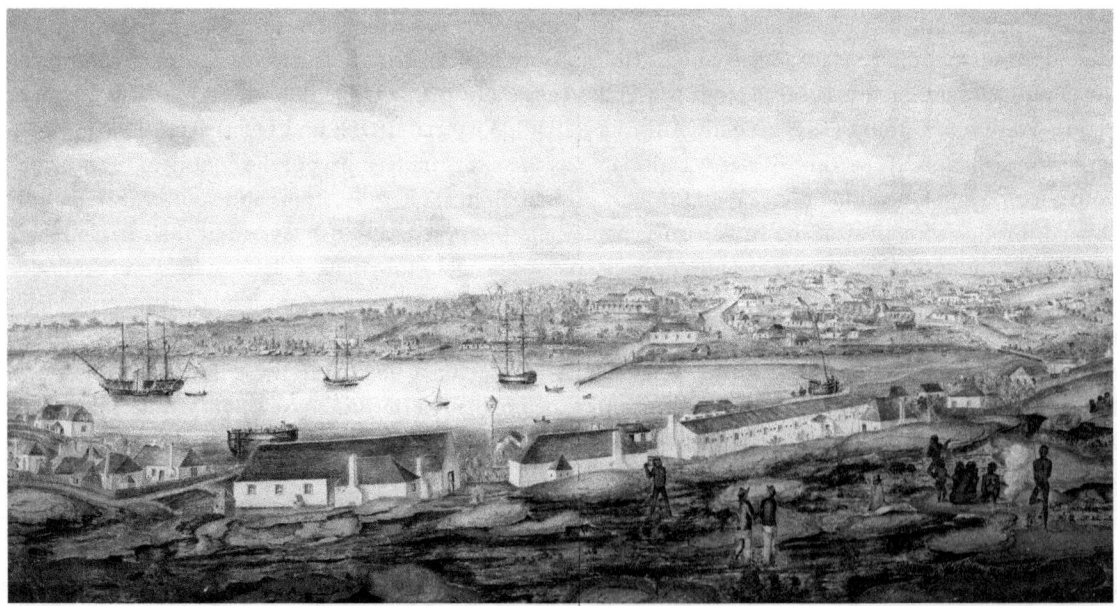

Figure 9.1 Prefabricated second hospital (the long range seen at the lower left), Sydney, viewed from the western side of Sydney Cove. Sydney General Hospital, Sydney, New South Wales, Australia; architect: Samuel Wyatt, 1790; artist: George William Evans (attrib.), *c.* 1803. Source: State Library of New South Wales

building cost £690 and was timber-framed and timber-clad with a copper roof, measuring some 20½ × 84 feet (6.25 × 25.6 m) and with walls 12 feet high (3.6 m) with "cross Partition and Porches."[10] Accompanying the prefabricated hospital were a large number of sick convicts: some 486—nearly two-thirds of the surviving convict population on board—were transferred to the hospital on arrival, and had to be accommodated in 100 tents around it.[11] Governor Phillip could express only dismay at the situation, writing, "I will not, sir, dwell on the scene of misery which the hospitals and sick tents exhibited when these people were landed ...."[12] The nursing staff were drawn from the female convict population and showed little care for their charges. Meager rations were given to patients, which they themselves were expected to prepare; indeed, convicts were often placed on hospital duty as a punishment for misdemeanors committed while on other assigned duties.[13] Although the new hospital was almost the same size as the old, it was an improvement as the building was raised on stumps with an internal timber floor. But it was not to last. Termites attacked the wooden stumps, and the hospital was rebuilt in October 1797 under the direction of Governor Hunter, this time on a new site nearby, and on stone foundations.[14] A hospital store and separate dispensary were also constructed, along with nearby living quarters for the surgeons that were built in brick.[15] The hospital and its subsidiary buildings were set in a fenced two-acre plot, within which vegetables were cultivated.

The Sydney hospital might have served that particular town, but it was not the only one in the New South Wales colony. Governor Phillip had established a small settlement for agricultural purposes late in 1788 at Parramatta, some 23 kilometers west of Sydney, soon after which one of the colony's assistant surgeons was dispatched to establish a hospital. The accommodation erected in 1789, although intended to be temporary, consisted of "two long sheds, built in the form of a tent, and thatched." Two years later, when still in use, it was described as "most wretched ... totally destitute of every convenience."[16] Its dire state was redressed by the building of a more permanent hospital in 1792 in brick, 80 feet long by 20 feet wide (24.4 × 6 m), but the continuing lack of lime for mortar meant that this building, too, soon deteriorated and was in constant need of repair.[17] With the completion of a military hospital adjacent to the parade ground at the Wynyard Barracks in Sydney late in 1797, a separate military medical system was established and military hospitals began to appear in many of the major settlements of the colony.

These early hospitals served everyone dependent on or in the employ of the Crown: convicts, military, and Navy seamen, treating every malady from venereal disease to dysentery. But the medical staff were not required to attend to the needs of those who were not supported by the Crown, such as free settlers or the local Indigenous inhabitants. There were no private medical practitioners at the time, and the limitations of Sydney's medical support are demonstrated by two midwifery cases. In 1805, Assistant Surgeon James Mileham was court-martialed for refusing to attend to a woman in labor at the Sydney General Hospital, as was Assistant Surgeon John Savage a few months later for "neglecting to attend" to another woman in labor, the wife of a settler, who subsequently died.[18]

A Public Edifice: Governor Macquarie and the "Rum Hospital"

The arrival to New South Wales of Lachlan Macquarie, who commenced as governor there in 1810, ushered in a new set of standards for the colony. Along with establishing a building code and a town plan, one of his first priorities was the construction of a new hospital. The prefabricated hospital, which had been relocated and refurbished during the last twenty years, was by then in "a state of total neglect."[19] In May 1810, Macquarie called for tenders to build a new facility, to be located on a ridge of high ground to the east of Wynyard on present-day Macquarie Street. The hospital was to be funded by creative means: the successful tenderers would be granted a monopoly to import rum to the colony over a three-year period, with the costs of building the hospital borne entirely by them. Given rum was the panacea used to ameliorate the suffering of most in the colony, it was an attractive deal: one of the principal surgeons, D'Arcy Wentworth, was part of the first acceptable tender until asked to withdraw by Macquarie.[20] The building became known as the "Rum Hospital" because of its unusual model of financing.[21]

The design, prepared in 1811, showed a grand two-story complex of three ranges strung along the street, surrounded by verandahs on all sides. The center range, the largest, was distinguished by a simple pediment and a series of wide steps leading to what appeared to be a central arched doorway (Figure 9.2). But the plan behind this grand facade was two pairs of large wards on each floor, with each pair conjoined by a stair and entrance hall; thus the implied central entrance was actually blind, bisected behind by a party wall between two wards. The two smaller ranges echoed the main plan in their arrangements of rooms, although they did not contain wards for patients. The plans were notable for the absence of any rooms for medical staff adjacent to the wards, and because the privies were inconveniently distant from the buildings (some later hospitals would be built with no provision for privies at all in the first instance). Each of the eight wards, either 58½ × 24 feet (17.8 × 7.3 m) or 61½ × 24 feet (18.7 × 7.3 m), were designed to hold twenty beds.

There is debate as to the authorship of the design. In 1810, the New South Wales colony had as yet no professional architects and its buildings were generally designed by military personnel, builders, or stonemasons. The Sydney General Hospital's design may have been proposed by John O'Hearne, the stonemason who worked with the successful tenderers, but it seems unlikely; it may have also been influenced by the Governor's wife, Elizabeth Macquarie, whose interest in architecture and influence over several Sydney

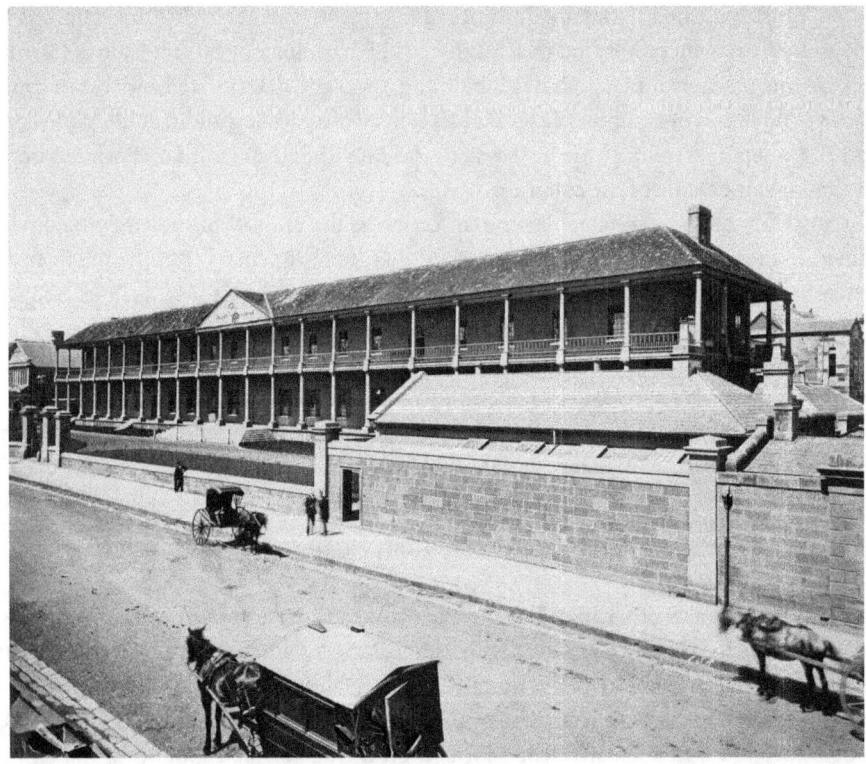

Figure 9.2 Central range of Sydney's general hospital, colloquially known as the "Rum Hospital," Macquarie Street, Sydney. Sydney General Hospital, Sydney, New South Wales, Australia; architect: unknown, 1811–16; photographer: Charles Percy Pickering, 1870. Source: State Library of New South Wales

buildings are well known.[22] The plans and elevations bore significant similarities to a design for a military barracks proposed by Macquarie's immediate predecessor, Acting Governor Lt. Colonel Joseph Foveaux, in 1809,[23] but also a credible similarity to the London Hospital designed by Boulton Mainwearing and built 1752–9. What is certain is that the designer's hand was amateur. The pediment, as built, was really a transverse gable, supported by the stacked Tuscan columns that supported the whole of the verandah, without further distinction: the designer could approximate a distinguished public building of the Georgian era, but did not understand how to correctly detail pediments and porticoes. Yet the building was the grandest structure in the fledgling Sydney settlement on its completion in 1816, even if its defective construction already needed attention.

Two smaller hospital buildings soon followed: a military hospital on Fort Street near Observatory Hill, completed 1815; and a convict hospital at Parramatta, completed 1818 (Figure 9.3), both of which were designed by Macquarie's aide-de-camp John Watts. The similarities were notable as both were two stories and used the same plan: two wards, conjoined by a stair, and flanked at the far ends of each ward by two small rooms that were accessed by the encircling verandah. The plan, like that of the Sydney General Hospital, was taken from standard plans for barracks, and would remain in use as a standard hospital plan until at least the 1830s in Australia.[24] Each building was surrounded by a double-story verandah accommodated under a spreading hipped roof.

Macquarie was focused on building New South Wales into more than just a penal colony, undertaking a significant building program in Sydney and other towns of the settlement. The benefits were twofold: not

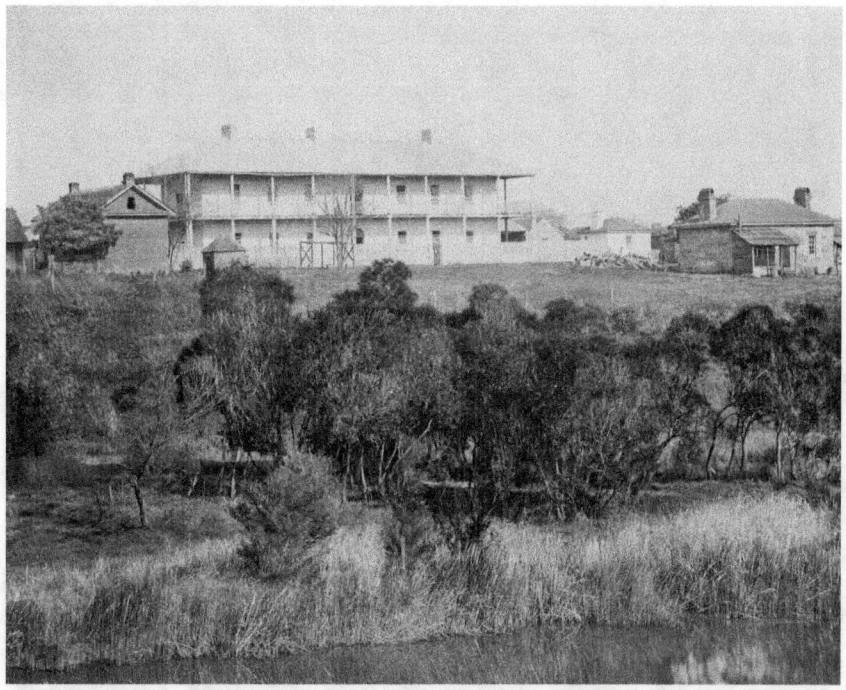

Figure 9.3 The Parramatta Convict Hospital is typical of early Australian colonial hospitals, with two identical wards per floor, surrounded by a verandah under a large hipped roof. Paramatta Convict Hospital, Parramatta, New South Wales, Australia; architect: John Watts, 1818; photographer unknown, c. 1870–1920. Source: State Archives and Records, New South Wales

only did the colony gain important improvements to its infrastructure, but it also made meaningful use of surplus convict labor in times when the free settler and government farms were unable to support them. More often than not, the buildings sought to reach a high architectural standard (for which Macquarie was roundly criticized back in London) and were permanent structures of brick or stone.[25] In terms of the provision of health facilities, Macquarie ensured that each major town had a hospital of a suitable standard. In his eleven-year reign as Governor, he oversaw the building, conversion, or substantial repair of ten hospitals, including at the New South Wales towns of Windsor, Liverpool, and Newcastle, and the Tasmanian settlements of Hobart and Launceston. While the hospital had been regarded as an essential requirement in early colonial Australia, Macquarie elevated it to the status of an important public building.

Before turning to other hospitals, there is one last New South Wales example of note: that of the Liverpool Hospital, completed in 1825 with the design conceived by the pardoned convict Francis Greenway, who served as Colonial Architect under Macquarie from 1816 until he was dismissed in 1822. The design, which has become one of the treasures of Australian colonial architecture, was distinctly different to the hospitals that had preceded it (Figure 9.4). Firstly, it departed from the standard plan, which had invariably placed the wards longitudinally, with the width of the building dictated by the width of the wards. At Liverpool, the wards were placed at ninety degrees to their usual position, giving the plan a depth of nearly 77 feet (23.5 m), and placed at the extremities of the building, meaning that the smaller rooms were sited toward the center of the building. The Liverpool design was also distinct because it eschewed the usual surrounding verandah, instead using an arcaded loggia on the ground floor along its west-facing front, and had a smaller east-facing rear entrance. But

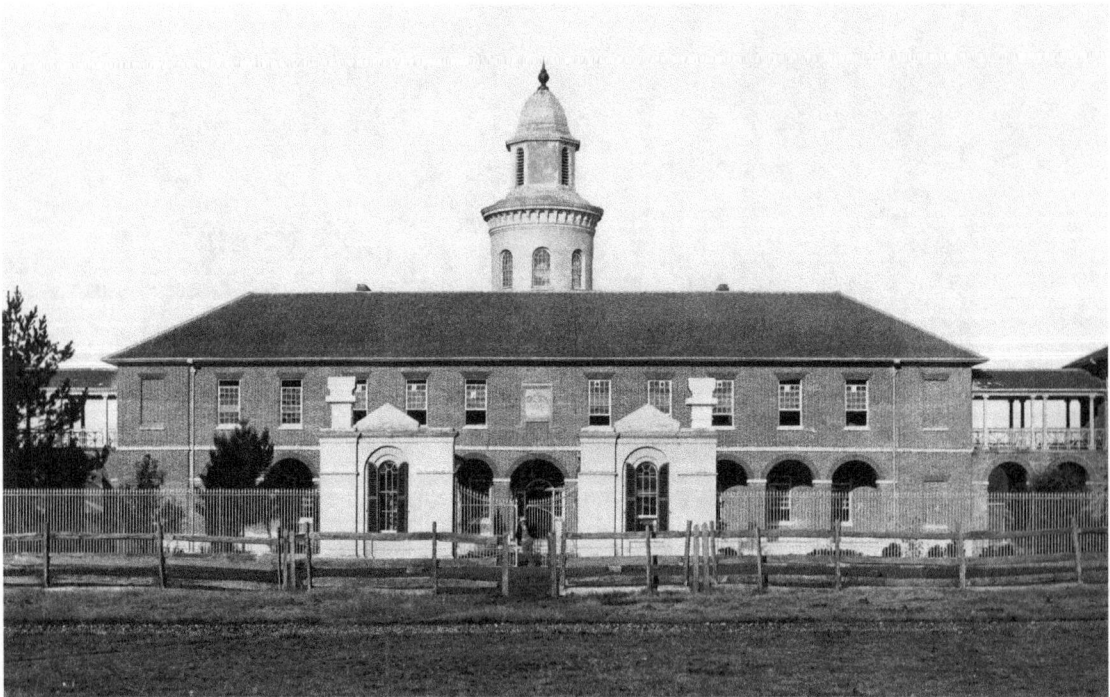

Figure 9.4 The Liverpool Hospital demonstrated for the first time in Australia architectural sophistication as yet unseen in a hospital. Liverpool Hospital, Liverpool, New South Wales, Australia; architect: Francis Greenway, 1822–5; photographer: unknown, *c.* 1880s. Source: City of Liverpool and District Historical Society

by far its most impressive element was the circular domed tower rising some 92 feet (28 m) from the center of the building. Whereas the Sydney "Rum Hospital" had sought grandeur in its attempt at Georgian design, Liverpool had attained it thanks to its refined brickwork and elegant tower. Although there is debate as to how much the design was changed after Greenway's dismissal,[26] there are elements that suggest his hand, in particular in the gatehouses that employ the Soanian motif of ringed brick arches which became somewhat of a Greenway signature, and the articulated tower. Greenway's connections to John Nash and inspiration derived from John Soane are well known.[27] The Liverpool Hospital may have been drawn from appreciation of Soane's Infirmary at the Royal Hospital, Chelsea (1810), and its tower, in part, from Christopher Wren's Great Hall at the same institution.[28] For the first time in Australia, here was a hospital that echoed the grand edifices of eighteenth-century hospitals in Great Britain.

Hospitals in Tasmania: Standard Plans and Regency Flourishes

Like the hospitals in and near Sydney, the provision of medical services in Hobart Town, in what is now Tasmania, had modest beginnings. The settlement, established in 1804 under the jurisdiction of New South Wales, struggled in its early days with the usual illnesses associated with close confinement, slack sanitary standards, and lack of fresh food; the hospital provided was a timber building close to the quay and able to hold up to eighty patients.[29] Despite Macquarie's concern as to the state of the accommodation as early as 1811, no permanent hospital would be constructed until 1820; in the meantime it moved from various timber huts into a number of leased houses.[30] The 1820 design, purported to be by Deputy Surveyor George Evans,[31] was a stone two-story building with two wards per floor, each of 18 × 28 feet (5.5 × 8.5 m).[32] The hospital extended under a skillion roof to the rear, in which smaller rooms and wards were contained; huts separated from the main building included a kitchen and "Lock-up House," which accommodated the insane in the daytime and the malingerers and those refusing treatment at night.[33] In all other respects it followed the design of Watts's Parramatta Hospital.

In a little over a decade, almost predictably the Hobart Hospital was considered overcrowded and dilapidated, with extensions and repairs undertaken to improve the accommodation.[34] By 1840 the building was considered unsalvageable: "The old hospital is decaying every day and before long must fall into a heap of ruins. Humanity and even economy requires a new one."[35] A new hospital, built on open ground in front of the old (and prompted in no small part by the outbreak of typhoid in 1839), was commenced the same year and opened in 1843 (Figure 9.5). It had been intended that the main building would be flanked by two wings, but these were not built due to the colony's economic downturn in 1842. The plan consisted of four wards on each of the two stories, with two wards paired on either side of the central stair. Each ward accommodated sixteen patients. Each pair of wards shared a party wall, in which stood a fireplace, meaning that the wards no longer occupied the full width of the building, and minimizing the opportunity for cross-ventilation. The front elevation was embellished by Regency touches such as the pilasters and breakfronts that gave interest and distinction to the facade, and which echoed the design of important public buildings in the town.[36]

At New Norfolk, some 35 kilometers inland from Hobart on the Derwent River, a convict invalid hospital was established in 1830. Designed by colonial architect John Lee Archer, it too used Regency styling, with its central two-story building punctuated by pilasters across its facade. Unlike hospitals in Australia that preceded it, this was a walled courtyard design where the single-story wards and other spaces formed a U-shaped building with all rooms facing into a central courtyard with no outward-facing windows.[37] A lunatic asylum built at the same time abutted its rear wall, the only connection between the two being the central, shared kitchen.[38]

Health and Architecture

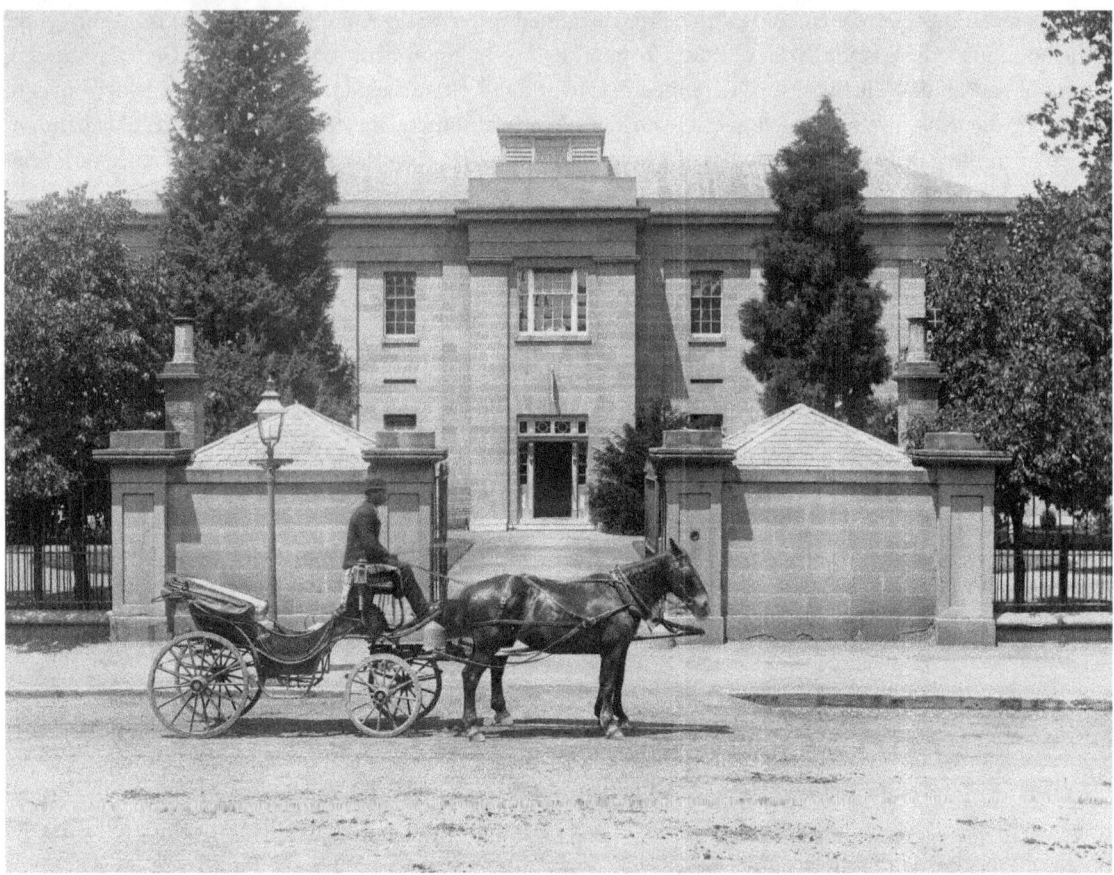

Figure 9.5 The use of the Regency style for the hospital aligned it with other prominent civic buildings in Hobart. Second Hobart Hospital, Hobart, Tasmania, Australia; architect: unknown, 1843; photographer: John Watt Beattie, *c.* 1880. Source: W. L. Crowther Library, Tasmanian Archive and Heritage Office

A Hospital for All: The Moreton Bay Hospital

The settlement of the Moreton Bay area as a penal colony for convicts sentenced to secondary punishment, in what is now Queensland but then was still considered to be part of New South Wales, saw the establishment of Brisbane Town in 1825. Although the settlement had a medical officer from its inception, it had no hospital. This was not from a lack of wanting one—plans were proposed for a hospital and a gaol in around 1825, but without a suitably experienced person to build them the project did not progress.[39] In 1826, there was a second attempt to realize the hospital, but it appears as though two sets of plans were proposed, and the design approved by Governor Darling in Sydney was not the one proceeded with, resulting in further conflict and raising the Governor's ire.[40] The hospital as built had the usual New South Wales hospital plan, with a large ward placed longitudinally on either side of the entrance and taking up the full depth of the building, and with wings extending from the rear on both sides. At some stage before 1835, the hospital was extended: two separate buildings, arranged symmetrically on either side of the hospital, were built to contain a medical officer's quarters and a small military hospital.[41] As a secondary site of punishment, the Moreton Bay settlement was completely closed to free settlers, but in 1840, when the penal colony was broken up and with settlers already established on the nearby Darling Downs, the demographic of its clientele changed dramatically. The hospital faced requests to accommodate patients who were not dependent on the Crown, creating a dilemma for the medical staff. With the proclamation of free settlement in 1842, the chief medical officer sought clarification from Sydney as to who could be treated and under what circumstances. The reply shows the transformation of the convict hospital system into a hospital for all patients, where government officers and others dependent on the Crown would continue to be treated gratis, and all others charged a daily fee for treatment.[42]

The provision of hospitals in the penal settlements of New South Wales (including modern-day Queensland) and Tasmania was considered a necessary aspect of the infrastructure that supported the colonies, particularly as the Crown had much of the population dependent on it for their care. The free settlers of those towns were generally treated for a fee in the convict or general hospitals, the hospitals themselves forming the foundation of the whole healthcare system there. But for the places which were not primarily or initially settled as penal colonies, the provision of hospitals was a more fraught situation.

Start, Stop, and State: Hospitals in the Free Settlements of Western and South Australia

The establishment of a British colony in the far west of the Australian continent, originally known as the Swan River Colony (now Perth, Western Australia), occurred in 1829 with the arrival of a convoy of ships, led by the *Parmelia*. The colony was established for the purposes of free settlement and, given the short time between it being mooted and the arrival of settler ships, it was founded more on optimism and ideal than on practical realities: little thought had been given to the formation of effective governance; and no preparation work was undertaken to manage the influx of expectant settlers.[43] But, from the outset, the government accepted a degree of responsibility for the provision of medical services and a hospital rather than rely on the charitable efforts of the settlement's leading citizens.[44] This may have been due to the influence of the colony's Governor Stirling, who had completed a tour of duty of New South Wales and would have been familiar with the necessities of providing medical care by the state in a fledgling settlement.[45]

Documents drafted on the *Parmelia* made it clear there were intentions to provide a hospital, but the reality was rather different. The first hospital was a tent erected soon after landing, which was relocated some months later to the newly laid out township of Perth.[46] This move did not imply plans to build a permanent hospital: instead, the authorities opened and closed a temporary hospital as the needs of the population required.[47] In June 1830, the hospital was housed in a hut rented from one of the settlers in June 1830, only to be closed and dismantled within some six months as the summer arrived.[48] The next iteration was some three years later, when the colonial surgeon Alexander Collie petitioned for support to open another hospital. This time it was located in a large room inside a house leased by Collie for a six-month period from September 1833, and at least offered a better standard of accommodation than the previous hospitals; it was distinguished by Collie treating a wounded Aboriginal woman during its existence. However, the lease was allowed to lapse a year later, possibly because of Collie's own ill health, which led to his death in 1835. The hospital thus closed with no provision of an alternative.[49]

Incredibly, it would take another six years for there to be sufficient impetus to establish another hospital in the colony. In mid-1840, colonial surgeon James Crichton petitioned Governor Hutt to open a hospital. While Crichton was successful, Hutt insisted on very strict economy, which saw the hospital established in stables refurbished for the purpose.[50] The limitations of this building were almost immediately apparent, as its siting meant it baked in Perth's heat without recourse to the cooling sea breezes; and the condition of its shingled roof meant that the hospital flooded whenever it rained.[51] This state of economy was enforced because the government's charity was meant to extend only to paupers and the destitute; in turn,

Health and Architecture

the disgraceful conditions meant only those with no choice at all attended the hospital. Other provisions for medical care in Perth comprised a hospital attached to the military depot on St. George's Terrace that served army personnel and others attached to the military contingent,[52] and a separate hospital for Aboriginal people, established in 1839.[53]

Predictably, by 1850, Perth's Colonial Hospital was neither fit for purpose nor in any habitable state, with its lease about to end. Community pressure to build anew came through a series of newspaper articles that detailed the dire conditions and the unfortunate fate of several patients left to their own devices, for the hospital had no night nurse.[54] With Western Australia about to receive its first cohort of transported convicts, dramatically increasing its population, the colonial government set aside a site for a new hospital late in 1850. It would take another four-and-a-half years to see the new hospital open and receiving patients. The new hospital was designed by James Austin, Superintendent of Public Works, in 1852. It was a handsome brick building of two stories, with solid brick corner rooms, between which were strung two-story verandahs on all four sides of the building (Figure 9.6). For a building of its size, it had comparatively few windows, with the expanses of brick wall broken up by subtle pilasters and arches, under an all-encompassing hipped roof.

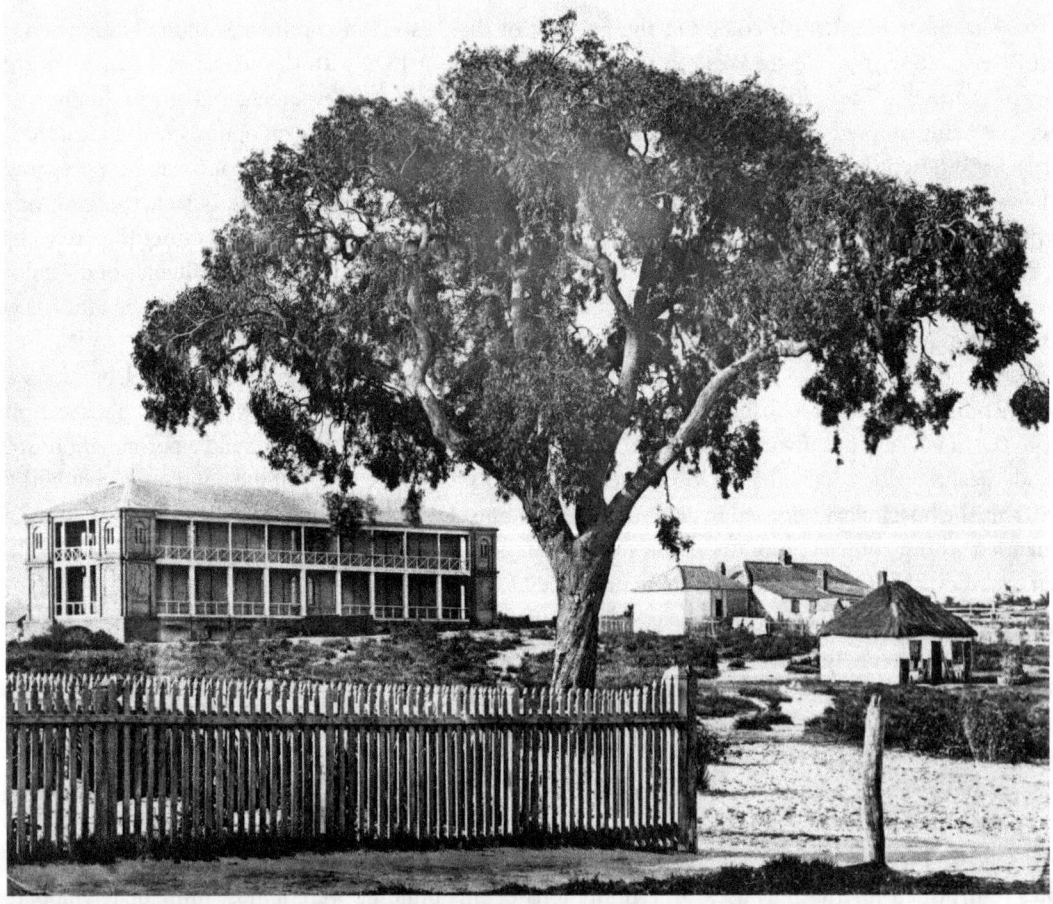

Figure 9.6 Perth finally realized a permanent hospital in 1852. The design is unusual for Australian hospitals in its use of the corner towers to bookend the verandahs. The Colonial Hospital, Perth; architect: James Austin, 1852; photographer: Alfred Hawes Stone, *c.* 1868. Source: State Library of Western Australia

The colony of South Australia was a free settlement established by private interests directly from London in 1836. Like the Swan River Colony (Western Australia), the immigrants who arrived to settle in the town of Adelaide and its surrounds imagined a bucolic, genteel, and ordered settlement; the reality was far different, with a lack of planning and basic infrastructure most apparent. Unlike the powerful positions other colonial governors held in Australian colonies, the administrative arrangements for South Australia saw power divided between the governor and the resident commissioner, the latter to ensure no interference in the business affairs or freedom of religion rights of the settlers. The settlers clearly wanted all the rights of a democratic society, but none of its responsibilities, for the provision of medical services and a hospital in Adelaide followed much the same sorry path as Perth. A colonial surgeon, Thomas Cotter, had been appointed at the outset of the venture in 1835; Governor Hindmarsh directed his surgeon to minister not just to "Officers of the Government and their families," but instead to focus his efforts primarily on the poor while receiving paying patients from those settlers who could afford to do so.[55] Yet no hospital or infirmary was established at the beginning of the settlement. In mid-1837, the dreadful conditions in which some of Cotter's patients were living finally prompted the foundation of an infirmary through the purchase of a partly finished building by the state, yet when opened as a hospital the building lacked basic amenities, being without privies. Within six months, with Government funds not forthcoming, the infirmary was in an appalling state, "without fuel, light or soap or the means of procuring them … [and] blankets and shirts that require washing."[56] By mid-1838, the infirmary was described in the press as "a disgrace to humanity" and Cotter's reputation besmirched.[57]

Efforts were made toward building a new hospital with the arrival of Governor Gawler. Gawler commenced the project in 1840, promising to pay half its construction costs on the understanding that the remaining funds would be provided through public subscription. However, the latter source of funds never materialized and it was years before the builder was paid. By early 1841, the hospital, designed by George Strickland Kingston, opened with two wards of twelve beds apiece, with four ancillary spaces containing a surgery room, dispensary, and two offices. The design was simple even by Strickland's standards, with no embellishments, no verandah (although one was added later), and with the wards and offices accessed from the exterior. A mere ten years later, the building was described as unfit for purpose and calls were made to build a new hospital.[58] This was finally achieved in 1855, with the opening of the second Adelaide hospital, a handsome two-story stone and brick building consisting of two solid bays punctuated by round-headed windows bundled in threes at either end, between which was an embedded arcaded loggia on each floor.[59] The hospital had male and female wards, each holding twenty beds, as well as an operating theater and various offices; within two years outhouses were built to accommodate a kitchen, a laundry, and a mortuary.[60]

The Melbourne Hospitals: Citizen-Led

Of all the settlements on the Australian continent, in terms of the provision of hospitals, that of Melbourne possibly most closely represented the state's preferred model of a citizen-led initiative. The initiation of settlement in the Port Phillip District (now Victoria) at Melbourne, nearly contemporaneous to Adelaide, commenced in 1835 by Tasmanian pastoralists who crossed Bass Strait to find new pastures and claim land without permission from the Governor of New South Wales, who claimed the territory.

The civil and military contingent that arrived in Melbourne in 1836 under Captain William Lonsdale to formally establish a sanctioned settlement came prepared. Although settlers had been in place for more than twelve months and had already appropriated land and built huts, the government officers were to survey the land and put it up for sale, and brought substantial cargo with them to enable this, including materials to build two houses, military barracks, and a hospital. All of these were erected in the government camp, slightly to the

Health and Architecture

west of the settler huts. The hospital, a small building probably only capable of accommodating a handful of patients, was said to be in a "miserable state" just eighteen months later.[61] It was soon moved to align it with the newly laid out streets of the town. But unlike hospitals in Perth and Adelaide, this hospital was strictly for those in the service of the government, including the very small contingent of convicts, and did not serve the wider population.

Melbourne's population grew rapidly with a series of land sales that attracted investors and settlers from 1837. The surveys that enabled the land sales demarcated the town, including the provision of a series of key public institutions, with land set aside for a hospital. By 1841, public meetings were being held to gather subscriptions for a hospital—a pro-active approach by the settlers, who did not intend to rely on the state for such provision. The first hospital was established in a small brick house that was rented for the purpose, and later moved to a two-story house.[62] As had occurred in Adelaide, the building of a permanent purpose-built hospital was achieved by the commitment of government funds for half of the construction costs, but, unlike Adelaide, Melbourne's citizens did manage to provide almost all the remaining funds through subscription. Although the land originally reserved for the hospital had been repurposed, the government made a new land grant, and the foundation stone was laid with great ceremony in 1846 to the design of Samuel Jackson (Figure 9.7).[63]

The hospital, opened in 1848, was a two-story stone Tudor Gothic design with a whimsical bow front above its entrance. The choice of style was a deliberate alignment with the highest status buildings of Melbourne's settlement. Whereas Melbourne's civic structures of the 1830s had been cast in a restrained Georgian mode,

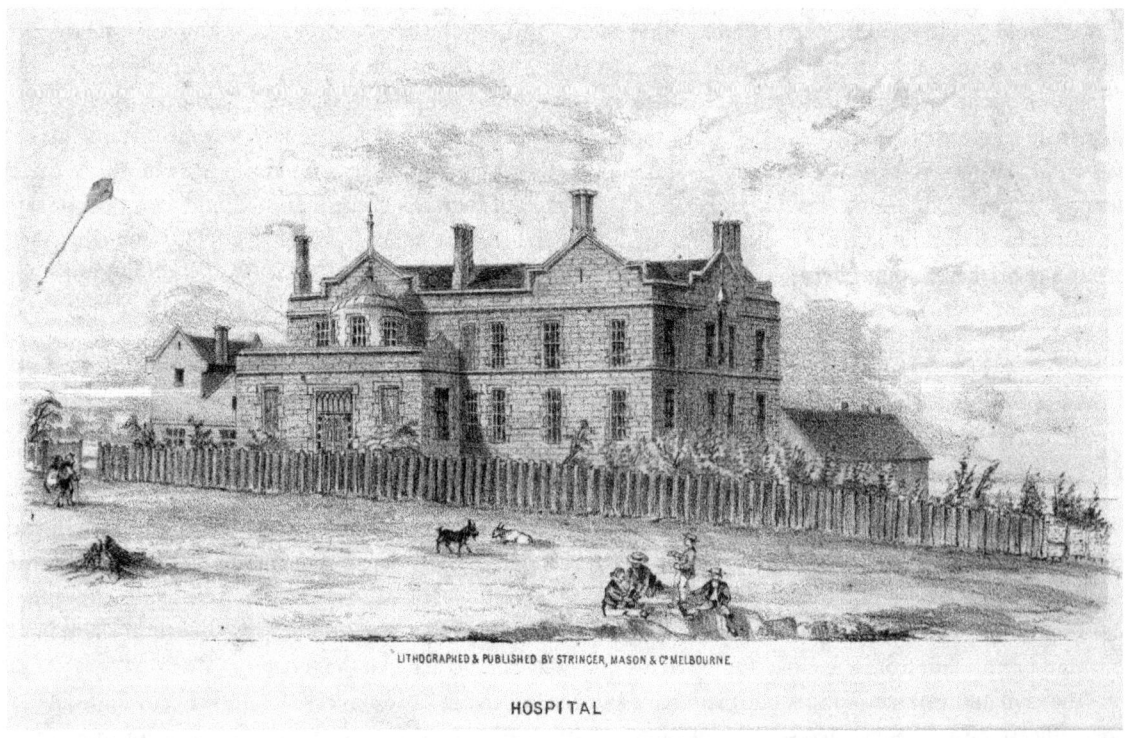

Figure 9.7 The Melbourne Hospital, with its Tudor Gothic style, represented the high aspirations of the town's citizens. Melbourne Hospital, Melbourne, Victoria, Australia; architect: Samuel Jackson, 1846–48; lithographer: Stringer, Mason & Co., *c.* 1850. Source: Pictures Collection, State Library of Victoria

those of the 1840s were more likely to use the Tudor Gothic, such as the new Law Courts of 1842–3, designed by the New South Wales's Colonial Architect. The stylistic choice was led by the example of the most important building in Australia, that of the New South Wales Governor's residence, designed in 1837 by Edward Blore. The Melbourne Hospital, through its architecture, declared itself to be a public building of taste and refinement and a worthy edifice distilling the citizens' hopes for the settlement.

Conclusions

The provision of hospitals in colonial Australia demonstrated the exigencies of establishing far-flung settlements. Without an indigenous or outpost trader infrastructure to appropriate, the colonies had to rely on what little provisions they brought or create from what materials were available in an unfamiliar and harsh environment. Hospitals were considered to be exceptionally important in the colonial settlements—the very survival of the colony relied on healthy individuals to work productively—and their erection was prioritized above all else. Yet the first hospitals built were vastly inadequate for the number and needs of the sick: conditions were dire and remained so for years. Hospitals were thus rebuilt multiple times in attempts to improve them.

The more permanent colonial hospitals were built in brick and stone and superficially resembled contemporary British examples. Yet, in comparison to the hospitals built in Britain, Europe, or North America at the time, Australian colonial hospitals were relatively unsophisticated efforts that offered basic patient accommodation and little more, and relatively plain architectural treatment. Examples like the Middlesex Hospital, London (1755) or the London Hospital (1752) showed in plan not only ward spaces, but a series of treatment, administrative, and service spaces, as well as internal toilets,[64] that were largely absent in the Australian hospitals.

Australia's early history of penal colonies ensured that the responsibility for the provision of hospitals was that of the colonial government. The designers of the earliest hospitals, and the doctors who staffed them, were generally military men and the buildings themselves took military barracks as their primary inspiration. It was not until Governor Lachlan Macquarie began his extensive building program in 1810 that hospitals were given any special architectural treatment, but from that time onward hospitals were more consciously designed as important public edifices equivalent to other major institutions in the colony. Stylistic choice had little to do with the identity of these buildings as hospitals; instead, style was used to consciously position the hospitals as important within a hierarchy of civic structures. The role of the state in the earliest settlements was understandable, given their penal colony status, but less so in the free colonies of Western Australia, South Australia, and Victoria. Although the expectation might have been that these colonies would found hospitals through the charitable efforts of their citizens, the reality was that this didn't occur and, at least in Perth and Adelaide, the poor provision of early hospital functions, and their short-lived existence, caused the state to step in to ensure an adequate and permanent hospital was established. Even in Melbourne, where the citizens were most active in creating a hospital, the state also provided an important catalyst to realize a permanent hospital.

The hospital, from the very first day of colonial settlement in Australia, was considered an essential public building. Arguably, it is the only building type in Australia considered an essential service and important public building continuously from 1788. Yet, Australian hospitals and the medical services around them were not just an import from Britain: the isolation and privation of the place, the necessities of colonial organization, and the increased role of the state in the establishment of a functioning society all had a profound impact on the hospitals and their designs.

Health and Architecture

Notes

1. The recent discovery of a depiction of a cockatoo by Dr. Heather Dalton (a distinctive non-migratory Australian parrot) in *De Arte Venandi cum Avibus* (The Art of Hunting with Birds), *c.* 1241–8, held in the Vatican Library, demonstrates trade connections between Australia and Europe. See Carolyn Webb, "Stone the Crows: Image of a Cocky Found in 13th Century Manuscript," *The Age*, https://www.theage.com.au/national/victoria/stone-the-crows-image-of-a-cocky-found-in-13thc-manuscript-20180625-p4znnt.html.
2. Stuart King and Julie Willis, "The Australian Colonies," in *Architecture and Urbanism in the British Empire*, ed. G. A. Bremner (Oxford: Oxford University Press, 2016), 318–19.
3. Governor Phillip, some two months before arrival at Botany Bay, ordered several ships from the fleet to form an advance party, including the *Supply* (which he joined), the *Scarborough*, and the *Friendship*, which would help prepare the settlement. In the end, the entire fleet arrived over a period of only three days. Arthur Phillip, *The Voyage of Governor Phillip to Botany Bay* (Sydney: Angus and Robertson, 1970), 20–3.
4. To understand the range of traditional structures created by Australian Indigenous peoples, see Paul Memmott, *Gunyah, Goondie & Wurley: The Aboriginal Architecture of Australia* (St. Lucia, Qld: University of Queensland Press, 2007); to understand further the Indigenous infrastructure of the Sydney region, see Bruce Pascoe, *Dark Emu* (Broome, WA: Magabala Books, 2018 [2014]).
5. C. J. Cummins, *A History of Medical Administration in New South Wales 1788–1973* (Sydney: Health Commission of New South Wales, 1979), 24–5.
6. James Semple Kerr, *Design for Convicts: An Account of Design for Convict Establishments in the Australian Colonies during the Transportation Era* (Sydney: Library of Australian History, 1984), 4.
7. Kerr, *Design for Convicts*, 4.
8. Ibid., 4.
9. J. Frederick Watson, *The History of the Sydney Hospital from 1811 to 1911* (Sydney: Government Printer, 1911), 3.
10. Invoice to Samuel Wyatt, as quoted by J. S. Kerr. Kerr, *Design for Convicts*, 4.
11. C. J. Cummins, "The Colonial Medical Service: I. The General Hospital, Sydney 1788–1848," *Modern Medicine of Australia* (January 7, 1974): 13.
12. Governor Arthur Phillip to Baron Sydney (Home Secretary), as quoted in Cummins, "The Colonial Medical Service: I," 13.
13. *Caring for Convicts and the Community: A History of the Parramatta Hospital* (Westmead, NSW: Cumberland Area Health Service, 1988), 14.
14. Report from Governor Hunter to Under-Secretary King, September 25, 1800. In *Historical Records of Australia* (Sydney: Library Committee of the Commonwealth Parliament, 1914), 562, 711.
15. Watson, *The History of the Sydney Hospital*, 7.
16. Account by Captain William Tench, November 1790, as quoted in *Caring for Convicts and the Community*, 13.
17. *Caring for Convicts and the Community*, 14.
18. Watson, *The History of the Sydney Hospital*, 9.
19. Cummins, *A History of Medical Administration*, 25.
20. Ibid., 25.
21. Macquarie was not the only governor to use taxes on the importation of spirits to support the costs of construction in New South Wales, as his predecessors King and Hunter had used them to fund the construction of gaols. See Kerr, *Design for Convicts*, 35.
22. See, for instance, Miles Lewis, "Pattern Books," in *The Encyclopedia of Australian Architecture*, ed. Philip Goad and Julie Willis (Melbourne: Cambridge University Press, 2012), 531.
23. Kerr, *Design for Convicts*, 47.
24. Ibid., 49.
25. Macquarie was subject to a formal investigation by Commissioner J. T. Bigge in which he was strongly criticized for his building program. See John Thomas Bigge, *Report on State of the Colony of New South Wales* (London, 1822).
26. See, for instance, Morton Herman's concerns about Greenway as architect of the building. Morton Herman, *The Early Australian Architects and Their Work* (Sydney: Angus & Robertson, 1954), 77–9.
27. Clive Lucas, "Greenway, Francis," in *The Encyclopedia of Australian Architecture*, ed. Philip Goad and Julie Willis (Melbourne: Cambridge University Press, 2012), 295–7.

28. This is illustrated in Herman, *Early Australian Architects*, fig. 32.
29. W. G. Rimmer, *Portrait of a Hospital: The Royal Hobart* (Hobart: Royal Hobart Hospital, 1981), 4.
30. Ibid., 4.
31. Kerr, *Design for Convicts*, 52.
32. Rimmer, *Portrait of a Hospital*, 5.
33. Ibid., 5.
34. Ibid., 19–20.
35. John Frederick Clarke, Deputy Inspector of Army Hospitals, 1840, as quoted in Rimmer, *Portrait of a Hospital*, 49.
36. Rimmer, *Portrait of a Hospital*, 49–50.
37. Kerr, *Design for Convicts*, 69.
38. Ibid., 77.
39. John H. Tyrer, *History of the Brisbane Hospital and its Affiliates* (Brisbane: Boolarong Publication, 1993), 2.
40. Ibid., 3
41. Ibid., 5.
42. Ibid., 26.
43. Margaret Pitt Morison, "Settlement and Development: The Historical Context," in *Western Towns and Buildings*, ed. Margaret Pitt Morison and John White (Nedlands, WA: University of Western Australia Press, 1979), 1–9.
44. G. C. Bolton and Prue Joske, *History of the Royal Perth Hospital* (Nedlands, WA: University of Western Australia Press, 1982), 1.
45. Ibid., 3.
46. Ibid., 3–4.
47. Ibid., 4.
48. Ibid., 5.
49. Ibid., 7.
50. Ibid., 8.
51. Ibid., 10–11.
52. It is difficult to ascertain information about the military hospital. It seems as though it, too, started in tent accommodation and was in operation by 1830. It was in a permanent building by 1848, when it was recorded on a town map for Perth. Bolton and Joske, *History of the Royal Perth Hospital*, 12.
53. See Considine and Griffiths Architects, *Royal Perth Hospital Precinct Conservation Plan* (Cottesloe, WA: Considine and Griffiths Architects, September 1995), 3–4.
54. Bolton and Joske, *History of the Royal Perth Hospital*, 13–14.
55. Rob Linn, *Frail Flesh & Blood: The Health of South Australian since Earliest Times* (Woodville, SA: The Queen Elizabeth Hospital Research Foundation, 1993), 53–4.
56. Thomas Cotter, as quoted in Linn, *Frail Flesh & Blood*, 55.
57. Ibid., 57–8.
58. Ibid., 61–2.
59. Ibid., 104–5.
60. "Adelaide—Hospitals," *The Manning Index of South Australian History*, State Library of South Australia, accessed August 20, 2018. http://www.slsa.sa.gov.au/manning/adelaide/hospital/hospital.htm.
61. George Tibbits and Angela Roenfeldt, *Port Phillip Colonial* (Clifton Hill, Vic.: Port Phillip Colonial, 1989), 13.
62. Ibid., 61.
63. "Laying the Foundation," *Port Phillip Gazette and Settler's Journal* (March 21, 1846): 2.
64. John D. Thompson and Grace Goldin, *The Hospital: A Social and Architectural History* (New Haven, CN and London: Yale University Press, 1975), 87–96.

PART III
TYPOLOGIES: PLACES OF HEALTH IN HISTORY

CHAPTER 10
HOUSE OF MISERICÓRDIA
HEALTHCARE AND WELFARE ARCHITECTURE IN SIXTEENTH-CENTURY PORTUGAL

Joana Balsa de Pinho

The confraternities of Misericórdia (Confrarias da Misericórdia), more commonly known as Misericórdias (Mercies) were first established in Lisbon in 1498 and rapidly spread throughout Portugal. Ultimately, they formed a network covering the entire Portuguese territory and became the most important welfare institution of the early modern age in Portugal. Indeed, the Misericórdias played a vital role in the Portuguese healthcare system of the time, for their territorial coverage, their critical institutional role in assisting the poor and the sick, and their political relevance in promoting local elites. In their field, the Misericórdias promoted different patrimonial practices, with particular manifestations that were directly related to their welfare nature, their devotions, and the dynamics of confraternal daily life. In fulfilling the various aspects of their charitable mission—namely, welcoming the poor and the sick, treating the unwell, burying the dead, and celebrating the liturgy—the Misericórdias needed a building to perform their activities. Depending on the local infrastructure and vocational requirements, the needy could be served by occupying preexisting autonomous spaces of another institution's buildings, by constructing entirely new buildings, or by adapting preexisting buildings. Despite their well-recognized historical importance as documented in the literature, these confraternities have seldom been studied in the artistic production field,[1] and certainly not with any rigor, principally because the historiography of art has always favored religious architecture in its multiple manifestations. Accordingly, this chapter systematically examines a range of sixteenth-century examples of this typology. The objective of this investigation is to understand the architectural and artistic characteristics of the Misericórdias as promoted by the confraternities during the first decades of their activity. Additionally, this study seeks to determine whether these characteristics are distinctive as compared to other buildings promoted by other civil and religious institutions, as well as the different constraints of this architecture.

Portugal in 1498: A Kingdom, Many Challenges

In social, economic, and politic terms, Portugal during the sixteenth century was at the height of its period of Discoveries. The expansionist movement led by the Portuguese, which later inspired the Spanish to follow suit, had begun during the prior century and was undergoing a process of consolidation. This movement presented many challenges to the kingdom—principally involving the political and social organization of a new and expansive territory encompassing four continents, which had myriad repercussions at different levels of society, culture, science, and the arts.[2] Interacting with new peoples and contact with previously unknown cultural realities raised new philosophical, scientific, and artistic questions that were fundamental for the definition and affirmation of Humanism and for changes in everyday life, such as increasingly multicultural cities and shifting alimentary habits.[3]

In 1498, Portugal's ruler, King Manuel I, pursued an expansionist and centralizing policy, following in the footsteps of his predecessors. He promoted legislative and administrative reforms that ultimately defined his reign.⁴ Social issues would also receive the attention of King Manuel I, specifically in the context of what was happening in other Iberian kingdoms and in Europe.⁵ In addition to diverse internal matters, the king was concerned with the international standing of his country, promoting numerous diplomatic missions.⁶

With the advent of the Discoveries, the social situation became increasingly complex; the urban population was rising and living standards in cities weakened, with deepening social inequalities and a mushrooming population of poor people. Likewise, dire forms of poverty emerged (i.e., shameful poverty) and previously unfamiliar circumstances resulted in the need for social reform and modernization.⁷ King João II, also with a political intent, initiated such reforms with the reorganization of assistance institutions, by merging small assistance units and their assets and income into larger institutions with greater capacity to respond to the challenges of early Modernity and operation under real protection. Likewise, the Regulation for Chapels and Hospitals was enacted, and a process of inventorying the patrimonial assets of these institutions was initiated in order to counteract waste and misappropriation, eventually leading to the creation of many property inventories.⁸ This process would culminate with the creation of the confraternities of Misericórdia.

The Misericórdias, although established in the sixteenth century, should be viewed and interpreted in a late medieval religious context. In Portugal, as in the rest of Europe, there was a proliferation of professional confraternities for the protection of their members, their families, and their devotees, with special emphasis on the confraternities of the Holy Spirit. The Misericórdias, however, were different from other confraternities in that they offered assistance to those most in need, even if they were from outside the confraternity. Later, in the seventeenth and eighteenth centuries, the Misericórdias coexisted with the popular confraternities of the Holy Sacrament and the Souls, in the context of directives promoted by the Catholic Reformation.⁹

The Confraternities of *Misericórdia*: Healthcare, History, and Art

The confraternities of Misericórdia, first established in Lisbon in 1498,¹⁰ rapidly proliferated, growing in number to about 250 in 100 years,¹¹ in large part due to the support that King Manuel I provided to this new charitable experience in the form of privileges, exemptions, alms, and donations to the confraternities, essential for their creation, development, and ongoing success in carrying out their mission.¹²

Therefore, due to the support provided by the king, the Misericórdias formed a vital geographic network that covered the entire Portuguese territory. In short, despite being administratively and economically independent from each other, these Portuguese confraternities represented the most relevant and well-structured institutional healthcare system in the country between the sixteenth and eighteenth centuries. Misericórdias coexisted with other assistance institutions, namely hospitals run by municipalities and other brotherhoods and religious orders. However, during the sixteenth century, the tendency was for these other institutions to pass to the administration of the Misericórdias, giving these a monopoly on the practice of assistance.¹³

In addition to this critical healthcare function, these confraternities were also important promoters of different patrimonial manifestations in their field, such as building or repurposing structures with distinct characteristics related directly to their mission, their healthcare activity, their devotional needs, and the dynamics of daily confraternal life.¹⁴ Importantly, distinctive works of art commissioned by the confraternities, which were displayed or used in public places and for events, further strengthened widespread public access to fundamental elements of the devotional and welfare program of the Misericórdias. In contrast with the artistic production promoted by or associated with parochial churches, monasteries, and noble families, the arts associated with the Misericórdias could be particular, both utilitarian in the context of the welfare practices of these brotherhoods, as well as more devotional. In the former category we have biers for burial ceremonies and everyday objects, such as tables and benches for the meetings of the brothers responsible for the management of the fraternity. Objects of devotion included those related to spiritual practices, such as a royal flag and the flags of the Passion of Christ.[15]

Moreover, their iconographic motifs were related to the welfare activities and the religious practices promoted by the brotherhood. Exemplifying the former are representations of Our Lady of Mercy, Visitation, and Works of Mercy, which refer to the welfare programs of the fraternity; and in the latter, the episodes from the Stages of the Passion of Christ, the spiritual program of the fraternity.[16] In this sense, the artistic collections of the Misericórdias, for their particularities, possess their own artistic identity—one that reflects a distinct institutional identity that the Misericórdia carefully developed and disseminated that is different from other religious and secular institutions.[17]

The Concept of the "House of Misericórdia"

Once established, the confraternities of Misericórdia provided help and healthcare for the sick and the poor, both in their own spaces and in other hospital institutions. and were designed to deliver healthcare outside the hospital context as it is traditionally understood. In this sense, the statutes of the confraternity, which regulated the activities and the organization of the Misericórdias (the so-called *Compromisso*), included a chapter dedicated to caring for the sick. Specifically, it explained that the confraternity should provide for four brothers to visit the poor and any imprisoned patients, bringing them medicine, clothing, food, and alms, and providing them with a place to stay.[18]

The existence of a physical space was highly advantageous for welcoming those in need and providing healthcare, but was also required for religious and administrative purposes. Thus, the singular characteristics of the art and architecture commissioned by the Misericórdias should be analyzed and understood in the broader context of the individuality and autonomy that the institution wanted to promote.

In this context, the Houses of Misericórdia should be considered in light of their healthcare-purposed architecture, while also examined in terms of their confraternal nature—being originally constructed or adapted during the early modern age in Portugal. Casa da Misericórdia (House of Mercy), a contemporary and generalized expression in the documentation of countless Misericórdias disseminated throughout the country, fittingly defines the architectural reality promoted by these confraternities. Indeed, this concept expresses the patrimonial identity of the confraternities (Figure 10.1).

This examination is based on available sixteenth-century archival documentation belonging to different Portuguese Misericórdias,[19] and a comparative analysis of building plans, spatial organization, and existing architectural elements. All told, this information enabled us to propose a more thorough grasp of the architecture of the Misericórdias than what had been previously established by scholars. The confraternities of Misericórdia would need a building that combined several spaces, usually interconnected, creating a specific organizational arrangement and spatiality. Notably, this structure or assemblage of multiple spaces would include a church or designated place to carry out the liturgical celebrations inherent to the daily life of the confraternities, a meeting house where the brothers that administered the confraternity could gather, a sacristy for church support, a cemetery for burying the dead, and an infirmary for helping the sick or providing respite for pilgrims. Other spaces would also be needed for archiving documentation, storing the bier or other liturgical equipment, and even a place to store grains and other foodstuffs.[20] Hence, this investigation defines the House of Misericórdia as referring to a building encompassing different spaces built for different purposes, including for healthcare, religious activities, and symbolic celebrations, where daily confraternal life took place, evidencing some shared characteristic elements of this experience, although

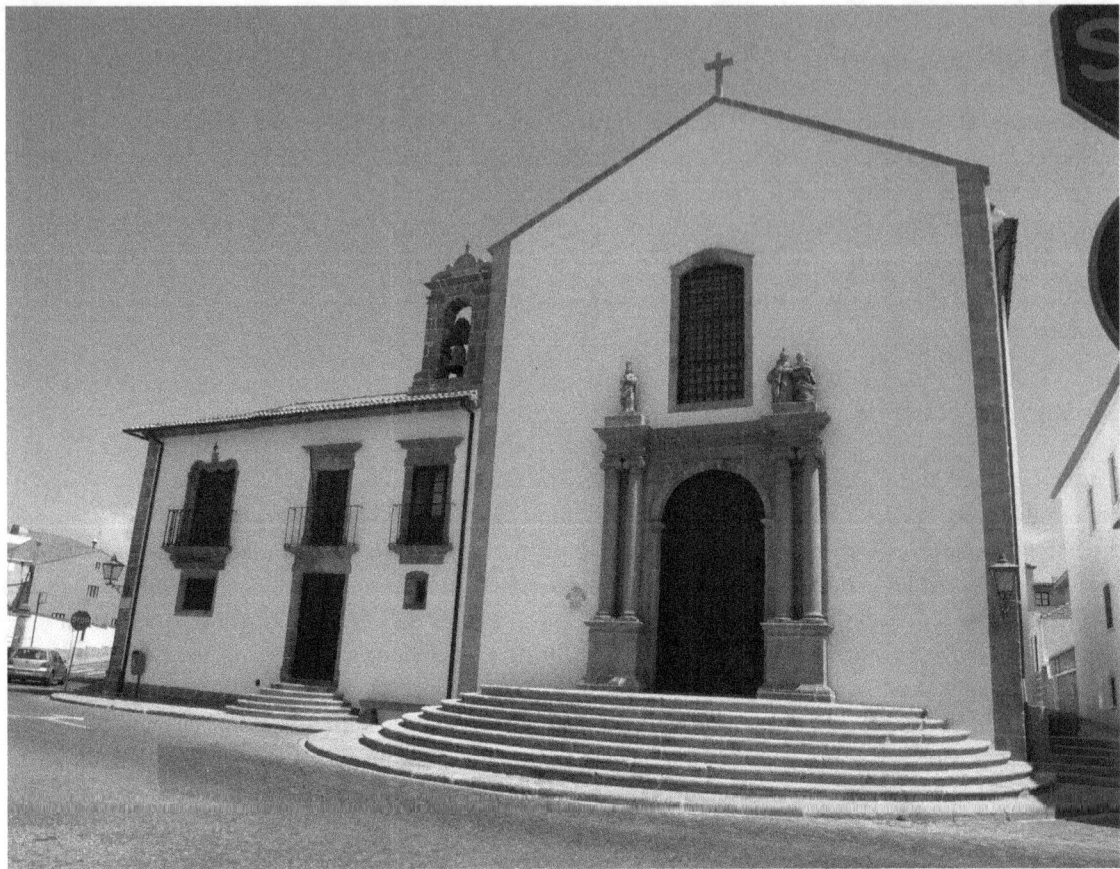

Figure 10.1 Vila do Conde House of Misericórdia. Photo: Joana Balsa de Pinho

not necessarily corresponding to a unitary project. In purely functional terms, the House of Misericórdia differs from other buildings (or architectural typologies) by bringing together a multiplicity of uses and for being the place where welfare, religious, and symbolic celebrations of these confraternities could take place. Nonetheless, although some specificities are recognized for buildings constructed by the Misericórdias,[21] existing monographs, touristic itineraries, heritage inventories, and even academic works often refer to them using simplistic terms, such as church, hospital, church and consistory, church and definitory, church and the brothers' meeting room, or church and annexes.[22] Such references, however, do not begin to describe the architectural reality of the Misericórdias or convey how the buildings were conceived, organized, and utilized so intensively throughout Portugal.

There are several reasons why this standardized nomenclature remains in use—the principal one pertains to the way research has been carried out to date. Specifically, the more detailed studies are almost always monographic, addressing a specific confraternity[23] rather than providing an overview and a generalization of the concepts. Another fundamental aspect refers to the modifications that the buildings have endured over the centuries. In many cases, architectural alterations, and sometimes even outright demolition, have given them a different configuration and reinforced an individualized vision.[24]

In other cases, the buildings that surrounded the church have disappeared, leaving only the religious space.[25] This attrition occurred in Constancia (1580–4) and Mogadouro (second half of the sixteenth century)

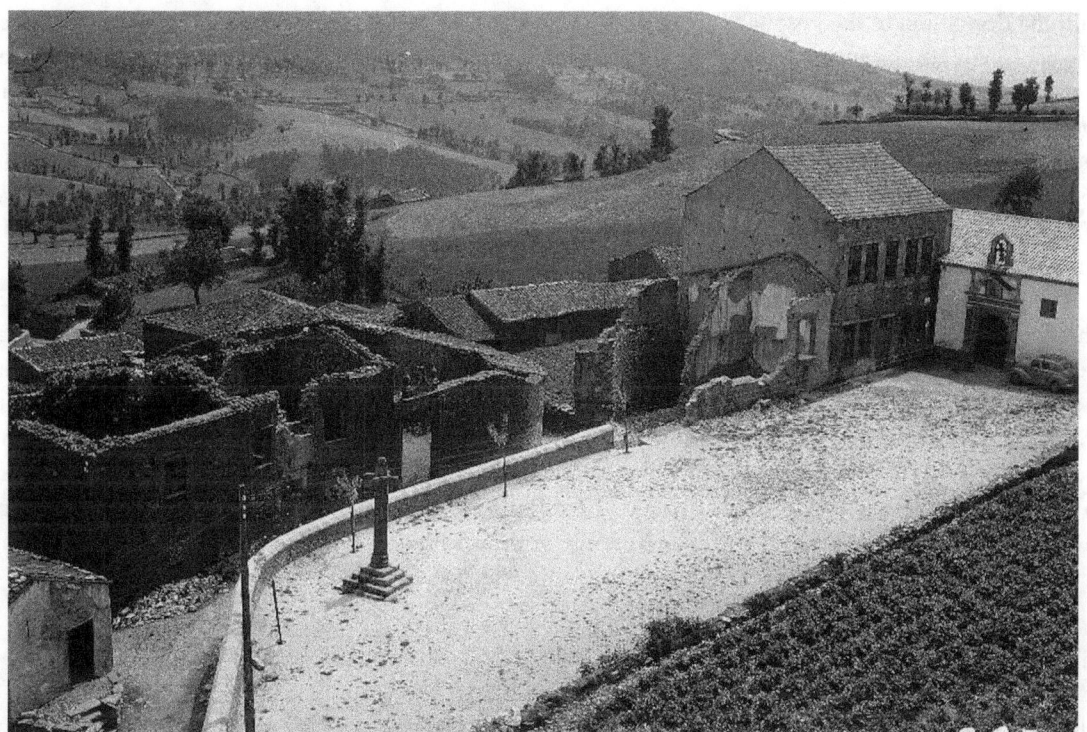

Figure 10.2 Old photo of Mogadouro House of Misericórdia (c. mid 20th century, before the demolitions). Source: Municipal Archive of Mogadouro

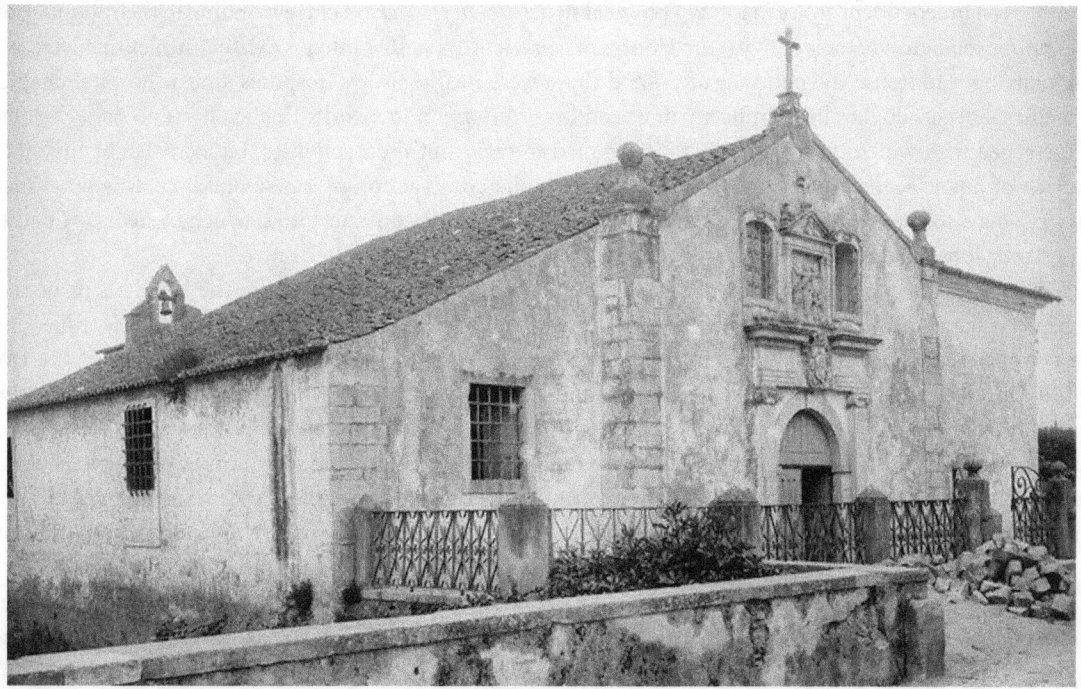

Figure 10.3 Old photo of Montemor-o-Velho House of Misericórdia (c. 1950, before the demolitions). Source: Information System for Architectural Heritage

with the demolition of the hospital located next to the church. The loss of one or more physical structures also contributes to the perceptual erosion of these architectural complexes, since the only thing that endures is the church. With the loss of the memory of the Misericórdias' welfare and administrative roles and the spaces to perform these roles, it is understandable that the remaining building, the church, determinates the nomenclature (Figure 10.3). As an example, a document from the Misericórdia of Colares (founded in 1623) that dates from the second decade of the seventeenth century is quite explicit in this regard: "*A casa da Misericórdia não he somente Igreja mas ha de ter muitas casas*" (The house of *Misericórdia* is not only a church, it includes many houses).[26]

Focusing unduly on the churches attached to Misericórdias leads us to consider it as religious architecture.[27] These compounds must be thought of in a different way, not only because of the absence of exterior architectural elements with religious connotations on many of these buildings but also because the existence of a church in the House of Misericórdia must be viewed more expansively. A building should not be considered religious architecture just because it incorporates a chapel or church. The same understanding must be accorded to the House of Misericórdia. All works of Mercy should be considered welfare acts, even "bury the dead" and "pray to God for the living and the dead." Other actions that happened in the church, such as the annual election of the brothers for the management of the confraternity or the celebration of masses before the weekly meeting of the brothers, constitute forms of legitimation and sanctification of these secular activities.

Misericórdias and Hospitals

Although it was primarily hospitals that took care of the sick and dying, the Misericórdias also had important healthcare functions to serve. The relationship between these two institutions is evident in three ways. First, some Misericórdias had their origins in medieval hospitals; rarely did the establishment of a Misericórdia emerge as an independent entity in its own physical structure. In the period corresponding to their foundation and the consolidation of their activity, the Houses of Misericórdia settled into preexisting spaces that were not originally built to house the confraternity—and these were nearly always hospitals and/or hospital chapels of medieval origin due to their similarity of use and institutional framework. This reality is no doubt related to the speed with which these confraternities wanted to carry out their activities, but can also be linked to the lack of financial means and the time necessary for the construction of a new building. This process of repurposing also emphasizes the importance of the activities of the confraternities, which by necessity had to have strong local institutional support (Figure 10.4).[28]

The most common cases of establishment into preexisting spaces are related to the hospitals or houses of Espírito Santo (Holy Spirit).[29] Their use during the initial period of activity of the Misericórdias and the permanence of the confraternity in these spaces are generally associated with the merger of the two institutions, whether in terms of incomes, assets, and charitable actions or via the transfer of administrative oversight from a Holy Spirit hospital to the House of Misericórdia.[30] This situation was so prevalent that it was the typology for most preexisting buildings—about half of them were based in houses or hospitals of the Holy Spirit. It is also worth noting that during their initial period of operations in the sixteenth century, the Misericórdias throughout Portugal also established, although in far fewer numbers, their operations in other already-existing hospitals or hospital chapels that were unrelated to the confraternities of Holy Spirit.[31]

A second relationship of note between the Houses of Misericórdia and infirmaries or hospitals that they occupied to care for the sick concerns the shift in administrative oversight. In many Portuguese cities and villages where Misericórdias were established, they began to take on a larger management role, including overseeing assets, income, legacies, and testamentary dispositions of medieval hospitals. Indeed, this role often extended to providing more direct human care and building management.[32] Because these hospitals pre-dated the establishment of the Misericórdias, and in some situations were geographically separated from

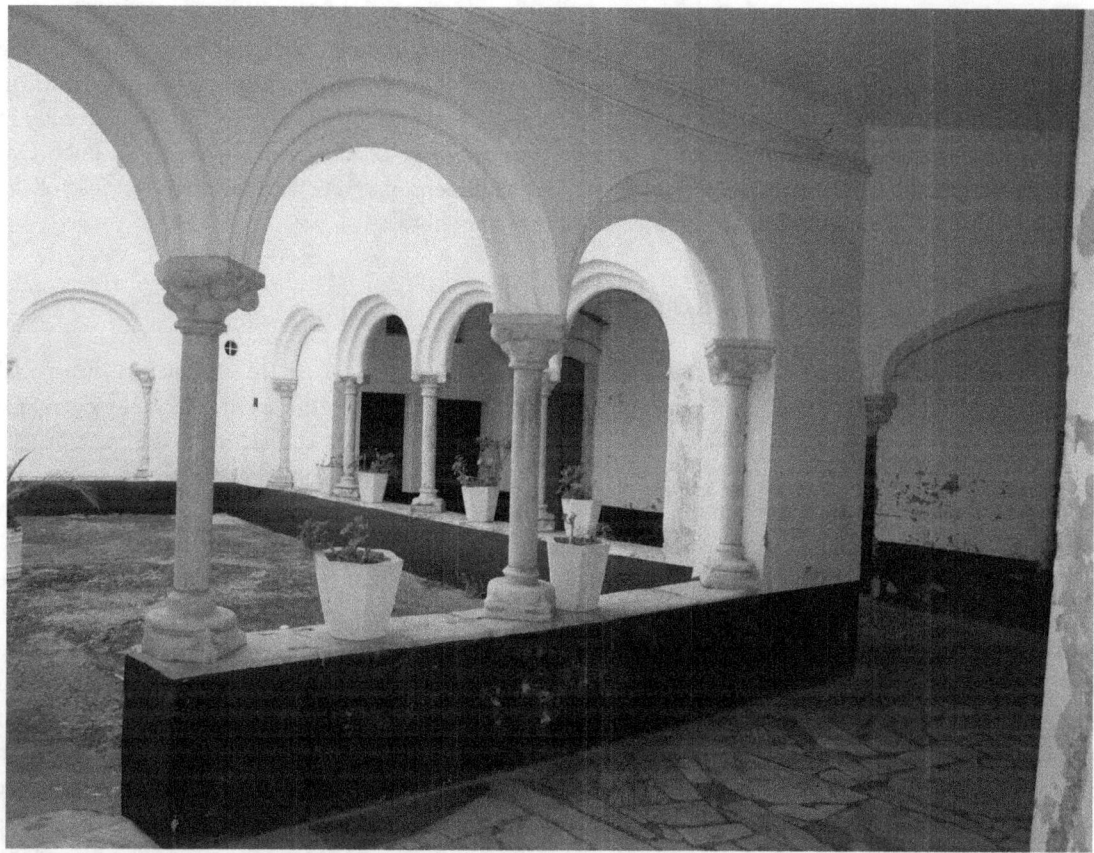

Figure 10.4 Renaissance cloister of the hospital of Estremoz. Photo: Joana Balsa de Pinho

them, some local Misericórdias were not integrated with those infirmaries, meaning that the functional and spatial design of these Houses of Mercy would include only church, sacristy, and meeting house.

This situation can be seen, for example, in Portel (1498), where the Holy Spirit hospital starting began operating in the second half of the sixteenth century, but which was not co-located with the headquarters building of the Misericórdia. Similarly, we see evidence of this arrangement in Arez (*c.* 1592), where the hospital was located next to the main church; in Évora (1499), with the hospital of Holy Spirit; in Beja (1499), with the hospital of Our Lady of Piedade; and in Braga (before 1513), with the hospital of St. Mark's.[33]

Thirdly, it is fruitful to examine the physical characteristics of the spaces used to care for the sick in the Houses of Misericórdia. In general, we see vestiges of a late medieval tradition, evidenced by their small size, simplicity of accommodation, and functional multiplicity. These structures also included spaces for both religious and administrative functions, thus conferring a triple functional dimension to the Houses of Misericórdia.[34] The complexity of the Houses of Misericórdia could be depending on several factors, principally whether or not the Misericórdia was attached to an existing hospital with its own facilities. It is also important to consider the matter of scale, since in most Misericórdias all these spaces within buildings were small, including the infirmaries themselves. Thus, while the buildings might be composed of several distinct spaces, they were not monumental in terms of overall size.

The visit by the Order of Santiago to Palmela in 1510 describes the village hospital as follows: "*a casa do hospital é uma casa grande térrea, de pedra e cal, e tem no meio um esteio de pedra e cal e é coberta de telha vã*" (the hospital house is a large one-story house, made of stone and lime, and has a stone and lime pillar in the center and is covered with vain tile); this house corresponds to the infirmary, which although considered to be a "large house," had only five beds.[35] Likewise, some material vestiges of a sixteenth-century hospital confirm these characteristics. In this context, we highlight the fifteenth-century Rosmaninhal Hospital, currently in ruins, which flanks the Misericórdia church. Despite its dreadful physical state, it represents an important source of information. To provide some idea of its size, its dimensions were approximated to those of the church, making it a space with about five rooms and a two-story house.[36]

The House of Misericórdia: Design, Space, and Elements

Accordingly, it is relevant to address some of the issues that exerted certain constraints on the spatial organization and functionality of the Houses of Misericórdia. For example, the sacristy is a religious space where liturgical objects and vestments are stored. Given the sacristy's intrinsic connection to the enactment of religious ceremonies, architectonically this connection is reflected in the proximity between the sacristy and the church. They are physically contiguous and thus can be viewed as functionally communicating with each other, as is common in religious architecture in general.

Another essential space of the Houses of Misericórdia is the meetinghouse, a room for the gathering of the twelve brothers elected annually to manage the confraternity, their assets, and activities. The meetinghouse, too, was both functionally and symbolically important, and designed architecturally to house the table and benches for the meetings of the brothers. This space was also very close to the church for two principal reasons: many of the civil acts the brothers directed were imbued with religious meaning, and their enactment was often preceded by the celebration of the Eucharist in which the brothers participated. In this context, in many of these sixteenth-century buildings the relationship between the meetinghouse and church would be reinforced via their close proximity so that the brothers could more easily attend various church celebrations (Figure 10.5). Specifically, when there was no actual structural connection between the meetinghouse and the church, a privileged link would exist—oftentimes a corridor or gallery outside the building, protected by a porch, representing a direct, differentiated access so that the brothers could reach the church in privacy.

The design of the various elements making up a House of Misericórdia did not follow any rigid architectural scheme beyond ensuring the provision of necessary religious, medical, social, and administrative functions. The church was the main structure due to its size in proportion to the other spaces and its sacred function. The location of the sacristy could be on either side of the church, according to how the building was situated and how it best served existing urban conditions. Likewise, the meetinghouse could be located in the same building as the sacristy, although sometimes occupying a different floor. Conversely, the meetinghouse has also been located in other zones of the building: in the axis of the church, next to the choir, or in the back of the main chapel. In general, however, research indicates that the most common location was at the side of the church (Figure 10.6).

In this context the three most standard models of spatial organization for the Houses of Misericórdia are:

- Parallel building design: dependencies (one or two floors) designed in parallel to the church, attached to one of its sides, almost always along the same internal organizational axis;
- Perpendicular building design: dependencies attached to one of the lateral elevations of the church, but with an axis of design and development perpendicular to that of the church, with the attached construction;
- Building design in axis: church and dependencies organized along a longitudinal axis. The dependencies are located in the back of the main chapel or near the choir.[37]

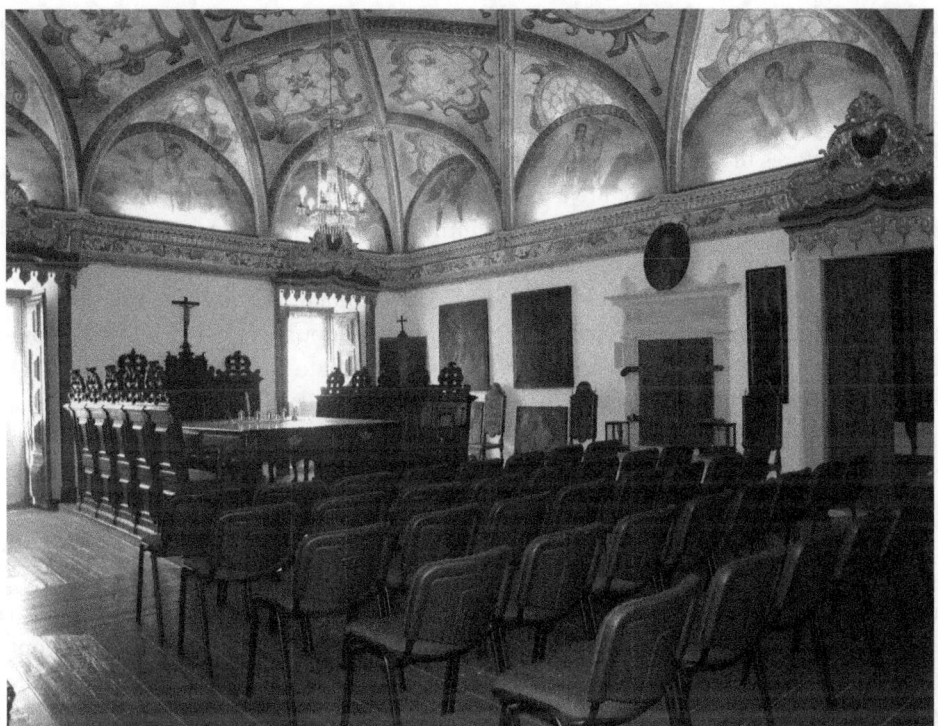

Figure 10.5 Meeting room of the brothers, Montemor-o-Velho House of Misericórdia. Photo: Joana Balsa de Pinho

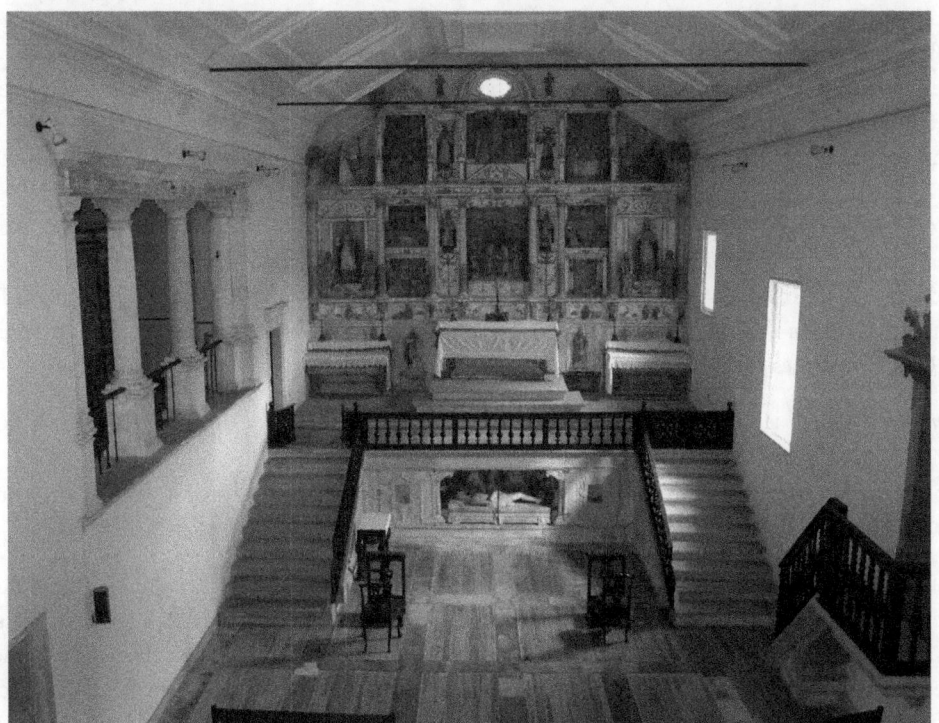

Figure 10.6 Church, Tentúgal House of Misericórdia. Photo: Joana Balsa de Pinho

Health and Architecture

As an urban phenomenon, the Houses of Misericórdia were built in towns of any size —sometimes well assimilated in the local urban infrastructure, but other times appearing as more solitary structures. In the latter instance, when the Misericórdia was not attached to other edifices, its volumetry tended to follow two different trends: one that reflected the articulation of the different spaces that composed the building, with distinct areas or independent structures that evidenced different functional purposes and constructive chronologies; and another where there was only one structure that housed all the dependencies that constituted the building. An important feature of the Houses of Misericórdia during the sixteenth century, which is also reflected in the external volumetry, is the absence of towers. The headquarters of a confraternity could not have had a bell tower because this was the prerogative of the main church; instead, many Misericórdias featured small belfries.

To the extent possible, the exterior facade of a building is often purposefully designed to communicate with the existing urban locality, as well as convey its functional intent to the population. In sixteenth-century Misericórdias there were two main types of facades: a traditional main facade situated on the same axis as the main chapel of the church, and a main lateral facade corresponding to one of the side facades of the building.[38] This latter variety has also been observed in female-cloistered convents, and although it is not possible to determine the reasons for its existence in the context of Misericórdias; it is likely that this architectural feature influenced the disposition of the remaining rooms of the House of Mercy, positioned against the church and privileging the organization in axis.

The main entryway for a House of Misericórdia is an element that presents a different aesthetic treatment, showing sculptural groups in relief, often coupled with inscriptions that relate to the nature of the confraternity, its activities, or its devotions. Commonly, they included representations of Our Lady of Mercy and the Visitation, displaying inscriptions such as: "Beati misericordes quia ipsi," "misericordiam consequentur" (Matt. 5, 7: Blessed are the merciful because they will obtain mercy), "Maria Mater Misericordiae" (Mary Mother of Mercy) or "Casa da Misericórdia" (House of Mercy).[39] These external inscriptions and representations were systemically and strategically employed to disseminate the Misericórdias' institutional identity via its external and visible face (Figure 10.7).

In the interior of the Houses of Misericórdia, the church space itself remained preeminent—serving as the sacred location where the sacred actions would be enacted. However, the election of the twelve brothers for the management of the confraternity was also deemed sufficiently relevant to take place within the church. The Misericórdia churches that remain today still serve as places of worship—although they evidence multiple changes to their original sixteenth-century specifications, especially at the level of altarpieces, mural decorations, devotional sculpture, and liturgical fixtures or furniture (such as choir and pulpits). The best-preserved aspect of a House of Misericórdia church is their planimetry or architectural arrangement. Typically, these churches feature a large planimetric diversity, and stand out as a space of architectural experimentalism (Figure 10.8).[40] Regardless of their interior diversity, however, two pervasive elements stand out:

- The *cruzeiro*, which is a high platform that precedes the main chapel or altarpiece and adjoining chapels (when they exist).[41]
- The presence of inscribed chapels or a simple altarpiece on the bottom of a wall of the church (Figure 10.9).

The combination of these two architectural elements in a single nave building became so ubiquitous that researchers have referred to it as the "Misericórdia type."[42] Nonetheless, a systematic analysis reveals a more complex reality for the architectural diversity of the Houses of Mercy. Despite the variety of schemes, there was a specific type linked to the church buildings of Misericórdias, based on these two elements described.

Another element of particular note is the tribune (*tribuna dos oficiais*), which designates the place or the equipment where the twelve brothers elected annually to manage the confraternity of Mercy and attended

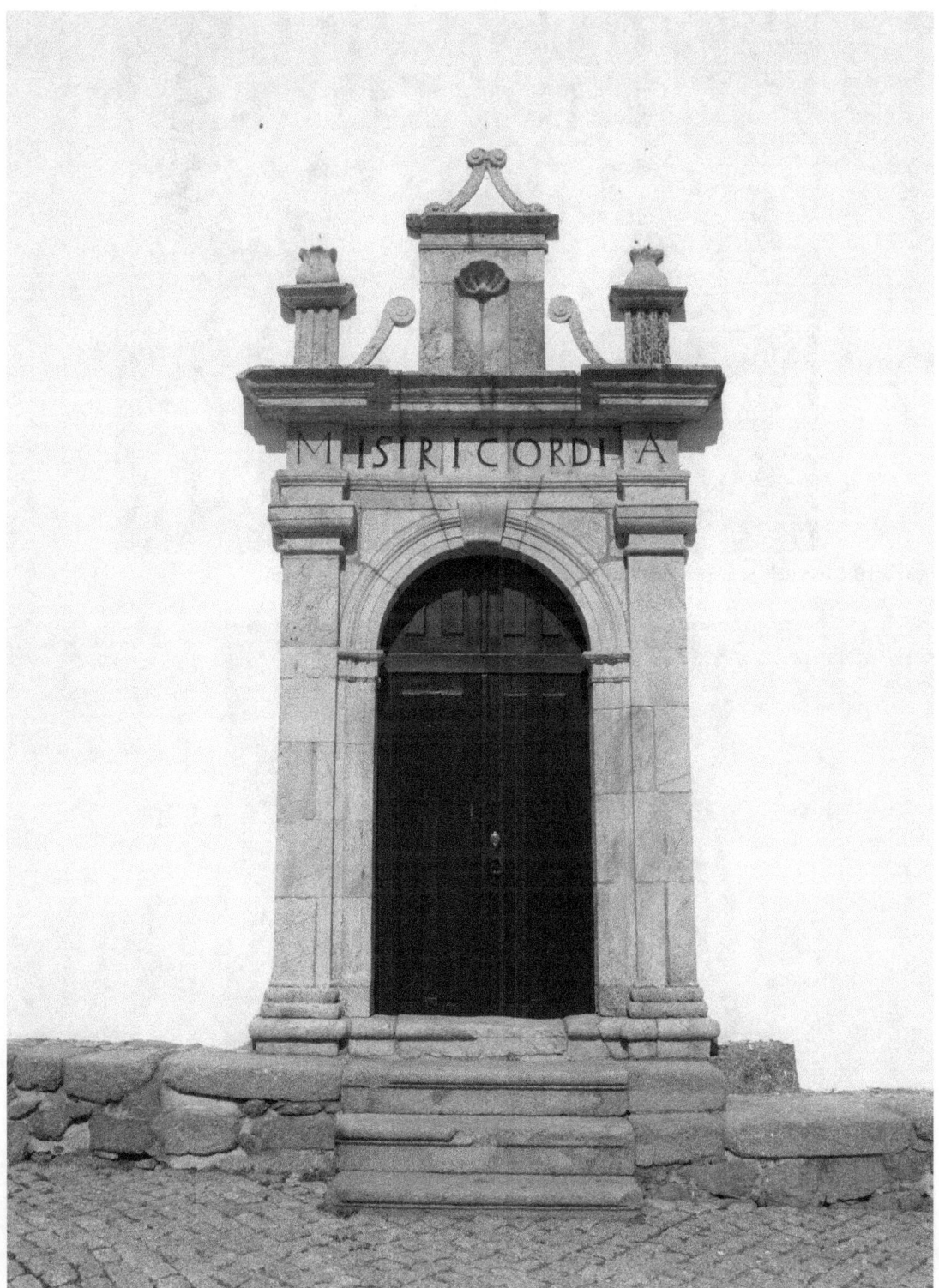

Figure 10.7 Exterior facade, Proença-a-Nova House of Misericórdia. Photo: Joana Balsa de Pinho

Health and Architecture

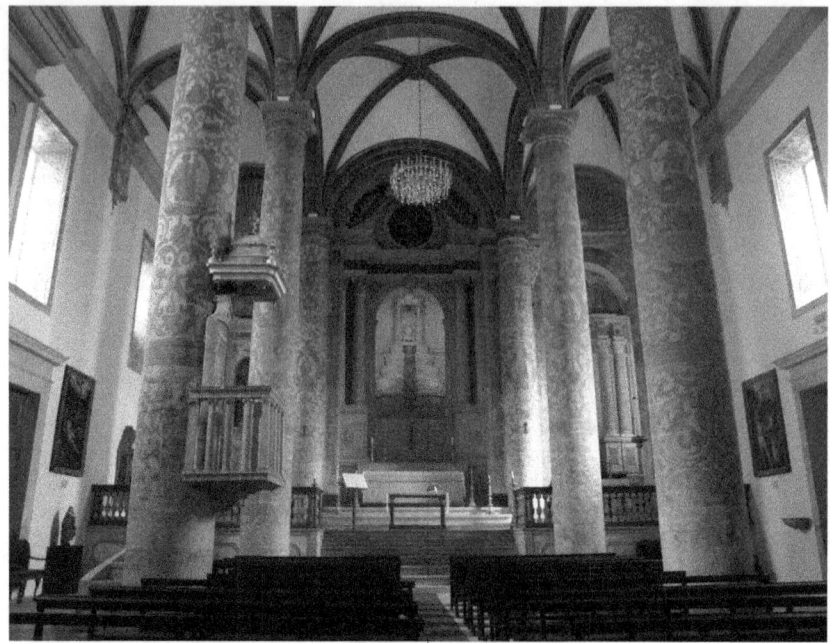

Figure 10.8 Church, Santarém House of Misericórdia. Photo: Joana Balsa de Pinho

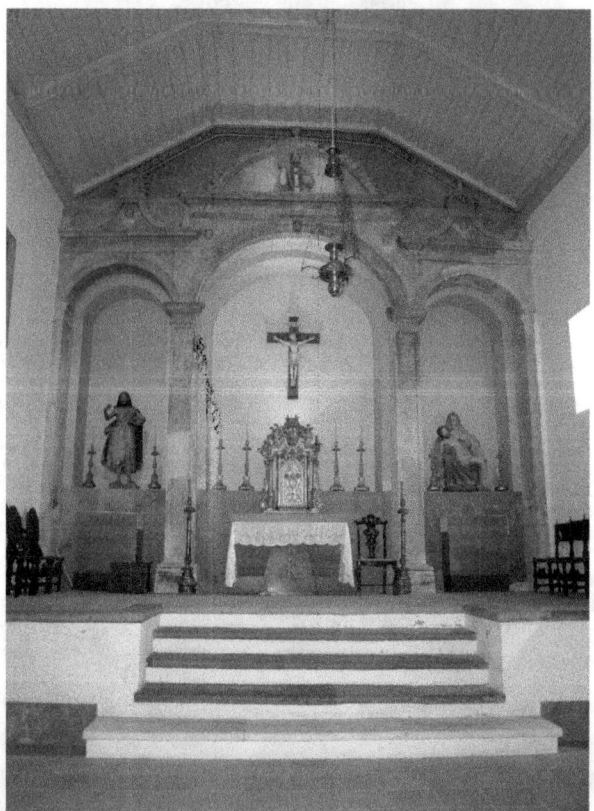

Figure 10.9 Church, Alcochete House of Misericórdia. Photo: Joana Balsa de Pinho

the celebrations held in the church. These tribunes, one of the most paradigmatic equipment of the House of Mercy, are assumed to be structures or appurtenances of social differentiation. One of its most characteristic morphologies is a row of chairs, although it could appear in other forms: a gap or a high structure attached to one of the church walls.

Conclusion

Beginning in the Age of Discovery, the Misericórdias, through their protracted and widespread territorial reach, served as the single most important welfare institution in Portugal during the sixteenth century, and survived well into the late eighteenth century. Forming a network encompassing the national territory, they existed as autonomous institutions serving the sick and the poor. They frequently partnered both structurally and functionally with preexisting hospitals, either leading this process or assuming the management of these hospital's activities and resources. The built heritage and artistic assets of the confraternities of Mercy, which are relevant as symbols of their own institutional practices and identity, stand as testimony to the critical role they played throughout Portugal. Importantly, the confraternities promoted a specific architectural archetype, which can be encompassed in the term "House of Misericórdia," which reflects an understanding of their architecture that differs from what has been discussed by experts in this field thus far, and refers to their unique patrimonial identity and their artistic specificity.

This investigation confirmed that there are specific elements that clearly stand out as common to the architecture of the Houses of Misericórdia. The first is more global in scale and is related to the building as a complex, not separated units. The other trait is more concrete and relates to the existence of specific iconography that we find in different manifestations in different places. These iconographic representations of Our Lady of Mercy, Visitation, and Works of Mercy appear in various iterations in sculpture, bas reliefs in portals and entryways, paintings in altarpieces, and tiles.

These two aspects that characterize the architecture promoted by the confraternities in the sixteenth century are complemented by other elements that reflect and support the daily life of the Misericórdias—their worship and devotional practices, their administrative role, and the delivery of welfare and healthcare services. Namely, there are three elements in the buildings constructed by the Misericórdias which show some relevance in the difficulty in defining their typological specificities: the *cruzeiro*, the shallow main chapel and collaterals or a single altarpiece, and the tribune for the brothers. These are considered relevant elements in this kind of architecture due to their persistent presence and distinctive elements regarding other religious or civilian buildings.

The House of Misericórdia can be conceptually defined as an architectural complex composed of several spaces essential to the development of the care activity promoted by the confraternities and their daily management. In this context, the functional characterization of each of these spaces is quite relevant. Indeed, it is the function assumed by each that helps to elucidate its architectural characteristics. And in considering the design of the building itself, we see artistic specificity—namely the spatial and functional articulation of spaces, the volumetry, the liturgical equipment, the decoration, and the iconography—all of which create an identity language common to many Houses of Misericórdia spread throughout Portugal and the Portuguese world in an authentic *journey of the form*.

Acknowledgment: This this research is part of the project "Hospitalis—Hospital Architecture in Portugal at the Dawn of Modernity: Identification, Characterization and Contextualization" (PTDC/ART-HIS/30808/2017), funded by FCT.

Health and Architecture

Notes

1. Compare the number of historical-artistic studies with those of a historical nature that are included in the literature review in Joana Balsa de Pinho, "A Casa da Misericórdia: as confrarias da Misericórdia e a arquitectura portuguesa quinhentista" (Ph.D. diss., University of Lisbon, 2012), 54–71.
2. Reijer Hooykaas, *O humanismo e os descobrimentos: na ciência e nas letras portuguesas do século XVI* (Lisbon: Gradiva, 1983); *Os descobrimentos portugueses e a Europa do Renascimento: XVII Exposição europea de arte, ciência e cultura*, 6 vols. (Lisbon: Presidência do Conselho de Ministros, 1983); Henrique Leitão, *Os Descobrimentos portugueses e a ciência europeia* (Lisbon: Alêtheia, 2009); Henrique Leitão (ed.), *360° Ciência descoberta* (Lisbon: Fundação Calouste Gulbenkian, Universidade de Lisboa, Museu de Marinha, 2013); *No tempo das feitorias: a arte portuguesa na Época dos Descobrimentos*, 2 vols. (Lisbon: Museu Nacional de Arte Antiga, 1992); *Sphera Mundi: arte e cultura no tempo dos descobrimentos* (Lisbon: Caleidoscópio, 2015); António José Saraiva and Óscar Lopes, *História da literatura portuguesa*, 17th ed. (Porto: Porto Editora, 2017); Hernani Cidade, *A literatura portuguesa e a expansão ultramarina: as ideias, os sentimentos, as formas de arte (séculos XV e XVI)* (Lisbon: Agência Geral das Colónias, 1943).
3. Cf. Annemarie Jordan Gschwende and K. J. P. Lowe, eds., *The Global City: On the Streets of Renaissance Lisbon* (London: Paul Holberton, 2015); José Eduardo Mendes Ferrão, *A aventura das plantas e os Descobrimentos Portugueses* (Lisbon: Instituto de Investigação Científica e Tropical, Comissão Nacional para a Comemoração dos Descobrimentos Portugueses, 1999).
4. *D. Manuel e a sua época: actas* (Guimarães: Câmara Municipal de Guimarães, 2004); Maria José Chorão, *Os forais de D. Manuel: 1496-1520* (Lisbon: ANTT, 1990); João José Alves Dias, *Ordenações manuelinas, 500 anos depois: os dois primeiros sistemas (1512-1519)* (Lisbon: BNP, 2012).
5. Cf. François Soyer, *A Perseguição aos Judeus e Muçulmanos de Portugal—D. Manuel I e o Fim da Tolerância Religiosa (1496-1497)* (Lisbon: Edições 70, 2013); José Pedro Paiva and Giuseppe Marcocci, *História Geral da Inquisição Portuguesa (1536-1821)* (Lisbon: Esfera dos Livros, 2013).
6. Pedro Soares Martínez, *História diplomática de Portugal* (Coimbra: Almedina, 2010); António Camões Gouveia, "Portugal e a Europa: a sociedade e as relações diplomáticas de Tordesilhas aos Pirenéus," *Revista ICALP* 15 (1989): 89–95.
7. About this complex social context, see Isabel Guimarães Sá, *As Misericórdias portuguesas de D. Manuel I a Pombal* (Lisbon: Livros Horizonte, 2001), and Isabel dos Guimarães Sá, *Quando o rico se faz pobre: Misericórdias, caridade e pobreza no império português 1500-1800* (Lisbon: Comissão Nacional para a Comemoração dos Descobrimentos Portugueses, 1997).
8. José Pedro Paiva (coord.), *Portugaliae Monumenta Misericordiarum*, vol. 3 (Lisbon: Centro de Estudos de História Religiosa da Universidade Católica Portuguesa, União das Misericórdias Portuguesas, 2002-4); *D. Manuel e a sua época: actas*.
9. With respect to the religious and confraternal ambience in which the Misericórdias were founded, see Ivo Carneiro Sousa, *V Centenário das Misericórdias Portuguesas* (Lisbon: CTT-Correios de Portugal, 1998); Ivo Carneiro Sousa, *A Rainha D. Leonor (1458-1525): Poder, Misericórdia, Religiosidade e Espiritualidade no Portugal do Renascimento* (Lisbon: Fundação Calouste Gulbenkian, Fundação para a Ciência e Tecnologia, 2002); Maria Helena da Cruz Coelho, "As confrarias medievais portuguesas: espaços de solidariedade na vida e na morte," in *Cofradías, gremios, solidariedades en la Europa medieval* (Estella, Pamplona: Governo de Navarra, 1992); and Maria Ângela Beirante, *Confrarias Medievais Portuguesas* (Lisbon: s.n., 1990).
10. On the foundation and diffusion of Confraternities of Misericórdia, see Sousa, *V Centenário das Misericórdias Portuguesas*; Guimarães Sá, *As Misericórdias portuguesas de D. Manuel I a Pombal*; Paiva, *Portugaliae Monumenta Misericordiarum*, vols. 1–3.
11. See Paiva, *Portugaliae Monumenta Misericordiarum*, vol. 3; and Sousa, *A Rainha D. Leonor (1458-1525)*, 62, 114.
12. See Sousa, *A Rainha D. Leonor (1458-1525)*, 12; Sá, *As Misericórdias portuguesas de D. Manuel I a Pombal*, 40-4; Fernando Silva Correia, *Origens e formação das Misericórdias Portuguesas* (Lisbon: Livros Horizonte, 1999), 558-60.
13. About the role of Misericórdias in the management of other welfare institutions, see Isabel dos Guimarães Sá, "A reorganização da caridade em Portugal em contexto Europeu," *Cadernos do Noroeste* 11, no., 2 (1998): 31-63; and Laurinda Abreu, "A especificidade do sistema de assistência pública português: linhas estruturantes," *Arquipélago: História*, 2nd series, VI (2002): 417-34.
14. On the role of Misericórdias as commissioners of works of art, see Pinho, "A Casa da Misericórdia," 109-44.

15. Ibid., 117–33 and 140–4.
16. Ibid., 133–40.
17. Ibid., 133–40.
18. See the statues of the confraternities of Mercy (Compromissos da Misericórdia) from the years 1498, 1500, 1502, 1516, Paiva, *Portugaliae Monumenta Misericordiarum*, vol. 3, 385–423.
19. For additional information about the archives consulted, see Pinho, "A Casa da Misericórdia," 37–8.
20. For the concept of House of Misericórdia, see Pinho, "A Casa da Misericórdia," 186–224.
21. See Rafael Moreira, "As Misericórdias: um património artístico da humanidade," in *500 Anos das Misericórdias Portuguesas: solidariedade de geração em geração* (Lisbon: Comissão para as Comemorações dos 500 anos das Misericórdia, 2000), 142–3; Paula Noé, *Património Arquitectónico: Igrejas de Misericórdia (version 1.0)* (Lisbon: Instituto de Reabilitação Urbana, Instituto de Gestão do Património Arquitectónico e Arqueológico, 2010), accessed November 15, 2018. http://www.monumentos.pt.
22. Only to quote some examples: José Ferrão Afonso, *A Igreja Velha da Misericórdia de Barcelos e cinco Igrejas de Misericórdias de Entre-Douro e Minho: Arquitectura e paisagem urbana (c. 1534-1635)* (Barcelos: Santa Casa da Misericórdia de Barcelos, 2012); Moreira, "As Misericórdias: um património artístico da humanidade"; Paiva, *Portugaliae Monumenta Misericordiarum*, vols. 1–10; Noé, *Património Arquitectónico*; several sheets of buildings of the Misericórdias that integrate the Informational System for the architectural heritage (SIPA, Sistema de Informação para o Património Arquitectónico), accessed November 15, 2018. http://www.monumentos.gov.pt; different texts at Natália Ferreira-Alves (ed.), *A Misericórdia de Vila Real e as Misericórdias do mundo de expressão portuguesa* (Porto: CEPESE, 2011).
23. See Paula Noé, "O Inventário do Património Arquitectónico das Misericórdias: ensaio tipológico: as Igrejas da Misericórdia do Distrito de Viana do Castelo," in Jornadas de Estudo, *As Misericórdias como Fontes Culturais e de Informação* (Penafiel: Câmara Municipal de Penafiel, Arquivo Municipal de Penafiel, 2001); and Paula Noé, "As igrejas de Misericórdia do distrito de Coimbra: ensaio de classificação tipológica," *Monumentos* 25 (September 2006): 198–207; José Ferrão Afonso, "Regressando a Alberti. As igrejas das Misericórdias de Entre Douro e Minho, de Vila do Conde a Penafiel: arquitectura e paisagem urbana," in II Jornadas de Estudos sobre as Misericórdias, *As Misericórdias quinhentistas* (Penafiel: Câmara Municipal de Penafiel, 2009), 123–51; the several buildings entries of the Misericórdias that integrate SIPA, accessed November 15, 2018. http://www.monumentos.gov.pt.
24. For example, in the Misericórdia of Tavira, the church maintains its sixteenth-century configuration, while the meeting room of the brothers dates from the eighteenth century, having its own main facade, unrelated to the church facade. There is a morphological and decorative difference between the two, which accentuates the architectural differentiation, leading us to consider them as two distinct buildings, rather than one with two different functional spaces.
25. Confront the differences that currently exist, included in the buildings entries, with the old descriptions that are found in the transcribed texts: Pinho, "A Casa da Misericórdia": Annex I and Annex IV (docs.), document 1—Alter do Chão; documents 1 and 8—Barcelos, document 1—Soure, document 1—Torrão, document 1—Lagos, document 1—Viana do Alentejo.
26. See the petition of the brothers for the beginning of the works, in Archive of the Misericórdia of Colares, ecclesiastic archives, B/IV/C/1/1 (cx. 1), transcribed in António Serôdio Lopes, *A capela da Misericórdia de Colares: uma capela palatina da Família Mello de Castro* (Lisbon: Fundação Ricardo Espírito Santo Silva, 2012), 143.
27. The identification of the architecture produced by the Misericórdias with religious architecture is also widely generalized in the bibliography. Just to quote a recent example, kit06—Churches of Mercy from the Heritage Kits collection states in the introduction: "We understand the religious architectural heritage of the *Misericórdias*, for the purposes of the use of this guide, the compounds of religious buildings (contemplating the buildings or structures built and their components) built by the Confraternities of the *Misericórdia* as their own headquarters" (Noé, *Património Arquitectónico*, 7).
28. Regarding the process of occupation preexisting spaces by *Misericórdias*, see Pinho, "A Casa da Misericórdia," 149–71.
29. The confraternities of the Holy Spirit are seen by some authors as direct predecessors of the Misericórdias, due to the numerous annexations that have occurred. However, there are significant differences between both in terms of organizational structure and religious and cultural functions. In our research, we have found that other confraternities have also been annexed to the Misericórdias (for example in Batalha, Montemor-o-Velho, Portel), and that there were some confraternities of the Holy Spirit in places that never had confraternities of Misericórdia, as well as places where both have been maintained simultaneously (e.g., Arraiolos, Alcácer do Sal, Évora, Portalegre, Portel, Santiago do

Cacém, Tavira, Torre de Moncorvo). On this subject, see Sá, *As Misericórdias portuguesas de D. Manuel I a Pombal*, 25–7; Sousa, *V Centenário das Misericórdias Portuguesas*, 51–6; and Pinho, "A Casa da Misericórdia," 154–60.

30. See the case of the Misericórdia of Vila Franca de Xira: the *alvará* of annexation of the hospital of the Holy Spirit to the Misericórdia of Vila Franca de Xira, dating from 1563, is very enlightening about this phenomenon and about the possible relation between these cases: "and because in the village there is a hospital of the holy spirit to welcome the poor, who is so poor that has no income of more than two thousand … whose administration has been from the city hall and because they are instituting the House of Mercy in the church of the Holy Spirit that is near the hospital, they ask to the king that for the better welcome of the poor, he decided that the administration of the hospital must go to the provider and brothers (of the Misericórdia) and in the way that has it in the cities of Castanheira, Azambuja, Benavente and many others of this kingdom" (see Pinho, "A Casa da Misericórdia," 556–7).
31. Sixteenth-century Misericórdias that settled in hospitals that were not run by confraternities of Holy Spirit: Barcelos, Estremoz, Freixo de Espada à Cinta, Moura, Santarém, and Serpa.
32. It is interesting to note the justification presented in the document related to the annexation of the confraternities of St. Peter and St. Domingos, from their hospital and grocery store, to the Misericórdia of Tentúgal: because by transferring part of their income to the monastery of Our Lady of Carmo "*ficou o hospital muito pobre e falto de muitas couzas necessarias pera a cura gazalhados dos enfermos e perigrinos*" (became the hospital very poor and lacked of many things necessary for the healing of the sick and perigrines) and "*por esta vila não ser muito grande pera poder todos os annos haver nove pessoas que se requerem no governo da dita confraria e treze no da Misericórdia*" (because this village is not very large so that each year there may be nine people to the government of the confraternity of St. Peter and St. Domingo and thirteen to the Misericórdia), it was decided that "*… trespassar-se assi a dita confraria e administração della na Mizericordia (como vossa magestade costuma conceder a todas as deste reino, onde ha similhantes hospitais) fica em grande bem dos proximos*" (the administration of the confraternity of St. Peter and St. Domingo passed to the confraternity of Mercy (as your majesty usually grants to all *Misericórdias* of this kingdom, where there are similar hospitals) in great good of the near ones) (Archives of the *Misericórdia* of Tentúgal, *Livro do compromisso, estatutos, privilégios e liberdades* [Book of commitment, statutes, privileges and freedoms] (1583, transfer of 1771), 59); see Pinho, "A Casa da Misericórdia," 220.
33. See Pinho, "A Casa da Misericórdia," vol. 3, for analytical-descriptive sheets of the referred Houses of Misericórdia.
34. See Pinho, "A Casa da Misericórdia," 199–226.
35. Document of the Visits of the Order of Santiago (1510), published in *Documentos para a história da arte em Portugal*, vol. 11 (Lisbon: Fundação Calouste Gulbenkian, 1972), 23, and in A. Matos Fortuna, *Misericórdia de Palmela: vida e factos* (Lisbon: Edição da Santa Casa da Misericórdia de Palmela, 1990), 74.
36. Pinho, "A Casa da Misericórdia," 218. However, between the eighteenth and nineteenth centuries, due to advances in medical practices during this period, many hospital buildings of medieval origin were remodeled and enlarged and others constructed from scratch, meaning that there are few material vestiges prior to this time. In short, most of the hospital spaces existing in the Houses of Misericórdia built in this period also present some complexity; relevant examples of this situation are the Houses of Misericórdia of Alandroal, Alcácer do Sal, Alcáçovas, Alcobaça, Alhos Vedros, Aljezur, Alter do Chão, Alverca, Arronches, Arruda dos Vinhos, Azambuja, Azinhaga, Barreiro, Borba, Cabeção, Cano, Castelo Branco, Estômbar, Fundão, Loulé, Mação, Redondo, Samora Correia, Sertã, Vila Franca de Xira.
37. To learn about the buildings that are exceptions to these models of spatial organization, see Pinho, "A Casa da Misericórdia," 278–80.
38. Relevant examples of this situation are the Houses of Misericórdia of Alenquer, Aljustrel, Arruda dos Vinhos, Benavente, Castanheira, Castro Verde, Castelo de Vide, Coimbra (primitiva), Lavre, Mação, Mogadouro, Montemor-o-Novo, Penas Roias, Ponte de Lima, Portalegre, Torres Novas, Tomar, Vila Nova da Cerveira, Vila Verde dos Francos, Viana do Castelo, Vinhais. About the possible context of these occurrences, see Pinho, "A Casa da Misericórdia," 298–302.
39. To review the complete catalog of these inscriptions and representations, see Pinho, "A Casa da Misericórdia," 319–20 and 323–7.
40. All types of planimetries and examples, in Pinho, "A Casa da Misericórdia," 330–2.
41. About the *cruzeiro*, see Pinho, "A Casa da Misericórdia," 340–52.
42. António Nogueira Gonçalves, *Inventário artístico de Portugal: distrito de Aveiro, zona sul* (Lisbon: Academia Nacional de Belas Artes, 1959), 104; Moreira, "As Misericórdias: um património artístico da humanidade."

CHAPTER 11
MAKING THE HOME A HEALING SPACE
SELF-CULTIVATING PRACTICES IN LATE IMPERIAL CHINA
Ying Zhang

Since the 1970s, when medical anthropologist Arthur Kleinman explained the Chinese medical system as composed of a professional sector, a folk sector, and a popular sector, much scholarly effort has been devoted to examining medical pluralism in late imperial China.[1] Recently, historians have highlighted the importance of non-medical experts, such as medical amateurs and the role of vernacular texts in shaping China's medical culture.[2] Medical amateurs did not make a living by practicing medicine, but they were well versed in medicine and had considerable social means with which to publish their medical works, which challenged the medical authority of physicians. Vernacular texts, such as encyclopedias, almanacs, various cheap printed handbooks, and novels, made medical knowledge accessible to a broader audience. Historians have also discussed how temples and pharmacies served as important sites for disseminating medical knowledge.[3] Yet, few studies have investigated the home as a major site for healing acts and technology. The existing scholarship on the history of domestic healing practices in late imperial China has focused on women's role as the major health provider in their homes. Francesca Bray uses a broadly conceived concept of technology to examine how reproductive technologies shaped gender relations through everyday practice within the household.[4] Charlotte Furth argues that elite women were influential decision-makers for healing choices in the domestic space.[5] When we highlight women's healing activities in the domestic space, we cannot ignore that the home was also a meaningful healing space for men. In late imperial China, the home provided a physical space for regulating bodily conditions for both men and women. Healing techniques used in the home bore strong moral connotations.

Starting from the late Ming (late sixteenth to early seventeenth century), all kinds of vernacular texts informed heterogeneous health-related practices in the home. Healing at home could mean many different things. It could herald the restoration of domestic ritual order, a demonstration of wifely virtue or filial piety, or the cultivation of virtue in daily practice (Figure 11.1). These various meanings suggest specific understandings of what constituted the domestic space and a cure, respectively.[6] In late Ming literati writings on "cultivating life" (*yangsheng*), as well as in many popular Qing (1644–1912) manuals on healing advice, we can observe a close connection between healing acts and moral performance as well as an emphasis on self-treatment and daily practices in the home. These texts introduced certain ways of arranging domestic spaces and artifacts and handling medicinal substances to make medicine a crucial component of a healthy life. The writings present these healing skills as part of daily activities in the household, the proper conduct of which led to a virtuous and even a prolonged life. These techniques first appeared as symbols of literati identity in the late Ming, and with the flourishing of popular prints in the Qing they spread further to a wider audience and became important means of accumulating merit. In this context, the home served not only as a physical space for daily healing practices but also as a locus for making reliable, beneficial medicines, and thus as a mechanism for increasing social prestige.

Based on earlier scholarship on medical pluralism, this article examines how the home was a crucial site of healing technology in late imperial China. It adopts Bray's definition of technology as a cultural construct that embodies material practices and artifacts as well as social relations. It also draws on her insight that

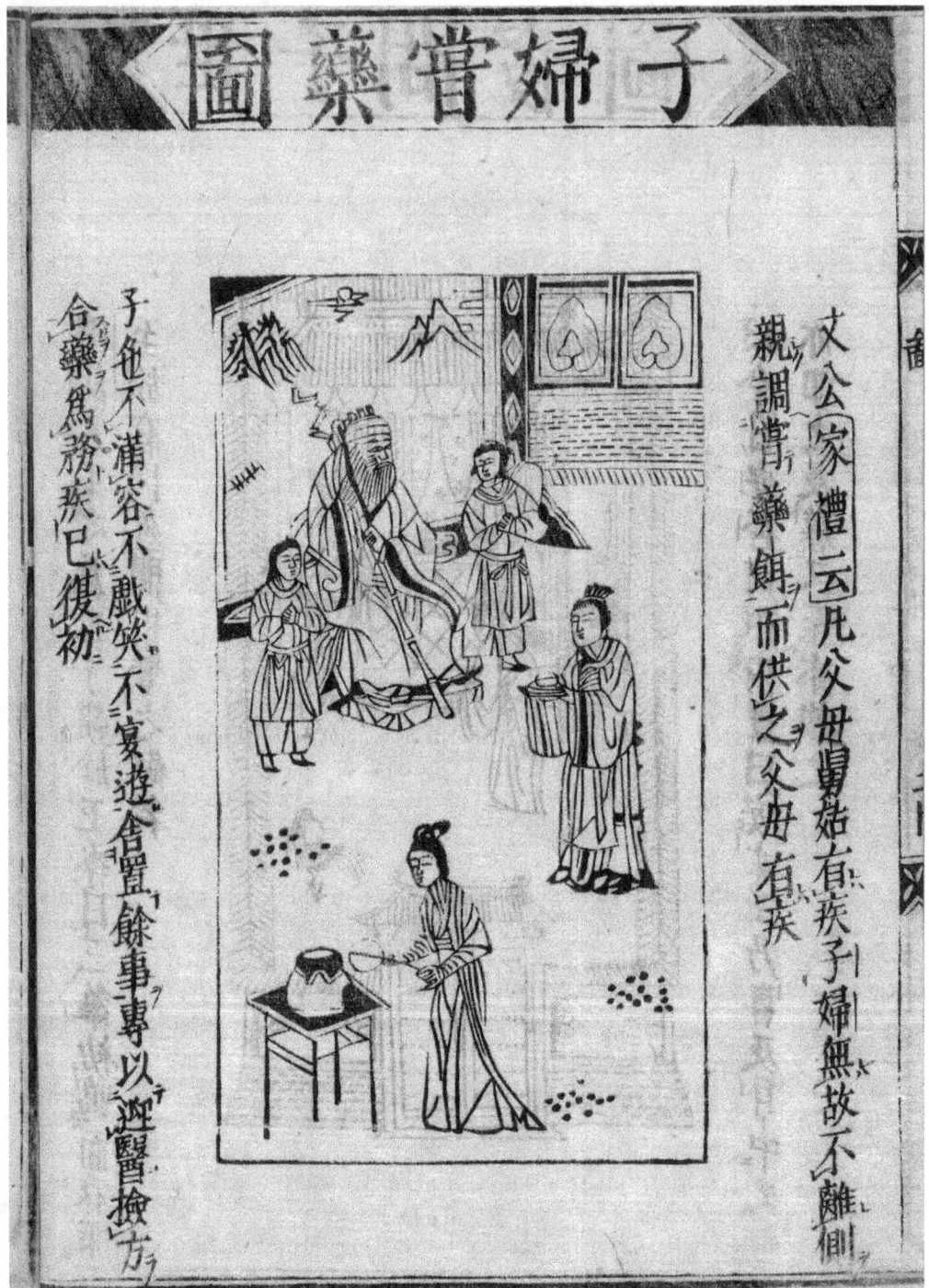

Figure 11.1 A page from a mid-seventeenth-century woodblock print showing a son and his wife preparing and tasting medicines in advance for their parents and parents-in-law in the home. Source: C. V. Starr East Asian Library, University of California, Berkeley

technological practices shaped the social identity of practitioners and the value of the artifacts they produced. Here, it specifically looks at the practice of making medicine in the home and the moral value of homemade medicines. It looks into vernacular texts related to the practice of "cultivating life" and "recipes" (*fang*) for household use to investigate these healing techniques in a domestic setting. It asks the following questions: How did the home constitute a meaningful healing space? How did the material setting of the domestic space shape the choice of healing techniques and the meanings of healthcare? How did the practice of self-treatment inform the social identity of the practitioners? And how did household healing relate to the broader social and cultural trends of the time?

Creating a Healing Space at Home

In the late Ming, "cultivating life" became part of the literati's daily activities, rather than mysterious skills held by religious practitioners.[7] It encompassed a wide range of practices and bodily techniques, including the appreciation of artifacts, reproductive technology, gymnastic practices, regulation of daily activities, cultivation of a positive mood, and dietary guidelines. Literati, and sometimes also alchemists of the period, wrote about related practices as a lifestyle that could distinguish themselves from people of other social strata. These texts introduce the practice of arranging domestic spaces and artifacts and making medicines oneself as essential to pursuing a healthy and pleasant life. These writings argue for a close connection between the proper conduct of daily activities and the pursuit of longevity. One representative text of this kind is the *Eight Essays on Cultivating Life* (*Zunsheng bajian*), which was written by the literati scholar Gao Lian (1573–1620) and published in 1591. Gao, an enthusiast of cultivating life and a renowned dramatist, divided his book into eight themes. The "Chapter on Peaceful and Pleasant Daily Activities" details methods of setting up spaces, furniture, utensils, and artifacts in the home. The "Chapter on Diet and Supplements" and the "Chapter on Divine and Secret Elixirs and Medicines" introduce ways to process food substances and make medicines.

In the "Chapter on Peaceful and Pleasant Daily Activities," Gao proclaimed the necessity of carefully arranging the home, an environment in which one can cultivate a peaceful and pleasant mental and physical state. He emphasized the importance of keeping a contented mind, working, eating, taking rest, sleeping, properly arranging and using furniture and utensils, enjoying the beauty of nature, observing the rules of the auspiciousness and inauspiciousness, and socializing with friends. Gao cited essays and poetry on these topics and also gave his personal advice, based on his own daily practices.[8] Gao also gave guidelines for setting up domestic spaces. He detailed the structure of pavilions, the setting of scholars' studios and teahouses, as well as the use of a series of household artifacts.[9] For example, he illustrated the construction of a "Pavilion of Pine Trees" in the garden for appreciating the exquisite beauty of being surrounded by pine trees, rare stones, bamboo, orchids, and plum flowers. He also introduced how to use twenty-four kinds of drugs to make a medicinal pillow that could cure all illnesses caused by wind, improve one's facial appearance, turn white hair black, promote the growth of new teeth, and improve hearing.[10] Indeed, Gao suggested that handling medicinal substances was an indispensable skill for living a healthy life.

Gao advised that among the many spaces a literati scholar should set up at his home was a medicine chamber (*yaoshi*). He proposed using a clean room located far from any domestic animals and locking it when it was not in use. Gao suggested setting up a desk for worshipping the famous physician Sun Simiao who lived in the seventh century, placing a large table for mixing medicines, preparing tools for grinding drugs, sieving powders and controlling fire, and using a cabinet and a box in which to store drugs.[11] This advice actually came from Gao's own experience of making medicine. In his short introduction to the "Chapter on Divine and Secret Elixirs and Medicines," Gao states that all the recipes were the personal collection he had gathered over the years for self-treatment.[12] Gao not only advocated making medicine for self-treatment but also mentioned how one could use self-made medicines to benefit others. In the section on utensils for travel, Gao advised his followers to take a medicine basket and fill it with proven recipes and ointments to "help people whenever needed."[13] Here, Gao made a moralistic claim for the significance of self-made medicine, but this point is overpowered by the more prominent theme of the connoisseurship of things, the practice of which marked literati identity in the late Ming.[14] Specifically, he recommended having a medicine basket decorated with red lacquer, which he claimed had a special, unworldly taste when a mountain dweller carried it.[15]

During the Qing, many sections of Gao's book found their way into vernacular texts, such as daily-use encyclopedias and manuals, which advertised the literati way of life as learnable and universally applicable to people of all walks of life.[16] Yet, these texts delivered a much stronger moral connotation: they often contained essays that urged people to follow moral norms and do good deeds. Lower-level literati and commercial printers avidly compiled all kinds of household manuals. On the one hand, these manuals illustrated an ideal of domestic life that was full of entertaining activities divorced from worldly concerns.[17] Yet few men could lead such a leisurely life, since elite males often needed to spend most of their time away from home, either serving as officials or, in those cases of not being able to obtain any official title, as private teachers or advisors, or even doctors.[18] On the other hand, these handbooks introduced many practical skills and knowledge for people to use at home, particularly medical recipes. These texts thus illustrated an ideal of domestic life for male literati and yet, at the same time, also served as a guide for household practices. In this context, making medicine at home became a domestic practice that was firmly associated with the accumulation of merit. Healing at home by taking self-made medicines meant a personal endeavor that testified to one's awareness of one's bodily condition and ability to self-manage in daily life, both of which demonstrated virtue and distinction from the uneducated masses. Healing at home also attested to one's mastery of practical healing knowledge that was accessible via a common readership of vernacular literature. With this knowledge, one could save the lives of others and thereby accumulate merit.

We can observe this emphasis on merit accumulation through daily domestic practice in the *Three Collections of Family Treasures* (*Jiabao sanji*), written by Shi Chengjin (1659–?). Shi was a prolific writer and philanthropist from Yangzhou, a city in which charitable organizations flourished in the seventeenth century.[19] This all-inclusive vernacular guide to quotidian practice was first published in the early eighteenth century and then reprinted in various editions under different titles throughout the eighteenth and nineteenth centuries.[20] Shi wrote his essays in the vernacular language in order to deliver moral lessons through texts that could reach the less well educated.[21] Besides providing moral teachings, the book was intended to serve as a daily-use encyclopedia for ordinary households. A large part of Shi's collection consists of essays explaining how to lead a peaceful, well-regulated, and pleasant domestic life. In the preface to a section titled "All about Human Affairs," Shi noted that the book was a product of his own domestic situation in a small house he built beside the Red Bridge, a famous site outside Yangzhou's city wall. He writes that, from his window, he could enjoy the natural beauty of the suburban setting and observe "human sentiments and the affairs of the world."[22]

Shi's essays identify trivial everyday matters as critical elements of a virtuous life. By doing things in the proper manner, one could demonstrate morality—and cultivate it. He used examples from his own daily practice to support his claims. In the preface of an essay titled "A Collection of Good Skills," Shi argued, "Among all the things in the world, some are good for one to be able to do, and some are not suitable for one to be able to do."[23] Among the former, moral behaviors were the principal ones, and the "miscellaneous matters of daily use, diet, and clothing in the household" were also part of moral practice. He continued: "One should do these things as much as possible, the more the better." He recorded those things that "I have done myself, which turned out to be effective," and expressed his hope that others could learn from him.[24] Among these skills were methods to determine the time, remove evil spells placed on one's house by a carpenter, protect paintings and calligraphy, wash one's hair and face, eat, sleep, and wash one's body, nourish one's eyes, ears, and teeth, and preserve and process food.[25]

Shi thus promoted a way of household life that required one to properly carry out daily activities in order to achieve health and cultivate virtue. As a kind of domestic practice, making elixirs to regulate bodily conditions evinced both self-awareness and self-control. Since Shi envisioned his book as a practical guide for everyday life, he included the "Secretly transmitted elixir for prolonging longevity," which contained detailed instructions for making elixirs, along with a group of simple recipes for self-treatment. He presented these recipes as suitable for prolonging life and treating common symptoms in ordinary households. The elixir recipe clearly recorded the trajectory of its transmission in a short quotation by Chen Xunzhai (c. 1600s–90s),[26] an amateur scholar of medicine, and two passages written by Chen's self-proclaimed "family brothers." The moral lessons these prefaces delivered and the literati way of life they illustrated facilitated the circulation of this recipe to a broad audience.

According to Chen Xunzhai, this recipe was originally created and used for years by the renowned late Ming scholar official Dong Qichang (1555–1636). The recipe initially circulated as a symbol of Dong's literary and political reputation among his followers in the late Ming and early Qing. In this small literati circle, to use and circulate this recipe already carried a strong moral connotation. Chen studied calligraphy under Dong, and finally asked him for the recipe after serving him for years. From his quotation, we learn that Chen devoted most of his time in his later years to studying classical medical texts, so when he fell severely ill at the age of seventy-five, he "looked for the substances, refined [them], and made the elixir" (*mi yao xiuzhi*) according to this recipe. After taking the elixir for several months, he was allegedly able to climb up Yuhua Mountain (in a suburb of Nanjing) faster than his friends, his white hair had turned black again, and he was able to walk faster than before. He stated that, since many of his relatives and friends asked for this recipe, he decided to publicize it in the hope of prolonging his own life as well as that of others. He stressed that, even though the drug was powerful, one must have "the drug's power and one's own moral power functioning in parallel" in order "to keep one's well-being."[27]

Chen's two "family brothers," He Lianggong and Fang Xiangxian (both c. seventeenth century), reaffirmed Chen's point on morality and prolonging longevity in their two prefaces written for the recipe.[28] Both of them expressed strong suspicion toward doctors. They gave examples in their prefaces of several doctors' failures in treating their family members: it was Chen who saved their lives at the last moment. They depicted Chen as a person who "understood the Way"—someone who, as a practitioner, used drugs correctly to regulate his own body. In their account, Chen's successful experience of cultivating life, attested by his black hair and good facial appearance, unquestionably indicated the reliability of the recipe, which is further supported with the "variety of techniques of processing drugs" clearly specified in the recipe.[29] Making medicines by oneself at home expressed a clear awareness and self-control of one's bodily condition, and the ability to learn from role models. Thus, using a home-healing option was seen as better and more effective than resorting to doctors. This elixir recipe possessed the moral imprimatur of both Dong and Chen, as well as concrete techniques with which to cultivate longevity. It thus became a gift that could be used to network with friends and relatives.

Chen Xunzhai was an active advocate and distributer of this recipe. The Ming loyalist Mao Xiang (1611–93) once wrote a short passage recounting how Chen brought him this recipe along with a letter of recommendation from his friend He Cide (c. seventeenth century). By then more than sixty years old, Mao's body was extremely weak and he had little confidence in doctors. He recalled that the two times he recovered from almost dying were not because he took medicine prescribed by a doctor, but rather because of fate. After Chen's visit, his two sons encouraged him to try the recipe, drawing on Chen's successful treatment of He Cide's uncle, as well as the moral power of the recipe's original creator, Dong Qichang, who had promoted Mao's writings in his youth. With Mao's approval, his sons collected the substances listed in the recipe and made the elixir themselves. After taking the elixir for less than a month, Mao reported an improved appetite.[30] Like Chen Xunzhai's "family brothers," he praised Chen for being quite unlike those doctors who only "showcased their techniques." He wrote that Chen had "deep compassion toward others and a strong belief in saving the world," and he "learns medicine according to the principles of the classics and history, and adjusts medicine with sympathy and in accordance with the rules of society."[31] Instead of focusing on medical expertise or any medical doctrine, all of these compliments present Chen as a morally apt practitioner of the true way of cultivating life, for which the processing of drugs and making elixirs in a correct way by oneself were essential.

The methods of making the elixirs this recipe introduced required much personal attention and piety throughout the whole process. Some ingredients in the recipe had to be carefully collected only at certain times of the year and in a ritualized manner. For instance, one needed to pick the leaves of *xixian cao* (*Siegesbeckiae*, pig pungent weed) in the fifth and sixth months of the year and the young leaves of mulberry trees—only from cultivated trees—in the fourth month. The person preparing the recipe's ingredients also had to collect the herb *nüzhenzi* (*Fructus ligustri lucidi*, Frivet fruit) in rural gardens on the day of the winter solstice, and only if they were black and kidney-shaped (Figure 11.2).[32] The instruction for processing each individual drug describes in detail the method of processing each ingredient under its name, which generally begins with where and how to collect the substance, followed by an explanation of how to clean, boil, steam, or dry it. It ends with the weight of the substance needed after processing. For example, for the second ingredient, *tusizi* (*Semen Cuscutae*, cuscuta seed), one needed to:

> Put [the *tusizi*] in a bowl of water and pick out the [seeds] that float up to the surface; wash away the soil and sand on the remaining ones with clean water, repeat this three to five times; dry the ones that drop to the bottom under the sun; pick out deteriorated ones and take only the hard, kidney-shaped ones that have a sprout on them. Soak them in clear yellow wine for seven days, steam for the duration of burning seven sticks of incense, and dry under the sun; then soak in a new batch of wine overnight, steam for the duration of burning six sticks of incense, and dry under the sun. Repeat this process nine times and record clearly. Dry thoroughly under the sun and grind into one *jin* of fine powder.[33]

These specific procedures reinforced the moralistic claim made by the prefaces: following these instructions strictly with piety demonstrated one's commitment to following the role model set by Dong Qichang and Chen Xunzhai. Including this recipe along with those short passages in his *Family Treasures*, Shi Chengjin highlighted exactly this image of literati life and underscored the manifestation of virtue in daily practice.

In sum, late Ming literati writings and Qing handbooks for cultivating life depict the home as an important site for people to maintain health. Late Ming scholars, such as Gao Lian, emphasized arranging domestic space and making medicines by oneself in the home as integrated dimensions of literati life. From the late Ming to the Qing, cultivating-life enthusiasts, such as Chen Xunzhai and Shi Chengjin, presented the practice of making medicine as a useful way to cultivate virtue. They claimed that one could maintain health by cultivating virtue in daily practices in the home, and advertised making medicines for self-treatment as a daily domestic practice that testified to one's awareness and self-control of bodily condition. They circulated recipes among themselves and to a broader audience via their writings. They also underlined the morality of circulating recipes to others. Shi's work illustrates a growing interest in collecting and circulating practice-oriented recipes for household use.[34] Through these recipes we find far more heterogeneous and rich healing practices than those introduced in the texts of learned medicine. In the eighteenth and nineteenth centuries, in addition to handbooks on cultivating life, all kinds of vernacular texts contained recipes with technical instructions for domestic healing practices.

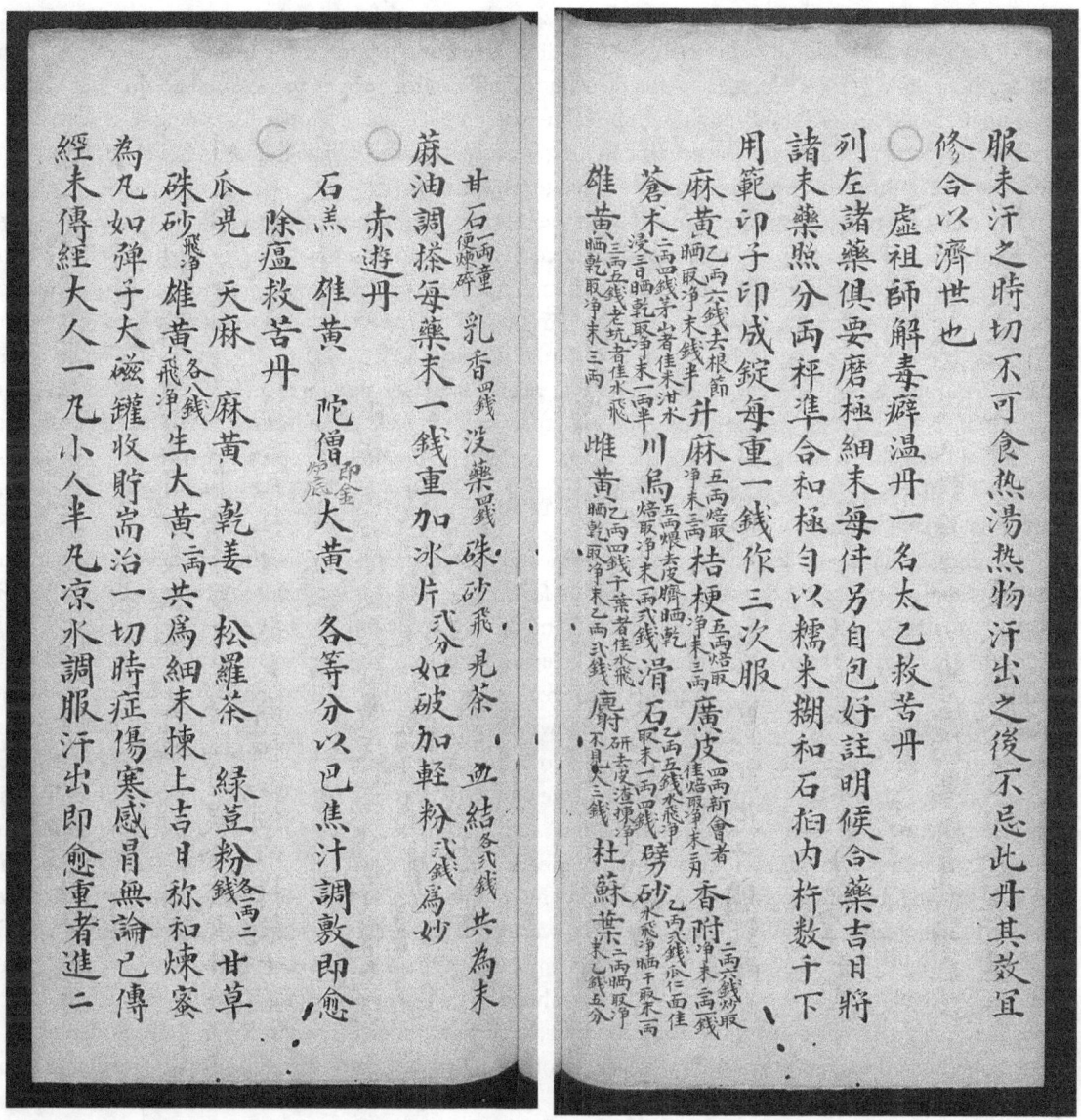

Figure 11.2 The pages showing the recipe of "Elixir for dispelling the plague and saving the suffering" in *Yifang bianlan*. Source: The Berlin State Library

Handling Substances and Utensils in the Household

The texts of the eighteenth and nineteenth centuries that promoted the practice of making medicine in the home suggested an even closer association between self-cultivation and a commitment to benefit others, which accumulated merit. Local elites engaged in all kinds of philanthropic activities, such as providing poor and disaster relief, burying the dead, operating foundling homes, and providing medical aid.[35] At the same time, people of varied social strata participated in merit accumulation as a result of the shared religious belief in reward and retribution. Practice-oriented recipes became more widely available through medical writings as well as popular commercial publications such as manuals and daily use encyclopedias. People from all walks of life, including physicians and medical amateurs, proposed the universal use of recipes in ordinary households. Their enthusiasm for distributing efficacious recipes to accumulate merit facilitated the circulation of these recipes through both print media and personal networks. The home thus served as a site for healing acts that involved the actual handling of all sorts of medicinal and household substances and utensils, which at the same time were moral and religious practices.

As we can see through the passages included in the "Secretly Transmitted Elixir for Prolonging Longevity," making medicine was tantamount to a moral practice in the domestic setting. Chen Xunzhai used the term "refine and make" (*xiuzhi*) to refer to his practice of making the elixir. This phrase was not randomly selected. In recipes intended for use at home during the late Ming and Qing, the words most frequently used to describe the process of making medicine were "to refine and mix" (*xiuhe*) and "to mix drugs" (*heyao*). The term "refine and mix" conveys a strong sense of personal endeavor related to personal refinement and self-cultivation (as in *xiushen*): the person mixing medicines needed to prepare himself well, clean himself beforehand, be sincere, and control the whole process of making the recipe. The potentially polluting presence of women, chickens, and dogs was prohibited during the process. This image of self-cultivation appeared in many practice-oriented recipes that circulated in the Qing.

For example, the "Recipe from the bare-foot immortal for pills made with fish maw to help insemination" in the late Qing manuscript *A Convenient Survey of Medical Recipes* (*Yifang bianlan*) tells the story of a person with the surname Zhou who "refined and mixed [medicine] according to the recipe" (*yifang xiuhe*) with sincerity.[36] This story validates the efficacy of the recipe by stating that, upon meeting an immortal on a mountain, Mr. Zhou "bowed and received it [i.e., the recipe]" and "refined and mixed [the medicine] according to the recipe." Here, "*xiuhe*" clearly refers to all the work, from processing individual drugs to mixing them together into a pill, which also conveys an associated sense of piety and self-cultivation. Mr. Zhou's sincere practice brought him good health. After taking doses for forty days he felt his "eyesight improved and his body strengthened with stronger sinews and bones," and later he had seven sons.[37] In a similar manner, but stating the intention of merit accumulation more clearly, one recipe with the title "Elixir for dispelling the plague and saving the suffering" in another late Qing manuscript concludes: "This elixir is extremely effective, and [one] should refine and mix [it] to benefit the world."[38] The phrases "saving the suffering" and "benefit the world" have a strong connotation of merit accumulation. These recipes suggest ways in which making medicine is a cognate of other types of activities involving ritual purity and right-mindedness, such as that of religious worship and self-cultivation. They also present making medicine according to their guidelines as a task anyone could do and even should do to benefit others. Distributing recipes or self-made medicines thus became a means of accumulating merit.

To make a medicine according to a recipe does not necessarily require one to buy all the ingredients from pharmacies. Many of the substances could have been found in the pantries of an average household. The majority of substances used in recipes from the manuscript *Book of Drugs and Demons* (*Yao sui shu*), a collection of folk recipes that probably circulated in Shandong province during the eighteenth and nineteenth centuries, comprised common foods. These included dried persimmon, cooked rice, raw ginger juice, large oranges, and chive juice. Or they were random everyday substances, such as "dirt from the scalp" or the "excrement of brown cows."[39] Even though a recipe asks only for household items, one needs to pay close attention to the procedure introduced by the recipe. For instance, a "Whole chicken ointment" in the *Survey* requires only a whole chicken, sesame oil, and the drug *huangdan* (*Plumbum Rubrum*, red lead) (Figure 11.3).[40] One would probably need only to buy the *huangdan* drug from a pharmacy to complete this recipe. The key to success in making the medicine was to choose, kill, clean, and process the chicken correctly:

Use an old red cock. One, two, or three years old is the best. Kill it with a bamboo knife. Withdraw its blood but keep the feathers. Cut open the belly and take out the gizzard, liver, intestines, and all the other organs. Wipe the blood from the chicken with a piece of paper or cloth. Avoid water and iron utensils. Put it into an earthen pot and boil it together with pure sesame oil, alternating between mild and strong fire. Boil and then take out the dregs. Squeeze out the oily liquid with a piece of rough cloth. Boil [the liquid] and constantly stir it with the branches of an elm tree, willow tree, mulberry tree, or locust tree until round droplets form in the water. Add in the roasted *huangdan* and mix well into an ointment.⁴¹

This paragraph describes the specific way to choose and clean the chicken, and gives instructions on how to further boil, filter, and stir the mixture and with what kind of implements. Adding the purchased *huangdan* was only the final step in a much more elaborate process that took place in the home.

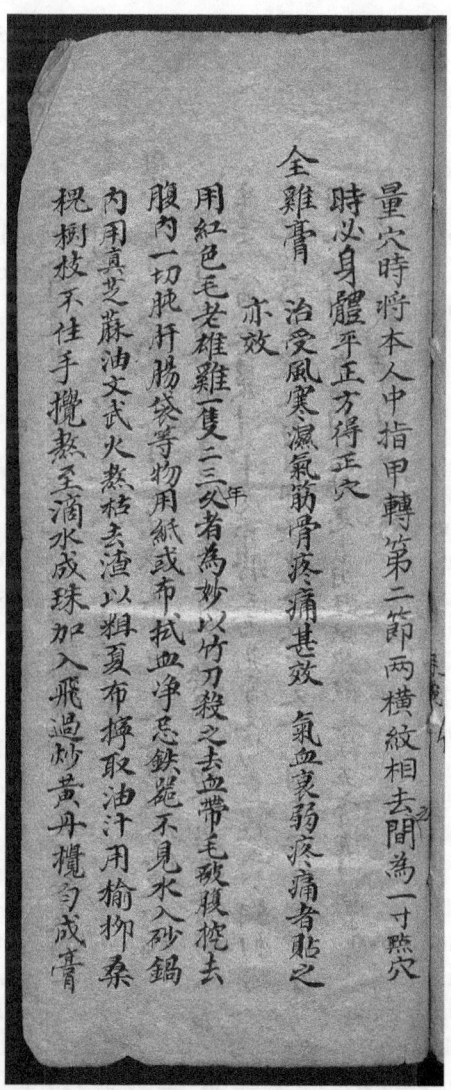

Figure 11.3 The page showing the recipe for "Whole chicken ointment" in *Jiye liangfang*. Source: The Berlin State Library

Health and Architecture

Not only were the substances used in these recipes readily available in a typical household, but so too were the utensils and tools they called for. In many cases, the recipe-making tools were the same kinds of food-processing utensils used at home. In the *Survey*, one recipe even recommends "using warmed shoes to heat the ointment plaster."[42] A recipe for treating vaginal bleeding instructs the reader to heat a "rice bowl" of cottonseed in an "earthen pot," and then place the cottonseed on the floor and cover it with the bowl.[43] A recipe to treat foot infections suggests using a piece of "roof tile" as the container for heating the powder.[44] A recipe from Wutai Mountain uses one "teacup" of water to boil the ashes from burned mulberry bark.[45] A recipe for hair dye explains that one should use a "needle" to spear a pine nut and hold it "on top of a candle flame" to extract the oil.[46] In another late Qing manuscript titled *A Collection of Superlative Recipes* (*Jiye liangfang*), we see some other household tools and everyday items as well, such as chopsticks, a rice pot, and chicken feathers.[47] All these examples illustrate how various household objects were doubly utilized to make medicines in the home.

Practice-oriented recipes thus presented the handling of drug substances and household utensils as a kind of household technique anyone could master. They legitimated related practices through a discourse of self-cultivation, rather than claiming medical expertise. Although many detailed technical descriptions might have originated from expert texts of earlier periods, the increasing appearance of these recipes in vernacular texts and their circulation as practical instructions for helping others rendered these recipes into a guide for household healing practices instead of being used solely for acquiring knowledge of drugs. Such a trend in reverse also encouraged the recording of even more details of healing technology through the textual form of the recipe. As a result, the home became a meaningful site for the application of healing techniques and for the reproduction of related technical knowledge in late imperial China.

Conclusion

From the late Ming to the Qing, commoners engaged in everyday home-healing practices in a world of medicine that was far from being the preserve of experts and the medical marketplace. In the late sixteenth and early seventeenth centuries, making medicines by oneself became a clearly articulated element of literati practice of cultivating life. Literature on cultivating life presents the practice of making one's own medicine as an important way to regulate one's bodily condition and secure a virtuous life in daily household practice. With the proliferation of vernacular texts in the eighteenth and nineteenth centuries, related practices then spread from literati to other social groups when practice-oriented recipes appeared in popular manuals and encyclopedias. Elite philanthropic activism and the religious belief of reward and retribution further contributed to what became a more widespread enthusiasm for the collection and distribution of recipes and self-made medicines. Recipes functioned as a guide for non-experts to follow at home and served as the major textual form in which healing techniques circulated.

With the greater availability of practice-oriented recipes through manuals, encyclopedias, and manuscripts, the home thus became a central site for healing acts and technology. The home served as a healing space in which people regulated their daily activities to cultivate virtue and maintain health. The home also provided a physical space for producing homemade medicines. Making medicine with one's own hands involved the skills to handle household substances and utensils, pay attention to detail, and follow instructions. It also required sincere piety, thereby linking following recipes with cultivating virtue. Recipes and the medicines they prescribed thus became culturally and socially significant artifacts. They represented a literati way of life, and circulated as gifts among scholars. They also circulated as a means of universal aid in the hands of people from all walks of life. Recipes introduced the techniques of making pills, ointments, and elixirs, and, even more broadly, the procedures to be used in healing. They presented these as skills for self-treatment that anyone could learn. Within the household, these healing techniques were thus no longer the exclusive purview of physicians, but technologies with which people cultivated virtue and constructed their social identity in daily practice.

Notes

1. Arthur Kleinman, *Patients and Healers in the Context of Culture: An Exploration of the Borderland between Anthropology, Medicine and Psychiatry* (Berkeley, CA: University of California Press, 1980), 24–70.
2. For example, see Yi-Li Wu's study on popular gynecology texts and Andrew Schonebaum's study on the intertextuality between medical and fictional texts. Yi-li Wu, *Reproducing Women* (Berkeley, CA: University of California Press, 2010); Andrew Schonebaum, *Novel Medicine: Healing, Literature and Popular Knowledge in Early Modern China* (Seattle, WA: University of Washington Press, 2016).
3. Yi-Li Wu shows that temples were important sites for the production of medical knowledge in the Qing. Bian He investigates the roles urban pharmacies played in constructing medical authority in the eighteenth and nineteenth centuries. Yi-Li Wu, "The Bamboo Grove Monastery and Popular Gynecology in Qing China," *Late Imperial China* 21, no. 1 (2000): 41–76; Bian He, "Assembling the Cure: Materia Medica and the Culture of Healing in Late Imperial China" (PhD diss., Harvard University, 2014).
4. Francesca Bray, *Technology, Gender and History in Imperial China: Great Transformation Reconsidered* (New York, NY: Routledge, 2013), 155–73; *Technology and Gender: Fabrics of Power in Late Imperial China* (Berkeley, CA: University of California Press, 1997), 273–368.
5. Charlotte Furth, *A Flourishing Yin: Gender in China's Medical History: 960–1665* (Berkeley, CA: University of California Press, 1999), 224–300.
6. Zhang Ying, "Household Healing: Rituals, Recipes, and Virtues in Late Imperial China" (Ph.D. diss., Johns Hopkins University, 2017).
7. Chen Hsiu-fen has studied how cultivating life became a favorite topic for literati writers and an accessible knowledge for common households in the Jiangnan region in the late Ming. This article further calls attention to the practice of making medicine an important part of cultivating life from the late Ming through the Qing. See Chen Hsiu-fen, *Yangsheng yu xiushen: Wan Ming wenren de shenti shuxie yu shesheng jishu* (Taipei: Daoxiang chubanshe, 2009).
8. Gao Lian, *Zunsheng bajian* (Yashang zhai, 1591), *juan* 7 and 8.
9. Ibid., *juan* 7, 28–35; *juan* 8, 8–19.
10. Ibid., *juan* 8, 10–11.
11. Ibid., *juan* 7, 34–5.
12. Ibid., *juan* 17, 1–2.
13. Ibid., *juan* 8, 35.
14. Craig Clunas, *Superfluous Things: Material Culture and Social Status in Early Modern China* (Honolulu, HI: University of Hawaii Press, 2004).
15. Gao Lian, *Zunsheng bajian*, *juan* 8, 36.
16. For a study on popular prints and their distribution networks in the Qing, see Cynthia Brokaw, *Commerce in Culture: The Sibao Book Trade in the Qing and Republican Periods* (Cambridge, MA: Harvard University Press, 2007).
17. For example, Shi Chengjin's book contains many essays that advise people to pursue happiness in daily life. See chapters such as "The Sources of Happiness" (*Kuaile yuan*) in *Family Treasures*. Shi and his relatives and friends, who wrote prefaces to these essays, stressed that learning to enjoy "genuine happiness" (*zhenle*) was essential for "nurturing good personality, improving fortune, and achieving longevity." Liu Zhengfu, "Kuaile yuan zongxu," in Shi Chengjin, *Chuanjia bao* (First printed 1739. Repr. eds. Jin Qinghui and Yan Mingxun. Tianjin: Tianjin shehui kexueyuan chubanshe, 1992).
18. Susan Mann discusses the sojourning life of elite men who were often exposed to infectious diseases in the nineteenth century. Susan Mann, *Talented Women of the Zhang Family* (Berkeley, CA: University of California Press, 2007), 184–5.
19. See Angela Leung's discussion of Yangzhou's charity organizations in the early Qing. Angela Leung, *Shishan yu jiaohua: Ming Qing de cishan zuzhi* (Taipei: Lianjing chuban shiye gongsi, 1997), 71–84.

20. For a list of editions published in the eighteenth and nineteenth centuries, see You Zi'an, *Shan yu ren tong: Ming Qing yilai de cishan yu jiaohua* (Beijing: Zhonghua shuju, 2005), 134–5.
21. See You Zi'an's discussion of Shi Chengjin's book as a meritorious book. You Zi'an, *Shan yu ren tong*, 131–41.
22. Shi Chengjin, "*Chuanjia bao er ji, juan zhi yi*," in *Chuanjia bao*, 419.
23. Ibid., 222.
24. Ibid., 222.
25. Ibid., 253–4.
26. This estimation of Chen's lifetime is based on Mao Xiang's (1611–93) account. When Mao Xiang was about seventy years old, Chen was eighty.
27. Chengjin, "*Chuanjia bao siji, juan zhi ba*," in *Chuanjia bao*, 1491.
28. He and Fang refer to themselves at the end of their passages as the "*jiadi*" of Chen Xunzhai, which probably indicates they were related to him by marriage.
29. Chengjin, "*Chuanjia bao siji, juan zhi ba*" in *Chuanjia bao*, 1493–4.
30. Mao Xiang, *Chaomin shiwenji*, printed 1661–1722 (Online source: Zhongguo jiben guji ku, Beijing ai ru sheng shuzihua jishu yanjiu zhongxin, 2009), *juan* 6, 65–7.
31. Ibid., *juan* 6, 65–7.
32. Chengjin, "*Chuanjia bao siji, juan zhi ba*" in *Chuanjia bao*, 1491–3.
33. Ibid., 1492.
34. I use the phrase "practice-oriented recipes" to refer to recipes recorded and circulated for domestic use that newly underscored the techniques and methods of making medicine. These recipes testify to a growing reliance on experience in the production of healing knowledge in the seventeenth century. For a discussion on the increasing emphasis on experience in formularies in medical case histories from this period, see Marta Hanson and Pomata Gianna, "Medicinal Formulas and Experiential Knowledge in the Seventeenth-Century Epistemic Exchange between China and Europe," *ISIS* 108, no. 1 (2017): 1–25.
35. Leung, *Shishan yu jiaohua*, 93–306; William T. Rowe, *Hankow: Conflict and Community in a Chinese City, 1796–1895* (Stanford, CA: Stanford University Press, 1992), 91–134; William T. Rowe, *China's Last Empire: The Great Qing* (Cambridge, MA: The Belknap Press of Harvard University Press, 2009), 119–21; Tobie Meyer-Fong, *What Remains: Coming to Terms with Civil War in 19th Century China* (Stanford, CA: Stanford University Press, 2013), 26–8, 128–32.
36. This unfinished manuscript gathers together miscellaneous recipes: simple declarative recipes are scattered among recipes that have long paragraphs describing the drug-making processes in detail. Many recipes in this manuscript contain detailed descriptions of the steps involved in making medicines and appear as practical instructions for ordinary people to use in their own homes. This manuscript was probably initially written before or during the 1820s by a person with the sobriquet Gaoyangshi. The manuscript was then updated by Gaoyangshi himself, Zhao Jinyun, or Xu Guoxiang, at least until the late Qing.
37. Gaoyangshi, *Yifang bianlan* (Nineteenth-century manuscript held at the Berlin State Library. Staatsbibliothek Berlin. Unschuld 8453), 9.
38. Anonymous, *Jiye liangfang* (Late Qing manuscript held at the Berlin State Library. Staatsbibliothek Berlin. Unschuld 8210), 89–90.
39. Pu Songling, *Yao sui shu* (Preface 1706, transcribed 1937. Manuscript held at Keio University).
40. The drug *huangdan* may have also been available in food markets. The author did not indicate where to find the substance. Many ointment recipes mention *huangdan* as the last ingredient added to the mixture.
41. Gaoyangshi, *Yifang bianlan*, 289.
42. Ibid., 290.
43. Ibid., 28–9.
44. Ibid., 253.
45. Ibid., 269.
46. Ibid., 18.
47. Anonymous, *Jiye liangfang*, 113, 170–1.

CHAPTER 12
FOR CARE AND SALVATION
LEPROSY HOSTELS IN PRE-MODERN JAPAN, c. 1200–1800
Susan L. Burns

On May 20, 2001, in the city of Nara in western Japan, local officials, residents, and journalists gathered to celebrate the restoration of a remarkable structure. Known as the Kitayama Jūhachikenko (hereafter, Kitayama Hall), it is the only pre-modern leprosy hostel that survives to the present (Figure 12.1). Originally constructed in the mid-thirteenth century, the Kitayama Hall was destroyed by fire in 1567. It was then rebuilt in its current location, not far from the original site, sometime between 1661 and 1675. In this location it continued to house sufferers of leprosy up until the mid-nineteenth century. In the early twentieth century, as leprosy became an international public health concern, Japanese advocates for quarantining leprosy sufferers to prevent the spread of the disease repeatedly referenced the pre-modern leprosy hostels, casting them as indigenous and prescient precursors to the modern leprosarium.[1] This view contributed to the passage of Japan's first modern leprosy law of 1907, which authorized the confinement of indigent leprosy sufferers. In 1931, the law was expanded to allow the confinement of any leprosy patient deemed a threat to public health. The result was a system of national leprosaria that continue to function today, housing a declining number of elderly recovered leprosy patients who, because of disability, loss of ties with families, and the stigma of their disease, were never able to return to life outside of these institutions. In the late 1990s, as Japan's leprosy policy began to be criticized as a violation of sufferers' human rights, some critics of the policy of quarantine invoked Kitayama Hall, arguing that it represented a humane and community-based approach to aiding leprosy sufferers. In contrast, others argued that any acknowledgment of the pre-modern practices of exclusion was simply a means to excuse the modern state's role in stigmatizing the disease.[2]

This chapter seeks to detach the Kitayama Hall and similar institutions from these modern debates over the ethicality of modern policies of leprosy prevention in order to explore how these institutions emerged and how they functioned over the course of Japan's long pre-modern period, from roughly 1200 to 1800. It draws upon textual and visual sources and modern architectural site reports to argue that the pre-modern leprosy hostels differed fundamentally from modern institutions of care and confinement. They were not founded to control infection, nor to treat or even to care for those with the disease. Rather, their establishment reflected the contemporary understanding of leprosy as a "karmic retribution disease." It was spiritual rather than bodily health that oriented these institutions, and they had the aim of facilitating the salvation not only of leprosy sufferers but also of those who offered them compassion. This was reflected in their architectural form: the leprosy hostels were based upon the architectural style of monastic dormitories and most were established on or adjacent to temple complexes.

Karma, Pollution, and Leprosy in Medieval Japan

The Japanese term for leprosy *rai* or *raibyō* derives from the Chinese *lai*. It was introduced to Japan beginning in the third century CE, as people, objects, and texts began to flow from the mainland to the Japanese archipelago. The Chinese character for *rai* appears in the earliest Japanese texts, compiled in the early eighth century, but there is no way to know whether it renamed an existing disease category or created a new one.

Health and Architecture

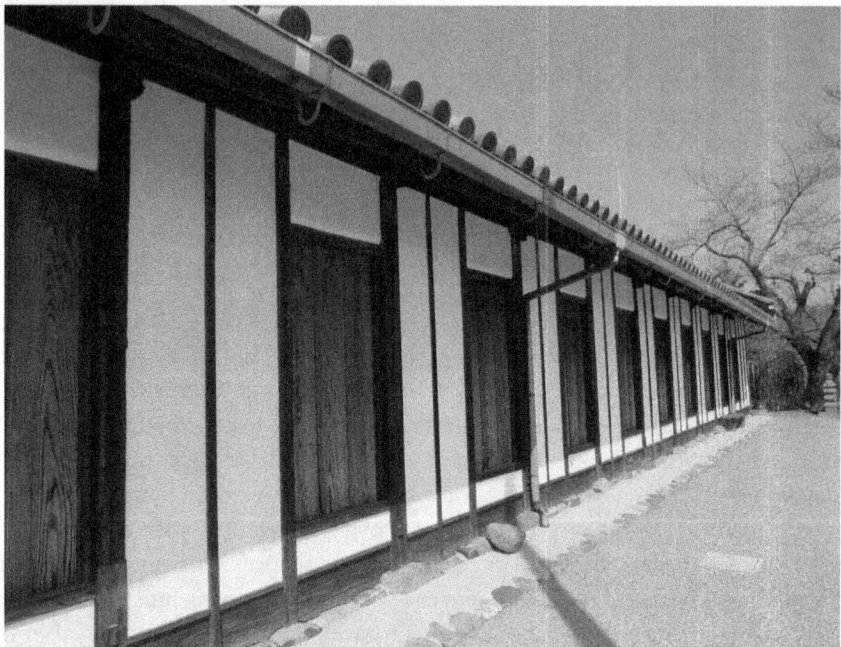

Figure 12.1 The restored Kitayama Hall. Photo: Susan L. Burns

Whatever the case, it seems likely that *rai* referenced a wider range of disfiguring diseases than just leprosy, which is defined by the presence of the mycobacterium *M.leprae*. One of the few extant medical texts from before 1600 describes multiple form of *rai* and attempts to distinguish those forms that were potentially treatable from those that were not, suggesting an awareness that *rai*, as it was then understood, was marked by different clusters of symptoms and progressed differently as well.[3] However, skeletons excavated from a medieval graveyard provide evidence that true leprosy was endemic in Japan. They reveal bone deformities that are associated with advanced cases of the disease.[4]

Within classical Chinese medical theory, diseases were understood to result from five atmospheric pathogens: Wind, Cold, Damp, Heat, and Dryness. Leprosy was understood to be a Wind disease. In the *Inner Canon of the Yellow Emperor* (*Huangdi Neijing*), a canonical text for Chinese medicine believed to date from the first or second centuries BCE, "leprosy wind" is explained as the result of Wind entering the body through the skin and harming *qi* (J: *ki*), the vital energy or "ether" believed to flow through the natural world and the human body. Its symptoms include sores, lesions, changes in skin color, and eventually the collapse of the nose and loss of fingers and toes.[5] Although the Japanese understanding of disease causality was profoundly influenced by Chinese medical theory until the rise of biomedicine in the mid-nineteenth century, it had little influence on the understanding of leprosy before 1600. Instead, it was the politicization of concerns about pollution (*kegare*) and the Buddhist concept of karma that informed the popular understanding leprosy.

Japan's early mytho-histories, such as the *Kojiki* (Record of Ancient Matters) and *Nihon shoki* (Chronicles of Japan), reveal that fear of sickness, death, and bodily fluids, particularly blood, had a prominent place among the people of western Japan from ancient times. However, beginning in the eleventh century, the imperial court, located in the capital of Heiankyō (later known as Kyoto), began to actively promote concern about pollution among its subjects.[6] The timing of this development is important: it occurred as the wealth and authority of the imperial court were being challenged by other powerful noble families in the capital.

Unique to the imperial family, however, was its longstanding role in performing rites of purification and expiation. As a means to maintaining authority, the court began to raise heightened concern for pollution, with the implication that the court alone could control it. Historian Niunoya Tetsuichi has argued that the imperial police force played a central role in promoting the new "pollution ideology." Its members began to patrol the center of Heiankyō in order to compel the removal of sources of pollution, by disposing of corpses, for example, but also by relocating the sick and dying away from the city center.[7] As anxiety about pollution grew, families stopped burying their dead close to home and instead discarded them in newly designated sites outside the capital, known as Toribeno, Rendaino, and Adashino.[8]

Buddhist doctrine, too, stigmatized sickness in general, and leprosy specifically. Buddhism was introduced from the continent to the archipelago in the third century CE, and the imperial state began to support it by establishing a network of temples in the eighth century.[9] Even so, the social and cultural influence of Buddhist doctrine was limited outside of elite circles until the aftermath of the civil conflict known as the Gempei War of 1180–5.[10] The war destroyed the capital, ushered in the political and economic power of the warrior class, and caused considerable suffering. In this time of turmoil, Buddhism found a newly receptive audience, leading to the founding of new sects and efforts to proselytize to ordinary people. Among several of the newly popular sects, the Lotus Sutra (Sanskrit: *Saddharma Puṇḍarika Sutra*, Japanese: *Myōhō renge kyō*) became an object of particularly intense veneration. Many sutras of Indian origin express the idea that illness was the result of the workings of karma, but the Lotus Sutra contained a particularly explicit claim: leprosy was a form of karmic retribution that occurred in this life, offering immediate bodily and therefore visible evidence of the consequences of wrongdoing.[11] For example, in describing the fate of someone who attacks a faithful Buddhist, one passage in the sutra states: "In existence after existence, he will have teeth that are missing or spaced far apart, ugly lips, a flat nose, hands and feet that are gnarled or deformed, and eyes that are squinty. His body will have a foul odor, with evil sores that run pus and blood."[12]

As fear of evil acts and pollution became intertwined and leprosy came to be viewed as the "karmic retribution disease," those with the disease were subjected to new forms of social exclusion. They became part of an expanding group of marginalized people known as *hinin* (literally, "non-humans"), who are often described as "outcasts" in Anglophone historiography. The origin of the *hinin* has long been an object of intense debate. In the late nineteenth and early twentieth centuries, speculation focused on the "difference" of these people, and it was suggested that they were the descendants of ethnic minorities, formerly enslaved people, or migrants from the continent. More recently, however, historians of medieval Japan have argued that they were the products of the "pollution ideology." That is, they were a heterogeneous and expanding group of people who were associated both with pollution and with its management.[13] By the fourteenth century, this group included certain types of itinerant entertainers and religious figures, gardeners, funerary workers, well diggers, roof thatchers, and leatherworkers, as well as the sick and disabled who had been abandoned by their families.[14]

It is difficult to identify when precisely the identification of leprosy with outcast status occurred, but literary and other sources suggest that it was firmly in place by the early thirteenth century. Social marginalization was accompanied by spatial marginalization: outcasts gathered in specific locations. In Kyoto, the steep path known as Kiyomizu-zaka ("Kiyomizu slope") that led to the Kiyomizu Temple in the southeastern part of the city became the site of the largest community of leprosy sufferers in the city. To some degree, this reflected economic expediency. Outcasts survived in part by begging, and pilgrims followed this path to the popular temple.

But more than just the convenience of alms-gathering was involved. The path that followed the incline of Kiyomizu-zaka led not only to the temple but also to Toribeno, one of the three charnel grounds located outside the city proper. Kiyomizu-zaka thus was a kind of borderland, situated at the border between the sacred confines of Kiyomizu Temple and the profane space of Toribeno. When someone died within the city, the outcasts at Kiyomizu-zaka were tasked with transferring the corpse to Toribeno. This stigmatized, if crucial, work reflected the belief that the outcasts, who were already in a state of pollution, were responsible for removing pollution from the pure space of the capital.[15] The association between leprosy sufferers and Kiyomizu-zaka was routinely depicted in illustrations of Kiyomizu Temple, particularly the images known as "pilgrimage mandalas." Pilgrimage mandalas were schematic visual maps of the routes to famous temples, which sought to illuminate the multi-layered significance of these sites for visitors and patrons.[16] One mandala on the environs of Kiyomizu Temple, the *Yasaka Hōkanji to sankei mandara* depicts the *torii* (a stylized wooden gateway that demarcates sacred space) that marked the starting point of Kiyomizu-zaka; at its foot sits a leprosy sufferer, his face covered with lesions and a basket for alms in his hand. Another shows two leprosy sufferers begging near a structure that historian Shimosaka Mamoru has described as a "long roofed hall" (*Chōtōdō*). Although this building is only partially visible, it is evocative of the form of the Kitayama Hall, which will be discussed later in this chapter.[17]

Eison, Ninshō, and the Economy of Salvation

The relationship of liminal space, Buddhism, leprosy, and a particular kind of structure that was apparent at Kiyomizu-zaka was replicated in the Kitayama Hall and other leprosy hostels that emerged over the course of the thirteenth century. The most important figures in the formation of these facilities were two Buddhist priests, Eison (also known as Eizon, 1201–90) and his disciple Ninshō (1217–1303). Eison was the founder of the Ritsu Precept sect, an offshoot of the Shingon sect, a form of esoteric Buddhism introduced to Japan from China in the ninth century. In the thirteenth century, in the wake of the Gempei War, the new faith-based Buddhist sects were advocating for the abandonment of monastic rules, including the requirement of celibacy for the clergy. In contrast, the followers of the Ritsu Precept sect promoted their revival, while also embracing a newly public role for the Buddhist clergy outside of monastic establishments. Eison and his followers venerated the Manjusri Bodhisattva (J: Monju), who was said to have taken a vow to aid the poor, disabled, and sick. Reverence for Manjusri inspired Eison and Ninshō to turn their attention to aiding outcast people, but this also earned them the patronage of political authorities in both Kyoto and Kamakura.[18] The latter was the site of the new warrior government headed by Minamoto Yoritomo, whose forces had prevailed in the Gempei War. Both cities were plagued by "disorder" in the new era, as the poor, the sick, and those fleeing violence flooded into them. In 1247 and 1250, concerned about the growing number of vagrants on the streets, authorities in Kamakura tried unsuccessfully to expel outcasts from the city.[19] Charity toward the outcasts thus served political as well as religious interests.

The involvement of Eison and Ninshō with leprosy sufferers and other outcasts began in the 1240s and continued for four decades. It took a variety of forms. On a single day in 1269, for example, it is recorded that they distributed rice, straw hats, sleeping mats, fans, chopsticks, and other goods to a gathering of 2,000 outcast people near Nara. Four years later, Ninshō is said to have provided rice porridge to the hungry of Kamakura for more than fifty days in succession.[20] Historian Janet Goodwin has described these and other activities as acts of "charity and public service," but this presentist description ignores the beliefs that informed the work of the two priests.[21] Contemporary records of the 1269 event describe it as a "rite in honor of the living manifestation of Manjusri."[22] In other words, the outcasts who received rice and other aid were cast as the embodiment of Manjusri in human form.

The legend of the Empress Kōmyō (701–60), the consort of Emperor Shomu, which was popularized in the medieval period, illuminates the spiritual logic that underlay this understanding of the leprosy sufferer.

It relates that Kōmyō, as an expression of compassion, offered to personally bathe 1,000 people, a pledge that reflects the medieval practice of funding the opening of medicinal baths on temple grounds as a compassionate act. According to the story, the thousandth person who presented himself to the empress was a leprosy sufferer whose body was covered with open, oozing sores. The empress, it is said, proceeded to wash him with care and even used her mouth to suck pus from the lesions on his body. When she was finished, a bright light emanated from the sick man, and he was revealed to be the Bodhisattva Akshobhya (J: Ashuku).[23] The efforts of Eison and Ninshō, based on this understanding of the leprosy sufferers, were thus not acts of charity in the modern sense of the term. Rather, they reflected a specific economy of salvation. The most stigmatized of diseases, leprosy was understood to be a guise that Ashuku or Manjusri might adopt to inspire (or perhaps to test) the compassion of the faithful. Compassion toward leprosy sufferers was regarded as a particularly potent means to gain "merit," in the Buddhist sense of the term, and reduce one's own karmic burden.

Buddhist Institutions of Care

The construction of leprosy hostels in the thirteenth century must be understood in the context of this economy of salvation, but these facilities also reflected other Buddhist-inflected institutions of care. Beginning in the late sixth century, members of the imperial court and the nobility sponsored the establishment of institutions known as *hiden'in* ("mercy houses") to house the impoverished and chronically ill, disabled people, and abandoned children and orphans. A related institution was the so-called *seyakuin* ("dispensary"), which seems to have provided medical care on what would now be termed an outpatient basis. Both were established on temple grounds. Shintennōji, a temple in what is now Osaka, housed both a mercy house and a dispensary, as did Kōfukuji, a powerful temple in Nara. In the late eighth century, two mercy houses were established in Kyoto with the support of the imperial court, one each in the eastern and western parts of the city. These institutions had largely ceased to function by the middle of the eleventh century amidst the growing political turmoil that culminated in the Gempei War.[24] No trace of these early institutions survives, but today a structure called Hiden'in stands on the grounds of a temple called Sennyūji located in eastern Kyoto, about 3 kilometers south of Kiyomizu Temple. According to temple records, in 1308, a mercy house was re-established in Kyoto near a temple called Ankyoji. Then, some time later, this institution was moved to Sennyūji, a temple closely associated with the imperial court.[25] It is unclear to what degree the Hiden'in that stands today resembles the mercy houses of the pre-modern period, but the current structure is a square wooden building, with partially plastered exterior walls, latticed windows, and inner doors for lighting and ventilation. It has a hip-and-gable style roof (*irimoya-zukuri*), which became popular only in the thirteenth century, and thus most likely was not a feature of the early mercy houses.[26] The Hiden'in is the type of structure often described in Japanese by the term *dō* ("temple hall"), a multipurpose structure that could be used for study, meditation, and even sleeping.

Other institutions that housed the sick were the so-called *mujōdō* (literally, "death halls," that is, hospices) of the medieval period. As the name suggests, these institutions were intended to house those near death. However, unlike modern hospices, the primary purpose of which is end-of-life care, these facilities were established to protect family members and others from exposure to pollution while also creating conditions that would facilitate the salvation of the dying person.[27] The first hospice was established in Kamakura after warrior officials ordered people to stop discarding the sick on the city's streets. It was part of temple complex known as Gokurakuji that was founded by Ninshō in the 1260s. According to a history of the temple compiled in 1561, the temple was established in an area then known as "hell valley." It was a site where corpses were discarded and where marginalized people gathered. Significantly, this reflected a spatial geography of exclusion similar to that of Kiyomizu-zaka. "Hell valley" was near a major route into the city that followed a natural incline that would later become known as Gokurakuji-zaka ("Gokurakuji slope").[28]

These institutions took their name, and presumably their practices, from a work entitled *Ōjoyoshu* (*Essentials for Rebirth in Paradise*), authored by the priest Genshin in 985. Genshin was a member of the monastic establishment at Mount Hiei outside of Kyoto, the center of the powerful Tendai sect. Written for a readership of Buddhist clergy, *Essentials for Rebirth in Paradise* described rites and practices intended to further the possibility of rebirth in the paradise known as the Pure Land. One chapter of *Essentials for Rebirth in Paradise*, entitled "Rituals for the End of Life," offers a description of how to establish a proper hospice. It directed that such a facility should be located in the northwest part of the temple compound, oriented toward the Pure Land, which was thought to be in the western direction. A statue of the Buddha was to be placed in the center, so that those near death could be positioned near it. Caregivers were tasked with cleaning up vomit and other waste but also with burning incense, providing offerings of flowers, and encouraging the "patient" to chant the name Amitabha (J: Amida), the Buddha associated with the Pure Land.[29] The thirteenth-century hospices were inspired by this monastic practice but extended it to laypeople. Texts from this period on end-of-life care make it clear that, while comfort was to be provided to the dying, the intent was not to prolong life but to make it possible for the patient to engage in prayer and penitence at the end of his or her life.[30]

Gokurakuji was heavily damaged in 1333–4 when the warrior government at Kamakura was overthrown, and although it was subsequently rebuilt, it was damaged by fire several times. Today, nothing of the original temple remains. However, evidence of the kind of structure that functioned as a hospice comes from a visual source that purports to show the temple at its height. Entitled "Map of the Confines of Gokurakuji" (*Gokurakuji kyōnai ezu*), it dates from the early modern period (Figure 12.2).[31] The hospice is depicted as part of a complex of buildings devoted to care, including a bathhouse, a leprosy hostel, and a clinic. Thus, the temple offered a range of services to leprosy sufferers, and perhaps others, too. The hospice is depicted in the typical form of a temple hall with the addition of a wrap-around veranda. Indeed, only the caption makes it possible to distinguish the hospice from the many other "halls" on the grounds of Gokurakuj. One can speculate that Gokurakuji's hospice may well have been similar to the Hiden'in that now stands on the grounds of Sennyūji, although the interior would presumably have been arranged according to the guidelines in *Essentials for a Rebirth in Paradise* and other manuals.

The multiple facilities at Gokurakuji represent the pinnacle of Ninshō's charitable endeavors. In contrast, the Kitayama Hall, established two decades earlier, was part of a less elaborate religious complex. According to a biography of Ninshō, he was inspired to establish the Kitayama Hall by the example of the Kōmyō empress who had founded a mercy house in the then capital of Nara in the eighth century.[32] The Hall was constructed near Hannyaji, a temple that had originally been established in 629 CE. However, Hannyaji was destroyed during the Gempei War, when the area around it became the site of a battle. Eison became involved in reviving the temple in the mid-thirteenth century and associated it with the veneration of Manjusri. It is recorded that Eison began raising funds for a statue of Manjusri in 1255 and that the statue was unveiled at Hannyaji in 1267.[33] Soon after, the Kitayama Hall was established nearby.

The establishment of both Hannyaji and the Kitayama Hall reflected Eison's and Ninshō's devotion to Manjusri, but their location is significant. They were founded near Nara-zaka, a site that had much in common with Kiyomizu-zaka, where the Kyoto outcast community was located, and with the "hell valley," where Gokurakuji would later be established. Nara-zaka is a hill located outside the old imperial capital of Nara, which after the removal of the court to Kyoto in 794 came to be dominated by powerful temples and shrines. Historian Kobayashi Shigefumi suggests that this area was once used as an execution grounds, and after a battle that took place during the Gempei War it was littered with corpses.[34] Thus, like Kiyomizu-zaka and the "hell valley" at Kamakura, this too seems to have been a place associated with pollution, and, like these

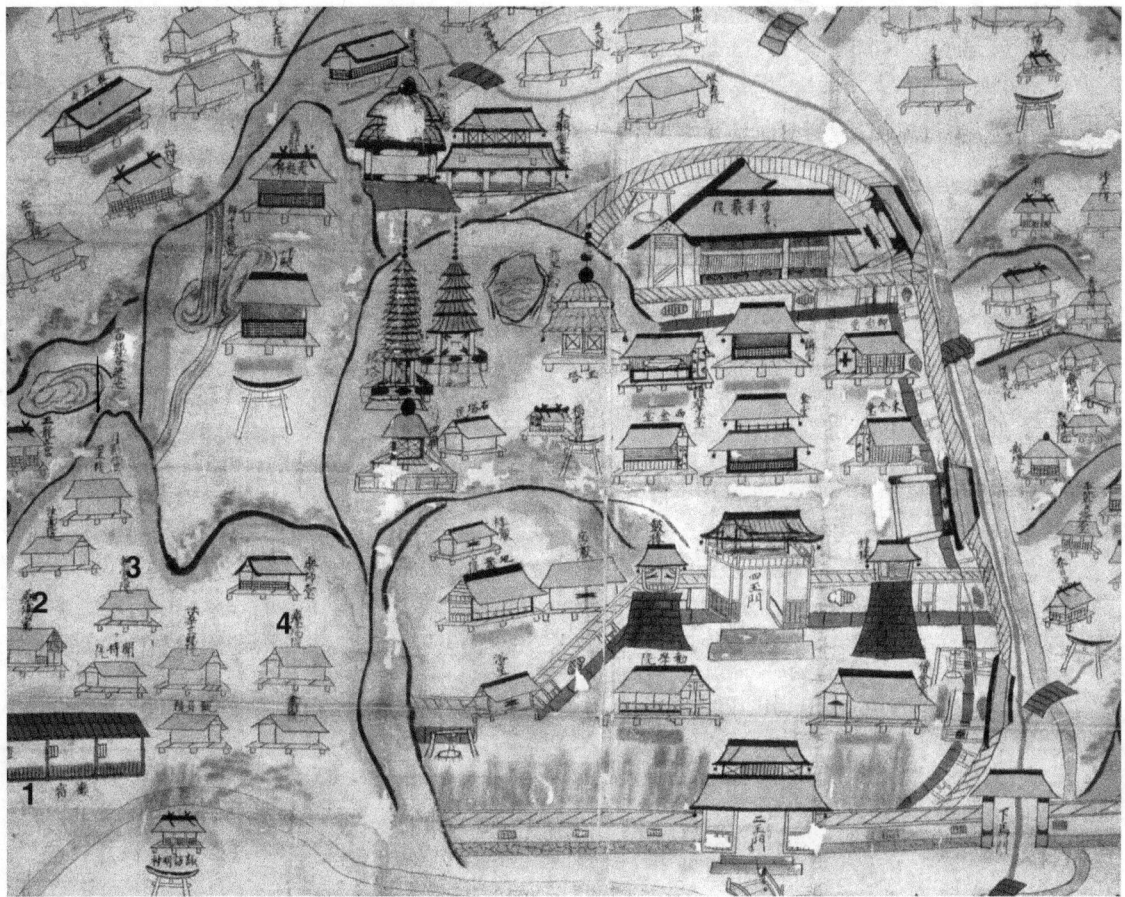

Figure 12.2 Facilities of care at Gokurakuji Temple: 1. leprosy hostel; 2. bathhouse; 3. hospice; 4. clinic. Detail from *Gokurakuji kyōnai ezu*, Edo period. Kokuritsu Hansenbyō Shiryōkan, eds., *Ippen Hijiri-e Gokurakuji ezu ni miru Hansenbyō kanja: Chūsei zenki no kanja he no manazashi to shogū* (Higashiyamamura: National Hansen's Disease Museum, 2013), 10

sites, Nara-zaka was also populated by a community of outcasts that included leprosy sufferers. As in Kyoto, the Nara-zaka outcasts were responsible for removing pollution from the nearby city of Nara, which in this case included disposing of the carcasses of the sacred deer that wandered the grounds of the Kasuga Shrine. There is another similarity as well: this would have been a good site for begging. Nara-zaka was traversed by the "capital highway" (*miyako kaidō*), a well-traveled road that connected the old and new capitals.[35] Thus, the three sites known to house organized leprosy hostels from the thirteenth century share similar symbolic topographies and social functions.

The Architecture of the Leprosy Hostels

The similarity of Gokurakuji, Kiyomizu-zaka, and Nara-zaka extends to the facilities for leprosy sufferers that were established on these three sites. The leprosy hostel shown in the "Map of the Confines of Gokurakuji" bears a marked resemblance to not only the recently reconstructed Kitayama Hall but also the depiction of the Hall in eighteenth- and nineteenth-century "picture maps" (*ezu*) of Nara and even the structure partially visible in the sixteenth-century mandala of Kiyomizu Temple. In all these sources, the leprosy hostels are represented as long, narrow buildings with multiple rooms and tile roofs. More information about the architecture of the leprosy hostels comes from a series of surveys on the Kitayama Hall that were published in 1920, 1928, and 1976.[36] The first of these was undertaken just before the Hall was designated a structure of historical significance by Nara Prefecture in 1921. By this time, the Hall, which had ceased to function as a hostel more than half a century before, was in a state of considerable disrepair, with flooring, roof tiles, sliding doors, and some of the exterior plaster walls all missing. Nonetheless, the detailed architectural plans included in the 1928 report and the follow-up analysis published in 1976 tell us much about the seventeenth-century structure and may offer some hints about the earlier building it replaced.

The term *ken* in the Japanese name of the Kitayama Hall, Jūhachikenko, is a traditional unit of measure used in architecture to denote the length between pillars. In the modern period, the length of a *ken* was standardized as 6 *shaku* or 1.818 meters, but in the pre-modern period there was variation in the actual length between pillars. Jūhachikenko literally means "hall of eighteen *ken*." However, the 1976 report reveals that the building was actually 19 *ken* in length and 2 *ken* wide. The length of the ridgepole was 37.42 meters and the width of the crossbeams was 3.939 meters. Thus, it seems that the builders were using a measure in which 1 *ken* was about 1.97 meters. The easternmost section (1 *ken*) of the building had a separate roof that was higher than the rest of the building, suggesting that it may have been a later addition (Figure 12.3).[37] The tiled roof of the structure was in the *kirizuma-zukuri* or gable style, which in temple architecture was relegated to minor buildings after the thirteenth century, after the hip-and-gable style (*irimoya-zukuri*) became popular.[38]

Kawata Nobuo, the author of the 1976 report, notes that the building resembles the style of monk and priest dormitories (*sōbō*) on the grounds of some of Japan's early temples.[39] A case in point is the structure known as the Tsumamuro that stands on the grounds of the temple Hōryūji in Nara. It is believed to have housed lower-ranking monks who worked as servants for higher-ranking members of the clergy housed in nearby buildings. The temple itself was established in 607 CE, but the Tsumamuro dates from later, with some

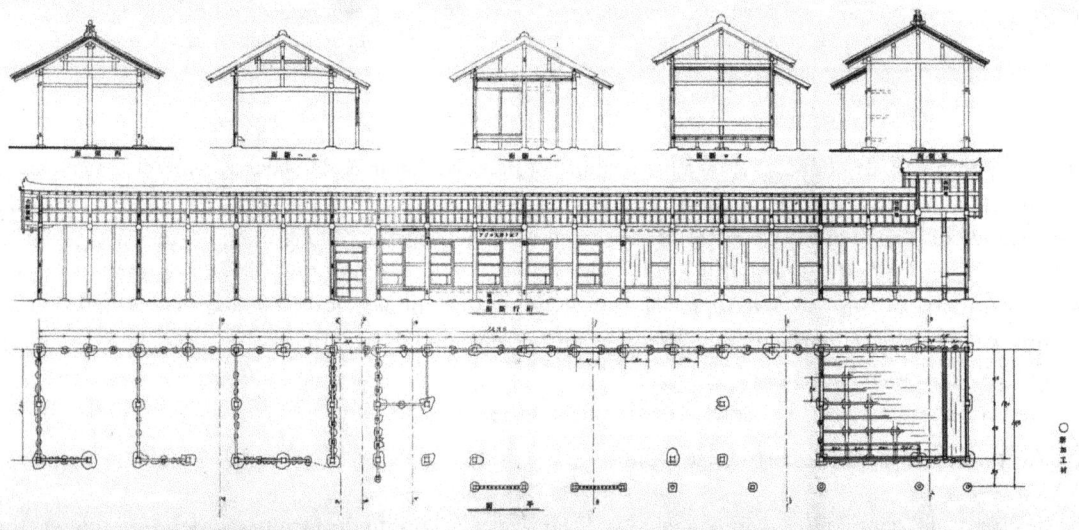

Figure 12.3 Architectural diagrams of Kitayama Hall, c. 1920s. Naimushō, ed., *Shiseki chōsa hōkokusho*, no. 4: "Nara-ken ka ni okeru shitei shiseki" (Tokyo: Naimushō, 1928), fig. 71

scholars suggesting the ninth century, others as late as the early twelfth century. It was subsequently rebuilt in the period after 1600. Like the Kitayama Hall, the Tsumamuro was 2 *ken* wide, but it was significantly longer, measuring 27 *ken*. It too featured a tiled *kirizuma-zukuri* roof.[40] The interior space of the Tsumamuro was evenly divided into nine 3-*ken* rooms. In contrast, the Kitayama Hall was divided into seven 1-*ken* rooms, four 2-*ken* rooms, and one 3-*ken* room. Thus, the rooms in the leprosy hostel were significantly smaller than those provided for the monks at Hōryūji. Kawata notes that the 1-*ken* rooms could have accommodated four tatami mats, and the 2-*ken* rooms, eight.[41] Given the commonplace understanding, then as now, that a single tatami mat provides a sleeping area for one person, the structure as a whole could have accommodated as many as sixty people. The small rooms of the Kitayama Hall would have housed no more than four people, while the far larger rooms of the Tsumamuro had a capacity of ten tatami mats and thus ten people. It is possible to speculate that the smaller rooms were designed for the comfort of the leprosy sufferers, whose poor health would have made communal living difficult. The rooms in both structures were windowless but they incorporated sliding doors, allowing for light and ventilation.

The single 3-*ken* room in the Kitayama Hall, located at the eastern end of the building, was comprised of a 2-*ken* section of the main structure and the 1-*ken* addition. The remnants of a dais in this room suggest that it was once a *butsuma*, a room that was used to house a Buddhist statue and thus a place where Buddhist services were held. Again, the presence of this room, given the Hall's close proximity to Hannyaji Temple, may have been an accommodation for the disabled residents of the Hall. Given that one tatami mat is considered seating space for three people, the ten tatami mats could have held thirty people at one time, about half the number of possible residents.[42] Another distinctive feature of the Kitayama Hall was the seventh *ken* space from the western end of the building. Although roofed, it was open on the north and south sides and seems to have functioned as a passageway, providing a shortcut through the long building, perhaps another form of accommodation.

The surveys reveal that the structure had once had a floor of rough wooden planks (*arayuka*), which would have been covered by tatami mats, and a wickerwork or woven ceiling of thinly split wood, bamboo, or some other flexible material (*ajirotenjō*). In the main part of the structure, the height from floor to ceiling was 2.107 meters, while the presumed addition had a height of 2.348 meters. The more elaborate cluster of buildings depicted in the plan for Gokurakuji suggests that the hostel itself was primarily used for sleeping, with nearby buildings designated for bathing, medical care, and end-of-life practices, and there is evidence that the Kitayama site, too, once housed outbuildings for cooking and bathing.[43]

Little is known about the lives of those who lived in Kitayama Hall, but its location, material form, and scant documentary evidence provide some clues. The resemblance to structures built as monks' quarters suggest that the hostels, like these buildings, were intended for long-term residence and functioned essentially as dormitories. Thus, they were unlike both the short-term hospices and the outpatient clinics. In the early modern maps of Nara, the Kitayama Hall is labeled in a variety of ways, including "lepers," "Kitayama," "eighteen-length hall," but also as "Ashuku Temple," evoking the Buddha that figured in the famous legend of Empress Kōmyō. It seems, then, that the Hall itself was viewed as a monastic-style lodging and those who resided there as akin to members of a monastic establishment, rather than "patients" within a medical institution.

The apparent Buddhist nature of the Hall notwithstanding, the association with pollution continued. Until the end of the seventeenth century, the outcasts of Kitayama-zaka continued to be responsible for the removal of the carcasses of the sacred deer from the city proper. Seventeenth-century sources suggest the procedure then in place: when a dead deer was discovered in the city, the magistrate notified the priests of a temple called Kōfukuji, and the temple then alerted both the residents of Kitayama Hall and the members of another marginalized group, called *eta*, who were associated with leatherwork, a stigmatized, if skilled, profession.

Health and Architecture

After the latter removed the valuable hide from the carcass, the members of the Kitayama community were charged with the disposal of the remains. However, it seems that the residents of the Kitayama Hall came to resent this work or found it overly burdensome, since they repeatedly complained about this requirement to the priests at Kōfukuji. In 1710 the temple officials, frustrated perhaps at their intransigence, turned responsibility for the Kitayama community over to another temple, Tōdaiji. At this point, the removal of the deer carcasses became the responsibility of the *eta*, and the leprosy sufferers at Kitayama came to be essentially a community of beggars.[44] Even so, the association with death and pollution lingered. In some early nineteenth-century maps, the Hall is pictured as standing adjacent to a crematorium, although there is no evidence that members of the Kitayama community were engaged in funerary work at this time.[45]

The significance of begging for the leprosy sufferers housed in the Kitayama Hall is suggested by a story, apocryphal perhaps, recorded in *Genkō shakusho*, a fourteenth-century history of Buddhism. It relates that, when a resident of the Kitayama became so infirm that he could no longer walk to the highway to beg for alms, Ninshō began to carry him there each morning, returning to retrieve him each evening. The point of this exercise was not simply to aid the leprosy sufferer by making it possible for him to continue to beg. Rather, by positioning him in a public site, Ninshō made the afflicted person into a visible display of the workings of karma in order to encourage reflection on the part of others.[46]

At some point after 1600, begging began to take a different form. Rather than begging at the roadside, members of the Kitayama community began to canvas for alms in nearby villages and within the city of Nara at times of celebration, such as during the New Year holiday and other seasonal festivals. In this period, the leprosy sufferers became known as *monoyoshi*, a term that means "felicitations" or "good fortune."[47] This apparently was the greeting they used to announce their presence as they moved from house to house seeking donations of rice and money. The greeting implied that charity toward the leprosy sufferers would bring good luck to the donor, a watered-down and secularized version of the economy of salvation that originated in medieval Buddhism.

Conclusion

This chapter has explored the founding, the material form, and the social and cultural significance of Japan's pre-modern leprosy hostels. Contrary to attempts over the course of the twentieth century to cast the hostels as the pre-modern predecessors of institutions of public health and social welfare, their establishment reflected Buddhist conceptions of sin, karma, merit, and salvation that came to overlay the "pollution ideology" that emanated initially from the imperial court. It was this nexus of political and personal concerns that ordered the location of the hostels on symbolically significant sites. The sloping paths at Kiyomizu-zaka, Nara-zaka, and Gokurakuji-zaka functioned as borders between sacred and profane spaces, between temple confines and charnel grounds. Maintaining the purity of the cities of Nara, Kyoto, and Kamakura became the job of the marginalized people known as *hinin*, whose numbers included leprosy sufferers, as well as others who were sick and disabled. They occupied the liminal space of these sloping paths, providing pilgrims and travelers with visible evidence of both the danger of immorality and the promise of the possibility of salvation.

The leprosy hostels established on these sites, like Buddhist hospices and mercy houses, provided some measure of care for those they housed, although their primary concern was not physical health but spiritual salvation. It is, then, not surprising the architectural form of the hostels drew directly upon a specific form of Buddhist architecture, the temple dormitories that were originally designed to house menial members of the clergy. Simple structures designed for communal living, the hostels stood on or near Buddhist temples. These were not medical facilities but religious institutions, designed for the public display of lives of prayer and penitence. That said, the Kitayama Hall, the only surviving leprosy hostel, reveals some significant modification of the temple dormitory model that may have been intended to accommodate the needs of ill and disabled residents, including a room for Buddhist services, smaller communal rooms, and an interior passageway. The designers and builders of the leprosy hostels were perhaps not indifferent to the needs of the leprosy sufferers these structures were to house.

Notes

1. See, for example, Sawa Riichiro, "Nihon saisho no raibyōin ni tsuite," *Kyōtō iji eisei shinbun* 100 (1902): 18. N.B. Japanese names follow traditional order of surname first followed by given name.
2. For a laudatory view of the Kitayama Hall, see, for example, "Kitayama Jūhachikenko no kengaku," Shiritsu Tsumizakakita Elementary School Homepage, 2012, accessed August 1, 2018. http://www.naracity.ed.jp/ele04/index.cfm/20,2946,15,323,html. For criticism of discussion of the pre-modern policies of exclusion, see, for example, the blog posted by Yabumoto Masako, a former newscaster for Nihon TV, "Fukakai. Kokuritsu Hansenbyō Shiryōkan," *Yabumoto Masako no burogu*, September 26, 2007, accessed August 1, 2018. http://ameblo.jp/yabumoto/entry-10048721209.html.
3. The text in question is Kajiwara Shōzen, *Ton'isho* (Tokyo: Kagaku Shoin, 1986), 534–45.
4. Suzuki Takao, *Hone kara mita Nihonjin: Kobyōrigaku ga kataru rekishi* (Tokyo: Kōdansha Sensho, 1998), 173–4.
5. Angela Ki Che Leung, *Leprosy in China: A History* (New York: Columbia University Press, 2009), 19–20.
6. On the issue of pollution in the capital, see Amino Yoshihiko, *Chūsei no hinin to yūjo* (Tokyo: Akashi Shoten, 1994), 25–63.
7. Niunoya Tetsuichi, *Kebiishi: Chūsei no kegare to kenryoku* (Tokyo: Heibonsha, 1986), 20–66.
8. Ōyama Kyōhei, *Nihon chūsei nōsonshi no kenkyū* (Tokyo: Iwanami Shoten), 390–2, cited in Janet R. Goodwin, "Outcasts and Marginals in Medieval Japan," in *The Routledge Handbook of Pre-modern Japanese History*, ed. Karl F. Friday (London and New York: Routledge, 2017), 399.
9. On the history of Buddhism in Japan, see Matsuo Kenji, *A History of Japanese Buddhism* (Folkestone: Global Oriental, 2007).
10. The Gempei War was fought between two warrior alliances, one headed by the Taira clan, which dominated the imperial court, the other headed by the Minamoto, based in eastern Japan. The Minamoto won the conflict and ushered in the era of warrior rule from their base at Kamakura.
11. Duncan Ryūken Williams, *The Other Side of Zen: A Social History of Sōtō Zen Buddhism in Tokugawa Japan* (Princeton: Princeton University Press, 2009), 109.
12. Burton Watson, trans., *The Lotus Sutra* (New York: Columbia University Press, 1993), 324.
13. Amino, *Chūsei no hinin*, 25–63.
14. For a lengthy list of those classified as *hinin*, see Thomas Kierstead, "Outcasts before the Law: Pollution and Purification in Medieval Japan," in *Currents in Medieval Japanese History: Essays in Honor of Jeffrey P. Mass*, ed. Gordon M. Berger et al. (Los Angeles: Figueroa Press, 2009), 289.
15. Kobayashi Shigefumi, "Kodai-chūsei no 'raisha' to shūkyō," in *Reikishi no naka no raisha*, ed. Fujino Yutaka (Tokyo: Miyuru Shuppan, 1996), 46–8.
16. On pilgrimage mandalas, see Talia Andrei, "*Sankei mandara*: Layered Maps to Sacred Places," *Cross-Currents: East Asian History and Culture Review* 23 (June 2017), 40–71, accessed August 3, 2018. https://cross-currents.berkeley.edu/e-journal/issue-23/andrei.
17. Shimosaka Mamoru, "Chūsei hinin no sonzai keitai: Kiyomizu-zaka Chōtōdō' kō," *Geino kenkyū* 101 (1990): 1–22.
18. On the Ritsu Precept sect, see David Quinter, *From Outcasts to Emperors: The Shingon Ritsu Sect and the Mañjúsrī Cult in Medieval Japan* (Leiden and Boston: Brill, 2015).
19. Andrew Edmund Goble, *Confluences of Medicine in Medieval Japan: Buddhist Healing, Chinese Knowledge, Islamic Formulas, and Wounds of War* (Honolulu: University of Hawaii Press, 2011), 16–17.
20. Kōno Katsuyuki, *Shōgaisha no chūsei* (Kyoto: Bunrikaku, 1987), 29–30, 49–50.
21. Janet R. Goodwin, *Alms and Vagabonds: Buddhist Temples and Popular Patronage in Medieval Japan* (Honolulu: University of Hawaii Press, 1994), 118.
22. Kōno, *Shōgaisha*, 49.

23. On the Empress Kōmyō legend, see Kobayashi, "Kodai-chūsei," 32–6.
24. Shinmura Taku, "Kodai ni okeru seyaku hiden'in nit suite," *Nihonshi* 343 (1976): 54–67.
25. This information comes from the website of Sennyūji: http://www.mitera.org/sannai/?id=16 (accessed August 1, 2018).
26. On this roof style, see the entry for "irimoyazukuri" on the JAANUS website, http://www.aisf.or.jp/~jaanus/deta/i/irimoyazukuri.htm (accessed August 3, 2018).
27. Fujiwara Yoshiaki, "Chūsei zenki no byōsha to kyūsai: Hinin ni kansuru isshiki ron," in *Rettō no bunkashi*, ed. Amino Yoshihiko et al. (Tokyo: Nihon Editāskūru Shuppanbu, 1986), 84–5. See also Shinmura Taku, *Shi to yamai to kango no shakaishi* (Tokyo: Hōsei Daigaku Shuppankyoku, 1989), 225–32.
28. Fujino Yutaka, ed., *Kanagawa no burakushi* (Tokyo: Fuji Shuppan, 2007), 23.
29. Fujiwara, "Chūsei zenki," 86.
30. For a discussion of medieval texts on end-of-life practices, see Shinmura, *Shi to yamai*, 235–42.
31. The plan is reproduced in its entirety in Kokuritsu Hansenbyō Shiryōkan, ed., *Ippen hijirie Gokurakuji ezu ni miru Hansenbyō kanja: Chūsei zenki no kanja he no manazashi to shōgun* (Higashimurayama: Kokuritsu Hansenbyō Shiryōkan, 2014), 10.
32. Sawa, "Nihon saisho no," 13.
33. Quinter, *From Outcasts to Emperors*, 95–8.
34. Kobayashi, "Kodai-chūsei," 47.
35. Ibid.
36. *Nara-ken shiseki shōchi chōsakai hōkokusho* 7 (Nara-ken, 1920); Naimushō, ed., *Shiseki chōsa hōkokusho*, no. 4: "Nara-ken ka ni okeru shitei shiseki" (Tokyo: Naimushō, 1928); Kawata Nobuo, "Jōdoji Jōdodō oyobi Kitayama Jūhachikenko kenchiku no jissoku hōkokusho," *Tōkyō geijutsu daigaku bijutsu gakubu kiyō* 11 (1976): 1–40.
37. Kawata, "Jōdoji Jōdodō," 11–12.
38. For more information on these roof styles, see the entry for "kirizuma-zukuri" on the JAANUS website, http://www.aisf.or.jp/~jaanus/.(accessed May 16, 2018).
39. Kawata, "Jōdoji Jōdodō," 14. For a discussion of and image of the architecture of monastic dormitories, see the entry for "soubou" on the JAANUS website (accessed May 16, 2018).
40. Ota Hirataro, *Hōryūji kenchiku* (Tokyo: Shokokusha, 1943), 118.
41. Kawata, "Jōdoji Jōdodō," 11.
42. Ibid., 12.
43. Naimusho, *Shiseki chōsa hōkokusho*, 88.
44. On the relationship between the residents of Kitayama and Kōfukuji and the conflict over the deer carcasses, see Buraku mondai kenkyūjo, ed., *Buraku no rekishi: Kinki hen* (Kyoto: Buraku Mondai Kenkyūjo Shuppanbu, 1982), 114–22.
45. See the maps reproduced in Nara Daigaku Sōgō Kenkyūjo, ed., *Nara Daibutsumae ezuya Tsutsui-ke kokusei ezu shūsei* (Nara: Nara Daigaku Sōgō Kenkyūjo, 2002), 25, 28.
46. Quoted in Kobayashi, "Kodai-chūsei," 38–9.
47. Yokota Noriko, "'Monoyoshi' kō: Kinsei Kyōto no raisha ni tsuite," *Nihonshi kenkyū* 352 (1991): 1–29.

CHAPTER 13
PURITY AND PROGRESS
THE FIRST MATERNITY HOSPITALS IN THE UNITED STATES
Jhennifer A. Amundson

Until the twentieth century, healthcare was almost always a matter of home care. This was perhaps especially true for the event of a child's birth. Maternity wards were uncommon additions to healthcare facilities, which were rare themselves before the eighteenth century. A few examples appear only beginning in the Middle Ages, including four seventh-century hospitals in Alexandria, which are the earliest known purpose-built facilities for childbirth, and one twelfth-century hospital in Constantinople with ten beds reserved for the care of women. The longstanding and global nature of traditional home-birth survived even longer in Western Europe: France established maternity care in extant hospitals before the eighteenth century, with England following suit by mid-century.[1]

Although they were ostensibly open to all, the maternity services provided by these institutions were only sought by women who were desperate: socially, rather than financially. At all points of the economic spectrum, women with adequate social circles saw birth as a natural event that unfolded within a social context rather than as a medical condition that required specialized attention. The appearance of the first specialty maternity (or lying-in) hospitals corresponded with neither change to these cultural preferences nor advance in medical technique. Rather, they manifest the aspirations of nascent medical professionals and social reformers that were mostly, although not entirely, aligned. Relatively unstudied in comparison with more architecturally striking institutional innovations of the nineteenth century that addressed other societal needs, such as prison reform and mental health treatment, lying-in hospitals are significant in part because they reveal the limits of overt innovation to improve a process as old as humanity itself. Thus, they complicate the generally accepted belief in a continual progress of science that is assumed in this admittedly technologically rich period. Modernist approaches to architectural history that presume a continued trajectory of improvement built on undeniable scientific advance, and correlate social benefit as an outcome of architectural innovation, are unable to contend with the reality of this specialty within the medical professions. Rather than expecting the appearance of a new building type to equate with innovation, seeing it as an imposition on adequate, or even preferable, traditions reveals a hidden human story and a more compelling history that addresses interests in social hygiene as much as public health. The first lying-in hospitals in America embody attitudes about gender and poverty that hinge on a collective interest in purity as a wide-ranging cultural value while also illustrating that not all allegedly progressive responses to tradition should be labeled as progress.

The Spaces of Childbirth

Through the nineteenth century in America, perhaps as few as 5 percent of births took place in institutional settings; the majority occurred among traditional networks of women joined by familial ties and neighborhood proximity, gathering within residences where bedrooms served as the standard spaces of care for the time of confinement—normally from the onset of labor until one month after delivery.[2] In substantial dwellings during the Colonial period, a dedicated "borning room" might be situated on the first floor, near the substantial thermal mass of a fireplace and easily adjacent to the hall that served a variety of residential functions. By the end of the nineteenth century, elites furnished elaborate birthing rooms in quiet, second-floor chambers with new commercially available apparatuses that enhanced the work of women in these spaces.[3] Impoverished people might have lacked the accoutrements of middle-class birthing rituals, but they benefited similarly from circles of female neighbors and relatives who were central to an event that unfolded in the cleanest corner of their small houses and tenements, tended by a midwife or the most experienced woman on hand.[4] Only the most destitute and isolated pregnant women—such as new widows, immigrants, wives of disabled or abusive men, and unmarried women carrying illegitimate pregnancies—sought substitutes for the networks of emotional, financial, and logistical support enjoyed by most. The out-of-home care available to them could occur in virtually any building but tended first toward actual residences and then to those that adopted residential design principles in their new construction.

In the most furtive option, entrepreneurial midwives of dubious reputation managed simple rooms among squalid tenements of impoverished neighborhoods.[5] At a much larger scale that boldly advertised both the dire need of the city's poorest citizens and the generosity of its richest, almshouses manifested Christian charity and social beneficence by providing shelter and assistance to a broad collection of the needy—poor pregnant women among them—but did so with a stinging judgment that made them a choice of last resort. A U-shaped, two-story brick building with scant architectural embellishment save for the cupola above its entry pavilion, the Philadelphia Almshouse (or "Bettering House") was founded in 1767 to shelter, feed, and care for all sorts of indigent people, an inventory that included "vagabonds, wrong doers, prostitutes," "people with venereal diseases," and "women in labor."[6] Its associated foundling hospital, where a woman could abandon the sign of her shame, confirmed its seedy reputation. In New York, beginning in 1799, needy women found assistance in a maternity ward within the city's small and plain almshouse. In 1816, it was relocated to the Bellevue estate, which was similar to Philadelphia Almshouse in its architectural character, as well as its multiple functions, including an orphanage, insane asylum, and prison that gathered those who suffered from every conceivable malady in one locus of desperation.

Open to all who sought what comfort they could offer, almshouses suffered from their association with the "vicious" poor, a result of the hardening of attitudes about poverty that had taken place by the time of the Revolution. Americans categorized the poor as either "virtuous"—those who *would* work but *could not*, due to a condition beyond their control—or "vicious"—those who *could* work but *would not*, due to some self-inflicted vice, such as sloth or drunkenness. This bias is evident even among those who administered the Philadelphia Almshouse, such as one chief resident physician of the 1820s who denigrated its "disgraced" occupants who (apparently by choice) circulated between the almshouse, county prison, and "dens of vice," bringing a stigma upon the virtuous who were "compelled here [to the Almshouse] to seek relief and support."[7] The one benefit of blending the bifurcated impoverished population was the capacity of the establishment to enhance order in the city by removing vagrants from its streets and inculcating them with correct behaviors and beliefs, especially through the work required of them to pay for their care.

Providing a more selective community in which to seek care, America's first voluntary hospitals opened in Philadelphia in 1751 and in New York in 1771,[8] both of them variations on the theme of multi-story, enlarged great-house type with central cupola that was prevalent throughout the Colonies for institutions ranging from colleges to statehouses (Figure 13.1). Although their general function was inspired by similar foundations in Europe that were, especially on the Continent, entirely supported by the state, American hospitals offered only medical care free of charge and required fees for board, lodging, and, occasionally and ominously, down payments on expected burial costs.[9] Although these charges were usually offset by charitable contributions from individuals and some financial assistance from state legislatures (a benefit that was not extended to almshouses), fees could be a barrier to access among the needy. Likewise, socially unconnected people suffered from the hospitals' selective system that allowed entry only to those patients with personal recommendations

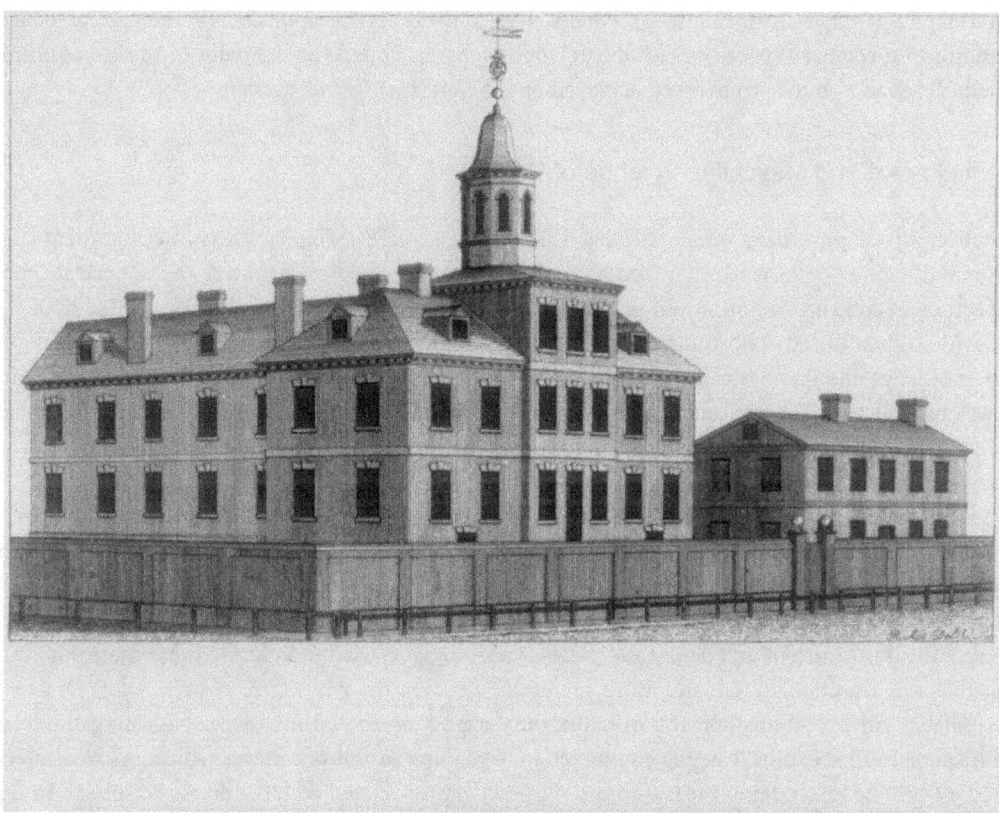

Figure 13.1 Pennsylvania Hospital (R. Scot, del. & sc.). Source: Library of Congress

from upstanding citizens (oftentimes subscribers and other financial supporters). This policy enhanced the somewhat higher reputations of hospitals over almshouses, burnishing them as more selective institutions that welcomed only the "worthy poor" and the "better sort" of people.

Although American hospitals excluded childbirth from standard medical services until the early nineteenth century, such care was offered earlier in the hospitals of large European cities.[10] In the eighteenth century, maternity care was named as one of five main departments of the Allgemeines Krankenhaus of Vienna (an Imperial establishment of 1693). By 1745, a well-established maternity ward at the Hôtel-Dieu, the oldest hospital in Paris (charitably founded but financed by the government and managed by a state-appointed General Inspector for Civil Hospitals and Jails as of 1690), also provided training for student-midwives.

Both at Paris and Vienna, the anticipated shame of patients was institutionalized in hospitals through their provision of private entries, basement locations, and procedures that allowed patients to seek treatment with complete anonymity. At the Allgemeines Krankenhaus, veiled women recorded their names on pieces of paper that would only be read in the case of their death.[11] An undesirable choice for pregnant women, these institutions and others like them in London and Edinburgh, were highly attractive to a new group of American physicians who found in them the training they could not receive at home. For decades, the establishment of lying-in departments in American hospitals lagged behind their European peers. Although the Pennsylvania State legislature approved a proposal for a lying-in ward as early as 1793, hospital commissioners in Philadelphia worried that the dissoluteness associated with pregnancies among the impoverished would taint the moral standing of their institutions—and themselves, as the officials responsible for them, by association.[12] The founding of specialized spaces for childbirth (such as that in Philadelphia, finally, in 1803) was ultimately not a medical advance, but a professional achievement of America's first obstetricians.

The Feminine Art and Masculine Science of Childbirth

This small group of physicians who specialized in maternity care recognized that an alignment of their professional discipline—not yet recognized as such by all in the medical field nor the American public—with a prominent civic institution would result in two primary benefits. First, maternity wards full of charity cases provided unparalleled opportunities for clinical experience—the most common means by which to gain medical knowledge among physicians who faced no requirement to attend school or even pass an exam, and which was unavailable in American medical schools.[13] Second, association with an institution legitimized these physicians' belief that their work was truly professional: so prized were these new positions attached to hospitals that doctors paid for them.[14]

Such signifiers of legitimacy were highly sought by the promoters of this new field that struggled to replace, and intrude upon, the longstanding traditions of home-birth. Educated abroad by necessity (if they desired and could afford formal education), the first American *accoucheurs* established practices in the 1760s. Their vocational label, a French word indicating "to go to childbed" that suggested an assisting role at bedside, was preferred to the more ancient and denigrating term, *man-midwife*, used to describe those male practitioners of work that was traditionally female. More preferable yet was the new term, *obstetrician*.[15] Drawn from the unassailably learned linguistic realm of Latin, the designation rooted the work of assisting childbirth in masculine pursuits of scientific learning conducted in masculine realms of colleges with surgical theaters and separated it from the folksy, feminine traditions of midwifery associated with the domestic sphere. In further pursuit of professional standing, these physicians founded university courses on midwifery and obstetrics in Philadelphia and New York in the 1760s that emphasized their differences by dividing the experiential training of female midwifes from the intellectual endeavor of male physicians who studied anatomy in classrooms.[16] Published in 1774 by Scottish anatomist and physician William Hunter, the first textbook on obstetrics, *The Anatomy of the Human Gravid Uterus*, was recognized a century later as having "[lain] the corner-stone of the science in giving to the profession a work which may be said to have been to obstetrics what that of Euclid was to mathematics."[17] Improving on the customs of the midwife, the first generations of obstetricians "elevated" what was now defined as a profession "to the position of a science, and opened the way to its rapid progress."[18] Within a few decades, millennia of women's work, defined as art, convention, craft, and at best, vocation, was replaced by a profession that claimed the certitude and progress associated with science.

Obstetricians embodied scientific expertise that introduced a new option for families with the social and financial means to invite a medical man to join and potentially enhance their birth-room experience. Unlike the folk remedies and intuitive rites of the midwife, an obstetrician could offer the potential of modern chemical drugs to treat pain and fever and novel instruments to ease a difficult labor into a safe delivery. Most often, they offered the promise of such intervention through a new knowledge base, but also through their apparent superior ability to act: it was commonly understood that nature had equipped men with quick-thinking minds that could address sudden problems when there would be, as Philadelphia obstetrician Joseph Warrington warned in *The Nurse's Guide* of 1839, "no time for consultation with books … no time for reflection." Such action that could not be expected of women, either by nature or experience.[19]

Yet obstetricians seldom were invited even to the threshold of these private realms and seldom found themselves with a role to play once they were (even more rarely) invited to enter. Almost always, a family that could afford to summon the physician had already gathered a traditional circle of women and summoned a midwife to oversee the labor. The physician stood at the edge of this assembly, unlikely to be called upon to intercede where nature took its course, feeling himself an awkward, "intimate intrusion into family affairs."[20]

Some physicians, including Scottish physician, professor of midwifery, and co-founder of the Royal Society of Edinburgh, Alexander Hamilton, accepted their redundant status, recognizing the greater capacity of friends to "inspire the patient with spirits and courage," interfering only to save the life of the woman or child, or to ease the woman from the sufferings of long labor.[21] Yet others felt a need to justify their presence, as well as their profession, through a more forceful participation, following the professional advice of Walter Channing, obstetrics professor at Harvard, to "do something [and not] remain a spectator merely, where there are many witnesses."[22] This pressure prompted them to intervene with unproven procedures, untried theories, or untested tools: efforts that were always hampered by the era's moral requirements to keep the woman's body out of sight. The entire process, from manual examinations before and during labor, to the delivery itself, was conducted beneath modest garments and bedclothes, the physician using his hands and tools without the aid of vision.[23] This puritanical approach was a foundation of medical training both in England and America, where students learned from books, diagrams, and manikins (in one creative Harvard classroom, a rag doll was thrust into a cadaver's womb). Unlike the shocking (but more instructive) *toucher* afforded to early nineteenth-century medical students in Paris, which allowed students to practice examining a real living woman through sight and touch,[24] the modest method practiced in America protected the woman's dignity and alleviated the "embarrassments" that were unavoidable realities for obstetricians, with the frequently contradictory effect of actually posing greater threats to women's health.[25]

In an era only beginning to understand germ theory, physicians' literal vocational blindness increased the likelihood of introducing unhygienic hands and tools into the process and disease into a woman's body.[26] As a result, the occurrence of infant and maternal injury, sickness, and mortality was higher in places where male physicians attended to the erstwhile feminine traditions of childbirth. Particularly worrisome was puerperal fever that struck within hours or days of birth. Most deadly in institutional settings, the disease and its resultant plagues made lying-in hospitals and maternity wards the focus of scrutiny and criticism through the nineteenth century.[27] No hospital escaped its ravages, although some were particularly notorious: at the Hôtel-Dieu and Maternité in Paris in the period 1819–20, almost one-quarter of women delivered of babies there fell ill to puerperal fever, with half of them dying.[28] Even after the nature of its contagions were first proven in the late 1840s, the idea that physicians themselves could be the source of puerperal fever was widely rejected.[29] Just as judgments of immorality hung about patients of the almshouse, expectation of morality and its associated cleanliness were assumed of medical professionals. As succinctly stated by preeminent physician Charles Meigs, Physician-in-Charge of the Lying-In Department at the Pennsylvania Hospital, "[The doctor] is a gentleman, and a gentleman's hands are clean." Rejecting growing evidence to the contrary, doctors clung to beliefs that their pure intentions and training must result in blameless action and that their station made it impossible for a physician to be a "walking pestilence."[30]

In lieu of their own professional interventions, physicians looked to manifold causes as the source of disease, including the mysterious workings of a woman's body and her mental state. Medical publications of the 1830s identified the wearing of corsets and general pursuit of pleasure as sources of unhealthy pregnancies and sickly children. Imperfect sanitation and ventilation of the birth environment could also be blamed, and were named as another responsibility that fell to the woman.[31] Even late in the nineteenth century, professionals advised women to maintain well-ventilated houses, since the air was a potential culprit of potential doom, carrying vapors that were suspected of causing puerperal fever.[32] A responsible mother would ensure that, during delivery and confinement, the lying-in chamber would be properly ventilated, kept clear of unnecessary visitors who "vitiate the air," and maintained at a cool temperature, which also affected the tending of the fire and the hanging of bed and window curtains.[33]

Health and Architecture

Such concerns reflect the centuries-old belief in the efficacy of miasmas to affect personal well-being. At the urban scale, the notorious Hôtel-Dieu in Paris was believed to be influenced by its proximity to the slow-flowing "impure Seine" that British obstetrician George Moore described as loitering "like a vagabond."[34] Congested neighborhoods were believed to play a role in the spread of moral impurities and physical contagions, which were also rife in the large, but crowded, wards of residential buildings, including prisons, asylums, almshouses, and hospitals, but with special concern for lying-in wards. At the Pennsylvania Hospital, physicians responded to each of four devastating epidemics of puerperal fever (1817, 1824, 1830, and 1835) by relocating the Lying-In Department to ostensibly healthier parts of the building due to assumptions that the building itself made women sick. After exhausting options in this experimental approach to purify the wards through changing their elevation and exposure to fresh air, the Lying-In Department was finally closed in 1854, out of frustration for the hospital's inherent unhealthiness.[35]

If Colonial buildings were observed to contribute negatively to patients' health, new construction could potentially be designed to affect a positive change. Physicians and architects alike focused on the theory that a healthy building should be designed to inhale adequate fresh air and to expel vitiated air. Ventilation was not a new concern per se, and efforts to facilitate the movement of air in hospitals are evident in French examples dating to the sixteenth and seventeenth centuries that employed cupolas to draw foul air away from wards and utilized cross plans to encourage breezes to sweep through wards. The 1622 Hôtel-Dieu of Lyons included a dome at its crossing to draw warm, foul air up and away from patients; in 1561 Philibert de l'Orme proposed a cross-shaped plan with large arcaded courts to ventilate the wards. Late eighteenth-century loges added to the Salpêtrière in Paris included openings in doors and ceilings to pull a draft. In America, the early hospitals in the colonies, including the original construction of the Pennsylvania Hospital in 1754, utilized cupolas as architectural motifs that also served as ventilators to expel foul air.[36]

The identification of poor air quality as a common cause in physical and social ailments among the poor was new to the nineteenth century, especially its early decades described as the "Age of Improvement," during which social reformers sought solutions to social problems including poverty, criminality, and ill health. Although physicians were correct in recognizing that puerperal fever disproportionally affected the women who were forced into voluntary hospitals and almshouses, they incorrectly correlated the sickness of the afflicted with their "confined [and] ill-ventilated" residences that made them susceptible to physical maladies as well as behavioral problems and character flaws.[37] A physician from the New York Hospital who, interestingly, held positions as City Inspector in 1842 and as General Agent of the Commissioners of Emigration starting in 1848 (a time of increasing immigration from Ireland and consequent anxiety among many Americans), aligned the "physical evils … which result from breathing corrupt air" with the "moral and mental degeneracy induced by it." Due to the reciprocal influence of mind and body, impure air deteriorated the blood, assailed the brain, and debased the morals and intellect.[38] Maladies inspired by foul air included ignorance, perverted judgment, intemperance, vice, cowardice, imbecility, and idiocy. The contagions spread by foul air thus took many forms, affecting both physical health and morality, contributing to the ailments that social reformers sought to solve through the foundation of new institutions of treatment, and that required architectural expression. Their goals to improve society through new institutions encouraged the construction of a variety of hospitals and asylums to provide architectural solutions to a host of social and personal ailments.

Lying-In Hospitals

Among these projects that sought to create environments that could ameliorate the suffering of mind and body, the first lying-in hospitals provided an environment that was intended to be free from puerperal fever and the immoral associations of large hospitals and almshouses. Serving the specific purpose of seeing a woman through the physically demanding process of birth and recovery in a controlled, sanitary environment, managers of lying-in hospitals also utilized the period of confinement and recuperation to instill virtuous behaviors, as defined by the predominately Christian, middle- and upper-class founders of the hospitals. These additional services were offered in the hopes that, unlike the degrading atmosphere of an almshouse, a lying-in hospital could "act as a bridge to lead the patients back to a life of virtue."[39] Focusing on the most materially and spiritually deprived, most lying-in hospitals served the virtuous poor exclusively, almost always requiring married or widowed status. To do otherwise would condone, if not encourage, immorality.[40]

First opened in rented rooms and residences that had been built originally for other purposes, the functions of most of the early lying-in hospitals were easily accommodated in unaltered bedrooms and salons utilized as delivery chambers and lying-in wards. Houses that stood within spacious yards were the preferred setting, as they ensured access to clean air and precisely replicated the ideal traditional environment for childbirth: homes that promised the lower mortality rates associated with middle-class births, whose safety was ensured by well-appointed and tidy quarters that allowed a free circulation of fresh air through the bed chambers. Even when the early institutions grew in capacity and sought purpose-built accommodations, their expansions maintained the planning principles of residential settings, only rarely and under certain conditions adopting civic architectural expressions.

Dozens of lying-in hospitals founded from the mid-eighteenth to the early nineteenth century in cities across Great Britain and its colonies followed this model.[41] In 1750, the City of London Lying-in Hospital for Married Women was founded in London House on Aldersgate Street, repurposing the former residence of the Bishop of London to accommodate up to twenty patients (Figure 13.2). It was replaced in 1773 with a purpose-built structure by Robert Mylne, its three Palladian pavilions maintaining the scale and character of a grand residence, even for a rather large building. Likewise, Queen Charlotte's Lying-In Hospital was first housed in a "spacious and substantial mansion" built in the 1790s on a site selected for its salubrious situation and expansive surroundings. Forty-two years after its founding, in 1855, it moved to a new two-story, residentially inspired structure that, in spite of its royal patronage, avoided architectural extravagance, emphasizing instead the architectural values of efficient ventilation and rigid economy. Accommodating fifty patients in small wards with three beds each, it was described by its builders only as "well proportioned" and "admirably ventilated," aligning with the building committee's commitment to "exercise the most rigid economy in not permitting any money to be spent in ornament whatever."[42]

Two outliers, both instituted in houses, then moved to new purpose-built buildings with civic scale, reveal the rarity of grand architecture for the building type. The enormous second building of the Dublin Lying-In Hospital (1748), a sweeping Palladian design by Richard Cassels, manifested the founder's shrewd use of architecture as a fundraising mechanism: the building's richness was an enticing setting for the concerts and other amusements planned for its grounds as a way to generate revenue for the operation of the hospital (Figure 13.3).[43] Almost a century later, the Melbourne Lying-In Hospital (1858) occupied a purpose-built structure designed with a character not dissimilar from private clubs being built in European cities (Figure 13.4). Its two-story U-plan featured a fine courtyard bordered by deep verandas to accommodate patient beds. The Italianate exterior complemented interior designs that included corridors and vestibules richly detailed in the Ionic Order. This grand design was the choice of the male physicians who partnered with an existing ladies' committee for the sake of fundraising for the hospital. While both groups desired to provide maternity care to needy women, the ladies' committee preferred the tradition of strengthening virtuous behaviors among admitted, worthy women; the doctors insisted upon access regardless of marital status to provide opportunities for clinical training. Unable to establish the institute on their own, the ladies acquiesced, allowing the men to run the institution, decide on admittance polices, and determine the architectural expression of professional pride.[44] Together, Dublin and Melbourne illustrate rare exceptions to the general rule of the

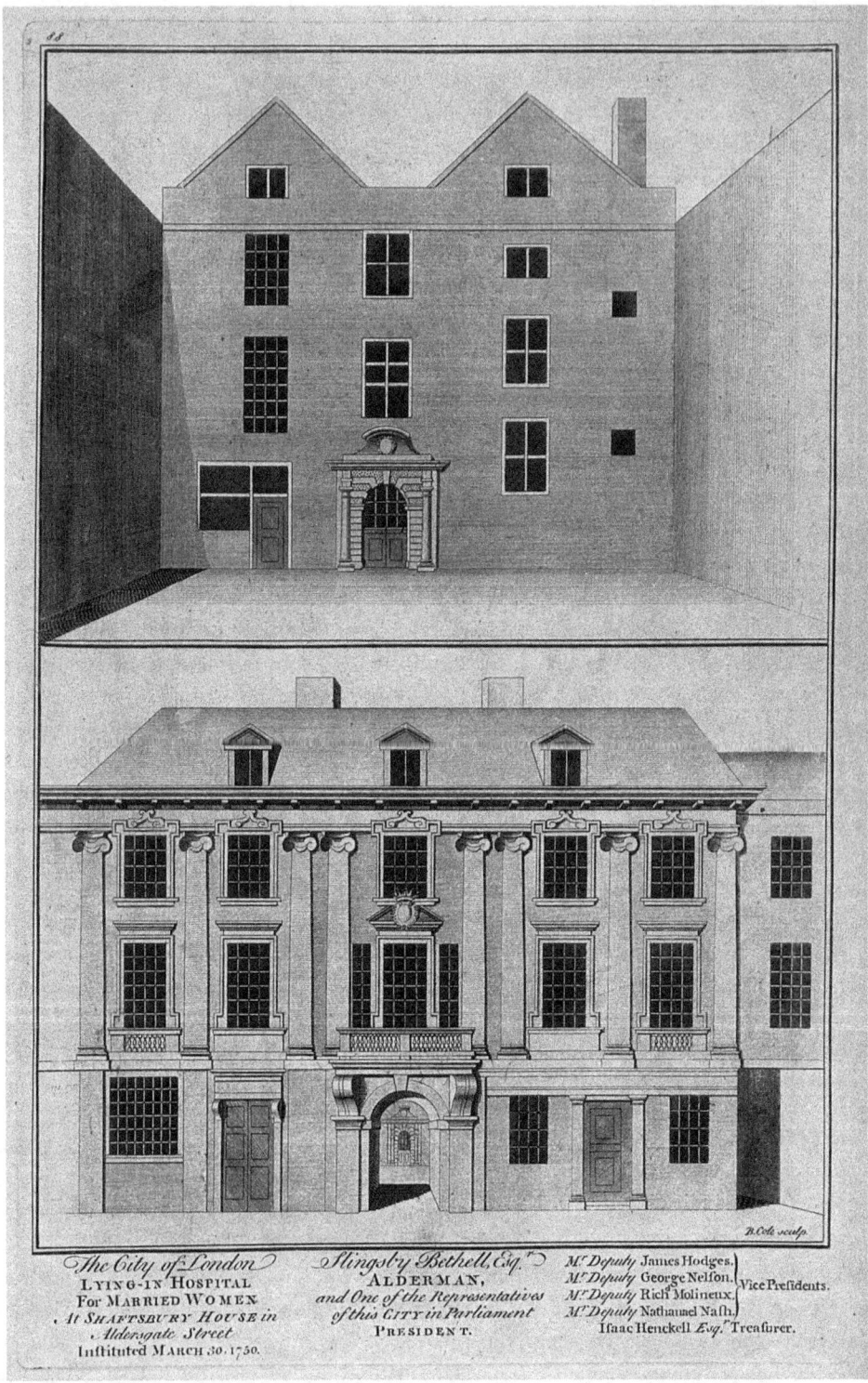

Figure 13.2 City of London Lying-in Hospital: views of the front elevation and courtyard. Engraving by B. Cole. Wellcome Collection. Attribution 4.0 International CC BY 4.0

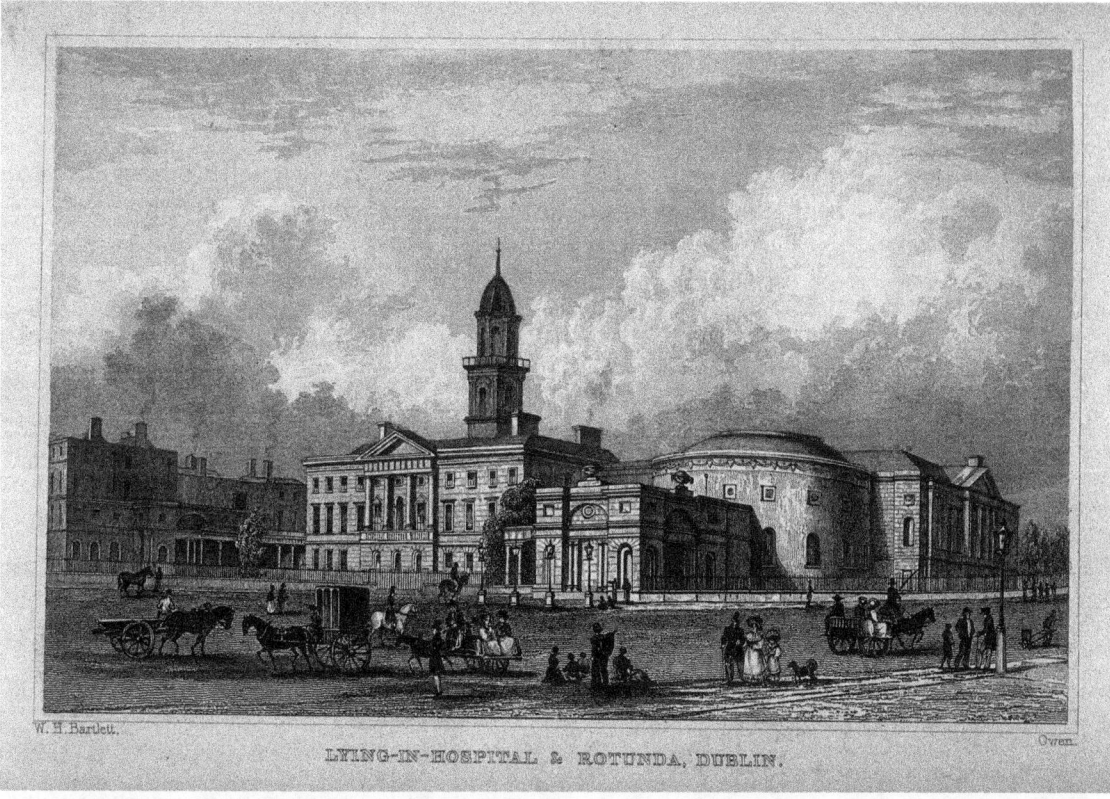

Figure 13.3 The Lying-in Hospital and Rotunda, Dublin, Ireland. Steel engraving by Owen after W. H. Bartlett. Wellcome Collection. Attribution 4.0 International CC BY 4.0

earliest lying-in hospitals in their architectural aspirations. These options reflect similar interests in two near-contemporary institutions in America, where traditionally female and male roles led to very different policies and architectural responses to the same functional problem.

Preston Retreat

Another unusual case, the Preston Retreat in Philadelphia was founded by a substantial endowment from a single person that supported the immediate construction of a purpose-built structure. Senator, banker, and physician Jonas Preston left $250,000 to provide free obstetric care for "indigent, married women of good character" who could avail themselves of an independent institution of the highest medical and social standards.[45] Thus it provided for a group of women who were unlikely to go to either the Pennsylvania Hospital or the Almshouse due to the lowly moral reputations and high rate of death of those institutions.

The Preston Retreat is also unusual as the product of a design competition. Further, its competitors were provided with documents that articulated current understanding of ailments connected with pregnancy and childbearing. Specially commissioned by Philadelphia's College of Physicians, the report offered observations on the function and relative health of European hospitals but could offer little in the way of new scientific insights to mitigate the unhealthfulness of lying-in hospitals. Instead, it advised architects to follow the design traditions of private homes, ideally by constructing a "village" of small pavilions to ensure the rapid

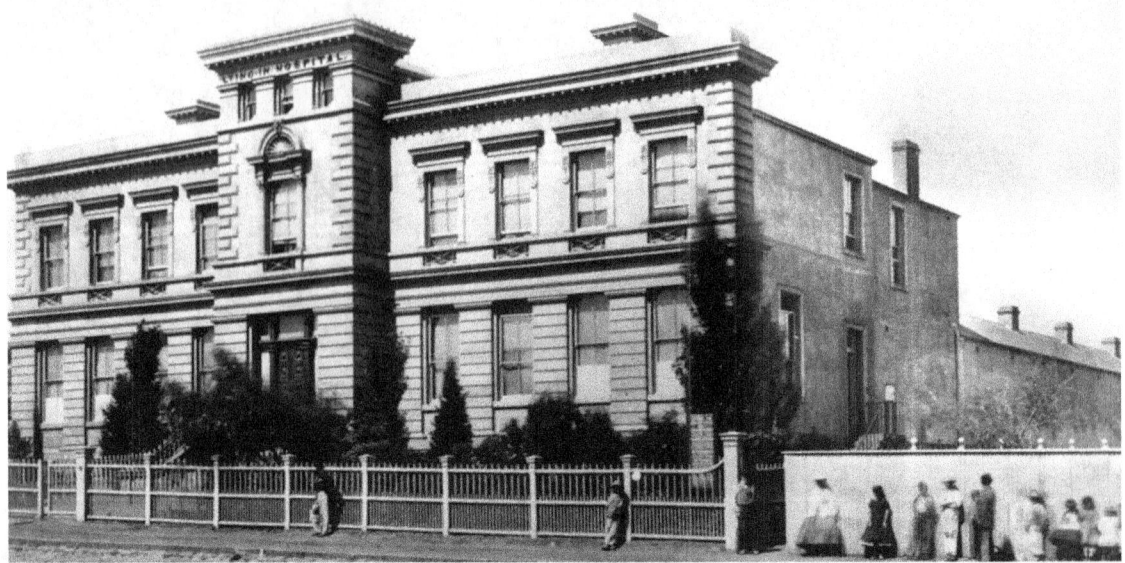

Figure 13.4 Melbourne Lying-in Hospital. Charles Nettleton, photog. (State Library, Victoria)

exchange of bad air for good.[46] Winner of the 1837 competition, Thomas U. Walter made marginal use of the Physicians' report and instead drew from his own studies of engineering treatises while aiming to serve his clients' aesthetic preferences.

Walter positioned the hospital on its broad 8-acre site (the size of two city blocks in Philadelphia), with a central unit of administrative functions flanked by wings comprising "truly separate and distinct" wards that each opened into a protected walkway that Walter likened to a sidewalk connecting "ordinary city houses". In the future, perpendicular wings with the same arrangement could be added, filling the site as social need demanded and finances would allow. Each ward utilized mechanical equipment that, by force of vacuum, ensured a continual introduction of clean air at a low point of the room, drawing it along the walls to a smooth, upward-sloping ceiling that would not allow the room to become "saturated with fœtid effluvia," nor "any secret impurity ever lurk about the angles and corners," and expelling it with harmful vapors from rooftop ventilators.[47] Walter's description of this "active ventilation on scientific principles," whereby exhaled air, made heavy by its composition with carbonic acid, was drawn upward, replaced by a "pure and wholesome atmosphere," reflected exactly the writings of engineer Thomas Tredgold, who explained in his 1824 publication on principles of warming and ventilating buildings the best way to expel "mixtures of azote, carbonic acid gas (carbon dioxide), and vapour" was through the design of ceilings that would "facilitate the ascent of the vitiated air to the outlet" through their domed, coved, or arched form.[48] Through this design the very structure of the hospital would function as an "important [auxiliary] in the medical treatment, as the perfect ventilation will ensure pure apartments."[49]

Just as unusual as the conditions of its design and construction, Preston Retreat is significant for being, with the exception of the special case of Dublin (which utilized monumental architecture to garner attention to the non-maternity fundraising and recreational functions), probably the earliest lying-in hospital designed with an intentionally civic expression in its scale and ornament (Figure 13.5). Stretching over 400 feet long in Walter's competition entry, the masonry vaulted structure featured two significant architectural elements punctuating the tripartite composition at the center and inspired by the Greek design for which Walter was

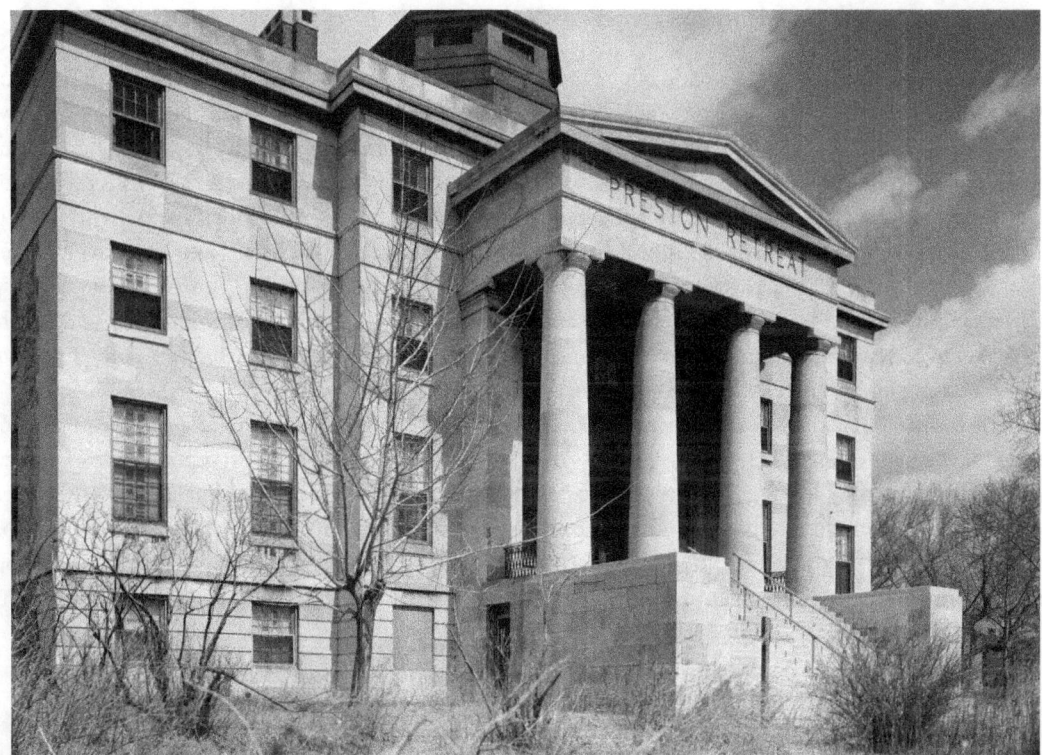

Figure 13.5 Preston Retreat, Philadelphia. Source: Library of Congress

so well known: an octagonal lantern (that also helped draw foul air out of the hospital) and a large marble Doric portico (with no such pragmatic justification). Although some critics condemned any such display as inappropriate to a charity establishment, surely a bold stylistic expression was anticipated by a board that hired one of the country's most prestigious architects to design their hospital. The committee revealed its priorities when budgetary constraints forced their decision either to execute the full scope of Walter's plan in simpler materials, or to build a smaller portion that maintained the rich details of his design. They easily determined on the latter: a smaller footprint with greater aesthetic presence.[50]

The architectural style of Preston Retreat projected the aims of its building committee and especially their view of its benefactor. The marble portico functioned as a distinct project commemorating the deceased Preston, whose institution is one of only two lying-in hospitals in this study that bears the name of a donor; notably, the other was a royal foundation. In good Republican fashion, the estate executor, Eli Price, reminded listeners at the cornerstone ceremony that the building was a "useful" monument in architecture; simple and in good taste, it manifested Preston's character. Price justified the adoptions of its expensive material as being commensurate with Preston's generous bequest that would inspire others to emulate his virtuous example to share their wealth in a likewise socially redeemable manner. The building added to Philadelphia's catalog of Grecian monuments dedicated to Republican virtue and achievement, and enhanced the city's reputation as "the Athens of America." Describing the portico as "commemorative of the civilization of the age," in which men ameliorated the suffering of "physically weak, but morally strong" women, and the hospital as gracing Philadelphia with "a moral beauty, still greater than … physical ornament," it is uncertain whether Price spoke of Preston Retreat or its patients.[51]

Health and Architecture

The New-York Asylum for Lying-In Women

Except for their shared mission to provide maternity care for worthy women, the New-York Asylum for Lying-In Women (Figure 13.6) diverged from that of Preston Retreat in almost every way. Funded by hard-won subscriptions (rather than the windfall of a generous bequest), it opened in an ordinary ward of a voluntary hospital in 1823. Within two years, it moved into rented quarters on Greene Street, a site chosen for its airy, high elevation. By the end of the decade, its Board of Managers deemed this "ordinary tenement" was "too small and inconvenient," and began fundraising for a new structure. Purchasing lots in a neighborhood on Orange Street, near Prince Street and central to the most needy population (unlike the Preston site, on a sweeping parcel at the edge of its city's westward development), the Board commenced and finished construction in 1831 on a building that in no way aspired to the grandeur of the marble-fronted, scientifically arranged monument designed by Philadelphia's most famous architect.[52]

Indeed, the fact that the word "architecture" never appears in the thirty-two years of annual reports available for the institution (1823–55) confirms its builders' intention to avoid stylistic pretentions. The scant textual descriptions that are available to enhance a single located view of the asylum describe the three-story building as an "edifice creditable to the benevolence of the community, and well fitted for the purposes intended." Measuring 45 × 60 feet (*c*. 13.5 × 18 m), it stood on a "high and airy" site with 15 feet of clear space all around for light and ventilation, and almost doubled the capacity of the original accommodations with its sixteen rooms for patients.[53]

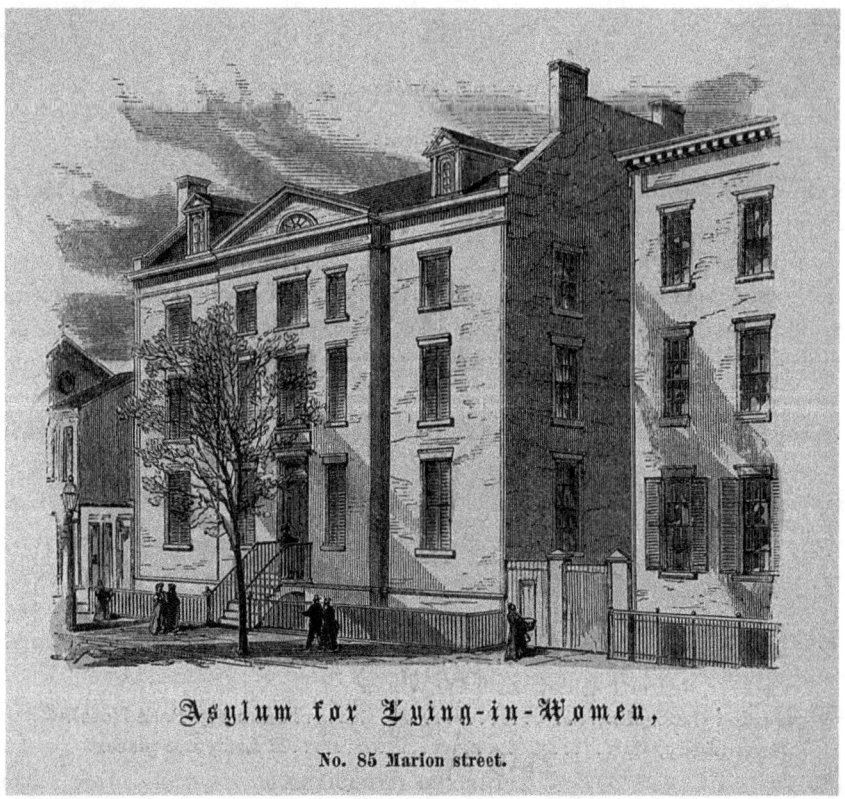

Figure 13.6 New-York Asylum for Lying-in-Women. Colored wood engraving. Wellcome Collection. Attribution 4.0 International CC BY 4.0

The functions housed within this simple building were similar to those in most lying-in hospitals. All admitted patients were "worthy," married women of good character.[54] After a screening to ensure her morality (and gauge her ability to pay for any portion of her care), a patient would be admitted, fed, housed, and delivered of her child; this process was guided by a midwife, with the house matron on hand. Only when facing a particularly challenging delivery would the matron call upon a consulting physician; medical students were not allowed in the house.[55] The intentional exclusion of scientific expertise and emphasis on the building's capacity as a refuge for women, and not training ground for young physicians, was underscored in the choice of naming the institution, which was never referred to as a hospital. The new mother was allowed to remain at the Asylum for a month to recuperate, during which time she provided care for other patients as directed by the matron, who was in charge of overseeing both daily operations and the vast majority of births. With this approach, the Asylum functioned akin to the workings of a typical—but very selective and highly honorable—almshouse, expecting labor from its virtuously poor inhabitants who could contribute to the workings of the asylum after delivery: a means of supporting the institution while teaching values and activities that would make the woman more useful to society upon her release. The matron could inculcate or strengthen behaviors in many of the well-screened patients who, in their confinement, proved their commendable deportment and suitability as wet-nurses. By providing "substitute mothers," the Asylum saved "valuable lives" of infants from wealthy families throughout the city.[56] Thus the Asylum served not just the immediate needs of unfortunates but also provided for their future employment while meeting a deep need among wealthy families.

Although many of these processes in the Asylum were common in other lying-in hospitals (although none other seems to have promoted its wet-nurse program as vigorously), its administration was unique in not only relying on a committee of respectable married women as an advisory board (as at Preston Retreat, where twelve women would "aid" the work of the male directors), but by being planned, established, and managed throughout its existence entirely by women. The Asylum's thirty-six-member board of female managers appointed two subcommittees: the Visiting Committee, which attended the Asylum two days weekly to interview prospective patients, determine if they had ability to pay (and, if so, what amount), discharge rule-breakers, and make sure enough Bibles were on hand; and the Inspecting Committee, which made unannounced visits to inspect the premises, its occupants, and review the management provided by the on-site matron who was in charge of the daily running of the Asylum. They also appointed a board of six superintending and consulting physicians—naturally, all of them male—to provide weekly patient visits and attend occasional challenging deliveries.[57]

The operations of the Asylum were tremendously successful, with a greater proportion of maternal survival than that of voluntary hospitals and almshouses. Whereas mortality rates among lying-in hospitals in London and Paris regularly reached into double-digits per 1,000 deliveries—including 14 at the British Lying-In Institution, 25 at Queen Charlotte's Hospital, and a horrifying 70 in a consortium of Parisian hospitals[58]—in its first 14 years, the Asylum saw only 8 deaths among the 950 women confined there. Through the years 1825–52, the Asylum recorded a total of 37 deaths, or about 1.25 percent of patients. When puerperal fever struck, as it did twice in three decades, the managers took drastic measures to cleanse the house and restore public confidence.[59] In annual reports, the managers attributed the success of their establishment to the blessings of God, but also recognized the advantages of the conventional approach to childbirth, recognizing "the traditional manner of birth in the place" as fundamental to the well-being of patients within it.[60]

In spite of their exemplary record, the all-female board could not stand on its own. Early in its history, recognizing that some people "doubted the propriety of trusting [such a charity] to the management of the ladies," the managers partnered with a "respectable" but unnamed "man of property and leisure" to assist in fundraising, purchasing the site, and supervising construction of the new building, and took pains to remind the public of his presence throughout the process.⁶¹ As of 1838, their annual reports included testimonies from their consulting physicians that reiterated the information already provided by the managers elsewhere. But these reports expressed the good management and social benefit of the Asylum with something a woman could not offer: a professional, male voice.

In addition to defending their accomplishments against gender bias, the managers also fielded complaints that their admittance policies were too restrictive. While defending the policy as maintaining the Asylum as a place of virtue and indicating that the city's poor laws provided adequate maternity assistance to the "vicious" poor at Bellevue, in 1830 they expanded services to serve women who either could not fulfill the moral expectations of the hospital's admissions test (e.g., being unmarried or unable to provide marital status, which was a frequent problem among immigrants), who did not want to leave their homes, or who were unable to do so.⁶² In their efforts to serve both the "worthy" and "unworthy," the managers revealed that even with a revolutionary administration addressing vulnerable women, judgments about poverty in America remained calcified, while the needs for such charitable work had only grown. A continuation of similar at-home services offered throughout Europe and already in other American cities (beginning in London in 1757 and Philadelphia in 1828), this "outdoor" service, in which at-home physician visits were provided free of charge beyond the walls of the Asylum, was very popular. In its first fifteen years, physicians tended to almost twice as many women at home than were confined within the Asylum, where they continued the policy of calling physicians only in difficult cases. It is noteworthy that, while the annual reports record scrupulous details about the low death rate in the Asylum, they provide no data about deaths that occurred in the outdoor charity, removed from the management of women.⁶³ It was only under the roof of the Asylum that the managers could ensure that the conduct and character of each of its patients would be as "uncontaminated" as the environment in which she was treated.

Conclusion

While offering a preferable option to giving birth alone and in squalid conditions, lying-in hospitals typically remained the choice of desperation, rather than of aspiration, for the minority nineteenth-century women who made use of them. Their impact was minimal beyond providing an important option for a small portion of American women and as training grounds for obstetricians whose focus was private practice, in which they may or may not have actually helped the women they treated. Although well intentioned, lying-in hospitals did not provide any fundamental improvement to the process of childbirth, which remained well served by vernacular traditions of residential design and longstanding social customs. Neither the architectural planning nor style of most lying-in hospitals was novel, unique, nor consistent enough to make them an identifiable building type, in the way that Kirkbride plans and the panopticon easily identify the functions of innovative nineteenth-century mental asylums and penitentiaries.

The lack of specialty architecture for the ordinary *and* extraordinary event of childbirth is worth consideration to reclaim a historic narrative that is not emblemized by monuments,⁶⁴ and distinguishes maternity architecture from contemporary efforts to reform the planning and function of other institutional buildings such as prisons and mental institutions, where scientific insights sometimes delivered on promises to ameliorate social and personal ills, with new architectural design strategies as its adjunct. Such was not the case with lying-in hospitals. Prior to the twentieth century, the architectural history of childbearing is more a story of accommodation than innovation, for any architectural invention was as much a willful impression on a satisfactory vernacular, as the presence of physicians was an almost always unneeded imposition of professional assistance on a natural process situated in a feminine sphere.

Notes

1. John D. Thompson and Grace Goldin, *The Hospital: A Social and Architectural History* (New Haven: Yale University Press, 1975), 10–20. For the common practice of home- or "social" childbirth, see Richard W. Wertz and Dorothy C. Wertz, *Lying-In: A History of Childbirth in America* (New York: The Free Press, 1977), 4–5.
2. This was true of virtually all medical procedures, including surgical procedures that could be accommodated by the strategic deployment of a kitchen table or ironing board. Morris J. Vogel, *The Invention of the Modern Hospital: Boston, 1870–1930* (Chicago: University of Chicago Press, 1980), 1; Jeanne Kisacky, *Rise of the Modern Hospital: An Architectural History of Health and Healing, 1870–1940* (Pittsburgh: University of Pittsburgh Press, 2017), 15.
3. Judith Walzer Leavitt, *Brought to Bed: Childbearing in America, 1750–1950* (New York: Oxford University Press, 1986), 96–7 and 106; Annmarie Adams, *Architecture in the Family Way: Doctors, Houses, and Women, 1870–1900* (Montreal: McGill-Queen's University Press, 1996), 111–15.
4. Leavitt, *Brought to Bed*, 36–7 and 76–7; Deborah Kuhn McGregor, *From Midwives to Medicine: The Birth of American Gynecology* (New Brunswick: Rutgers University Press, 1988), 36; Wertz and Wertz, *Lying-In*, 3–5.
5. Vogel, *The Invention*, 12–13.
6. This was the second Almshouse in Philadelphia; the first was built by Quakers on Walnut Street in 1731 and limited to members of their own sect. William H. Williams, *America's First Hospital: The Pennsylvania Hospital, 1751–1841* (Wayne, PA: Haverford House, 1976), 17 and 99–101.
7. Dr. A. B. Campbell quoted in Charles Lawrence, *History of the Philadelphia Almshouses and Hospitals* (n.p., 1905), 199; Williams, *America's First Hospital*, 12; and James Leiby, *A History of Social Welfare and Social Work in the United States* (New York: Columbia University Press, 1978), 43–5.
8. Founded and funded by private citizens and philanthropic organizations, voluntary hospitals admitted patients with a wide variety of ability to pay, but denied entry to patients with chronic and incurable diseases, and also the vicious. See Kisacky, *Rise of the Modern Hospital*, 18, and Williams, *America's First Hospital*, 1.
9. Lawrence, *History of the Philadelphia Almshouses*, 49–50.
10. The Pennsylvania Hospital was typical in admitting only women whose pregnancies were complicated by other afflictions. The New York Hospital began serving childbirth needs in 1801, when it became the new home of a lying-in hospital that had operated for two years in a house at No. 2 Cedar Street. Weill Cornell Medicine Samuel J. Wood Library. "Lying-In Hospital," https://library.weill.cornell.edu/lying-hospital (accessed December 22, 2017).
11. Thompson and Goldin, *The Hospital*, 112–13, 119.
12. Penn Medicine, "A Brief History of Obstetrical Care at Pennsylvania Hospital," History of Pennsylvania Hospital, accessed December 11, 2018. http://www.uphs.upenn.edu/paharc/timeline/1801/tline10.html.
13. Williams, *America's First Hospital*, 39.
14. Ibid., 131. This approach to make hospitals teaching centers was not universal; in Boston, the lying-in ward was opened with no plans for it to double as a teaching facility, out of respect to not adding to the shame of women there. Wertz and Wertz, *Lying-In*, 87.
15. The term *obstetrician* was coined by an English physician; derived from Latin, "to stand before." Wertz and Wertz, *Lying-In*, 29–38 and 66–7.
16. In Philadelphia, William Shippen (trained in London and Edinburgh) established the first systematic series of lectures on midwifery in America, soon enforcing what would become gendered expectations by first training women in midwifery and men in anatomy, then limiting lectures to male students. Leavitt, *Brought to Bed*, 38–9. This gendered division was not present in the earliest programs in Europe, such as that in Edinburgh, which taught men and women. G. J. Barker-Benfield, *The Horrors of the Half-Known Life: Male Attitudes toward Women and Sexuality in Nineteenth-Century America* (New York: Harper & Row, 1976), 81.
17. T. Gaillard Thomas, "A Century of American Medicine, 1776–1876: Obstetrics and Gynaecology," *American Medical Science* 72 (July 1876): 133–4.
18. Thomas, "A Century of American Medicine," 133–4. The lingering association of women's work clung to the function of attending childbirth, so much so that obstetrics lagged far behind other fields of medicine: the Medical Act of 1858, passed by the British Parliament, entirely ignored childbirth as unworthy of the attentions of a true medical man. See also Frances E. Kobrin, "The American Midwife Controversy: A Crisis of Professionalism," *Bulletin of the History of Medicine* 40 (1966): 350–63.
19. Joseph Warrington, *The Nurse's Guide* (Philadelphia: Thomas, Cowperthwait and Co., 1839), ii–iii. Especially in the face of the sudden demands of difficult childbirth, mere experience was inferior to "the man of education

20. William Allen Pusey, *A Doctor of the 1870s and 80s* (Springfield, IL: Charles C. Thomas, 1932), 106; quoted in Leavitt, *Brought to Bed*, 100.
21. Alexander Hamilton, *A Treatise on the Management of Female Complaints and of Children in Early Infancy* (New York: Samuel Campbell, 1792), 174; quoted in Leavitt, *Brought to Bed*, 102.
22. Walter Channing, *A Treatise on Etherization in Childbirth* (Boston: William D. Ticknor, 1848), 229; quoted in Leavitt, *Brought to Bed*, 43.
23. Warrington, *The Nurse's Guide*, 45. Well after its founding in 1847, the American Medical Association maintained that adequate knowledge pertaining to obstetrics could be obtained from descriptions, plates, and manikins, and touch under a sheet. Barker-Benfield, *Horrors of the Half-Known Life*, 62; Jonah Spaulding, *The Female's Guide to Health* (Skowhegan, ME: Sentinel Office, 1837), 96–7.
24. Diana E. Manuel, ed., *Walking the Paris Hospitals: Diary of an Edinburgh Medical Student, 1834–1835* (London: Wellcome Trust Centre for the History of Medicine at UCL, 2004), 59.
25. Some believed that women's willingness to have incomplete examinations in the name of modesty was "evidence of the dominion of a fine morality in our society." Charles D. Meigs, *Females and Their Diseases; A Series of Letters to His Class* (Philadelphia: Lea and Blanchard, 1848), 18–19.
26. Scattered data suggest that mortality rates were worse among physician-assisted births, both in homes and hospitals, than among midwives in homes. Leavitt, *Brought to Bed*, 56–7; Wertz and Wertz, *Lying-In*, 18. Recent studies have confirmed the efficacy of midwives in childbearing. Nina Martin, "Does a Larger Role for Midwives Mean Better Care?" *NPR Investigations* (February 22, 2018), accessed May 23, 2018. https://www.npr.org/2018/02/22/587953272/does-a-larger-role-for-midwives-mean-better-care?utm_source=facebook.com&utm_medium=social&utm_campaign=npr&utm_term=nprnews&utm_content=20180222.
27. Henry C. Burdett, *Hospitals and Asylums of the World: Their Origin, History, Construction, Administration, Management and Legislation* (London: J. & A. Churchill, 1891), 99.
28. Between 1819 and 1820, of 4,924 persons delivered at the Maternité in Paris, 1,177 were attacked by puerperal fever, and half died. Likewise, at the Midwifery Institute of Vienna, across fourteen months in 1833 and 1834, 511 women fell sick out of 2,218 and 158 died. George Moore, *An Enquiry into the Pathology, Causes, and Treatment of Puerperal Fever* (London: Samuel Highley, 1836), 10, 149, and 169.
29. Hungarian physician Ignaz Semmelweis was one of the first to discover the connection between infection and disinfected hands by observing in Vienna that the mortality rate among patients of medical students—who tended to multiple patients without washing their hands—exceeded that among midwives who cared for only one patient at a time by 437 percent.
30. Meigs, *Females*, 585. Meigs was one of the country's most powerful voices against the empirical evidence emerging in the 1840s. Wertz and Wertz, *Lying-In*, 120–1; see also Leavitt, *Brought to Bed*, 154, and Moore, *An Enquiry*, 150–3.
31. Moore, *An Enquiry*, 198–201 and 177–8; *The American Lady's Medical Pocket-Book, and Nursery-Adviser* (Philadelphia: James Kay, 1833), 16 and 113.
32. William Potts Dewees, *A Treatise on the Diseases of Females* (Philadelphia: Carey, Lea, & Blanchard, 1837), 382–3 and 419; Pye Henry Chavasse, *Advice to a Wife on the Management of Her Own Health* (Toronto: Hunter, Rose, 1879); quoted by Adams, *Architecture in the Family Way*, 111–13. Scottish obstetrician and physician-*accoucheur* to Queen Victoria Robert Ferguson encouraged patients from healthy neighborhoods to stay at home where there was bound to be purer air changed more frequently than to resort to city hospitals. Robert Ferguson, *Essays on the Most Important Diseases of Women: Part I: Puerperal Fever* (London: John Murray, 1839), 98–103.
33. *American Lady's Medical Pocket-Book*, 132–3; Thomas Bull, *Hints to Mothers for the Management of Health during the Period of Pregnancy and in the Lying-In Room* (New York: Wiley & Putnam, 1842), 127.
34. Moore, *An Enquiry*, 196–7.
35. Williams, *America's First Hospital*, 131.
36. Thompson and Goldin, *The Hospital*, 37, 57, 97, and 127; Kisacky, *Rise of the Modern Hospital*, 45.
37. Fleetwood Churchill, *Observations on the Diseases Incident to Pregnancy and Childbed* (Dublin: Martin Keene and Son), 297. Noting that puerperal fever was more rampant in hospitals than "Among dense and immoral population of

large cities," where it was also common, he encouraged treatment at home, so that the poor "may not generate disease and contaminate each other, by being cheaply crowded together." Moore, *An Enquiry*, 198–201.
38. John H. Griscom, *The Uses and Abuses of Air* (New York: J. S. Redfield, 1850), 145–51.
39. Burdett, *Hospitals and Asylums*, 234.
40. In 1817 the Board of the Pennsylvania Hospital stated that "The relief granted should hold forth no temptation to increase the number of those applying for it, or in the most distant way to encourage vice or idleness." Pennsylvania Hospital Archives quoted in Williams, *America's First Hospital*, 126.
41. These include the Lying-In Hospital in Brownlow Street, Long Acre (1749), the City of London Lying-In Hospital at London House, Aldersgate Street (1750), the General Lying-In Hospital, Bayswater (1752), and the Westminster Lying-In Hospital, Surrey Road, Westminster Bridge (1765). One early example in America followed this British model precisely: opened in 1832, the Boston Lying-In Hospital was an alternative to the maternity facilities established at the Massachusetts General Hospital in 1821. It moved from its adapted residence into a "magnificent edifice" with fifty beds in 1854. Thomas Ryan, *The History of Queen Charlotte's Lying-In Hospital* (London: Hutchings and Crowley, 1885), ix; Frederick C. Irving, "Highlights in the History of the Boston Lying-In Hospital," *Canadian Medical Association Journal* 54 (February 1946): 175.
42. Ryan, *The History of Queen Charlotte's Lying-In Hospital*, 20–1 and 28–9.
43. Opened in March 1745, the original site was a "large house" in George's-Lane (now South Great George's-street), situated in a spacious yard, with twelve rooms. William Wilde, "Illustrious Physicians and Surgeons in Ireland: Bartholomew Mosse, MD, Surgeon," *Dublin Quarterly Journal of Medical Science* 2 (1846): 565–96.
44. The hospitals' first iteration opened in 1856 in a rented house that accommodated seventeen patients. Janet McCalman, *Sex and Suffering: Women's Health and a Women's Hospital* (Baltimore. Johns Hopkins University Press, 1999), 4–14.
45. Jonas Preston, May 12, 1835, included in the "College of Physicians Report," printed in W. Robert Penman, M.D., "The Public Practice of Midwifery in Philadelphia," *Transactions and Studies of the College of Physicians, Philadelphia* 37, no. 2 (1969): 124–32.
46. The ultimate directive of the report was that "All lying-in establishments ought to be made as far as possible, conformable … to the private dwelling." "College of Physicians Report," printed in Penman, "The Public Practice of Midwifery," 126–7. Their suggestions reflected a growing popularity of pavilion hospitals, first in Europe and in the United States by the middle of the nineteenth century. See Kisacky, *Rise of the Modern Hospital*, 15, 22, and 37; Thompson and Goldin, *The Hospital*, 118 and 127.
47. Thomas U. Walter, Specifications for Preston Retreat, Box 14, 122-M-204, Walter Archives, Athenaeum of Philadelphia.
48. Specifications for Preston Retreat, Box 14, 122-M-204, Walter Archives, Athenaeum of Philadelphia; Thomas Tredgold, *Principles of Warming and Ventilating Public Buildings, Dwelling-Houses, Manufactories, Hospitals, Hot-Houses, and Conservatories* (London: Josiah Taylor, 1824), 70–1, 73.
49. Eli K. Price, *The Address Delivered at the Laying of the Corner-Stone of the Preston Retreat, July 17, 1837* (Philadelphia: John Richards, 1837), 5.
50. Walter offered a total of five options: the condensed version ranged from $30,500 to $54,500; the expanded version of the plan ranged from $72,000 to $121,500; the addition of the projecting portico built of marble added $14,640 to the design. Specifications for Preston Retreat, Box 14, 122-M-204, Walter Archives, Athenaeum of Philadelphia.
51. Price, *The Address Delivered*, 6–8 and 10.
52. "Minutes," *Annual Report of the Managers of the New-York Asylum for Lying-In Women*, March 13, 1828 (New York: Gray and Bunce, 1828), 61 (hereafter *Annual Report*); *Annual Report* (1829), 4 and 9; "Minutes," *Annual Report* (1830), 106.
53. *Annual Report* (1831), 8.
54. Weill Cornell Medicine Samuel J. Wood Library, "New York Asylum of Lying-In Women," accessed December 22, 2017. https://library.weill.cornell.edu/new-york-asylum-lying-women; *Annual Report* (1829), 7–8.
55. The Asylum's founders believed that exposing its patients as medical specimens would disincline worthy women to seek its services. Virginia A. Metaxas Quiroga, *Poor Mothers and Babies: A Social History of Childbirth and Child Care Hospitals in Nineteenth-Century New York City* (New York: Garland, 1989), 25.
56. *Annual Report* (1831), 5
57. *Annual Report* (1828): 15–20.
58. These statistics represent the period 1820s–60s. Florence Nightingale, *Introductory Notes on Lying-In Institutions* (London: Longmans, Green, and Co., 1871), 6.

Health and Architecture

59. Outbreaks of puerperal fever are indicated in *Annual Reports* for 1838 and 1841, when the Managers record closing the house and spending significant funds to cleanse it after losing three and four patients, respectively. *Annual Reports* (1829–52), passim.
60. *Annual Report* (1837), 5.
61. *Annual* (1833), 5; *Annual Report* (1829), 9–10.
62. *Annual Report* (1832), 3; (1831), 6–7.
63. The 1847 *Annual Report* referred to the "so small number of deaths" within the outdoor charity. Yet because the outdoor service depended on individual physicians to conduct themselves as they would in their private practices, there is no reason to believe that their maternal survival rates are anything like the great achievement of the indoor charity provided on Marion Street. The outdoor, extended services probably functioned as successfully as home-births had for eons, and as safely as private obstetricians had for the last several decades.
64. For more on this theme, see Gail Lee Dubrow, *Restoring Women's History through Historic Preservation*, ed. Gail Lee Dubrow and Jennifer B. Goodman (Baltimore: Johns Hopkins University Press, 2003), 3.

PART IV
ARCHITECTURE: DESIGNING SPACES OF HEALING

CHAPTER 14
HEALTH AS HARMONY
THE *PELLEGRINAIO* CYCLE OF SANTA MARIA DELLA SCALA IN SIENA
Maggie Bell

Beginning in the eleventh century the hospital of Santa Maria della Scala in Siena provided medical care and assistance to the local and traveling poor. The hospital grew organically over the centuries, absorbing almost half of the buildings around the piazza it shares with the cathedral of Siena. By the mid-fifteenth century, similar to other massive civic hospitals at the time, the Scala was a sprawling complex allowing for varying types of care that included treating the sick, caring for foundling children, distributing alms, and housing pilgrims and poor travelers. The hospital today remains a maze of rooms and passages indicative of extensive building initiatives over the centuries, both demonstrating the Scala's financial and political might and its adaptations to changing societal needs and standards of care.

The Scala's built structure was central to the hospital's institutional identity and self-image, evident in its most important fifteenth-century artistic intervention—eight monumental frescoes in the central male ward known as the *pellegrinaio*, or "pilgrim's hall," depicting the mythologized history of Santa Maria della Scala and scenes of its daily activities (Figure 14.1). This cycle was painted between 1439 and 1444 during a time of significant architectural development that enabled the hospital to accommodate its many charitable and medical functions. Four of the scenes represent the history of the hospital on one wall and its charitable works on the other. The frescoes are expansive—all but one (*The Banquet for the Poor*) are about 450 centimeters in height and fill the wall under each bay. This large size makes the elaborate architectural settings, which dominate at least half of the visual field in each fresco, all the more impressive. These structures, though imaginatively depicted, overflow with quotidian details that would have called to mind specific aspects of the Scala and its urban surroundings, reminding viewers of the physical structure in which they were standing.

This chapter identifies the role of the *pellegrinaio* frescoes within the distinct yet overlapping fifteenth-century discourses on architecture and medicine, which coalesced in the phenomenon of the institutionalized hospital. The following analysis relies on two guiding principles: first, that the *pellegrinaio* must be understood as a complete environment, in which viewers were encouraged to draw meaningful connections across the room between images on the ceiling and walls. This was a common way of "reading" painted rooms in the fifteenth century, particularly frescoes in sacred and civic spaces, and would have been equally operative in the hospital.[1] Second, that the frescoes actively theorize the relationship between architecture and medicine, rather than merely reflect written texts. These images were painted on the cusp of an increasingly systematic interest in architectural theory, six years before Leon Battista Alberti (1404–72) finished his famous treatise on architecture, *De re aedificatoria*, in 1452. This chapter proposes that in the *pellegrinaio* frescoes, as in the writings of Alberti and Antonio di Pietro Averlino (1400–69), known as Filarete, architecture is given ethical, societal, and cosmic significance. The treatises of Alberti (1452), and Filarete (*Trattato di architettura*, 1460–4) serve as comparanda due to their extensive treatment of the relationship between health and architecture.[2] Like these texts, the frescoes are a work of idealized fiction, grounded in reality while presenting the world as it should be, made possible through architectural intervention. This chapter explores the way in which these particularized images of the hospital are connected to broader theories about the relationship between architecture and medicine, which is made clear in references throughout the fresco cycle to the concept of harmony—a fundamental principle in architectural design and medical theory at the time. This imagery, which would

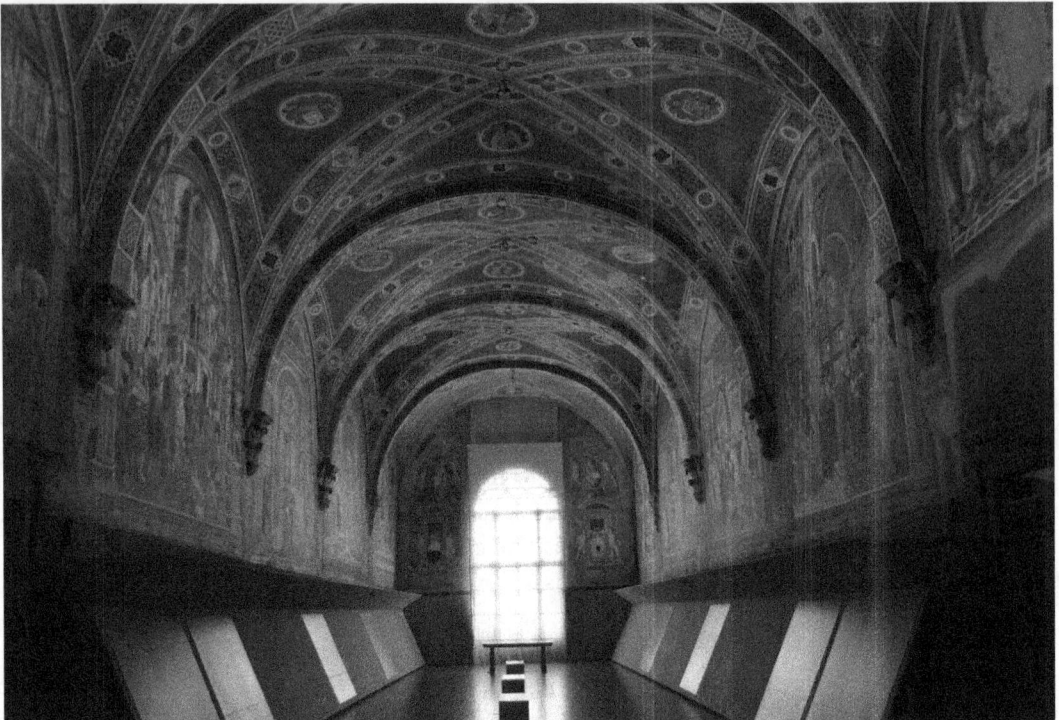

Figure 14.1 *Pellegrinaio*, full view. Photo: Maggie Bell

have been legible to the hospital's diverse population, grounds abstract concepts about the salutary effects of harmonious design in the brick-and-mortar structure of the Scala.

Historical Circumstances of the *Pellegrinaio* Fresco Cycle

The *pellegrinaio* was built in 1328, perpendicularly to the facade of the Scala and centered in the hospital's sprawling structure. Located on the "acropolis" of the city, patients or beneficiaries of the hospital's charity, such as pilgrims and the poor seeking alms, would have walked up one of Siena's main thoroughfares and traversed the busy piazza that the hospital shared with the cathedral to enter the Scala using one of the main portals.[3] Of all the spaces of hospitality, the *pellegrinaio* was one of the most accessible from the piazza. Such accessibility was permissible due to the fact that it was a male ward—women and children were housed in secluded and closely monitored quarters. Because the *pellegrinaio* was one of the more readily visible spaces in the hospital, it was a fitting location for the vast fresco cycle that painted a laudatory picture of the Scala's history and activities.

Although the term "*pellegrinaio*" suggests a place for pilgrims, little is known about specific occupants of the ward since the patient records from this period are lost. Nevertheless, other archival sources suggest that the *pellegrinaio* sheltered people in varying states of health.[4] According to the Scala's fifteenth-century financial records and statutes written in 1305, two different names were used for spaces that housed hospital inmates: the *pellegrinaio*, referring to a place for poor pilgrims and travelers, and the *infermeria*, a place for the infirm.[5] Payment documents for the frescoes in question designate the decorated hall as a *pellegrinaio*,[6] though in another entry for the now-lost frescoes by Pietro di Giovanni Pucci, the terms *infermeria* and *pellegrinaio* seem to refer to the same space.[7] While it is possible that these terms were used interchangeably, it is not necessarily useful to create hard distinctions between the functions of the *pellegrinaio* and *infermeria*, since pilgrims often fell into both categories, having traveled great distances outside of their traditional support networks.[8] That pilgrims and the sick shared spaces of care is supported by accounting documents indicating that cloth merchants purchased the old fabric belonging to pilgrims who had died in the *pellegrinaio*, suggesting that people who were cared for in this space suffered, at least in some cases, from life-threatening conditions.[9]

Along with caring for the poor, sick, and travel-weary, the Scala provided integral services to the wider city of Siena by offering aid to those who could not support themselves, and by functioning as a place of employment and commerce. Often the "children of the hospital" would return as lay brothers or sisters, working in a caregiving capacity or helping to manage the hospital's vast properties.[10] Numerous artists and artisans also worked for the hospital, especially in the decades around the painting of the *pellegrinaio* frescoes when the hospital underwent architectural improvements and expansions.[11] The Scala additionally functioned as a bank and marketplace, as well as a center of civic and religious ceremony and spectacle.

The Scala's high-profile role in the city suggests that the *pellegrinaio* frescoes were intended to impress a wide range of European visitors, some of whom, such as Pope Eugenius IV, were influential and wealthy. The complex iconography encompassing biblical, hagiographical, political, medical, and architectural imagery was likely organized by the rector Giovanni di Francesco Buzzichelli and an adviser.[12] There are four groups of payment entries for the *pellegrinaio* frescoes between 1440 and 1444, which were likely meant to work in concert with one another, though they are often treated as independent interventions in modern scholarship.[13] First, on June 20, 1440 the vaults of the *pellegrinaio* were frescoed with saints and Old Testament figures.[14] Second, in October of 1440, the window wall of the *pellegrinaio* was painted with scenes that have been lost due to the expansion of the ward in the sixteenth century.[15] Third, in 1441 scenes depicting the life of Tobit, a common theme for the decoration of hospitals and charitable institutions, were painted in the first bay of the *pellegrinaio*, and now only exist in disparate fragments.[16] And finally, between 1440 and 1444, the Sienese artists Domenico di Bartolo, Vecchietta, and Priamo della Quercia received payments for the eight wall frescoes, which survive today in restored condition: Vecchietta on November 30, 1441 for the scene of *The Vision of Sorore*, along with the Tobit frescoes,[17] Priamo on April 18, 1442 for *The Investiture of the Rector by Beato Agostino Novello*,[18] and Domenico on January 23, 1444 for five scenes: *The Care of the Sick, The Distribution of Alms, The Care and Marriage of Foundlings, The Liberation of the Hospital and Indulgence of Pope Celestine III*, and *The Expansion of the Hospital*. On April 2, 1444, Domenico was paid for the last scene in the ward, *The Banquet for the Poor*.[19] Almost all of these scenes, particularly those depicting acts of care, refer to recognizable, if idealized, spaces within the Scala.

The Third Bay: Expansion of the Hospital and Depictions of Harmony

The architecture of the Scala is thematized most straightforwardly in the fresco *The Expansion of the Hospital* (Figure 14.2), which occupies what would have been the third and central bay of the ward prior to its sixteenth-century extension. Painted by Domenico di Bartolo in 1443, the inscription along the bottom of the image reads "*Chome avendo ricevuta limosina per potere accresciare la casa di muraglie e di letti e venendo el veschovo con … quanti canonaci fece assorore nuova limosina*" (How having received alms in order to extend the walls and [number of] beds in the hospital, and, coming with many canons, the bishop made a new donation to Sorore).[20] The figure of the rector, identified in the inscription as the legendary shoemaker and hospital founder known as Sorore, emerges from under the scaffolding. He removes his hat as he receives a sack of money from a messenger sent by a man on mounted on a mule, likely the ecclesiastical benefactor. This transfer occurs above a pair of workmen: a bricklayer gathering his material, and a stonemason holding a

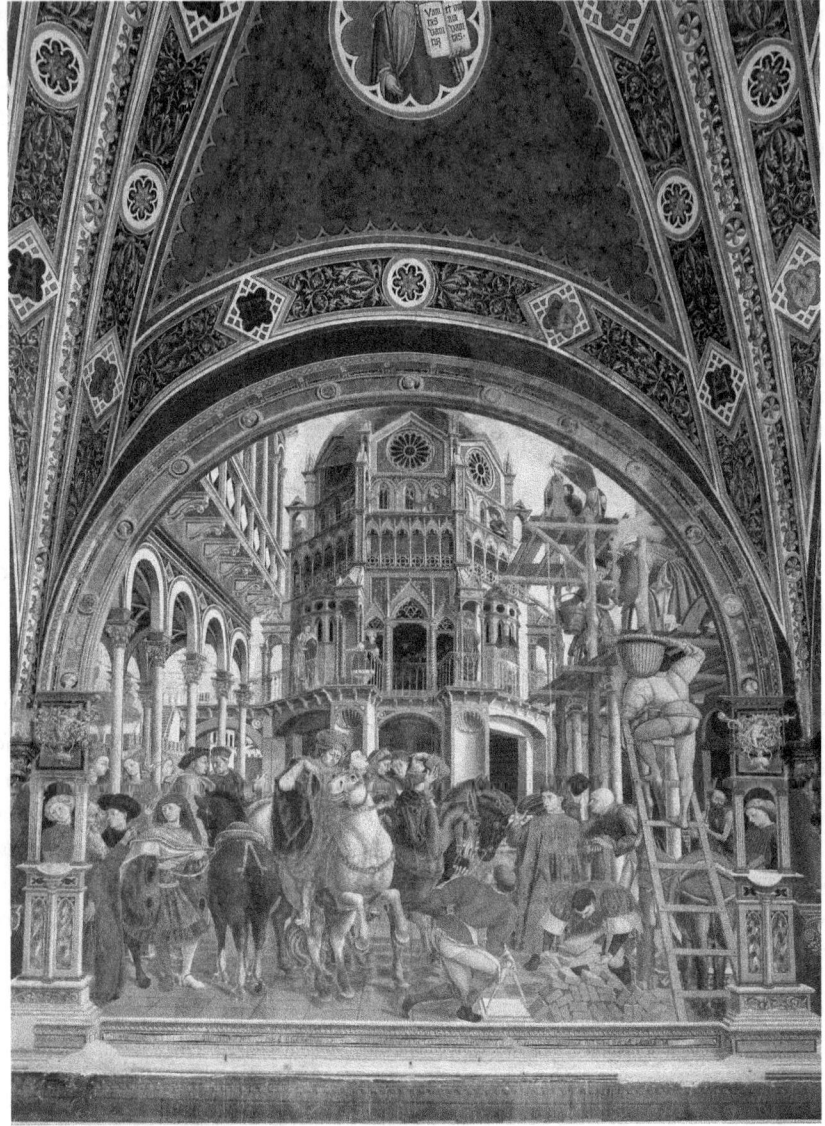

Figure 14.2 Domenico di Bartolo, *The Expansion of the Hospital*, 1443. Source: Comune di Siena, photo by Bruno Bruchi, 2013

large compass whose work is interrupted by a rearing horse.[21] Together these figures represent the patronage and labor required to build the hospital. The fruits of their efforts occupy the right third of the image, though the facade of the Scala is shown covered in scaffolding—its identity as a charitable institution indicated by the mendicant figure standing in the main portal. Surrounding the worksite are spectacular structures that anticipate the grandeur of the finished hospital. A monumental eight-sided building with rose windows and delicate pointed arches fills the center of the fresco and likely refers to the former baptistery of Siena, which stood between the Scala and the cathedral before it was demolished in 1296.[22] The classicized two-story loggia, also competing for the viewer's attention, may refer to the bishop's palace located to the right of the cathedral, which would have still existed at the time the fresco was painted.[23]

The Scala was not the only fifteenth-century hospital to decorate its walls with images of its own foundation and construction, and the few surviving examples of these scenes are supplemented by written accounts. In his *Trattato di architettura* (1460–4), Filarete vividly describes a ceremonial construction scene from the fresco program in the Ospedale Maggiore in Milan, which he designed for Francesco Sforza around 1456. In a fictitious dialogue with his patron, he outlines the appearance and significance of these frescoes:

> When the place where the hospital was to be built in the name of Christ was laid out, a solemn procession of the archbishop and all the clergy was ordered. [After the clergy followed] the duke Francesco Sforza with the most illustrious Bianca Maria ... who came with the populace of Milan in procession to the designated place where the first stone was to be laid. When we arrived at the aforementioned place, I and one of the deputed laid the stone. It was ordered placed in the foundations. On it were written the century, the day and the month, that is April 4, 1457 ... I also [put] in an earthen vase in which there was a leaden box containing ... certain carved medals of the heads of noteworthy men ... [Then] my lord, the pontiff, and I laid this stone with all the aforementioned things. In order to create a notice for mankind, something like a sign or, better, a boundary stone was erected ... He wanted all these things commemorated and painted in the portico.[24]

As Filarete describes them, the frescoes convey the charity and power of the hospital's benefactors as being imbued in the foundation of the institution through the inaugural construction ceremony. The act of building is ritualized in the laying of the foundation stone, conflating the Ospedale Maggiore and the community it serves with the Sforza family. The moment is enshrined in the frescoes, visually and physically enmeshed with the walls of the hospital itself.

The fresco cycle in the main ward of the Hospital of Santo Spirito in Sassia, Rome also includes foundation scenes painted between 1476 and 1478 by a team of unknown artists, which celebrate the history of the hospital and establish its benefactor Sixtus IV as a holy builder and new founder of Rome.[25] In one of the frescoes, the pope observes the renovation of Santo Spirito, standing in the foreground of a busy construction site. The Latin inscription reads: "Having called the best architects, and a great number of workmen from all over, he constructed the hospital itself with much care."[26] Sixtus's public identity was centered on his success as a builder, and the frescoes link spiritual virtue and salvation to the production of architecture, made clear in the fresco *Sixtus IV Presents His Works to God*, added to the hospital cycle in 1485, in which Sixtus kneels while angels hold out a model of Santo Spirito.[27]

As in the frescoes at the Ospedale Maggiore and Santo Spirito, the *Expansion* scene in the *pellegrinaio* confronts the viewer with activities that are typically invisible, creating cognizance of the hospital as a built work. In doing so, meaning becomes attached to the generative processes of architecture. The depiction of the ecclesiastical benefactor offering a donation to the rector identifies the patron's beneficence as foundational to the structure and was a call to other possible donors to similarly support the ongoing construction of the Scala in the mid-fifteenth century. On a broader level, the *Expansion* scene is integral to understanding the *pellegrinaio* cycle as a whole. The exposure of the hospital's architectural development invites viewers, guided by the complex imagery of the surrounding frescoes, to find meaning in the hospital structure as such.

Depictions of Harmony in the Third Bay

The decoration in the vault above *The Expansion of the Hospital* lends spiritual gravity to the building activity depicted below. The vault is divided into four sections, each containing a solitary roundel of an Old Testament figure on a blue starry background—Tobit and Job, arranged head-to-head along the axis of the ward, while Solomon and David, also head-to-head, are located respectively above *The Expansion of the Hospital* and

Health and Architecture

The Care and Marriage of Foundlings, situated on opposing sides of the *pellegrinaio*. This grouping above the *Expansion* scene was not incidental.[28] Given the identities of these figures, associated alternately with sacred architecture and miraculous healing, the vault decoration of the third bay identifies the Scala's construction as stemming from an ancient and divine imperative to build virtuously, and visually concretizes the relationship between architecture and healing.

Solomon, clearly identified as "Il savio Salamone" or Solomon the Wise, presides over the *Expansion* scene holding a text displaying the words *vanitas vanit[atum] et omnia vanitas* (vanity of vanities and all is vanity)— his first spoken words in the book of Ecclesiastes (Figure 14.3). His position over the construction of the hospital is logical, given his celebrated role in biblical history as a builder of cities, palaces, and the

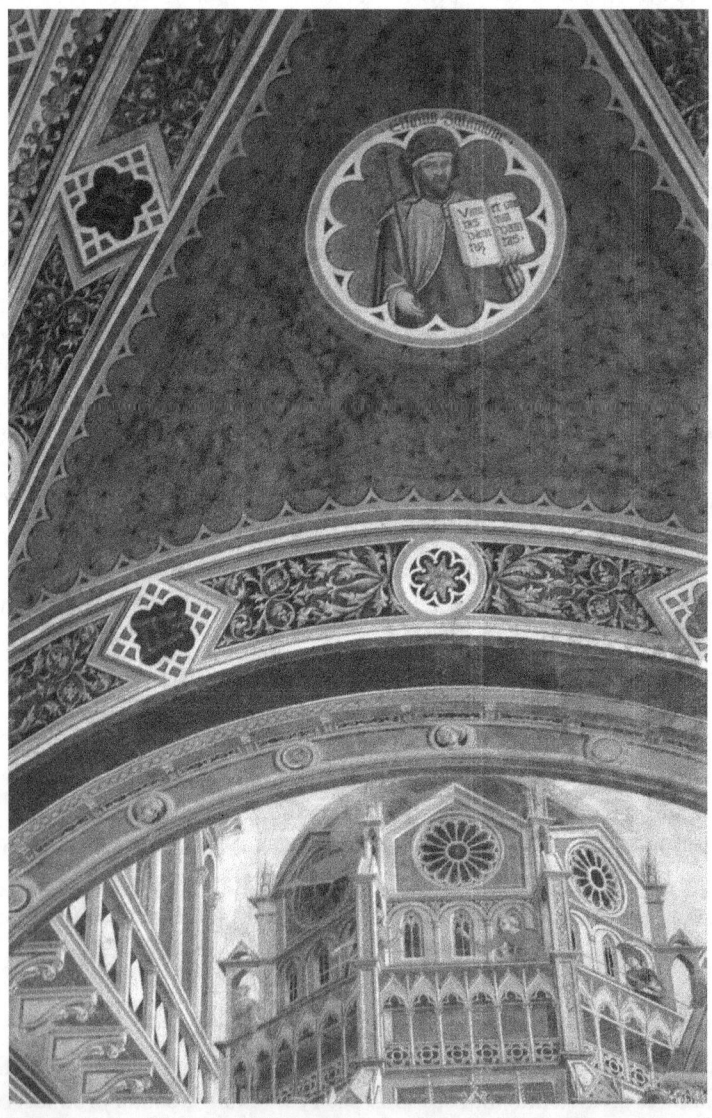

Figure 14.3 Agostino di Marsilio, Gualtieri di Giovanni, and Adamo di Colino, *Solomon* in vault above *The Expansion of the Hospital*, 1439–40 (detail). Photo: Maggie Bell

first Temple in Jerusalem. In period sources, Solomon is lauded for his prudent spending and the judicious use of decorative features in the structures he built.[29] The text in his hands alludes to his role as an effective patron, motivated by his love of God rather than the vanity of earthly glory. The most famous example of such an architectural monument was his Temple, which was praised for its beauty and hailed as the model of the Christian church—a sacred place in which heaven is revealed on earth.[30]

The reference to Solomon's architectural legacy may have had particular meaning for pilgrims traveling along the Francigena who stopped to rest at Santa Maria della Scala. In looking at the *Expansion* scene, perhaps from a prone position in a bed, the pilgrim would have seen the image of Solomon directly above the large octagonal building in the center of the scene. This eight-sided structure suggests the original baptistery of Siena, though in association with Solomon it doubles as a manifestation of his Temple. In the Middle Ages, despite biblical descriptions of the Temple of Jerusalem as a rectangular building, it was often represented as an octagonal domed structure, likely due to confusion with the Dome of the Rock.[31] The motif appears again in a 1446 fresco by Vecchietta in the Old Sacristy of the Scala's church, depicting Solomon praying to the Holy Spirit in the Temple. It is conceivable that the Scala would have associated itself with this divinely inspired structure emblematic of the Holy Land, given that the hospital was not only a place that housed and cared for pilgrims, but a pilgrimage destination in its own right that held a vast collection of Byzantine relics.[32]

In the segment of the vault opposite the *Expansion* scene, David, Solomon's father, appears as the consummate composer of psalms, identified by his harp. Below in the fresco *The Care and Marriage of Foundlings* by Domenico di Bartolo, are two wedding musicians in the balcony, one of whom plays a harp, echoing David's musical attribute (Figures 14.4 and 14.5). Given that he was the original impetus for the Temple that Solomon completed, David also served as a model patron of architecture. This role is evident in images such as a Florentine panel painting by Pesellino from 1445, in which David supervises the construction of the Temple while holding his harp (Figure 14.6).[33] The proximity of David to Solomon and the *Expansion* scene introduces a conceptual link between music and architecture in line with well-established Renaissance thought.[34] In his treatise, Filarete makes the theoretical relationship between architecture and music clear: "[The architect] should also know geometry so that the things he does can be measured with good and perfect measure and by rule … He also needs music so that he will know how to harmonize the members with the parts of the building. They should all be harmonized like the notes of a song."[35] In addition to providing a conceptual, if metaphorical, model for architectural design, music was generally believed to have healing potential. Depicted in the hospital ward, David may have called to mind the moment when he played his lyre for a tormented Saul, who was "refreshed and was made better, for the evil spirit had departed from him (1 Samuel 16:23)."[36]

The figures of Tobit and Job, who appear in the vault between David and Solomon, further highlight the healing potential of harmonious architecture, serving as reminders of the good works that the Scala's structure facilitated. In the *pellegrinaio* Tobit and Job, whose unwavering faith and charitable activities were ultimately rewarded with a return to health, would have acted as exempla of pious suffering.[37] The exemplary good works of Tobit and Job are echoed in the four *pellegrinaio* frescoes illustrating the daily responsibilities of the hospital. These activities take place in specialized spaces like the large ward in *The Care of the Sick*, the women's and children's quarters in *The Care and Marriage of Foundlings*, and the chapel in *The Distribution of Alms*, which shows one portal welcoming the needy into the hospital, and the other allowing them to return, satiated, to the city.[38] Tobit and Job, when read in conjunction with Solomon and David, suggest that the care provided by the Scala was made possible by the hospital's virtuous architectural endeavors. This connection is made more significant by the fact that in the 1430s and 1440s, the Scala was constructing increasingly specialized spaces, such as a pharmacy, a *barberia* for dental surgery and hygiene, and an additional *pellegrinaio*.[39]

Health and Architecture

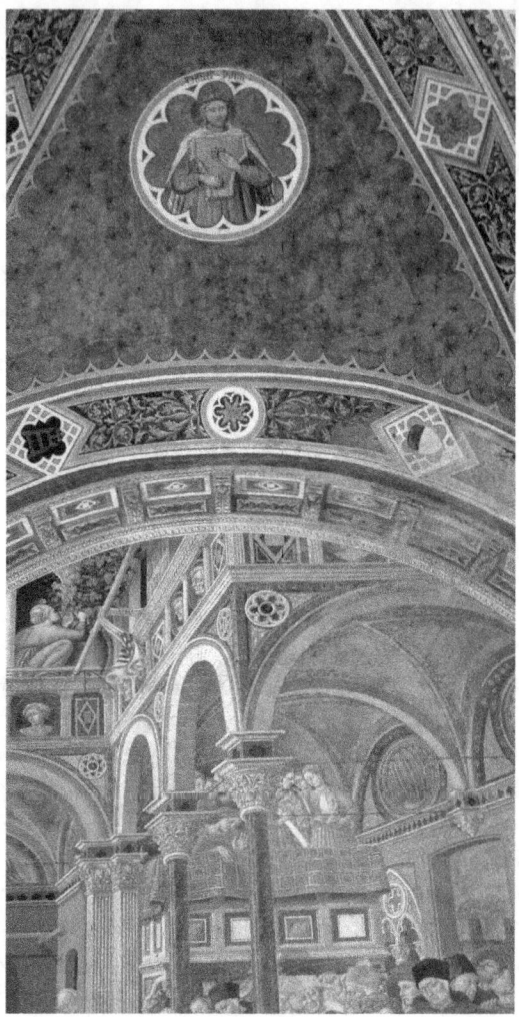

Figure 14.4 Agostino di Marsilio, Gualtieri di Giovanni, and Adamo di Colino, *David* in vault above *The Care and Marriage of Foundlings*, 1439-40 (detail). Photo: Maggie Bell

The *Expansion* scene references the ongoing architectural activity at the hospital, and the crouching figure holding a large compass suspended over a stone tablet is of particular interest. Dressed as a workman, his off-kilter pose in response to the rearing horse contrasts with the rigidity of the measuring device that has slipped off the right edge of the slab. The instrument is shown flush with the picture plane close to the viewer's space, giving it an emblematic aspect (Figure 14.7). The unconventional compositional importance of the compass, which rarely appears in images of construction from this period, suggests that it is not merely a prop in the *Expansion* scene, but rather is a meaningful element that commented on both the labor and design involved in producing the structure.[40]

The compass appeared elsewhere in medieval and early modern images, often as the attribute of the allegorical figure of Geometry, which had a prominent position in Sienese visual culture. For instance, just across the piazza in the cathedral of Siena, Nicola Pisano's 1265–8 pulpit includes a female figure representing Geometry seated with the other Liberal Arts at the base of the central supporting column, giving structural

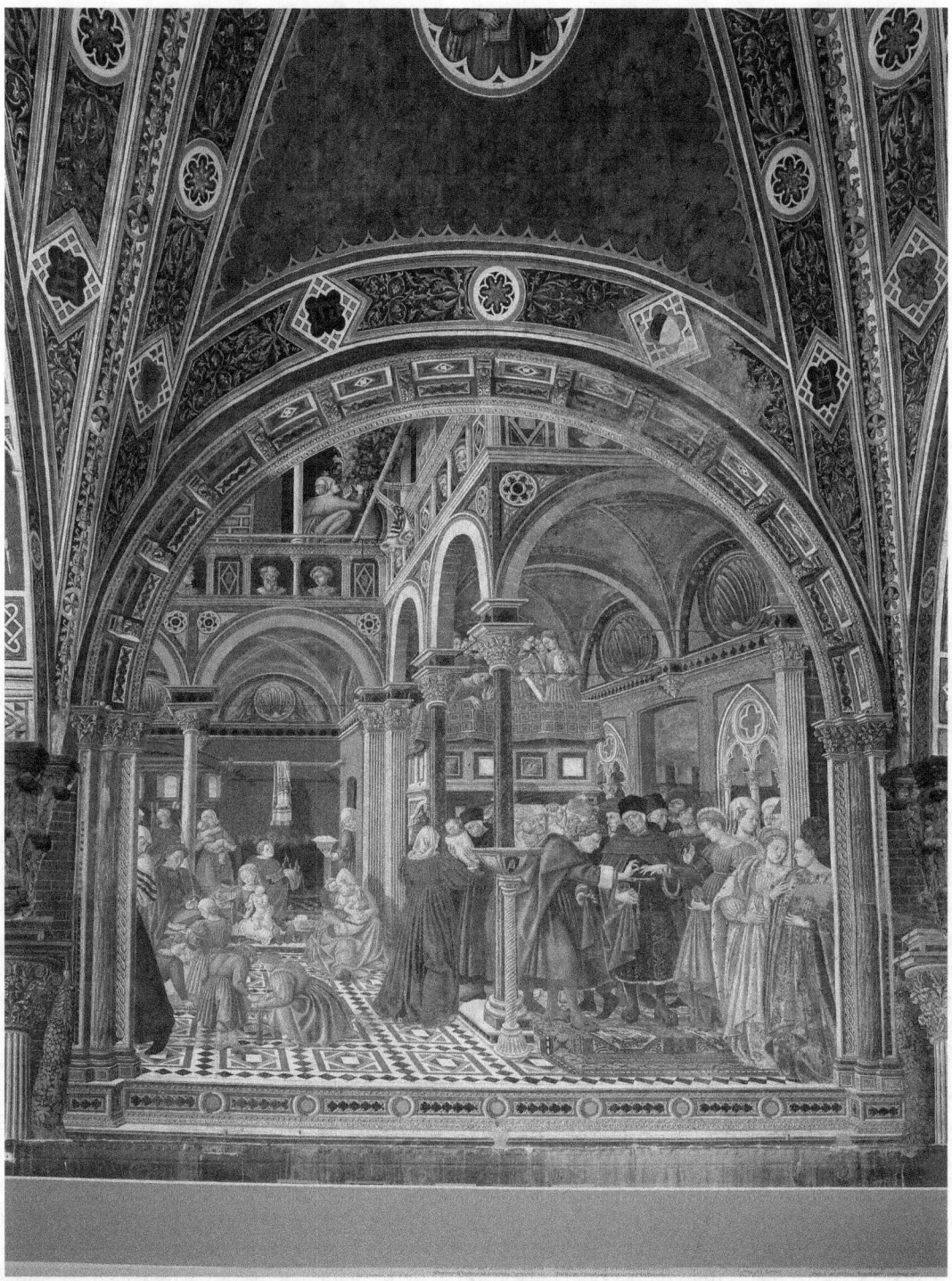

Figure 14.5 Domencio di Bartolo, *The Care and Marriage of Foundlings*, 1441. Source: Comune di Siena, photo by Bruno Bruchi, 2013

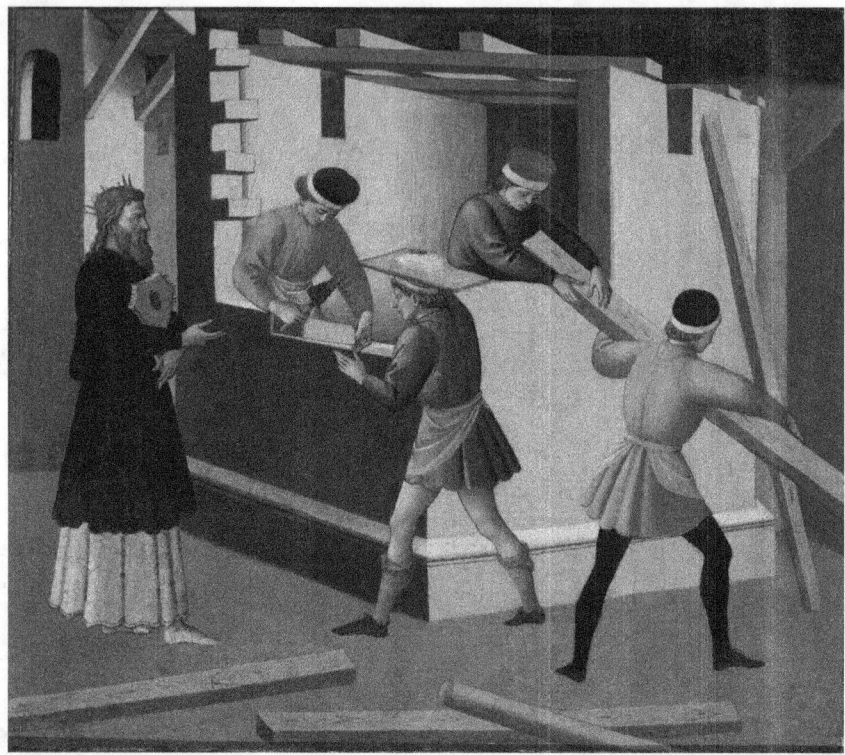

Figure 14.6 Pesellino (Francesco di Stefano), *The Construction of the Temple of Jerusalem*, 1445. Source: Harvard Art Museums/Fogg Museum, Friends of the Fogg Art Museum Fund, Accession no. 1916.495

and intellectual integrity to the sermons delivered above them. A personification of Geometry also appears in the border of Ambrogio Lorenzetti's *Effects of Good Government* (1338–9) in the Sala dei Nove in the Palazzo Pubblico. The figure is seated in a quatrefoil frame, holding a tablet in her left arm on which she rests the point of a compass.[41] In the fresco above her formidable walls extend toward the viewer, and a team of builders constructs a new palazzo while citizens enjoy the comforts of a peaceful, prosperous, and well-fortified city. Given the carefully considered allegorical machinations of the fresco cycle in the Sala dei Nove, it is conceivable that placing the figure of Geometry underneath builders at work was meant to underscore the order-producing nature of architecture, something that was of central concern to the Sienese government in the fourteenth and fifteenth centuries.[42] Viewers familiar with these and other such figures of Geometry may have read the compass in the *Expansion* scene as an allusion not only to the precise measurements necessary for designing and constructing buildings but also to the civic harmony that well-designed buildings could produce.

The compass also entered into the discourse and visual vocabulary of architectural design and labor. In discussing practices of architectural design, Filarete identifies the compass as an indispensable tool, stating "a spherical body cannot be done correctly without a compass … All bodies are measured and constructed with these two instruments [the compass and the square]."[43] In the margin of the text a drawing of a compass, splayed across a tablet, adds visual punctuation to the importance of the instrument.[44] In the same section, he emphasizes the role of drawing as the foundation for architecture, and spends a great deal of time discussing how to render buildings in one-point perspective in order to reveal any logical inconsistencies in the design that would distort the physical structure.[45] The compass also appears regularly in images of the Maestri di

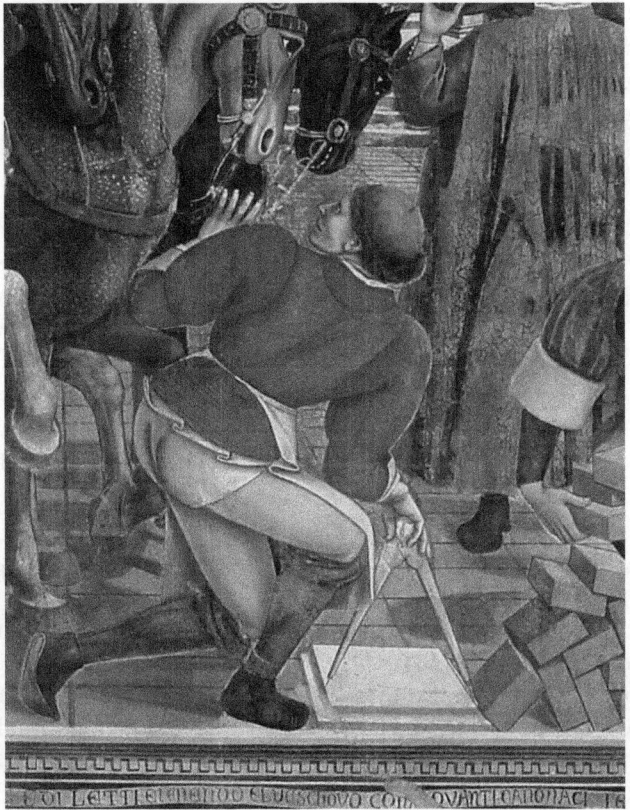

Figure 14.7 Domenico di Bartolo, *The Expansion of the Hospital*, 1443 (detail). Source: Comune di Siena, photo by Bruno Bruchi, 2013

Pietra e di Legname, or the guild of stonecutters and woodworkers, which was active in Florence and Siena.[46] In the *pellegrinaio*, the depiction of the mason working with the compass may have referred directly to the members of the Maestri di Pietra e di Legname who worked in the hospital during and after the years that the frescoes were painted.[47]

The stonemason in the *Expansion* scene introduces the concepts of proportion, balance, and harmony associated with the image of the compass in various visual traditions and ties these concepts to the architectural foundation of the Scala. Beyond making conventional reference to the aesthetic quality of the building, these notions take on special meaning in the context of a hospital—a structure meant to heal bodies whose infirmities were believed to be caused by internal imbalances. As will be shown below, the representation of harmony appears elsewhere in the fresco cycle as a conceptual thread that ties architecture to healing, suggesting a conscious attempt to situate the physical structure of the Scala within concurrent medical discourses that also identified the concept of harmony as central to well-being.

Harmony, Medicine, and Architecture

References to harmony appears regularly in the medical discourse of the fifteenth century, shaped by writings from diverse historical contexts, such as Galen, Hippocrates, and Avicenna among others, which both Alberti and Filarete mined as foundational sources for theories of salutary building.[48] At the core of Galenic thought was the principle that a healthy human body required the balance of four elementary qualities—hot, cold, wet, and dry—that composed the humors: melancholic, choleric, sanguine, and phlegmatic. In turn, the configuration of humors shaped the "complexions" of individuals, which indicated personality, talents, and propensity for diseases.[49] An imbalance in the humors could cause behavioral and physical changes, evidenced in external symptoms such as discoloration of bodily fluids. Drawing on Hippocrates, Galen states in his *A Method of Medicine to Glaucon* that when diagnosing fevers, "the urine occurring in these fevers teaches you the phases of the whole disease."[50] Such a diagnostic technique is underway in the fresco *The Care of the Sick*, located in the fifth bay of the *pellegrinaio*, in which a physician and his assistant assess the urine of an emaciated man on a stretcher in the left-hand side of the image, suggesting that the Scala wanted to advertise its adherence to current medical practice.

Maintaining internal humoral balance depended on external, or "non-natural," factors that could be both preventive and curative. These included ambient air, food and drink, exercise and rest, sleeping and waking, evacuation and repletion, and the passions of the soul, or emotions.[51] Of particular concern in both architectural and medical treatises was establishing a comfortable environment devoid of extremes and with access to clean air, water, and moderate temperatures. Alberti and Filarete recommend that cities be constructed within reasonable distance to water, in winds that are not too strong but that nevertheless refresh the air. Alberti notes that moderate temperatures must be maintained indoors, stating that

> account should also be taken of the seasons, so that rooms intended for summer use should not be the same as those intended for use in winter … Care must be taken to prevent the inhabitants' moving from a cold place to a hot one, without passing through some intermediate zone, or from a warm place to one exposed to the cold and the wind. This can be very detrimental to the body's health.[52]

This concept is echoed in the medical *consilie*, or advice manuals, written by fifteenth-century doctors concerned with the effects of their patients' environments on their health. For example, physicians to the chronically ill Pius II advised the Sienese pope to build his palace in such a way that he could moderate his bodily temperature.[53] Similar measures were taken in the construction of large institutionalized hospitals in the late Middle Ages, and the Scala was no exception. The frescoed *pellegrinaio* is a long and high-ceilinged space similar to the wards of Santa Maria Nuova in Florence, the Ospedale Maggiore in Milan, and Santo Spirito in Rome, with an identical adjacent ward constructed in 1439.[54] This design was believed to be most effective in allowing for appropriate airflow, while also facilitating the spiritual care of patients, who could observe Mass performed at the end of the ward.[55] Such a space is represented in *The Care of the Sick*, which depicts an expansive ward with high ceilings, illuminated by large windows with open shutters allowing for the circulation of light and air.

In Book XV of the *Trattato*, Filarete confirms that the primary salutary function of architecture is to provide a moderate and clean climate. He asserts that it is imperative for the architect to study medicine, stating that one might think this is because of "our comparison with the human body, but I do not say it for this reason. I say this because the architect should see to it that he builds in a healthy place. Thus he who inhabits the building will not become ill, because the architect had not thought of locating it in good air."[56] Filarete seemingly dismisses the medical relationship between a harmonious (proportional) structure and a harmonious (healthy) body, though this assertion feels almost ironic. Until this moment in the treatise, Filarete has relied heavily on anthro-centric anatomical analogies based on the concept of internal harmony, aligning a well-proportioned healthy body with beautiful and functional architecture. He develops this analogy to its full extent, likening the design and construction of a building to the gestation and birth of a child; comparing ill-proportioned buildings with "deformed" bodies; and discussing the care of a building as analogous to caring for a human body in order to prevent illness and death.[57]

In contrast, Alberti suggests that the beauty of a building derived from its harmonious "lineaments" could affect the well-being of the viewer or inhabitant. He clarifies this dynamic in his discussion of *concinnitas*, starting by saying that "beauty is a form of sympathy and consonance of the parts within a body, according to definite number, outline, and position, as dictated by *concinnitas*, the absolute and fundamental rule in Nature."[58] Alberti identifies certain "numbers" (*numerus*) that order all things including biological phenomena.[59] These numbers, which also govern music and the human body, can be harnessed by architects to create "delight":

> The very same numbers that cause sounds to have that *concinnitas*, pleasing to the ears, can also fill the eyes and mind with wondrous delight … Architects employ all these numbers in the most convenient manner possible, they use them in pairs, as in laying out a forum, palace or open space.[60]

Despite Alberti's Platonic conviction that beauty derives from universal numbers, he is nevertheless interested in the physical sensory implications of experiencing harmonious buildings. In his treatise on the soul, *Della tranquillità dell'animo* (1441–2), Alberti describes the pleasing effects of the cathedral of Florence, derived both from its harmonious beauty and moderate internal climate:

> And certainly this temple has in itself grace and majesty; and as I have often thought, I delight to see joined here a charming slenderness with a robust and full solidity so that, on the one hand each of its parts seems designed for pleasure, while on the other, one understands that it has all been built for perpetuity … Here is the constant home of temperateness, as of springtime, outside, wind, ice and frost; here inside one is protected from the wind, here mild air and quiet.[61]

The *pellegrinaio* frescoes similarly address the salutary effects of architecture on two levels, as both regulating environmental extremes and tempering the passions of the soul. In the first place, the vast and airy ward depicted in *The Care of the Sick*, which would have mimicked the *pellegrinaio*, emphasizing the Scala's regulation of climate and airflow according to conventional wisdom about healthy building practice. At the same time, allusions to healing music and the processes of design and construction based on proportional measurement draw attention to the hospital's underlying harmonious orientation, suggesting the therapeutic role of visual and aesthetic experience.

Santa Maria della Scala as Healing Architecture

It is important to linger for a moment on the site-specificity of the frescoes, which were designed for a permeable space of care and healing meant to house a large number of inmates that included the poor, sick, and peregrinating. The frescoes themselves are monumental, covering the walls and ceilings of the ward, and depicting the hospital's history and various specialized spaces of care. The particularity of these scenes, set within the Scala's wards and courtyards, links universal and abstract theories of harmony presented in the fresco cycle to a physical site. This is a common rhetorical strategy employed in the texts of Alberti and Filarete, who each offers concrete examples from history, scripture, or contemporary life to illustrate their arguments. Here, however, the commentary provided by the frescoes could be compared in real time to a brick-and-mortar *exemplum*. Through the visual strategies employed in the *pellegrinaio* cycle, the Scala is conceived of as an embodiment of ideal medical and architectural practice, innately harmonious and grounded in biblical precedent, producing a salutary experience only described in theoretical texts.

The *pellegrinaio* frescoes both identify the Scala as a healing structure and actively contribute to the healing efficacy of the ward. The figures alluding to medical, musical, and architectural harmony offer one thread among a tapestry of interpretive possibilities within the cycle. Viewers are confronted with engaging visual material that presents complex narratives and allegories that would have elicited different interpretations from the Scala's diverse population. To identify individual figures, much less to draw connections among the frescoes required an investment of time and attentiveness on the part of the viewer that was considered conducive to healing. Frances Gage has written about the prevalence of a belief in the therapeutic power of art in the early modern period.[62] In one sense, beautiful things could inspire delight and ease a troubled spirit. The fifteenth-century Neo-Platonic philosopher Marsilio Ficino (1433–99) wrote ardently about this aspect of music, which he felt mimicked the movements of the soul, and could actively correct spiritual, and therefore physical, imbalance.[63] In another sense, the arts could provide healthful recreation for the mind. The Sienese physician Ugo Benzi (1376–1439), who was professor of medicine at the Studio in Siena, recommended that a melancholic youth observe "beautiful and entertaining decorations" to restore his humoral balance.[64] Given the close working relationship between the Scala and the Studio, which typically supplied the hospital's resident physicians, it is very possible that Benzi's belief in the curative function of "beautiful decorations" may have had an impact on the Scala's artistic endeavors.[65] Alberti similarly addresses the positive effects of art in his treatise *On Painting* (*Della pittura*) (1427), describing the pleasure that can be produced by gazing at a painting (*historia*) for an extended period of time:

> But a *historia* that you can deservedly both praise and admire will be such that it shows itself so agreeable and rich in certain stimuli [as] to attract for a long time the eyes of the instructed spectator, or even illiterate, with a certain sense of pleasure and emotion of the mind. The first thing, in fact, that brings pleasure in a *historia* is richness itself and a variety of objects. As, in fact, in food and music, new and extraordinary things always delight, not only perhaps because of all other reasons but also and above all for the fact that they differ from those old and customary [things], so the mind feels pleasure exceedingly in every variety and abundance of objects.[66]

The *pellegrinaio* frescoes, themselves examples of the monumental history paintings that Alberti describes, offer various and diverting details that absorb the viewer's attention. At the same time, the frescoes anchor the viewer in the physical reality of the ward by depicting episodes from the daily life of the Scala in recognizable, if idealized, places. The cycle invites viewers to draw connections among the frescoes across architectural space, creating a dynamic, therapeutic engagement with the images and the very walls they decorate. In doing so, the *pellegrinaio* frescoes do not merely comment on the Scala's architecture, but rather act architecturally themselves, directly impacting the viewer's experience of the ward by enhancing through visual means the space's healing potential, already imbued in its structure through harmonious design and construction.

The architectural function of the *pellegrinaio* frescoes is particularly interesting in light of the fact that, while the Scala underwent significant architectural growth during the mid-fifteenth century, much of the hospital's structure, including the *pellegrinaio*, had been built in the previous century.[67] This means that, despite the visual emphasis placed on the concept of harmony, the Scala itself did not adhere to an overarching rational grid scheme like the Ospedale Maggiore in Milan, designed in 1456 by Filarete. In fact, the architect writes in his treatise after having visited Santa Maria della Scala and Santa Maria Nuova in Florence, another medieval hospital, that their designs were not useful as models, and left much to be improved upon.[68] On the one hand, then, the *pellegrinaio* frescoes could be understood as an attempt to argue for the harmonious rationality of the Scala's architecture and its healing efficacy, despite the reality, in a way that was in line with the intellectual fashion of the period. On the other hand, or perhaps concurrently, the frescoes themselves fulfill the function of healing architecture, turning the *pellegrinaio* into a visually harmonious and pleasing space conducive to healing.

Conclusion

As previous research has revealed, the architectural design of early modern Italian hospitals was considered central to their healing efficacy, particularly in terms of ensuring access to light and airflow. Beyond considerations of ambient conditions, the question of a hospital's harmonious design had potential therapeutic implications, restoring internal balance and health for those housed within them. The association between well-formed (i.e., proportional) buildings and healthy bodies was explicitly theorized in fifteenth-century treatises on architecture—described with particular clarity in the section of Filarete's treatise dedicated to his plans for the Ospedale Maggiore in Milan—and became increasingly visible in the plans for hospitals built later in the century, which were based on regular grid patterns with long nave-like wards surrounding open courtyards.

While the medieval hospital of Santa Maria della Scala in Siena was not built according to such a rationalized model, this chapter argues that the Scala nevertheless wanted to present an image of itself as participating in mid-fifteenth-century discourses surrounding the relationship between architecture and health through self-representation in the monumental *pellegrinaio* fresco cycle. In the first place, the frescoes draw attention to the Scala as a work of architecture through elaborate fictive buildings that dominate the visual field and make reference to actual spaces within the hospital. Secondly, representations of architecture, music, and medicine, all practices guided by a pursuit of proportion and balance, appear in the *pellegrinaio* frescoes. When considered together, these images provide a commentary on the Scala's built form, identifying the physical walls as the products of virtuously harmonious design and construction, which in turn produce bodily health and social harmony. As a theoretical text of sorts, the *pellegrinaio* frescoes achieve what written treatises could not by allowing viewers to compare the visual exposition of medical and architectural theory in relation to a concrete example that they could experience in real time.

In a broader view, the *pellegrinaio* cycle demonstrates the deeply entwined relationship between frescoes and architecture in fifteenth-century Italy. In addition to self-referentially commenting on the hospital through the inclusion of certain motifs, the format of monumental frescoes would have required viewers to engage with the ward in a dynamic way, moving and looking from one fresco to the next in order to draw meaningful connections among them. The inherently spatial and bodily nature of the viewing experience of a fresco cycle is made additionally powerful in a space of healing. In the case of the *pellegrinaio* cycle at Santa Maria della Scala, infirm viewers may have found relief in the variety of figures, narratives, and architectural forms depicted on the walls, latently reinforcing the healing capacity of the structure itself.

Notes

1. On the interpretation of painted spaces, see Anne Dunlop, *Painted Palaces: The Rise of Secular Art in Early Renaissance Italy* (Pennsylvania: Pennsylvania State University Press, 2009), 89.
2. Throughout I will use Leon Battista Alberti, *On the Art of Building in Ten Books*, trans. Joseph Rykwert, Neil Leach, and Robert Tavernor (Cambridge, MA: MIT Press, 1988), and Antonio di Piero Averlino, *Filarete's Treatise on Architecture: Being the Treatise by Antonio di Piero Averlino, Known as Filarete*, trans. John R. Spencer, 2 vols. (New Haven: Yale University Press, 1965).
3. Beatrice Sordini, *Dentro l'antico ospedale: Santa Maria della Scala, uomini, cose e spazi di vita nella Siena medievale* (Siena: Protagon, 2010), 321. The 1305 statutes of the hospital mention the comings and goings of visitors, suggesting the wards had long functioned as semi-permeable spaces. Luciano Banchi, *Statuti volgari de lo spedale di Santa Maria Vergine di Siena* (Siena: I. Gati Editore, 1864), section XLV.
4. In addition, the fifteenth-century patient records from the Ospedale della Misericordia in Prato, which functioned similarly to the Scala, reveal that inmates were admitted for a variety of reasons, from wounds to "chronic poverty."

Giulo Paolucci and Giuliano Pinto, "Gli 'infermi' della Misericordia di Prato (1409–1491)," in *Società del bisogno: povertà e assistenza nella Toscana medievale*, ed. Giuliano Pinto (Florence: Salimbeni, 1989), 101–29.

5. There is some debate as to the interchangeability of these terms. Fattorini suggests that the bookkeeping would have been precise, and *pellegrinaio* and *infermeria* would not have been used to refer to the same space (155), though Gallavotti thinks the distinctions are less clear (156). See Daniela Gallavotti Cavallero, *Lo spedale di Santa Maria della Scala in Siena: vicenda di una commitenza artistica* (Pisa: Pacini, 1985), 156; Gabriele Fattorini, "Domenico di Bartolo: pittura di luce e pittura fiamminga: per una definitive rivalutazione del ciclo del Pellegrinaio," in *Pellegrinaio dell'ospedale di Santa Maria della Scala*, ed. Fabio Gabbrielli (Arcidosso: Effigi, 2014), 155.

6. The payment record for Domenico di Bartolo reads that he "was given on January 24, 1000 lire for five scenes [*storie*] painted in the Pellegrinaio" (Ane dati a di' xxiiii di giennaio 1443 [stile senese, i.e., 1444] lire mile, sonno per cinque storie a' dipinto nel pellegrinaio). Archivio di Stato di Siena, Spedale 520, fol. 99r, 1443/4.

7. Pietro is paid "for two scenes painted at the end of the *infermeria* on the window wall at the head of the chapel of the pellegrinaio" (Per due storie dipinte nell'infermeria da piedi nella faccia della finestra a capo la cappella del pellegrinaio). Archivio di Stato di Siena, Spedale 519, fol. 203r, 1440.

8. Paolucci and Pinto observe that the Misericordia in Prato provided medical care for pilgrims who arrived with injuries or illnesses. Paolucci and Pinto, "Gli 'infermi' della Misericordia di Prato," 124.

9. "Batista di giovanni *ligritiere* owes on March 16, 11 *lire* and 10 *soldi* for an assortment of old cloth purchased from the *pelegrinieri* of those [clothes] that remained in the pellegrinaio belonging to the poor pilgrims who had died" (Batista di giovanni ligritiere die dare perisino ad xvi di marzo lire undici soldi dieci sono per una sortarela di pani vechi chonpri da pelegrinieri di queli rimasti al pelegrinaio di poveri pelegrini si so[no] morti). Archivio di Stato di Siena, Ospedale 519, fol. 174v, 1439/40.

10. Mariella Carlotti and Bernhard Scholz, *Ante gradus: quando la certezza diventa creativa: gli affreschi del Pellegrinaio di Santa Maria della Scala a Siena* (Florence: Società editrice fiorentina, 2011), 40; Gabriella Piccinni and Laura Vigni, "Modelli di assistenza ospedaliera tra Medioevo ed Età Moderna: quotidianità, amministrazione, conflitti nell' ospedale di Santa Maria della Scala di Siena," in *La Società del bisogno: povertà e assistenza nella Toscana medievale*, ed. Giuliano Pinto (Florence: Salimbeni, 1989), 138.

11. Sordini, *Drento l'antico ospedale*, 106.

12. Elda Costa and Laura Ponticelli, "L'iconografia del Pellegrinaio nello spedale di Santa Maria della Scala di Siena," *Iconographia* 3 (2004): 125.

13. The ceiling frescoes are often grouped with the Tobias frescoes because of their more archaic style (though little remains of the Tobias frescoes to substantiate this), and their Old Testament themes. See Costa and Ponticelli, "L'iconografia del Pellegrinaio," 11; Carl Brandon Strehlke, "Domenico di Bartolo" (Ph.D. diss., Columbia University, 1986), 106.

14. "Paid on August 7, 1440, eighty-four *soldi a lire* 3 *soldi*, and this is for painting six vaults in the *pellegrinaio* and the church …" (Ane dati a di xii daghosto 1440 soldi ottantaquatro a lire iii soldi e questa sono per dipentura di sei volte del pelegrinaio e dela chiessa …). Archivio di Stato di Siena, Ospedale 519, fol. 187r.

15. "Paid on October 27, 1440 32 lire and 0 soldi for two scenes painted at the end of the infirmary on the wall with the window at the end of the chapel of the *pellegrinaio* as commissioned by Giovanni our rector" (Ane dati a di xxvii d'ottobre 1440 lire trentadue soldi 0 sono per due storie ci dipensse nela fermaria da pie in nela facia dela finestra a chapo la chapella del pelegrinaio dachordo chomisso Giovanni nostro rettore). Archivio di Stato di Siena, Ospedale 519, fol. 203. See also Gallavotti, *Lo spedale di Santa Maria della Scala*, 156.

16. Archivio di Stato di Siena, Ospedale 519, fols. 523 (for da Velletri) and 533 for Vecchietta. See Gallavotti, *Lo spedale di Santa Maria della Scala*, 156; Costa and Ponticelli, "L'iconografia del pellegrinaio," 116.

17. "Master Lorenzo di Piero, painter, to receive on November 30, 1441 seventy florins and four lire for painting a scene of Sorore in our *pellegrinaio*" (Maiestro Lorenzo di Pietro dipentore die avere a dì XXX novembre 1441 fior. settanta a libr. quattro fior. e' quali sono per dipentura duna storia a dipento di Sorore … e per dientura di tre storie dipese a chapo larcho del pellegrinaio de la infermaria de la storia di Tobia). Archivio di Stato di Siena Ospedale 519, fol. 533. Transcribed in Costa and Ponticelli, "L'iconografia del Pellegrinaio," 116.

18. "Master Priamo di Pietro is owed on April 18, 0200 lire: they are for a painted scene in our *pellegrinaio* of the story of saint Agostino Novello, when he gave the habit to the rector of the hospital" (Maiestro Priamo di Pietro die avere a dì 18 d'Aprile lire dugento: sono per una storia a dipento nel nostro Pelegrinaio de le storie di santo Aghustino Novelo, quando dè l'abito a' Rettore de lo Spedale). Archivio di Stato di Siena, Ospedale 519, fol. 545. Transcribed in Costa and Ponticelli, "L'iconografia del Pellegrinaio," 126.

19. "Master Domenico di Bartolo, painter, was given on January 24, 1000 lire for five scenes [*storie*] painted in the Pellegrinaio: one depicts the care of the sick, the other the alms, the other the marriage of the [foundling] girl, the other the indulgence of the Pope, the other the growth of the hospital's walls" (Maiestro Domenico di Bartolo, dipentore—ane dati a di' XXIIII di giennaio 1443 lire mile, sonno per cinque storie a' dipinto I' nel Pelegrinaio: l'una disegna el ghoverno degl' infermi; e l'altra, la limoxina, l'altra el maritare de le fanciulle; e l'altra, de la 'ndulgentia del Papa; e l'altra l'achre'sciare lo spedale di muraglie: per fior: cinquanta l'una). Archivio di Stato di Siena, Ospedale 520, fol. 99."[Domenico] was given on April 2, 1444 seventy lire ... they are for two scenes: one that represents the alms in the courtyard, and the other above the gate of the church, that is a Madonna of the Misericordia. The wise citizens who govern the hospital judged these scenes" (Ane dati a di' ij d' Aprile 1444 fior: settanta di lire quarto l'uno, so' per due storie; l'una che disengnia la limosina de la Chorticiela; et l'altra sopra la graticola di chiexa, cioe' una Nostra Donna di Misericordia; le quali due storie giudicharo e savi citadini al ghoverno de lo Spedale). Archivio di Stato di Siena, Ospedale 520, fol. 99.
20. Costa and Ponticelli suggest that the inscription is original to the fresco because it stylistically corresponds to other fresco inscriptions from the same period. Costa and Ponticelli, "L'iconografia del Pellegrinaio," 117.
21. This device may also be a divider, a tool identical in function to a compass but with a sharpened end used to incise stone. Because of the formal and functional similarities, for the sake of clarity I will refer to this device throughout as a compass.
22. Sordini, *Dentro l'antico ospedale*, 51.
23. The bishop's palace, or *vescovado*, was torn down in 1660 to expand the piazza along the south side of the cathedral. Wolfgang Loseries, "Der Dom im städtebaulichen Zusammenhang vom mittleren 14. Bis zum 20. Jahrhundert," in *Kirchen von Siena*, 3.1, 1.2 (Munich: Bruckman, 2006): 693–4; Costa and Ponticelli, "L'iconografia del Pellegrinaio,"1 34.
24. Filarete, *Treatise on Architecture*, 146. For an Italian transcription, see Filarete, *Antonio Averlino detto il Filarete: trattato di architettura*, trans. Anna Maria Finoli and Liliana Grassi, 2 vols. (Milan: Il Polifilo, 1972), 319–21. Friedhelm Scharf also notes the connection between Filarete's description of the frescoes in Milan and the *pellegrinaio* cycle, suggesting that both serve a propagandistic function. Friedhelm Scharf, *Der Freskenzyklus des Pellegrinaios in S. Maria della Scala zu Siena: Historienmalerei und Wirklichkeit in einem Hospital der Frührenaissance* (Hildsheim: G. Olms, 2001), 133.
25. See Eunice D. Howe, *Art and Culture at the Sistine Court: Platina's "Life of Sixtus IV" and the Frescoes of the Hospital of Santo Spirito* (Vatican City: Biblioteca Apostolica Vaticana, 2005), 76.
26. Accitis undique optimis architectis conductoque magna fabrorum multitudine hospitale ipsum magno studio aedificat. Howe, *Art and Culture at the Sistine Court*, 103.
27. Howe, *Art and Culture at the Sistine Court*, 91.
28. On the "ubiquity and multivalence of Biblical lore" as an interpretive framework in fifteenth-century artistic production, see Amy Bloch, *Lorenzo Ghiberti's Gates of Paradise: Humanism, History, and Artistic Philosophy in the Italian Renaissance* (New York: Cambridge University Press, 2016), 8.
29. Both Filarete and Alberti reference David and Solomon several times in their treatises, identifying them as ideal patrons capable of acquiring fine material and attracting the best architects and builders. Leon Battista Alberti, *On the Art of Building in Ten Books*, trans. Joseph Rykwert (Cambridge, MA: MIT Press, 1988), 39; Filarete, *Treatise on Architecture*, 246–53, 260, 264.
30. Bloch, *Lorenzo Ghiberti's Gates of Paradise*, 256.
31. Carol Herselle Krinsky, "Representations of the Temple of Jerusalem before 1500," *Journal of the Warburg and Courtauld Institutes* 33 (1970): 5.
32. Sordini, *Dentro l'antico ospedale*, 78. Gabriella Piccinni and Carla Zarrilli, *Arte e assistenza a Siena: le copertine dipinte dell'Ospedale di Santa Maria della Scala* (Ospedaletto, Pisa: Pacini editore per Santa Maria della Scala, 2003), 19.
33. This panel is one of four, though the origin and function are uncertain. It may have been part of a larger series on the Life of David. Everett Fahy, "Italian Painting before 1500," *Apollo* 107, no. 195 (1978): 377–88.
34. This is illustrated in an anecdote in which the composer Guillaume Dufay created a motet, *Nuper rosarum flores*, based on the ratios of Solomon's Temple on March 25, 1436 for the celebration of the consecration of Santa Maria dei Fiori in Florence. The composition aurally demonstrated the perfectly harmonious measurements of the biblical structure and identified the newly consecrated cathedral as a continuation of David and Solomon's original project. Bloch, *Lorenzo Ghiberti's Gates of Paradise*, 254.

35. Filarete, *Treatise on Architecture*, 99.
36. Colum Hourihane, *King David in the Index of Christian Art* (Princeton: Princeton University Press, 2002), xxi.
37. Because both Old Testament patriarchs cared for the needs of the sick, dead, and dying, their lives were popular subjects in hospital decoration, including the fragmentary frescoes in the first bay of the *pellegrinaio* depicting scenes from the life of Tobit. See Samuel L. Terrien, *The Iconography of Job through the Centuries: Artists as Biblical Interpreters* (University Park, PA: Pennsylvania State University Press, 1996), 73.
38. This last space was the Capella delle Reliquie, whose function is identified by the rear view of the balcony from which the hospital's relics were displayed. The chapel became the Cappella del Manto in 1441. Loseries, "Der Dom im städtebaulichen Zusammenhang vom mittleren 14.," 691–2; Sordini, *Dentro l'antico ospedale*, 92–5; Gallavotti, *Lo spedale di Santa Maria della Scala in Siena*, 106, 418; Scharf, *Der Freskenzyklus des Pellegrinaios*, 253; Petra Pertici, *The Fabric of History: Power, Prestige and Piety in Siena in the Pellegrinaio of Santa Maria della Scala* (Siena: Betti, 2015), 51.
39. Sordini, *Dentro l'antico spedale*, 120–1; Piccinni and Vigni, "Modelli di assistenza ospedaliera tra Medioevo ed Età Moderna," 145–6; John Henderson, *The Renaissance Hospital: Healing the Body and Healing the Soul* (New Haven: Yale University Press, 2006), 4, 14–25, 39, 45, 88, 337.
40. This assertion comes from extensive comparative study of construction scenes from the fifteenth century, facilitated by the Photo Library of the Kunsthistorisches Institut in Florence.
41. Randolph Starn, *Ambrogio Lorenzetti: The Palazzo Pubblico, Siena* (New York: George Braziller, 1994), 93.
42. The civic approach to architecture in Siena was highly regulated by the *Ufficio dell'ornato*, a body dedicated to monitoring the city's building activity. For more on the *Ufficio dell'Ornato*, see Berthold Hub, "'Vedete come e bella la cittade quando e ordinata': Politics and the Art of City Planning in Republican Siena," in *Art as Politics in Late Medieval and Renaissance Siena*, ed. Timothy B. Smith and Judith B. Steinhoff (Farnham: Ashgate, 2012), 72.
43. Filarete, *Treatise on Architecture*, 297. For an illustration of the compass, see the facsimile in vol. 2, fol. 174r. For an Italian transcription, see Filarete, *Antonio Averlino detto il Filarete*, 641: "A volerlo fare sperico non giusto si può fare sanza sesto, cioè tondo. E questo è l'altro strumento sanza il quale non si potrebbe fare; e sta in questa forma come a ciascheduno è noto. E questi sono e' due strumenti coi quali tutti i corpi si misurano e fanno, come è detto di sopra, benché d'essi ne derivi molti sanza i quali ancora male si farebbe."
44. See Filarete *Treastise on Architecture*, vol. 2 (facsimile), Book XXII, fol. 174r.
45. Filarete, *Treatise on Architecture*, 81.
46. For the exterior of Orsanmichele, the Florentine guild commissioned a *predella* relief from Nanni di Banco (1413) for the niche of the Quattro Coronati, the guild's patron saints, which shows a stonecutter's workshop with a divider hanging on the wall. Siena had a guild of the same name that also honored the Quattro Coronati, and may have used similar imagery for its own self-representation. The Quattro Coronati are mentioned in the guild statutes of the Maestri di Pietra senese, Archivio di Stato di Siena, Arti 47, fol. 1r.
47. Master stoneworkers were hired frequently by the hospital in the years that Buzzichelli was rector. See Archivio di Stato di Siena, Ospedale 520, fols. 32r (1442), 34v (1442), 116r (1444).
48. Katherine Park, *Doctors and Medicine in Early Renaissance Florence* (Princeton: Princeton University Press, 1985), 60.
49. Frances Gage, *Painting as Medicine in Early Modern Rome: Giulio Mancini and the Efficacy of Art* (University Park, PA: The Pennsylvania State University Press, 2016), 48; Angus Gowland, "Medicine, Psychology and the Melancholic Subject in the Renaissance," in *Emotions and Health*, ed. Elena Carrera (Leiden: Brill, 2013), 192.
50. Galen, *On the Structure of the Art of Medicine; The Art of Medicine; On the Practice of Medicine to Glaucon*, trans. Ian Johnston, The Loeb Classical Library, 523 (Cambridge, MA: Harvard University Press, 2016), 373.
51. Peregrine Horden, "A Non-Natural Environment: Medicine Without Doctors and the Medieval European Hospital," in *Hospitals and Healing from Antiquity to the Later Middle Ages*, ed. Peregrine Horden (Burlington, VT: Ashgate, 2008), 135.
52. Alberti, *On the Art of Building in Ten Books*, 23.
53. Antonia Whitley, "Concepts of Ill Health and Pestilence in Fifteenth-Century Siena" (Ph.D. diss., University of London, 2004), 206.
54. Sordini, *Dentro l'antico ospedale*, 120.
55. Henderson, *The Renaissance Hospital*, 58.
56. Filarete, *Treatise on Architecture*, 199.
57. "I will [then] show you [that] the building is truly a living man. You will see what it must eat in order to live, exactly as it is with man. It sickens and dies or sometimes is cured of its sickness by a good doctor. Sometimes, like man,

it becomes ill again because it neglected its health. Many times, through [the cares] of a good doctor, it returns to health and lives a long while and finally dies in its own time. There are some that are never ill and then at the end die [suddenly]; others are killed by other people for one reason or another." Filarete, *Treatise on Architecture*, 13.
58. Alberti, *On the Art of Building in Ten Books*, 302–3.
59. "That Nature is composed of threes all philosophers agree. And as for the number five, when I consider the many varied and wonderful things that either themselves relate to that number or are produced by something that contains it—such as the human hand—I do not think it wrong that it should be called divine … Then again the physicians are all agreed that many of the most important things in Nature are based on the fraction of one ninth. For one ninth of the annual solar cycle is about forty days, the length of time, according to Hippocrates, that it takes the fetus to form in the uterus." Alberti, *On the Art of Building in Ten Books*, 305.
60. Alberti, *On the Art of Building in Ten Books*, 305.
61. Quoted in Helen Hills, "Architecture and Affect: Leon Battista Alberti and Edification," in *Representing Emotions: New Connections in the Histories of Art, Music and Medicine*, ed. Penelope Gouk and Helen Hills (Burlington, VT: Ashgate, 2005), 91.
62. Gage, *Painting as Medicine*, 52–5.
63. Gage, *Painting as Medicine*, 53.
64. Gage, *Painting as Medicine*, 54.
65. On the relationship between the Studio and the Scala, see Whitley, "Concepts of Ill Health," 130–5.
66. Leon Battista Alberti, *On Painting: A New Translation and Critical Edition*, trans. Rocco Sinisgalli (Cambridge: Cambridge University Press, 2011), 276.
67. On the thirteenth-century building projects of the Scala, see Sordini, *Dentro l'antico ospedale*, 42–9.
68. "He placed me on the task of making a drawing. First he asked me if I had seen the hospitals in Florence and Siena, and if I remembered how they looked. I replied yes. He wanted to see a rough sketch of the foundations and I drew him one as best I remembered. I drew the hospital in Florence for him. However, it did not seem as suitable to him as he would have liked and he doubted if the others could be improved [enough to satisfy our needs]." Filarete, *Treatise on Architecture*, 137.

CHAPTER 15
UTERUS HOUSE
INCUBATING OBSTETRICS IN EARLY MODERN BOLOGNA
Kim Sexton

When Bologna's renowned university was founded in 1088, its fame rested primarily on the study of law and the liberal arts, while medicine was the field for which the universities of Salerno, and later Padua, were celebrated. Counter-Reformation restrictions on scientific and intellectual inquiry precipitated a decline for Bologna's great Studium from the preeminence it had long held in Europe as a leader in liberal education.[1] Yet, even as enrollments plummeted, the Emilian capital produced widely recognized experts in emerging modern sciences, including mathematicians like Giovanni Cassini (1671–1712), who left Bologna in 1669 to direct Louis XIV's new astronomical observatory in Paris; and surgeon Giovanni Antonio Galli (1708–82), a pioneer in modern midwifery and the founder of an obstetrics school in his own home in the 1730s. His residence is known to historians as the Casa Nascentori, a sixteenth-century *palazzetto* on Via Drapperie located in the heart of Bologna's busy market area (Figure 15.1). While built in the 1520s by the Nascentori, a family of glassmakers, for their business and domicile, this edifice can claim a meaningful position in the history of healthcare architecture.

Galli was a surgeon, man-midwife, and trainer of midwives of both genders. In his teaching, he employed an unprecedented array of obstetrical wood, clay, wax, and papier-mâché models as well as devices with moving parts (*macchine*)—some two hundred pieces in all—which he commissioned from Bolognese sculptors and modelers.[2] For such a professional to manage a school of midwifery in his own residence and to use anatomical models in the process is a rare, but not entirely isolated, occurrence in European medicine. Extraordinary scientists in Bologna, such as Galli and Cassini, came into their leading professional roles not solely via university curricula but also through private academies. Structurally, these organizations were private in that they sprang from personal initiatives, but they were public as well, inasmuch as they were open to anyone with the skill, desire, and time to join.[3] Galli's obstetrical school was a type of private academy, and, as with other such circles, its "headquarters" was the leader's residence. To situate Galli's residence within the history of healthcare architecture, his Casa Nascentori might be compared with the meeting places of other private academies to gauge how "public" his house-school was. But, while some six hundred or so private academies came and went in Italy between 1525 and 1700, their meeting places are rarely seriously studied, at least in part because they do not readily lend themselves to conventional methods of architectural analysis. Most groups—like Galli's—met in respectable, but unremarkable, residences. They could change meeting locations rather frequently in the often short duration of their existences. The visual and physical traces of these intellectual networks also constituted themselves in ephemeral contact zones such as streets and squares as members came and went from meetings.

Of particular interest in this architectural puzzle is a novel description of Galli's house-school by philosopher and scientist Francesco Maria Zanotti, who became president of the Institute of the Sciences in 1766. In 1755, Zanotti wrote that "the most illustrious school of [his] house [was] dedicated to begetting, frequented by surgeons and the most enterprising midwives."[4] He gushed further, "you can see from his private chambers that he once dedicated the enclosed space to the female uterus."[5] Through the language of embodiment, his characterization almost identifies Galli's house as a women's health center, but to think that women actually

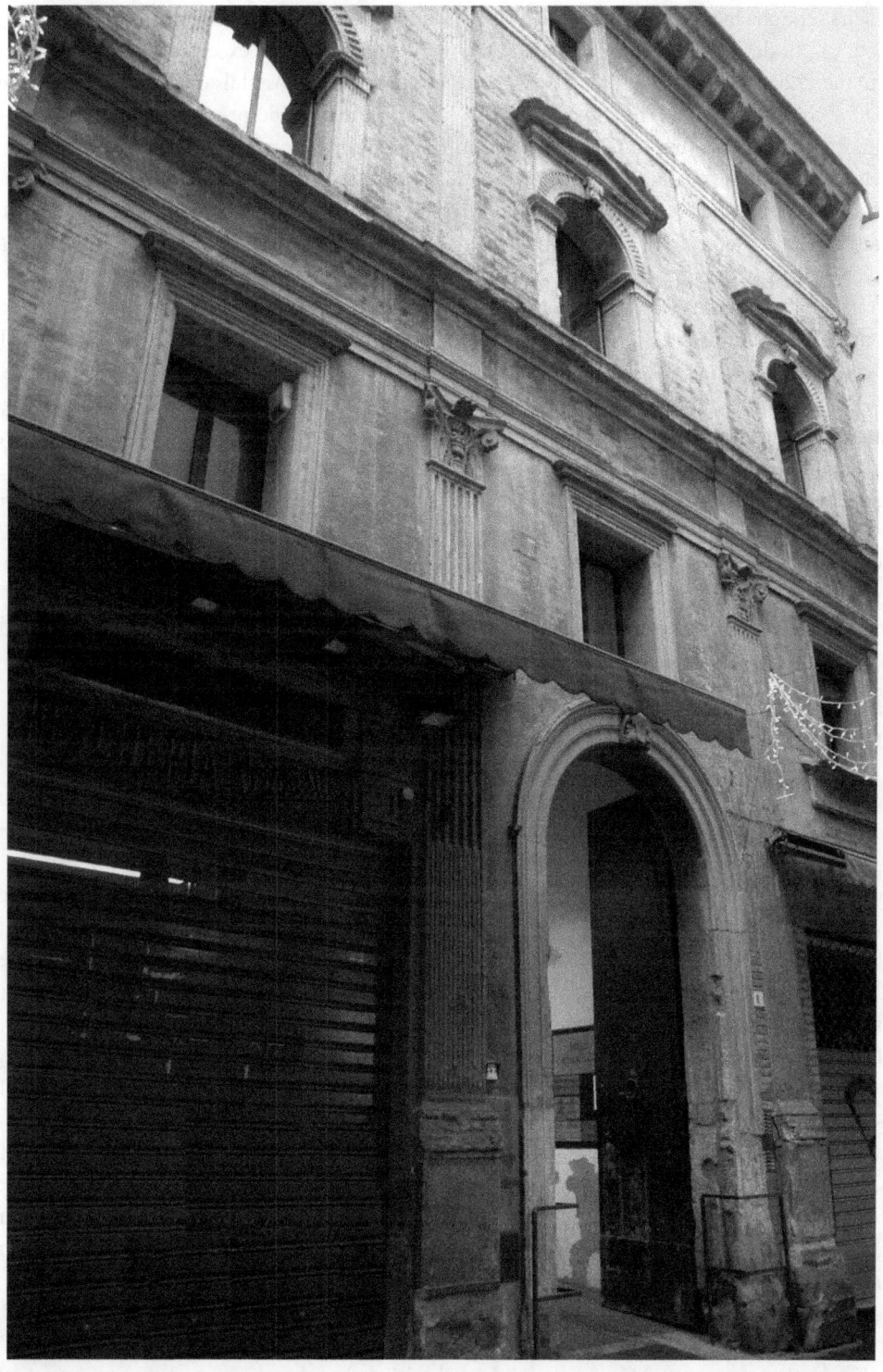

Figure 15.1 Casa Nascentori, Bologna (via Drapperie, 8), *c.* 1527–50 Photo: author

went to Galli's school while pregnant or to give birth would contradict nearly everything historians of Europe know about premodern parturition. This history holds that, with a few exceptions, women gave birth at home until the 1920s, at which point wealthy women started going to hospitals on account of newly available anesthesia for childbirth. Even then, hospital births did not become widespread until after the mid-century point. Still, Zanotti's description of Galli's house is intriguing. On the one hand, it was a private house—the typical setting for childbirth—but, on the other hand, it was more than a home at a time when maternity wards (*ospizi per partorienti* or simply *maternità*) were first emerging in some Italian cities.[6] Galli's "house dedicated to begetting" emerged at a transitional time in the design of healthcare facilities, a time for which we are in the process of defining the norm.

Research I have recently conducted on Galli's house-academy in Bologna has turned up records of renovations to the plumbing, heating, and windows of his house. Galli supervised these changes himself, and they could relate to the residence's transformation into "a most illustrious school," including the remote possibility that Galli received "patients" there. His school was a place where midwives of both genders gathered for the latest in experimental and demonstration-based lessons, and these activities required a laboratory of sorts. Discussion of the physical form of Galli's house leads to questions of interest for architectural historians of healthcare facilities, questions that this chapter seeks to address. Above all, what exactly did Zanotti and others *see* in Galli's house? What did they literally behold when looking at the building, and what kind of facility was it conceptually that excited them so? Even though Galli's residence was healthcare architecture without professional architects, it stands in the field of design at a critical juncture in medical history—that is, between medieval natural philosophy and modern science—and it responded to specific contextual issues in Bologna, which were related to the social and cultural roles of private academies.

Shifting Thresholds

Galli's obstetrical school—being housed in a private residence, run by a male doctor, and based on empirical pedagogies that deployed as many as two hundred wax and clay anatomical models and operable *macchine* (Figure 15.2)—occupied a position in an unaccustomed relationship between old and new healthcare establishments. In pre- and early modern Italy, medical education and practice operated in domains that were more distinct and separate than they are in the present day. Training was theoretical and took place in universities; doctors visited the sick at home, unless they were poor, in which case physicians treated them in hospitals.[7] The architectural precedent for European hospitals was the monastery. In fact, convents often literally served as hospitals. Their cloisters, prayer spaces, and large halls (refectories, dormitories, etc.) found practical uses in the service of healing, and their design for seclusion from the outside world and regulated, collective organization of living offered a logical precedent.[8] For similar reasons, the monastery was likewise the model for many university colleges in Europe.

Childbirth, however, presented a different set of circumstances from ordinary healthcare. While life-threatening, parturition was not a disease, and, like the sick, women wanted to be in domestic settings when they gave birth. They wanted a female midwife to attend to their needs. Man-midwives were rare until the eighteenth century and remained uncommon even afterward except in England and its colonies.[9] Surgeons, the vast majority of whom were male, were called in only when critical births threatened the life of the mother or baby. Female midwives trained future practitioners of the art on the job at the bedside of women in labor. Women who did give birth in hospitals—for instance, in Paris's twenty-four bed "maternity ward"—were often on the margins of society.[10] Many were unmarried, while others were poor, victims of domestic violence, or at risk of acute and life-threatening deliveries. The stigma of illegitimate pregnancy in particular, which would only worsen in the nineteenth century, tended to taint the reputation of hospitals and, by association,

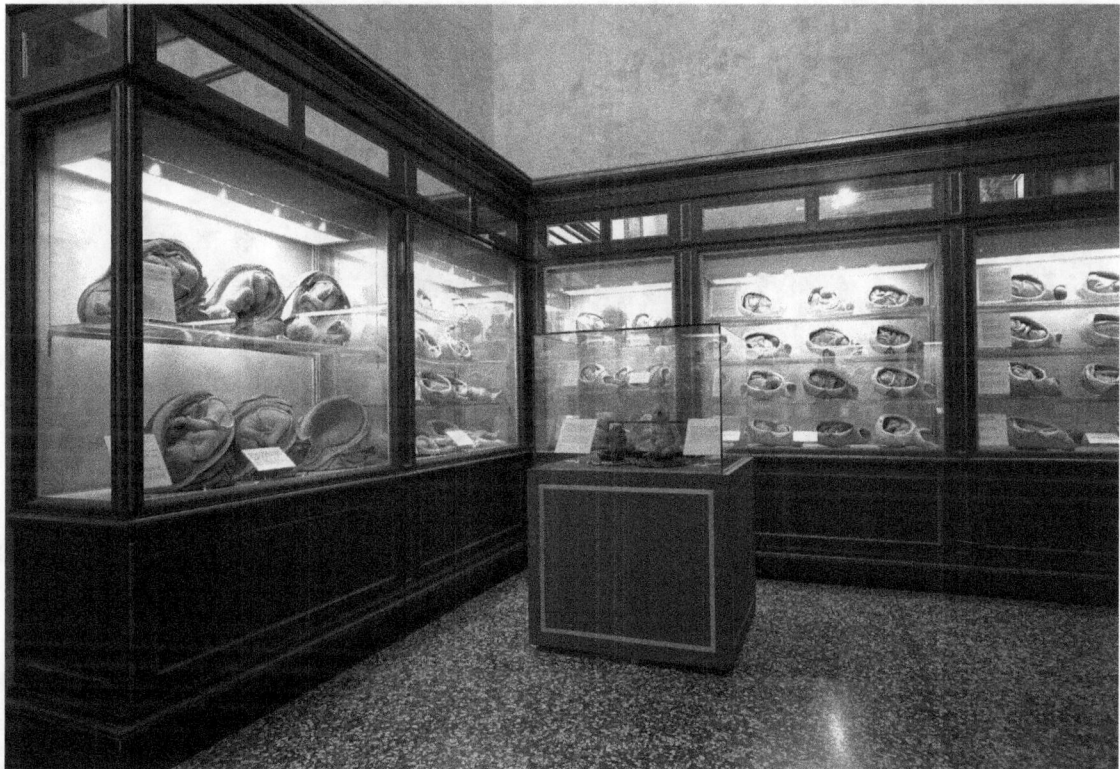

Figure 15.2 Obstetrical models made for Giovanni Antonio Galli between 1734 and 1746/50 by Anna Morandi and Giovanni Manzolini and others, as installed in the Museo di Palazzo Poggi, Bologna Photo: Phillip Bond/Alamy Stock Photo

all who gave birth there.[11] Galli and his house-school thus juxtapose old and new concepts in premodern healthcare—midwife and surgeon (or man-midwife), domestic residence and training facility, prosthetic wombs (models, etc.), and flesh-and-blood trainees—to emerge as a compelling counterweight to received social and architectural histories of hospitals.

Galli's house-academy was betwixt and between historical moments in healthcare in other ways as well. Primary among these was its origin in the milieu of private academies, rather than in the domain of university clinics or home birthing. More than sixty private academies thrived in Bologna from the sixteenth through eighteenth centuries.[12] By the late seventeenth and early eighteenth century, academies dedicated to science facilitated the real and sometimes culturally risky work of empirical research. Most universities, including Bologna's, still taught received knowledge from Renaissance treatises based largely on classical texts. It was not unusual, however, for professors, including surgeons like Galli, to not only hold a university chair and deliver scheduled lectures but also to organize a private academy in which they met with truly committed men of science, literature, or history—whatever the focus of a given circle was. Galli's school was exceptional in that the focus on childbirth ensured that many of his students were women. Female membership in other private salons is not unknown, but they were male-dominated networks.[13]

Galli's academy would become closely associated with another novel betwixt-and-between institution in Bologna: the Institute of the Sciences, established in 1714 (Figure 15.3).[14] The Institute specialized in the experimental sciences, and for that reason competed with the university, where natural philosophy was taught through theoretical methodologies. Here, too, scholars were often both professors at the university

Health and Architecture

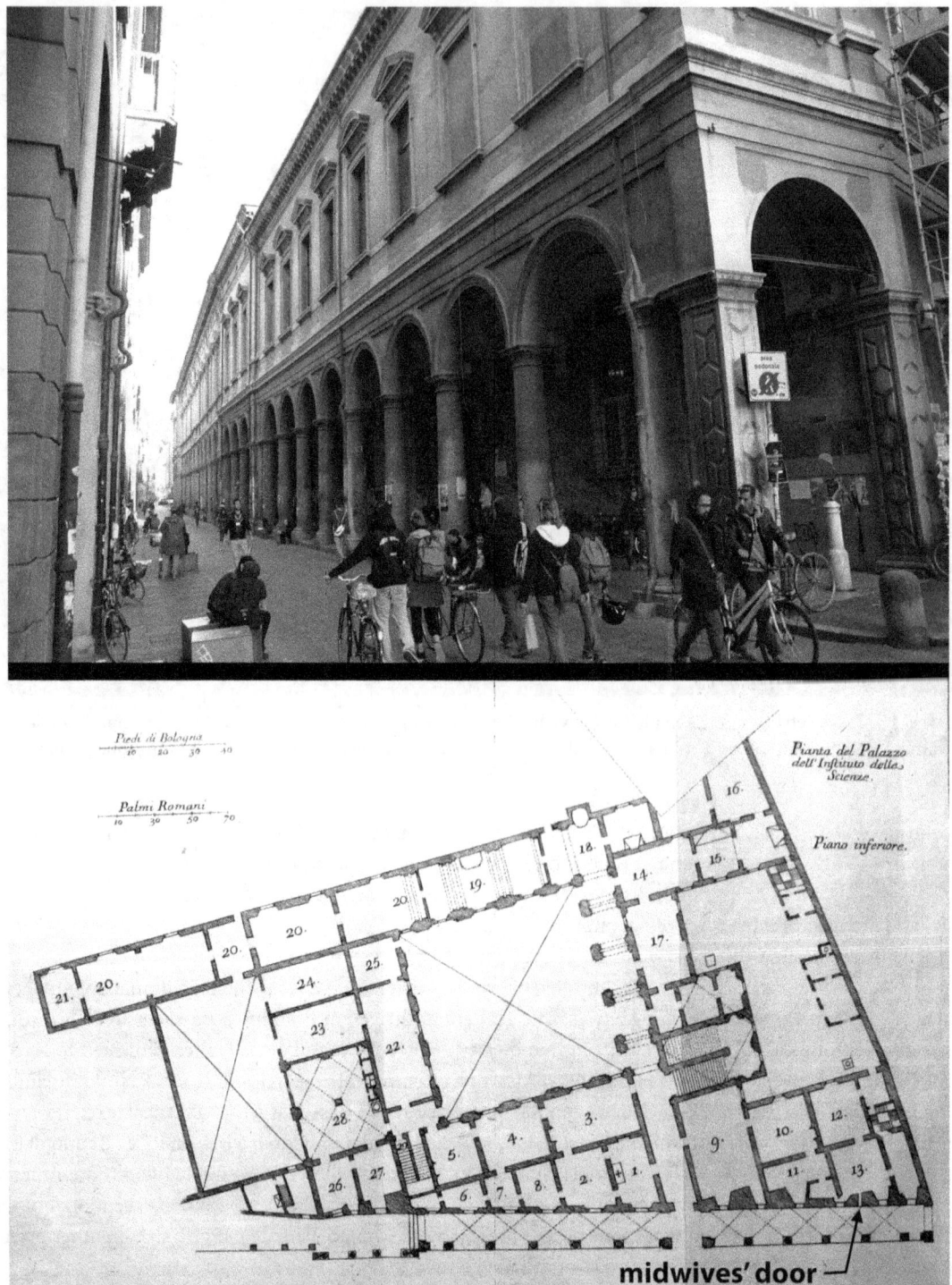

Figure 15.3 Palazzo Poggi, Bologna, 1549–60, with alterations after it became home to the Institute of the Sciences in 1711. Above, the facade on via Zamboni; below, plan of the ground floor, rooms 12 and 13 contained the obstetrical models. Photo: Kim Sexton; plan: Angelleli, *Notizie dell'origine, e progressi dell'Instituto delle scienze di Bologna*, 1780

and members of the Institute of the Sciences, as Galli was, as were some rare female scientists like Laura Bassi (1711–78).[15] Lastly, science academies, including Galli's school, and the Institute of the Sciences were essential organizational elements in the transition between the traditional practices of premodern healing on the one hand, and the medicalization of healthcare on the other. The trajectory is very familiar to historians, and its impact on women's healthcare is well known: From its start in the late eighteenth century, the professionalization and codification of medicine led to the establishment of modern disciplinary fields, such as obstetrics, and the marginalization of women, especially midwives, in healthcare practices.[16]

Galli's obstetrics academy was technically not the first school for midwifery in Europe, but it became a model for many that came after. The term "obstetrics" is anachronistic for the eighteenth century, but it is used on occasion in this chapter to refer to the plurality of people involved in pre- and postnatal care and delivery.[17] The first training center for *accoucheuses* may well have been that founded in 1531 by barber-surgeon Ambroise Paré within the Hôtel-Dieu hospital in Paris, an impressive complex containing 279 beds, 24 of which, as noted, were designated for childbirth.[18] Midwifery schools attached to hospitals or university clinics became more widespread in the eighteenth century, first in Northern Europe and later in Italy. In 1728 Turin's Ospedale Maggiore established the first Italian training facility on the premises of a hospital. The earliest obstetrical schools connected to Italian universities did not arise until 1818 in Pavia and 1819 in Padua.[19] The spatial contiguity of a school coupled with a clinic was especially advantageous to male surgery students and man-midwives, because it gave them access to experience with actual deliveries. In Italy, the presence of a man in the birthing chamber met with an especially strong and enduring cultural resistance compared to elsewhere in Europe.[20] But the low social status of pregnant women in hospitals eroded the threshold of this taboo, making their bodies available to the medical touch and gaze of male and female health providers alike.[21]

In most places in Italy, anatomical uterine and fetal models had to suffice as surrogates for pregnant women in the flesh. But to say that the models "sufficed" as substitutes for bodies reveals a presentist bias against the power of early modern objects representing human anatomy. Eighteenth-century audiences viewed the materials of production—especially malleable media like wax and clay—and the sex of the maker, when female, as adding an organic dimension to its presence. As cultural historian Lucia Dacome put it, "the very act of wax-modelling resonated with long-term views of generation that regarded offspring as the result of the impression of soft matter."[22] Physicians were known to describe real fetuses as similar to wax in their vulnerable softness and to urge utmost care during deliveries, so that doughy newborns were not inadvertently disfigured by inept midwives and surgeons.[23] Even if an obstetrical school like Galli's was not a clinic with real women as patients, contemporaries were likely to see life, rather than inert, scientific objecthood, in the natural simulacra that filled its rooms.

It was a combination of the two hundred models installed in Galli's residence—his *suppellettile* or "furnishings," as they were known (Figure 15.2)—and the demonstrative teaching methods facilitated by this equipment that made the surgeon's house-academy so famous.[24] The "hall of deliveries" (*Salle des Accouchemens*), as French astronomer Jérôme Lalande called a large room in Galli's house, was "one of the most singular things in Europe for the study of anatomy."[25] The exquisite and numerous models crafted by Anna Morandi and her husband, Giovanni Manzolini, among others, made Galli's set-up "amazing," dazzling, and marvelous, as well as a source of pride for the entire city, according to science illuminati such as Jacopo Bartolomeo Beccari (1682–1766).[26] The Bolognese surgeon's example convinced other doctors in Italy to commission similar equipment—often directly from Bolognese sculptors and modelers—and to start schools in their own homes or in hospitals. Such was the case with surgeon Giacomo Bartolomei, who, in the 1760s, managed a school in his own residence in Siena. He supplied it with obstetrical models made in Bologna, like those he had seen when he visited Galli in 1762.[27] Already in 1773 the university in Siena had begun to purchase Bartolomei's models; by 1783, his collection numbered forty terra-cotta pieces.[28] Like professors who led private academies, Bartolomei had permission to give lessons in his house and in the hospital, but he came to prefer the university hospital, where bones and cadavers were easily available and where a delivery might happen at any hour.[29]

Bartolomei was far from the only specialist inspired by the fame and excellence of Galli's *supellex*. The surgeon Francesco Febbrari in Modena commissioned fifty-two obstetrical models from Bolognese sculptor Carlo Mondini for his *studio ostetrico*, which may have been in his house.[30] In Padua, Luigi Calza (1736–83), who studied with Galli and worked in Bologna, ordered a similar set of models in 1765/9 from Bolognese artists Giovan Battista Manfredini and Pietro Sandri. Calza's school was attached to the city's university clinic. Florentine doctor Giuseppe Galletti, who had visited Galli's collection in 1761, did not credit the famed surgeon with the expertise behind a collection of gynecological models he commissioned for the midwifery school at the Ospedale di S. Maria Nuova, which irked Bolognese professor of obstetrics Giambattista Fabbri (1806–74).[31] Even as far away as Rome, the science-minded Cardinal Francesco Saverio de Zelada (1717–1801) ordered thirty-six pieces in 1799 from Mondini for the Ospedale di S. Spirito, where they would be used in the education of midwives.[32] Still farther afield, and seemingly completely unaware of Galli's school, the Roman surgeon Antonio Santimorosi operated an obstetrical school in Macerata by 1789, where he instructed both male surgery students and midwives. Santimorosi had devised a unique artificial uterus of leather and waxed silk, in which he would insert preserved fetal cadavers in order to demonstrate certain embryotic operations.[33] As in many cases, sources do not situate Santimorosi's *camera ostetrica* in a specific locale, be it a university, hospital, or residence. Amid these progressive educational initiatives, historians must not lose sight of the hundreds of private houses in which women continued to both teach midwifery and put it into practice in the delivery of babies and prenatal consultations.

The Architecture of Galli's Residence in the Context of Private Academies

To come to grips with the design of Galli's residence as an early, or a localized, chapter in the history of healthcare architecture first entails a close examination of the design of the building and its location in the city of Bologna in relation to other buildings where learning about female anatomy and problematic childbirth took place. When Galli opened his obstetrical school in around 1734, it occupied one half of the tidy sixteenth-century Casa Nascentori.[34] The house and location suited his school's purposes, but he clearly did not have the building designed *for* his obstetrical academy. In fact, he only rented half of the building, as his father Angelo Camillo Galli had before him.[35] The building, having been constructed by the Nascentori family of glassmakers with their business in mind, had two shop spaces on its street front, a long, vaulted corridor leading to the interior courtyard, and residential apartments upstairs. It therefore falls within the typology of a *palazzetto*, a small palazzo accessible to an upper-middle-class clientele with some pretentions. The applied pilasters on its facade speak to a modish, but not cutting-edge, awareness of contemporary stylistic currents. Despite the normalcy of the architecture, there are many ways in which Galli's circle of obstetrical professionals may have externalized their presence through their building.

One fundamental strategy in "advertising" the school's presence lay in the selection of a location in downtown Bologna (Figure 15.4). While Galli appears to have been passive with regard to the exact position, he did retain the house his father rented when he could have sought other premises. The Nascentori had selected wisely for their own commercial activity, in that the house stands not only on the busy north–south Via Drapperie in the city's bustling market area but also anchors the two-block-long Via Pescherie Vecchie, the east terminus of which is right at the facade of the Casa Nascentori. Clearly, Galli did not shrink from public visibility. On the contrary, he embraced it. Indeed, the location was only two blocks away from the city's

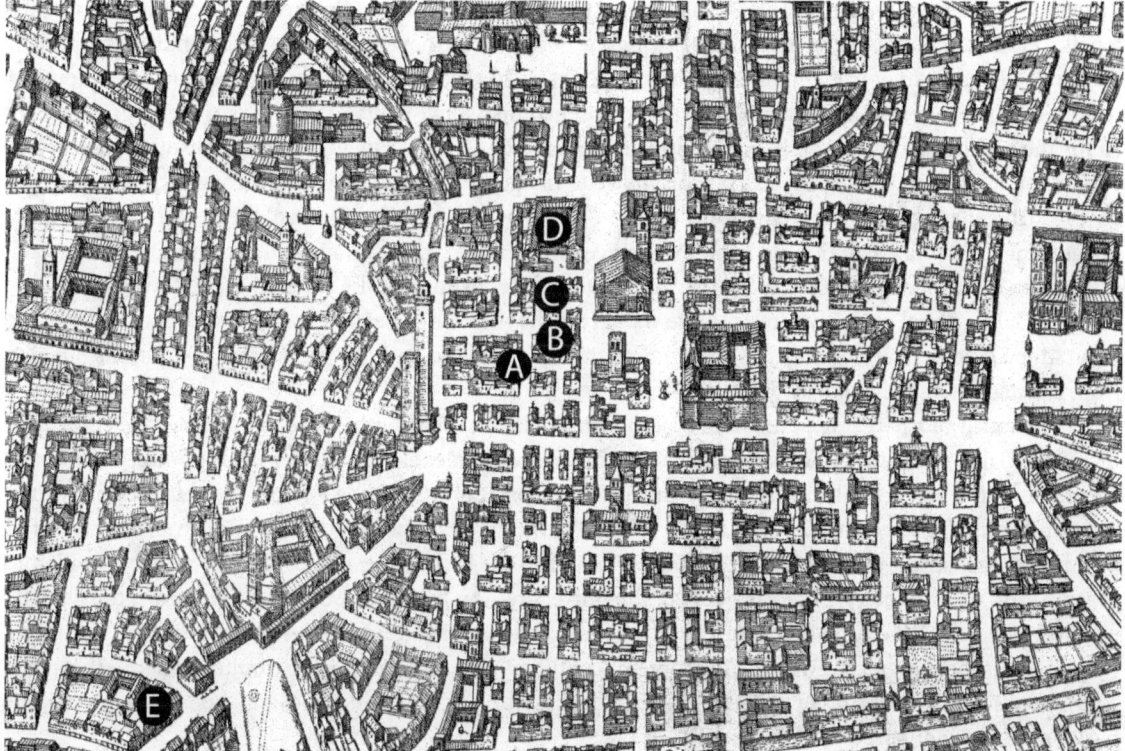

Figure 15.4 The geography of early modern medicine in central Bologna, showing the location of key schools and hospitals. A. Antonio Galli's house-academy (Casa Nascentori); B. Santa Maria della Vita; C. Santa Maria della Morte; D. the Archiginnasio; E. Institute of Sciences (Palazzo Poggi). Image: after Georg Braun and Franz Hogenberg, *Civitates orbis terrarum*, vol. 4 (Cologne, 1588); photo: author

center of government on the Piazza Maggiore. Equally important, it seems, was proximity to old and new medical service establishments. Within two blocks of Galli's residence stood the city's largest hospital, Santa Maria della Vita, founded in 1289 to assist pilgrims and the sick. Not far away was the similarly named hospital of Santa Maria della Morte, founded in 1347 for the sick poor. The architecture of these two hospitals was monastic, making use of cloisters, refectories, and large dormitories. Finally, only a few doors away stood the imposing Archiginnasio, erected in 1562–3 to serve as the new university center and provide lecture halls for courses in natural science and anatomy. The architecture of most educational buildings at the time, including the Archiginnasio, belonged to a cortile-centered residential typology (i.e., two to three stories, a handsome facade, and a porticoed courtyard). In contrast to the nearby hospitals, the early modern Archiginnasio was similar to Galli's Casa Nascentori, only much grander, based, as it was, on the *palazzo* of the elite citizenry.[36] In terms of location, the surgeon had shrewdly elected to hold on to a position in the city that ensured his new school was shored up by both venerable monastic and modern medical facilities, all the while being highly visible to the consuming and governing public.

About a century before Galli opened his school, the city's celebrated Anatomy Theater (1637–49) was installed in the Archiginnasio. The new arrival contributed to making the environs a growing center of medical renown. Ensconced within a remodeled lecture hall, the Anatomy Theater was a performative space and, just as the name proclaims, a setting in which anatomical lessons were reenacted for mixed audiences of city magistrates, clergy, university scholars, and ordinary citizens. Public dissections of male and, less frequently, female bodies took place there, most often during the period of Carnevale, a timing which indicates that such "lessons" were a form of pre-Lenten entertainment. This held true even if professors and doctors conducted serious debates there, as Laura Bassi did in 1732. The encompassing totality of such events, perhaps especially so for the rare female professor, is even illustrated in a famous Insignia degli Anziani Consoli.[37] They began with great pomp with professors, star pupils, and celebrity guests making their way through the streets of the city, ensuring that large numbers of citizens were aware of the occasion. The climax of the ritual in the Anatomy Theater makes it clear that, despite being in a university building, this famous hall was not a laboratory for research in experimental science, as private academies or the Institute of the Sciences were. Nevertheless, the fact that Galli's school was only a five-minute walk from the Anatomy Theater meant his school's presence and reputation could benefit not only from neighbors that included old and new healthcare institutions but also from popular interest in medical discoveries.

While much of the real experimental research in the later seventeenth and early eighteenth centuries—including Galli's midwifery studies—took place in private academies assembled in private homes, Galli would eventually move his school into an elite "institutional" palazzo at the edge of the city after twenty-three years in the city center. In 1758, he had his school, including his models and *macchine*, transferred to the palazzo of the Institute of the Sciences (Figures 15.2 and 15.4). At the time, the forty-three-year-old academic organization was still not yet officially part of the university. The Institute's building, still known today by its original name, the Palazzo Poggi, began its existence in the sixteenth century as a private palazzo. Additions were made as the Institute grew.[38] The fundamental outlines of its architecture were quite similar to the larger Archiginnasio. Like many other early modern residences in Bologna, including Galli's house, these were not particularly individualized designs.

In spite of its conventional appearance, the Galli residence might still have advertised the presence of the specialized medical school it housed and, in the process, helped market early advances in obstetrical sciences to the public. Some Bolognese academies did assert their identity through the architecture of their places of assembly, thereby establishing a precedent for others, like Galli, to follow suit. The Palazzo Bocchi, the "Domus Academiae" of a literary salon, is one precocious example (1546–60). It was designed equally as the home of Achille Bocchi (1488–1562) and the headquarters of his group, the Accademia Ermatena.[39] The building verbalized the academy's purpose through inscriptions and sculpted emblematic imagery on its facade as well as published architectural "portraits."[40] Another was the Palazzo Marsili (1653–81), meeting place of the Academy of the Unquiet, a circle of experimental philosophers (mathematicians, physicists, physicians, and anatomists), and home to their leader, naturalist and military commander Luigi Fernando Marsili (1658–1730). The professional equipment and specialized library required by this group was such that, in 1705, Marsili had an observatory tower (*specola*), on which telescopes could be mounted, added to the family palazzo (Figure 15.5). He was the only leader of a Bolognese academy to build one.[41] The tower etched the activities and ambitions of the science academy onto the skyline of southern Bologna. Through architectural objects, inscriptions, and representations, buildings housing private academies aspired to be part of public life.

The premises of the Palazzo Marsili proved too limiting for the Academy of the Unquiet, and in 1711 the group became the founding organization of the Institute of the Sciences, the progressive think tank that would eventually welcome Galli's obstetrical academy, after some internal resistance, in 1758.[42] Marsili had all the equipment, books, and instruments transferred from his residence to the Palazzo Poggi, newly acquired for this purpose, and a monumental *specola* added to the building in 1723–5.[43] Bologna's Torre della Specola represents the Palazzo Poggi's first decisive step away from its conventional residential mold. If a facade or a tower could summon a private academy, represent it, promote it, and mediate access to it, it could also help

Uterus House

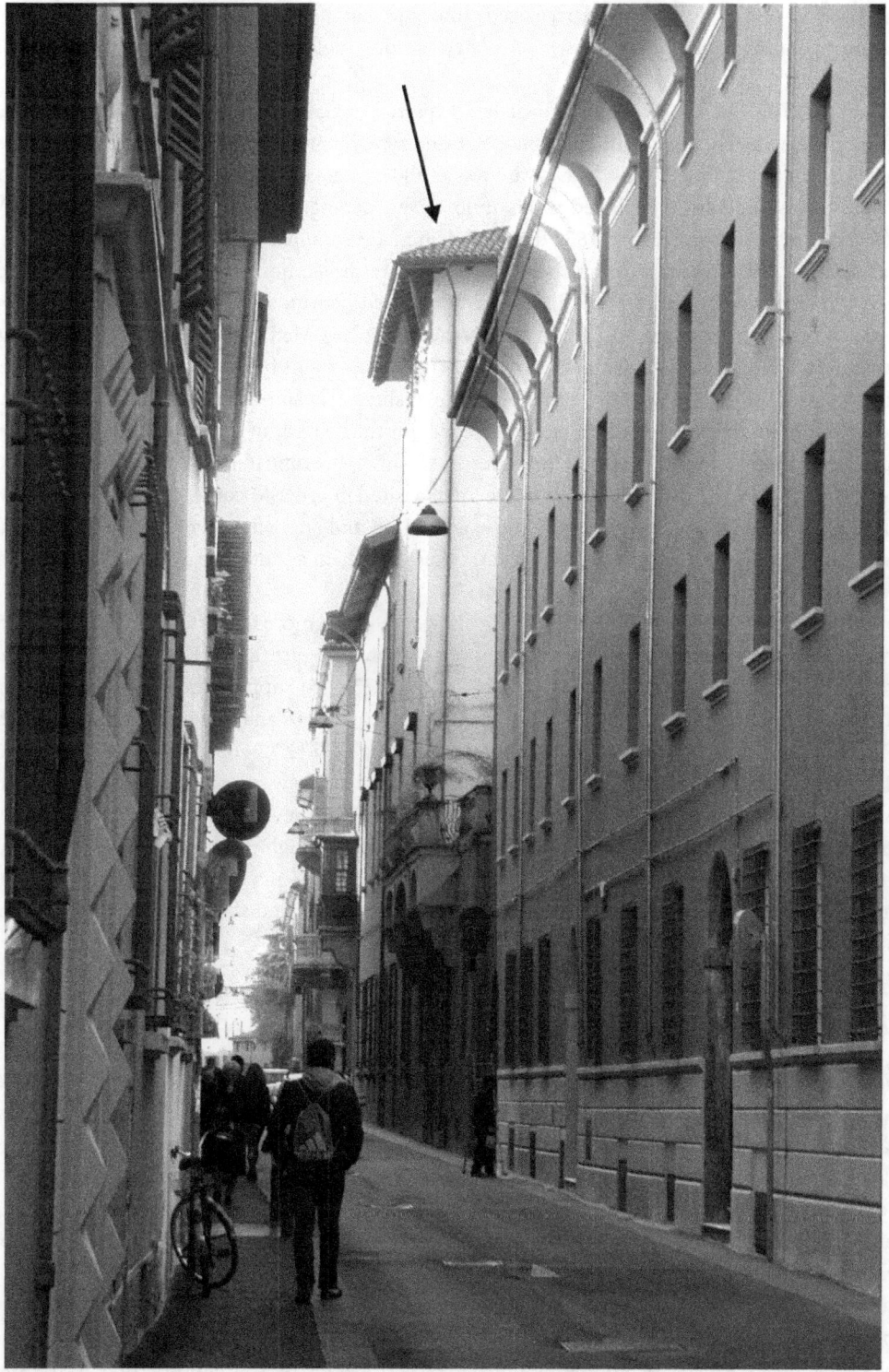

Figure 15.5 Palazzo Marsili, Bologna (via D'Azeglio 48), 1653–81, rebuilding of an earlier palazzo on the site, sometimes attributed to Francesco Dotti. The arrow points to the remains of the observatory tower. Photo: Kim Sexton

create an evocative and a symbolically experienced atmosphere in the public space around a building.[44] While lacking an arrogant tower or a purposefully articulated facade, Galli's residence was not without possibilities in this regard.

One might assume that the "internal knowledge" explored in Galli's obstetrical school was pointedly not destined to make an ostentatious, public display. But one factor that rendered Galli's unassuming residence visible and known as a "uterus house" was awareness of the contents it harbored, that is, the numerous clay and wax obstetrical models he deployed in his innovative teaching. In fact, Bolognese anatomist Michele Medici (1782–1859) could still rave in 1857 that Galli had made the *suppellettile* the "ornament and delight of his private house."[45] Medici's enthusiasm for Galli's healthcare-driven house must have been inspired either by collective memory or by Zanotti's earlier description (cited above), since Galli's school had moved into the palazzo of the Institute of the Sciences a hundred years earlier. Medici was not alone in praising Galli's female anatomical models as the "ornament and delight" of the surgeon's house. Contemporary physician and physicist Luigi Galvani (1737–98) also found Galli's furnishings "beautiful and elegant."[46] Moreover, while Francesco Febbrari in Modena waited a couple of decades for the delivery of fifty-two obstetrical models from sculptor Carlo Mondini, the artist enjoyed their presence in his own home in Bologna, calling them "décor for his house."[47] He wrote that many scholars and foreigners visited in order to contemplate the hidden wonders his work revealed to them and left satisfied. The examination and appreciation of relatively small table-top pieces like Galli's models helped give his rooms and others like them an intimate domesticity more typical of a cultural salon than a classroom or anatomy theater.[48]

Interior "decoration" with anatomical models did, however, have a more famous—and more architectural—local precedent in the Anatomy Theater's skinned atlas figures (Figure 15.6). Known as the *Spellati* ("the Skinned Men"), the two wooden statues were installed in 1733–4 to support the canopy of the professor's *cathedra*, the perch from which he presided over public dissections and anatomy lessons. While these depict correct male musculature, as designed by wax-modeler Ercole Lelli (1702–66) and sculpted by Il Lucchese (1680–1750), they were not teaching tools.[49] Rather, they occupied a new sphere in which medicine and high art joined forces to form a classical order of science. As noted above, the Anatomy Theater was a space for the performance of knowledge rather than the practice of medicine, so a high rhetorical register for the language of architecture in this setting was quite suitable. As with a decor consisting of obstetrical models, many early modern viewers appreciated the revelation of interior organic worlds and the coexistence of verisimilitude, scientific fact, and beauty.

Externalizing Obstetrics

Galli, who had been a professor of surgery at the University of Bologna since 1736, was eligible to lecture in the Anatomy Theater, but the interior of his residence-school is the starting point for an alternative analysis of healthcare architecture for education through surrogate bodies. Like the pregnant, embryo-sheltering female bodies that inspired the descriptions of Zanotti and Medici, Galli's house contained the nearly two hundred lifelike obstetrical models crafted by Morandi and Manzolini. The installation of these anatomical models today in the Palazzo Poggi, the home of the Institute of the Sciences to which they, along with the school itself, were transferred, may offer some idea of how this equipment would have transformed a domestic space into a healthcare laboratory (see Figure 15.2). Before their transfer into the Palazzo Poggi, these sculpted and modeled objects were both ornaments, at least in the eighteenth-century understanding of the term, and novel apparatuses, capable of simulating normal and critical birthing situations. They were essential to demonstration-based teaching methods.[50] When in 1755 Zanotti praised Galli's "house of begetting," he also

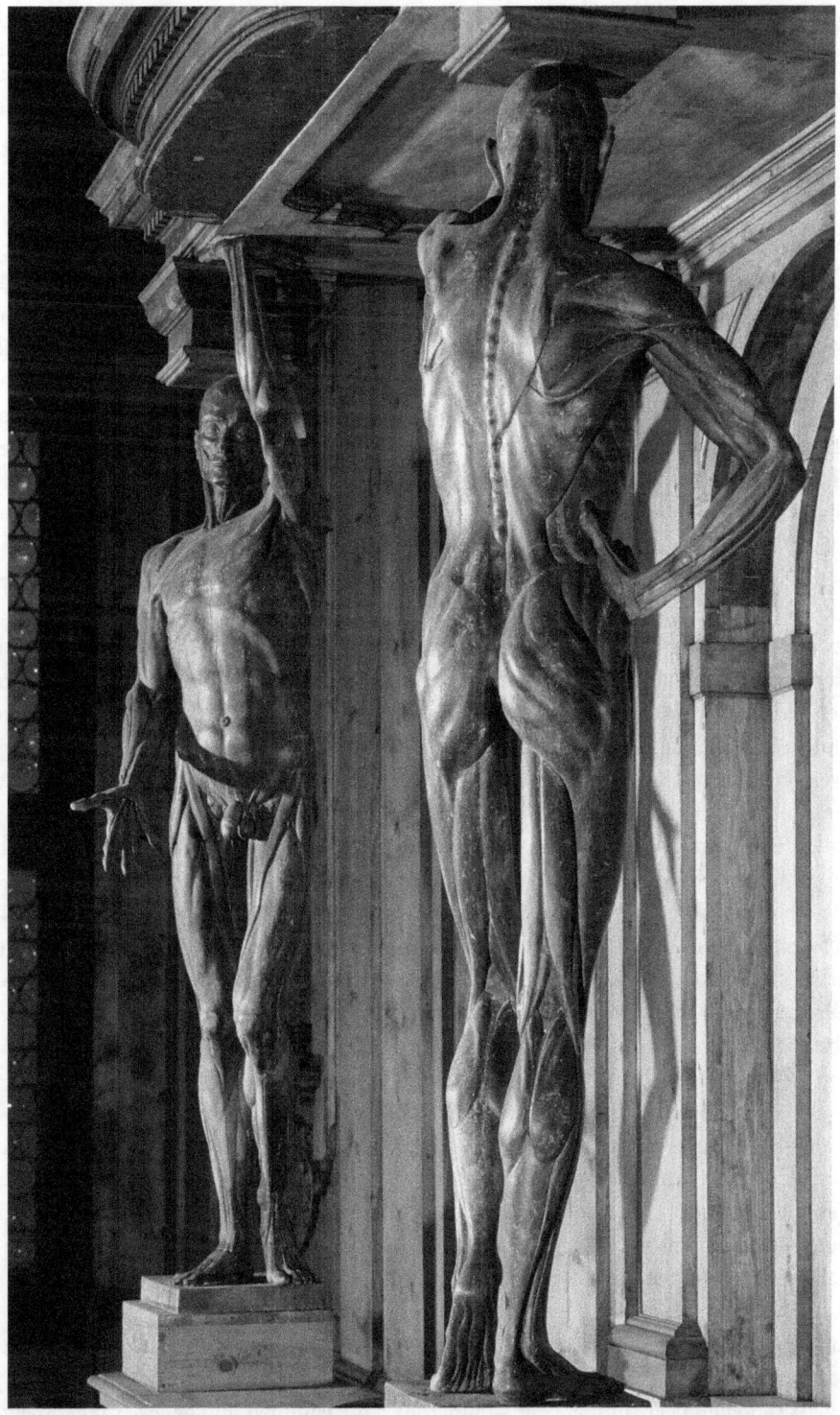

Figure 15.6 The *Spellati*, 1638–49, by Antonio Levanti, skinned atlas figures in the Anatomy Theater in the Palazzo dell'Archiginnasio, Bologna. Photo: Raffaello Bencini/Alinari Archives, Florence

offered admiring insights into the pedagogical advances taking place in Galli's residence: "Nor did he enhance significantly this part of medicine [i.e., obstetrics] through the art of speaking, but rather in another way altogether … he taught by means of numerous representations [the models], formed out of earth or other materials through wondrous art, not without great expense. Here all ways of giving birth appear."[51] A detailed description of some of the models follows in Zanotti's text. Co-opting the language of pregnancy and birthing, he juxtaposed the modern teaching of the medical arts through *seeing* the body and its parts with the old and inferior way of verbal discourse—i.e., that which still took place at the university.

The visibility of Galli's obstetrical group and the female corporeal proxies depended in part on the commercial origins of his palazzo, built as it was to suit the business needs of the Nascentori glassmakers. Unnoted in previous architectural histories of the building, a notary by the name of Antonio Moratti owned the property when Galli's father leased half of it in 1720. For four years, the elder Galli proceeded to make several repairs to the dwelling (see Figure 15.1).[52] The building had not been designed with healthcare in mind, obviously, when Galli's school moved into the building in 1734. In 1743, after almost a decade in residence, Galli himself started to make improvements to the house, changes which may indicate that the premises were proving inadequate to the demands the obstetrical academy placed on it. Details of these renovations—both Galli's and his father's—were recorded because they were the cause of a dispute between the younger Galli and Moratti in 1748–9. The notarial proceedings describe structural changes as well as alterations of some of the rooms and their furnishings; unfortunately, no floor plans of the building survive before or after these interventions.[53]

Links between Galli's alterations and the needs of his academy, including a desire for public recognition, seem clear and logical. The differences between the remodeling projects of father and son suggest that the latter's projects were directly related to the activities of the school. This is not surprising on the face of it, but the thoroughness of the changes indicates the house was more laboratory than dwelling. For instance, the litigation reveals a priority placed on greater illumination and improved heating and aseptic conditions.[54] The documents mention the remaking of a conduit through which water passed for the kitchen. Specimens in liquids could form part of an obstetrics teaching studio, so services for handling them with efficiency and tidiness would have been desirable.[55] Places with armoires ("luoghi coi armarij"), which could have held obstetrical models, are also mentioned.[56] Galli's Sienese counterpart, Giacomo Bartolomei, expressed appreciation for armoires in which to store anatomical models properly, but, for him, these were to be found in the university clinic, not necessarily in his own home.[57] Without Bartolomei's option of making use of a hospital, Galli adapted his house to the necessary furnishings rather than the furnishings to the house. It is not impossible that Galli had these repairs and modifications done for the sake of his own comfort, but they suggest the professional efficiency of a building designed for medical work.

The renovated Casa Nascentori not only sheltered Galli's school, but it helped externalize it as well. Several of Galli's alterations enhanced not only the illumination within the building but also visibility from exterior to interior. He remodeled a large salon (*sala*)—possibly the one mentioned by Lalande and Beccari—and described it as opening onto a galleria, possibly a courtyard arcade (Figure 15.7) or the entrance corridor.[58] At least one upper suite of rooms had a loggia and a lower one received large glazed windows.[59] He closed one loggia "to make better use of the space," but added glazed windows with iron bars, suggesting proximity to the public and a need for security.[60] Two rooms near the street received six windows. While these need not have been at ground level, four large, now closed, openings in the entrance corridor (Figure 15.7) could account for at least some of the six.[61] All of these qualities suggest a transformed residence, one even more public than the original glass shop had been, in that Galli's numerous large windows and galleries potentially invited the gaze of curious citizens to penetrate farther into the interior.

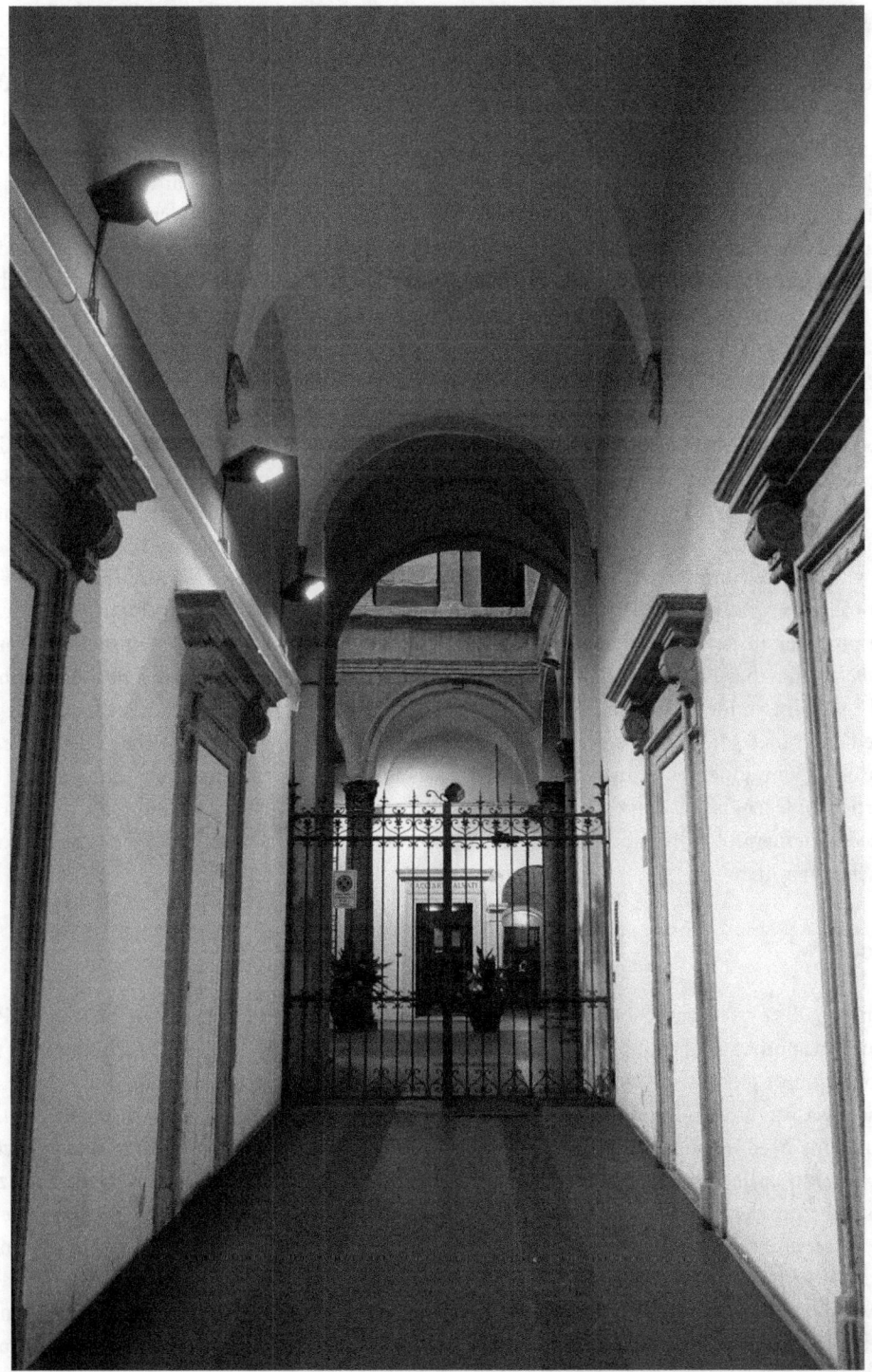

Figure 15.7 Casa Nascentori, Bologna, *c.* 1527–50, passage from street to courtyard, with later alterations. Photo: Kim Sexton

Health and Architecture

While undoubtedly prompted by multiple concerns, the nature of the extensive remodeling could not help but enhance the marketing of obstetrical science to the public, including pregnant women anxious about their futures. Nevertheless, a certain amount of mystery must have still shrouded this interior-oriented, uterine enclosure. A letter Galli wrote in 1757 to Flaminio Scarselli, secretary to the city's ambassador to Rome, reveals that Bolognese Senator Sigismondo Malvezzi had never laid eyes on the *suppellettile*, nor had wax-modeler Ercole Lelli for that matter, the latter on account of his jealous antagonism toward Anna Morandi, creator of many of the obstetrical models.[62] The equipment was therefore probably not overly conspicuous from the street.[63] But the sheer number of models, coupled with the increased fenestration, must have yielded some enticing sights for attentive and curious passersby, creating a "shop" that hawked both medical knowledge and promises of safer parturition.

The focus on water, heat, and light raises the question of whether Galli's residence could have functioned as a clinic actually visited by patients seeking care. If so, it was certainly a most precocious space. At minimum, the renovations Galli ordered for the Casa Nascentori transformed it from a home into a "facility," one comfortable and practicable for numerous students and midwives, whose learning and practice were intimately connected in life-and-death situations beyond the threshold of this private academy. But similarities between Galli's domicile and those domestic settings that actually sheltered pregnant women until they gave birth would have already blurred the lines between school, clinic, and dwelling. For example, some midwives hosted unmarried pregnant women in their own homes, maintaining *pensioni* for this purpose for clients who could afford to pay.[64] This longstanding type of arrangement had a traditional healthcare provider in her own home, overseeing a "patient" from pre- to postnatal care. Conceivably, the *accoucheuse* may have taught other women the techniques of midwifery in her house with her flesh-and-blood pregnant residents as the obstetrical "models." In such instances, school, clinic, and dwelling were indeed combined into a single premodern healthcare space. Viewed against the historical backdrop, Galli's house-academy emerges as an evolutionary phase of this discreet arrangement. His was one in which the proportion of learners was larger, a medical "professional" was the teacher, and the expectant mother was replaced with manifold, disembodied, but lifelike simulacra of her anatomy and the possible conditions that threatened her life.

Conclusion

In 1758, when Galli's obstetrical school was absorbed into the Institute of the Sciences in the Palazzo Poggi, the event was not an apotheosis of the uterus house as a gynecological hospital. Galli did obtain the right to decide how his collection of models was to be arranged in its new home, which, he stipulated, was to be precisely the same as it was in his own home.[65] The presence of Galli's academy and his obstetrical *suppellettile* in the Institute had long been resisted, because many leading professors did not view birthing as a science worthy of their space. Moreover, welcoming Galli's students meant the presence of women in the Palazzo Poggi, including some from the lower social orders.[66] The pioneers of obstetrics had to reach a compromise with the leadership, a resolution that entailed the creation of a separate entrance, a small door ("piccola porticella") through which the handmaidens of female medicine came and went (see Figure 15.3).[67] Thus, Galli's private academy was swallowed up by a larger palazzo, a pompous edifice gendered male, not unlike the university's Palazzo dell'Archinnasio. The installation of Galli's academy in the Institute was in every way as asymmetrical as the emerging practice of modern obstetrics. Indeed, it is ironic that the exceedingly diminutive door for midwives actually stood out as an anomalous figure among the long, repetitive bays of the Palazzo Poggi's portico, like a dormant cell, invisible but in plain sight, like the homes where women gave birth in the dark privacy of their own rooms.

Galli's example of a house-based, school-centered academy may have been more common than historians have realized, but it was not a model with a long future for healthcare delivery as such. The convention of doctors making house calls to their patients' dwellings, for instance, was certainly more widespread and enduring than that of healthcare providers living and practicing in their own residences. In the world of obstetrics, the latter arrangement had a continuing chapter in the houses of midwives who offered *pensioni* to unwed mothers. On the whole, however, the first steps toward the medicalization of midwifery in Italy were to be found in maternity homes (*ospizi per partorienti*) in the late eighteenth century.[68] Trained midwives and surgeons were available not *in* the ward, but in attached obstetrical schools, a small step closer to a home-and-clinic setting.[69] Architecturally, however, the *ospizi per partorienti* were still based on the medieval monastery; in fact, some were literally part of a convent.[70] Hence, they did not contribute to the design history of healthcare facilities. Indeed, the organizational and architectural design of old and new healthcare facilities would long coexist together.

Galli's midwifery school, housed in half of a small palazzo, expands definitions of healthcare architecture for the premodern era in that it, while being a dwelling, was more laboratory than domicile. This and other early modern residences likely played a larger role in the history of medical buildings than is generally thought to be the case. Galli's house also suggests that historians might look for architectural concepts that gestated in minds not of architects, but of forward-looking scientists like Francesco Zanotti. Zanotti's enthusiastic description of Galli's uterus house holds precocious intimations of later theoretical horizons, including notions of architectural *caractère*, or buildings as sexed beings. The decor of obstetrical models may constitute the novel ornament for a new architectural order of science, and this too can be seen as anticipating architectural innovations to come. Conceptually speaking, new chapters in the history of healthcare architecture for the premodern period may, like Galli's school, be found on the edges of discipline.

Notes

1. David A. Lines, "Reorganizing the Curriculum: Teaching and Learning in the University of Bologna," *History of Universities* 26, no. 2 (2012): 1–59; Francesco Ceccarelli and Pier Luigi Cervellati, *Da un palazzo a una città: La vera storia della moderna Università di Bologna* (Bologna: Il Mulino, 1987).
2. See the concise biographies in Claudia Pancino, *Il bambino e l'acqua sporca: Storia dell'assistenza al parto dalle mammane alle ostetriche (secoli XVI–XIX)* (Milan: Franco Angeli, 1984), 97–102; and Lucia Dacome, *Malleable Anatomies: Models, Makers, and Material Culture in Eighteenth-Century Italy* (Oxford: Oxford University Press, 2017), 167–70.
3. Jürgen Habermas, *The Structural Transformation of the Public Sphere: An Inquiry into a Category of Bourgeois Society*, trans. T. Burger (Cambridge, MA: MIT Press, 1991), 35–7; Bronwen Wilson and Paul Yachnin, eds., *Making Publics in Early Modern Europe: People, Things, Forms of Knowledge* (New York: Routledge, 2010), 1–21.
4. "Sic ludum domi habet pariendi pulcherrimum, e quo chirurgi obstetricesque experientissimae prodierunt," from Francesco Maria Zanotti, *De Bononiensi Scientiarum et Artium Instituto atque Academia commentarii*, vol. 3 (Bologna, 1755), 88.
5. "… quippe qui in privatis suis aedibus muliebri utero conclave quondam dicavit," ibid.
6. In Italy, these modern maternity homes were tainted by some of the same social stigmas as hospitals. See Nadia Maria Filippini, "Gli ospizi per partorienti e i reparti di maternità tra il Sette e l'Ottocento," in *Gli ospedali in area padana fra Settecento e Novecento*, ed. Maria Luisa Betri and Edoardo Bressan (Milan: Feltrinelli, 1992), 395–411.
7. John Henderson, *The Renaissance Hospital: Healing the Body and Healing the Soul* (New Haven, CT: Yale University Press, 2006), 3–69.
8. John D. Thompson and Grace Goldin, *The Hospital: A Social and Architectural History* (New Haven, CT: Yale University Press, 1975), 10–40.
9. Adrian Wilson, *The Making of Man-Midwifery: Childbirth in England, 1660–1770* (Cambridge, MA: Harvard University Press, 1995), 1–7; Nadia Maria Filippini, "The Church, the State and Childbirth: The Midwife in Italy

during the Eighteenth Century," in *The Art of Midwifery: Early Modern Midwives in Europe*, ed. Hilary Marland (London: Routledge, 1994), 152–75, esp. 153–7 and 167.
10. Ernest Coyecque, *L'Hôtel-Dieu de Paris au Moyen-Age. Histoire et documents*, vol. 1 (Paris: Champion, 1889), 73.
11. Filippini, "Gli ospizi per partorienti," 400.
12. Michele Medici, *Memorie storiche intorno le accademie scientifiche e letterarie della città di Bologna* (Bologna: Sassi nelle Spaderie, 1852).
13. Achille Bocchi's daughter, Costanza, whom he educated in Greek and Latin poetry, was a member of his literary academy, the Accademia Ermatena, in the sixteenth century; see Medici, *Memorie storiche*, 36–7.
14. Marta Cavazza, *Settecento inquieto: Alle origini dell'Istituto delle Scienze di Bologna* (Bologna: Il Mulino, 1990), 31–78.
15. Monique Frize, *Laura Bassi and Science in 18th-Century Europe: The Extraordinary Life and Role of Italy's Pioneering Female Professor* (Berlin: Springer, 2013), 47–70.
16. Michel Foucault et al., *Les machines à guérir: Aux origines de l'hôpital moderne* (Brussels: Mardaga, 1979); Pancino, *Il bambino e l'acqua sporca*; Nadia Maria Filippini, "Assistenza al parto nel primo Ottocento: Appunti sull'intervento istituzionale," in *Le culture del parto*, ed. Ann Oakley (Milan: Feltrinelli, 1985), 63–73; Gabriella Berti Logan, "Women and the Practice and Teaching of Medicine in Bologna in the Eighteenth and Early Nineteenth Centuries," *Bulletin of the History of Medicine* 77, no. 3 (2003): 506–35.
17. Filippini, "Assistenza al parto," 65.
18. Coyecque, *L'Hôtel-Dieu*, 73.
19. An overview of eighteenth-century schools for midwifery can be found in Pancino, *Il bambino e l'acqua sporca*, 92–126; concisely in Filippini, "Gli ospizi per partorienti," 402. For more on Turin, see T. M. Caffaratto, *Storia dell'Ospedale S. Anna di Torino (Opera di Maternità)*, supplement to *Annali dell'Ospedale Maria Vittoria di Torino* 63, no. 7–8 (1970), also Pancio, *Il bambino e l'acqua sporca*, 93–7; for Daniela FranchettiPavia, *La scuola ostetrica pavese tra Otto e Novecento* (Milan: Cisalpino, 2012).
20. Filippini, "The Church, the State and Childbirth," 168–9.
21. Filippini, "Assistenza al parto," 65.
22. Lucia Dacome, "Women, Wax and Anatomy in the 'Century of Things,'" *Renaissance Studies* 21, no. 4 (2007): 522–50, quote on 528–9; Dacome, *Malleable Anatomies*, 130–62.
23. Dacome, "Women, Wax and Anatomy," 531–5; Dacome, *Malleable Anatomies*, 177–80.
24. The sources consulted for this chapter favor using the term "suppelletile," or "suppellettile" in the singular, while the English translations ("furnishings," "ornaments," or "goods") are frequently plural. The plural is found in Italian without a substantial change in meaning. On Galli's models, see Marco Bortolotti and Viviana Lanzarini, *Ars obstetricia bononiensis: Catalogo ed inventario del Museo Ostetrico Giovan Antonio Galli* (Bologna: CLUEB, 1988), 17–19; Karen Newman, *Fetal Positions: Individualism, Science, Visuality* (Stanford: Stanford University Press, 1996), 44–59; Viviana Lanzarini, "La scuola ostetrica di Giovan Antonio Galli e la sua collezione didattica," in *Nascere a Siena: Il parto e l'assistenza alla nascità dal medioevo all'età moderna*, ed. Francesca Vannozzi (Siena: Protagon, 2005), 25–34, esp. 26–8; Dacome, *Malleable Anatomies*, 163–91.
25. Jérôme Lalande, *Voyage d'un François en Italie, Fait dans les années 1765 & 1766*, vol. 2 (Venice, 1769), 34. For other European admirers, and some detractors, see Dacome, *Malleable Anatomies*, 180–1.
26. Biblioteca Universitaria di Bologna (hereafter BUB), Ms. 243, Lettere di Jacopo Bartolomeo Beccari a Flaminio Scarselli, Letter of November 6, 1751, as cited by Dacome, *Malleable Anatomies*, 163.
27. Francesca Vannozzi, "Una palestra per la didattica ostetrica: Il ricovero di maternità," in *Figure femminili (e non) intorno alla nascita: La storia in Siena dell'assistenza alla partoriente e al nascituro, XVIII–XX secolo*, ed. Francesca Vannozzi (Siena: Protagon, 2005), 225–43, at 237–8.
28. Vannozzi, "Una palestra," 237, 239.
29. Ibid., 237.
30. Febbrari had studied medicine in Bologna under Galli from 1765 to 1769 and worked there in 1773–6. The models he ordered were not delivered until sometime between 1801 and 1815, to Febbrari's sister and heir, Angiola, so presumably to her house. Giambattista Fabbri, "Antico museo ostetrico di Giovanni Antonio Galli, restauro fatto alle sue preparazioni in plastica e nuova conferma della suprema importanza dell'ostetrica sperimentale; con appendice," *Memorie della Accademia delle scienze dell'Istituto di Bologna* 2, ser. 3 (1872): 129–66, at 154–5; more recently, Bernardo Fratello et al., "Una collezione settecentesca del Museo di Anatomia dell'Università di Modena e Reggio Emilia. I modelli ostetrici realizzati in terracotta da Giovan Battista Manfredini," *Museologia scientifica memorie* 2 (2008): 215–20.

31. Fabbri, "Antico museo ostetrico," 151–3; Pancino, *Il bambino e l'acqua sporca*, 106–7.
32. Giambattista Fabbri, "Rendiconti accademici, Sessione ordinaria, 16 Gennaio 1873," *Bullettino delle scienze mediche* 15, ser. 5 (1873): 383–5, at 384–5; Vannozzi, "Una palestra," 239.
33. Fabbri, "Rendiconti accademici," 384–5; Alfonso Corradi, *Dell'ostetricia in Italia dalla metà dello scorso secolo fino al presente* (Bologna: Gamberini e Parmeggiani, 1874), 25.
34. Marco Bortolotti, "Insegnamento, ricerca e professione nel museo ostetrico di Giovanni Antonio Galli," in *I materiali dell'Istituto delle Scienze, Catalogo della Mostra* (Bologna: Accademia delle Scienze, 1979), 239–47, at 240.
35. See below, n. 51.
36. See the discussion in John Alexander, "The Educational Buildings of Pius IV: Variations upon a Building Type in Urban Monuments," *Landscape and Urban Planning* 73 (2005): 89–109.
37. On the Carnevale setting, see Giovanna Ferrari, "Public Anatomy Lessons and the Carnival: The Anatomy Theatre of Bologna," *Past & Present* 117 (1987): 50–106, esp. 80–7. In addition, Paula Findlen, "Science as a Career in Enlightenment Italy: The Strategies of Laura Bassi," *Isis* 84, no. 3 (1993): 441–69, at 452–3 and fig. 1 for a reproduction of the insignia.
38. Renato Roli, "Il Palazzo Poggi, il Palazzo Malvezzi, la Biblioteca," in *I luoghi del conoscere: I laboratori storico e i musei dell'università di Bologna*, vol. 2, ed. Franca Arduini et al. (Bologna: Banca del Monte, 1988), 18–31.
39. Giancarlo Roversi, *Palazzi e case nobili del '500 a Bologna: La storia, le famiglie, le opera d'arte* (Casalecchi di Reno: Grafis, 1986), 36–56; Manfredo Tafuri, *Venice and the Renaissance*, trans. J. Levine (London: MIT Press, 1989), 62–3.
40. Kim Sexton, "Academic Bodies and Anatomical Architecture in Early Modern Bologna," in *Architecture and the Body, Science and Culture*, ed. Kim Sexton (London: Routledge, 2017), 139–56, at 142–3; Johann Karl Schmidt, "Zu Vignolas Palazzo Bocchi in Bologna," *Mitteilungen des Kunsthistorischen Institutes in Florenz* 13, no. 1–2 (1967): 83–94, figs. 1 and 2; Daniela Monari, "Palazzo Bocchi: il quadro storico e l'intervento del Vignola," *Il Carrobbio* 6 (1980): 263–72.
41. Enrica Baidada, "Notizie sull'origine e lo sviluppo della Specola bolognese e della sua strumentazione negli archivi cittadini," in *Gli strumenti nella storia e nella filosofia della scienza*, ed. G. Tarozzi (Bologna: Litosei, 1983), 129–38, at 131–2; Sexton, "Academic Bodies and Anatomical Architecture," 143–6. The old Palazzo Davia on Via Cesare Battisti boasted a *specola*, but its remains are not as conspicuous as that of the Palazzo Marsili.
42. Cavazza, *Settecento inquieto*, 64–75.
43. Ceccarelli and Cervellati, *Da un palazzo a una città*, 14–22; Sexton, "Academic Bodies and Anatomical Architecture," 144–6.
44. Henri Lefebvre, *The Production of Space*, trans. Donald Nicholson-Smith (Oxford: Basil Blackwell, 1991), 39.
45. "suppellettile, della quale avea egli fatto ornamento, e delizia della sua privata casa," from Michele Medici, "Elogio di Gian-Antonio Galli," *Memorie della Reale Accademia delle Scienze dell'Istituto di Bologna* 8 (1857): 423–50, at 425.
46. Cited by Dacome, "Women, Wax and Anatomy," 527.
47. See above, note 30, and Fabbri, "Antico museo ostetrico," 154–5.
48. Dacome, "Women, Wax and Anatomy," 526–7.
49. Gualtiero Tonelli, "Sul teatro anatomico dell'Archiginnasio. Chi furono i padrini?" *Strenna storica bolognese* 28 (1978): 381–400, at 394.
50. Dacome, *Malleable Anatomies*, 171–4.
51. "Neque vero sermonibus tantum hanc medicinae partem amplificavit, sed etiam re … idque proinde imaginibus quamplurimis, e terra, aliave materia, mira arte conformatis, non sine magno sumtu, instruxit. Hic omnes pariendi modi apparent," in Zanotti, *De Bononiensi Scientiarum*, 88.
52. Archivio di Stato di Bologna (hereafter ASB), Uff. Registro, Copie degli atti notarili, vol. 466, fols. 309r–v and 316r–322r.
53. Ibid., fols. 309r–322v; and ASB, Uff. Registro, Copie degli atti notarili, vol. 467, fols. 35r–46v; vol. 478, fols. 496r–497v.
54. ASB, Uff. Registro, Copie degli atti notarili, vol. 466, fol. 314r.
55. Vannozzi, "Una palestra," 241; Dacome, *Malleable Anatomies*, 163–4.
56. ASB, Uff. Registro, Copie degli atti notarili, vol. 466, fols. 314r, 371v.
57. Vannozzi, "Una palestra," 238.
58. ASB, Uff. Registro, Copie degli atti notarili, vol. 466, fol. 314v; Lalande, *Voyage d'un François*, 34; and above n. 26.
59. Ibid., fol. 314r.
60. Ibid., fol. 314v.
61. Ibid.

62. Rebecca Messbarger, *The Lady Anatomist: The Life and Work of Anna Morandi Manzolini* (Chicago and London: The University of Chicago Press, 2010), 79–84.
63. BUB, Ms. 72, vol. 1, lettera 6, fol. 100v.
64. Romolo Griffini, "Sul progetto di regolamente organico dell'ospizio provinciale degli esposti e delle partorienti di Milano," *Annali universali di medicina* 206, no. 618 (December 1868): 465–563, at 489. Filippini notes that the custom was very old, and the medical establishment in the nineteenth century sought in vain to limit it ("Gli ospizi per partorienti," 405).
65. Galli rejected the first room they proposed as "poco vantaggiosa" in BUB, Ms. 72, I, lettera 6, fols. 101r–102r. Also, ASB, Assunteria di Studio, Requisiti dei Lettori, busta 40, cartella 17, "Relazione alle SS.rie VV, Ill:me ed Ecc.se degli Assunti di Studio," as cited by Dacome, *Malleable Anatomies*, 182.
66. Bortolotti, "Insegnamento," 240; Dacome, *Malleable Anatomies*, 182.
67. Giuseppe Gaetano Bollette and Giuseppe Maria Angelleli, *Notizie dell'origine, e progressi dell'Instituto delle scienze di Bologna e sue accademie … nuovamente compilate* (Bologna: Istituto delle Scienze, 1780), 84; Dacome, *Malleable Anatomies*, 180–4; Messbarger, *Lady Anatomist*, 82.
68. Filippini, "Assistenza al parto," 66–9; Filippini, "Ospizi per partorienti," 395–411; Filippini, "The Church, the State and Childbirth," 161–4.
69. In a short time, the new schools became the domain of male surgeons at the expense of midwives. See Filippini, "Assistenza al parto," 65–6; Filippini, "Ospizi per partorienti," 402–3.
70. Filippini, "Ospizi per partorienti," 397, 402, 408–10.

CHAPTER 16
HEALING BY DESIGN
AN EXPERIENTIAL APPROACH TO EARLY MODERN OTTOMAN HOSPITAL ARCHITECTURE

Nina Macaraig

"Hospital patients should never be imbued with the idea that they are sick; health should be constantly before their eyes," commented Frank Lloyd Wright in a 1948 interview on modern hospital design.[1] Ironically, in the subsequent decades architects moved further and further away from the restorative environments that the ancient Greeks had already emphasized in their approach to medical treatment, which generally took place in healing shrines (*asclepieia*) dedicated to Asclepios and situated in idyllic surroundings.[2] Instead, modern architects allowed functional efficiency to become their sole guiding principle, resulting in buildings that privilege doctor and machine over patient and increase the already stressful experience of illness or accident: symmetrical, blocky structures of intimidating proportions, with endless, labyrinthine hallways. Since the 1980s, however, the medical establishment has once more begun to show interest in the architectural environment in which health is delivered, particularly following Roger Ulrich's groundbreaking paper on how surgical recovery may be affected by the patients' interaction with their environment.[3] Since then, increased attention has been paid to the ways in which buildings and gardens can either support or undermine the healing process—a turn summarized by the concept "healing by design."[4]

It is through the lens of the latter concept that this chapter will examine the architecture of early modern Ottoman hospitals from a new perspective. The Ottomans emerged in northwestern Anatolia in the late thirteenth century, as one of several Turkish-Islamic principalities which by then had pushed back the eastern border of the Byzantine Empire as far as its capital, Constantinople. They swiftly expanded their territory both east and west with Sultan Mehmed the Conqueror (r. 1444–6 and 1451–81) taking Constantinople (present-day Istanbul) in 1453 and thus setting the scene for building an empire. It was under the long and stable reign of Süleyman II (r. 1520–66) that the Ottoman Empire experienced its largest territorial extent, and turned truly into a world power, holding lands from Northwest Africa to Vienna, and from the Near East to the Indian Ocean. An important aspect of Ottoman rule throughout the imperial territory—from its humble beginnings in Anatolia, to its final demise shortly after the First World War—was the elite's prolific architectural patronage and the construction of monuments that heralded their power and legitimacy, not only by means of a distinct architectural style marked with central domes and pencil-like minarets but also by way of providing charity to the populace in the form of infrastructure, water supply, places of prayer for Muslims, employment opportunities, food, and healthcare.

While Gönül Cantay's work on Seljuk and Ottoman hospitals on the territory of modern-day Turkey has provided a valuable corpus and taxonomic survey of monuments that can serve as basis and vantage point,[5] Miri Shefer-Mossensohn has taken a step further and considered especially Ottoman hospital gardens in relation to "healing by design."[6] She provides a brief discussion of the buildings' experiential qualities and their contributions to the type of integralistic therapy linked to Galenic humoralism,[7] as practiced by the learned doctors of the Ottoman *darüşşifas*.[8] In her own words, Shefer-Mossensohn's aim is "*not* to focus on the architectural aspects of these buildings as such, but rather to discuss how contemporary Ottomans perceived

Health and Architecture

[them] as revealed by chronicles, biographical dictionaries, and pictorial miniatures."[9] Therefore, there is still a need for a detailed discussion of Ottoman hospital architecture in terms of its spatial qualities—such as the variety of the users' sensory experiences, as well as the aspects of orientation, connection, scale, and symbolic meaning.

This chapter will therefore take as a starting point the present knowledge of "successful" hospital architecture, as it rests on "evidence-based design." The latter is a design practice that takes into account the measurable physiological and psychological effects that an environment has on the people who are exposed to it.[10] Departing from this knowledge, I will examine the architecture of a group of early modern Ottoman hospitals (Figure 16.1) in order to understand how these buildings appealed to the senses, promoted well-being, and assisted in the therapeutic process.[11] The present purpose here is *not* to demonstrate how "advanced"

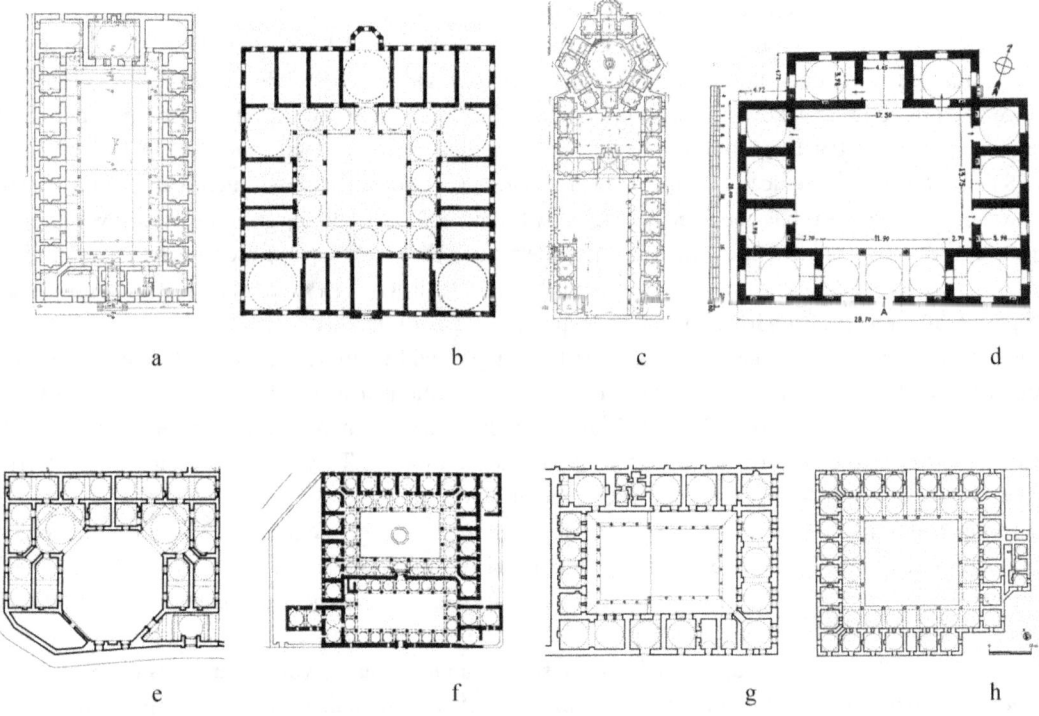

Figure 16.1 Ground plans of the Yıldırım Darüşşifası (a), Fatih Darüşşifası (b), Hospital of Bayezid II (c), Hafsa Sultan Darüşşifası (d), Haseki Sultan Darüşşifası (e), Süleymaniye Darüşşifası (f), Atik Valide Darüşşifası (g), Sultanahmed Darüşşifası (h). Please note that scales are not consistent. Sources: (a) Ekrem Hakkı Ayverdi, *Osmanlı Mi'mârîsinin İlk Devri, 630–805 (1230–1402)* (Istanbul: İstanbul Fetih Cemiyeti, 1966); (b) Ekrem Hakkı Ayverdi, *Osmanlı Mi'marîsinde Fâtih Devri, 855–886 (1451–1481)* (Istanbul: İstanbul Fetih Cemiyeti, 1989); (c) İ. Aydın Yüksel, *Osmanlı Mimarisinde II. Bâyezid Yavuz Selim Devri (886–926/1481–1520)* (Istanbul: İstanbul Fetih Cemiyeti, 1983); (d) Nihad Yörükoğlu, *Manisa Bimarhanesi* (Istanbul: İsmail Akgün Matbaası, 1948); (e) Aptullah Kuran, *Sinan: The Grand Old Master of Ottoman Architecture* (Washington, DC: Institute of Turkish Studies, 1987); (f) Godfrey Goodwin, *A History of Ottoman Architecture* (London: Thames & Hudson, 1992); (g) Kuran, *Sinan*; (h) Zeynep Nayır, *Osmanlı Mimarlığında Sultan Ahmet Külliyesi ve Sonrası (1609–90)* (Istanbul: İTÜ Mimarlık Fakültesi, 1975)

Ottoman medical institutions and practices were when measured against the late twentieth-century rise of holistic and integralistic medicine in Europe and the United States. Rather, the value of this somewhat anachronistic employment of contemporary architectural design concepts—much like the application of contemporary cultural or sociological theory to the study of primary sources—lies in their utility for forging a more interpretative and user-centered approach to this otherwise neglected group of Ottoman architectural monuments.[12] Such a user-centered approach may also be achieved by viewing the monuments within the context of three burgeoning fields in Middle Eastern and Ottoman history: the history of the senses (which the below section on "Sensory Experiences of Hospital Users" takes into consideration), the history of emotions, and the history of the environment—all three of them offering paths for further inquiry.[13]

The limitations of the present approach should be evident: Ottoman users of *darüşşifas* left barely any historical record describing their perceptions, and neither did the architects themselves seem to have recorded their thoughts on how their monuments were to affect the patients. While the relevant endowments' title deeds do record basic data about the buildings, as well as more detailed information about the staff, their matter-of-fact tone and often-lapidary nature make it difficult to tease out the built environment's effects on its users. For instance, the *vakfiye* of the Atik Valide Mosqye Complex refers to the hospital in a typically pithy manner: "A *darüşşifa* [hospital] consisting of high and beautiful rooms and cells which the founder built next to the *imaret* and bequeathed to all kinds of patients for their treatment and medication. Because all of these buildings are well known in the area, there is no need to describe and define them."[14] Still, because of the endowment deeds' prescriptive character, conceptions about the ideal, rather than actual, circumstances of healthcare can be inferred, and relevant exemplary passages are therefore referenced below throughout the footnotes. More informative textual primary sources can be encountered in the eyewitness accounts of Ottoman and European travelers recording their impressions about these institutions. The most telling evidence, however, are the formal and (as far as they can still be determined) functional characteristics of the structures themselves.

Ottoman Hospitals and their Architectural Form

Between 1400 and 1700, elite patrons, ranking from the sultan at the top to a provincial governor in Tunisia at the bottom, erected and endowed eleven hospitals, mostly as a dependency of a mosque complex that also included a *mekteb*, medrese, han, *imaret*, hamam, and so on. It should not be surprising that these buildings constitute a rather unified group in terms of design, functional units, and general formal characteristics. As can be deduced from their ground plans (Figure 16.1), all of them have a minimal number of entrances and often a limited number of windows within a forbidding exterior wall. All are self-contained, inward-looking units, even if they may be attached to another dependency or service building, such as a han or *imaret* (see, for example, the Atik Valide Darüşşifası, Figure 16.1g). All feature a central courtyard, and in some cases more than one (see, for example, the Süleymaniye Darüşşifası, Figure 16.1f). For most of these hospital buildings we know that this courtyard had a central pool or fountain, making it likely that others whose structure was either transformed or demolished also included such a water element. All have at least one row of covered small rooms, which would have served as patient rooms, surrounding the central courtyard(s). Most have a colonnaded, dome-covered portico that mediates between the outdoor space of the courtyard and the indoor space of the rooms. Many feature at least one room distinguished in size and positioning from the others, or a large, open niche (*eyvan*) (see, for example, the Hafsa Sultan Darüşşifası, Figure 16.1d). In several cases, one can still discern wet spaces such as latrines or small integrated hamams (see, for example, the Süleymaniye Darüşşifası, Figure 16.1f).[15] In terms of function, the hospitals needed to provide spaces for the inpatients' quarters, a "pharmacy," a storage area, a kitchen, some kind of administrative office, a prayer area, and the above-mentioned wet spaces.[16] (Where latrines are missing from the hospital's building program today, one may assume that chamber pots were used and emptied into latrines of other mosque dependencies close by,[17] or that they did indeed exist, but were converted and rendered unrecognizable during subsequent structural modifications.) In those cases where the hospital also functioned as a teaching institution, a "classroom" was also required.[18] Moreover, while none of them have survived in their original shape, based on textual sources beautiful gardens in the courtyard were also a crucial component of *darüşşifa* architecture.[19]

Although the Hospital of Bayezid II and the Haseki Sultan Darüşşifası boast more complex polygonal arrangements (Figure 16.1c and 16.e), hospital courtyards and the building's outer perimeter are usually rectangular. The plan of a row of portico-fronted rooms surrounding a central courtyard with a water feature is, of course, a signature staple of Ottoman architectural planning. Conceptually simple because of its modular nature, yet extremely flexible and multi-functional, it accommodated various types of schools, caravanserais, *imaret*s, and the like. The flexible and adaptive capacity of the architectural scheme in a way reflects that of the food served in the *imaret*s: in particular, the customary rice and wheat soups could be stretched with water or thickened with solid ingredients and even meat, depending on the number of beneficiaries, the funds available, and the significance that the patron assigned to the quality of the dishes.[20] Innovation in the architectural form of Ottoman hospitals between the fifteenth and seventeenth centuries was found not so much in the overall concept, but rather in the details and adjustments made to suit the specific stipulations of the patron, or the monument's site within the urban fabric.

As for the site, hospitals were usually part and parcel of a sizable mosque complex, and thus the decision concerning their location was pre-determined by the complex's site and boundaries within a given city. The construction of a mosque complex required the permission of the incumbent sultan, who in the decision-making process had to rely on the expertise of his imperial court architect in terms of site selection and design. An important factor in choosing a suitable location appears to have been the desire to develop certain urban areas so as to make them attractive to potential Muslim residents: wherever a major mosque complex provided employment, infrastructure, a place of worship, food from its *imaret*, communal hygiene through the nearby bathhouse, education, healthcare, and so on, an increase in population could be expected. Such was the case, for example, with the Atik Valide Mosque Complex. Its construction caused the once sparsely populated hills beyond the village of Üsküdar on the shore of the Bosphorus to attract many more people to settle there, resulting in a population increase by one-third according to the geographer Mehmed Aşık, writing in the 1590s.[21]

The scope of this chapter does not permit a detailed discussion of the architectural form of each of the eleven hospitals that falls under the scope of this study, an endeavor that has already been accomplished by Gönül Cantay as far as those monuments located in Thrace and Anatolia are concerned;[22] however, descriptions of the grand Süleymaniye Darüşşifası, erected by Süleyman the Magnificent (r. 1520–66) as part of his mosque complex in Istanbul in the 1550s, and of the small Hafsa Sultan Darüşşifası in Manisa, erected in 1539 on behalf of the same sultan's mother (d. 1534), shall illustrate the range of possible forms and adaptations within this architectural scheme.

The Hafsa Sultan Darüşşifası is a rather modest structure, which according to endowment documents employed seventeen medical and eight administrative staff to take care of no more than twenty patients—a ratio of staff to inpatients that likely was an ideal never achieved in real practice.[23] As part of a group of buildings belonging to the Hafsa Sultan Mosque Complex, once surrounded by a perimeter wall, it is located north of the mosque and the (vanished) *imaret* and west of the hamam (Figure 16.2). The independent hospital building forms a rectangular block of 28.7 × 24.7 meters, including a protruding row of rooms at the rear, with the walls displaying a mixed brick-and-stone masonry crowned by a sawtooth cornice and a tiled roof. The domes rest on octagonal brick drums, have a shallow profile, and are also covered with tile, rather than the

Healing by Design

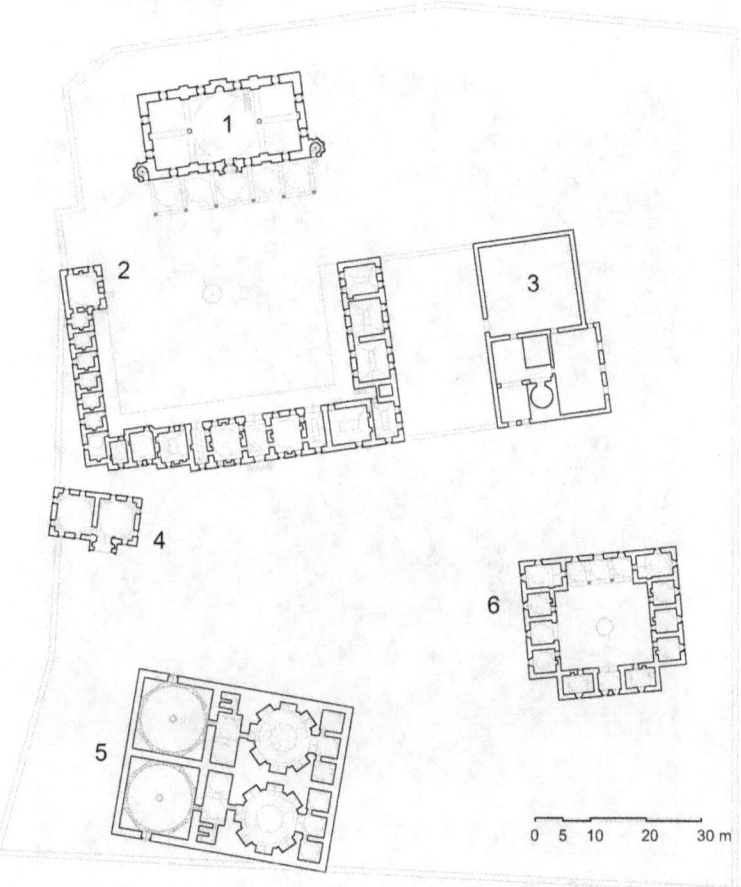

Figure 16.2 Overall plan of the Hafsa Sultan Mosque Complex, Manisa. Necipoğlu, *The Age of Sinan*, 54

lead-sheets that would come to cover the much higher-profiled domes we associate with imperial architecture of the "classical" period. It is entered through a small gate marked by a marble doorjamb with a depressed arch, an inscribed panel and a blind pointed arch within the masonry (Figure 16.3).[24] Each of the four facades is broken up by four windows. Since the hospital lay enclosed behind a wall, the need for separation from the urban fabric by means of a blind facade would not have been as acute as it would have been, for instance, in the hustle and bustle of Istanbul.

Upon entering, the visitor finds himself in a portico made up of three dome-capped units (Figure 16.4), with two columns supporting the three pointed arches opening up into the central courtyard (17.3 × 13.75 m). The portico also gave access to the two larger rectangular rooms in the southeast and southwest corners, which may have served administrative and treatment functions. Both to the left and the right, a row of square, domed rooms (3.98 × 3.98 m), with fireplaces and windows, housed the patient rooms, which were of typical proportions. Opposite the entrance, across the courtyard, which is now entirely paved but for a new fountain and likely had contained a garden and original water feature, an *eyvan* serves as indoor-outdoor space, flanked by two rectangular rooms—without a by-now discernible function—that reflect

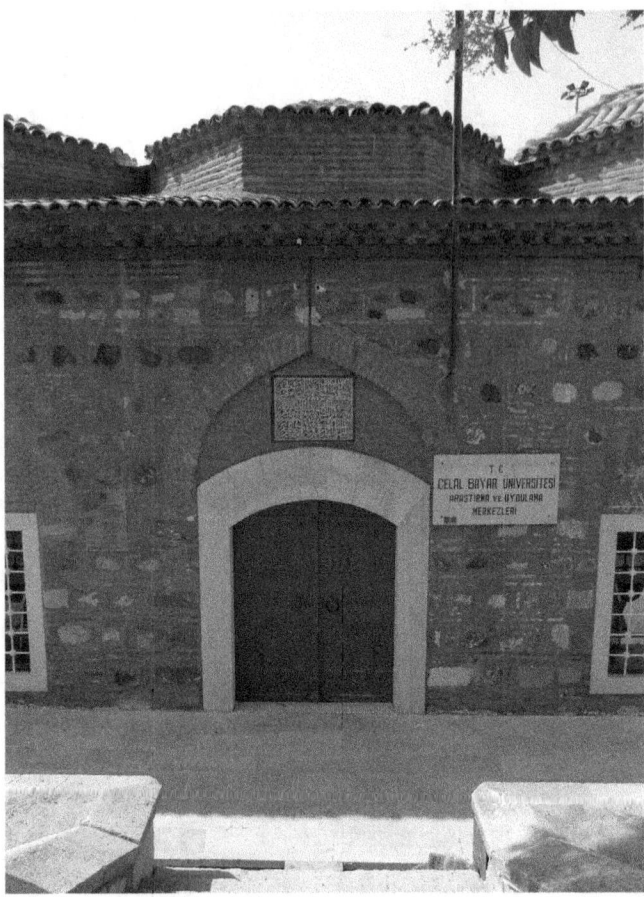

Figure 16.3 Entrance of the Hafsa Sultan Darüşşifası. Photo: Nina Ergin

those in the northeast and northwest corners. The surrounding portico, which I have argued constituted a signature of Ottoman architecture, has here been reduced to a three-bayed porch at the entrance and the *eyvan* opposite. Did the architect, Mimar Acem Ali, not feel a need for a larger indoor-outdoor space, or perhaps a no longer extant wooden structure may have created additional shaded areas within the courtyard?

In contrast to the small and provincial Hafsa Sultan Darüşşifası with its decidedly local building characteristics, the Süleymaniye Darüşşifası—designed by the famous imperial architect Mimar Sinan[25]—presents a large-scale, two-story monument with two courtyards (Figure 16.1f), which by dint of its carefully cut ashlar masonry, form, and location clearly makes up an integral part of the imperial mosque complex.[26] It is located on a sloping area in the northwestern corner of the complex, between the medical school (*tıp medresesi*) where the doctors working in this and other imperial *darüşşifa*s were trained,[27] and the *imaret*'s service building (Figure 16.5). The inscribed main entrance on the narrow street between the hospital and the medical school punctures a forbidding wall that is almost blind, except for a second smaller and simpler entrance into the irregularly shaped outer service courtyard to the southwest, which contains the bakery and the patients' hamam. Like the entrance to the Hafsa Sultan's hospital, this one consists of an outer pointed arch encircling a recessed pediment with space for the epigraphic panel and the actual door capped by a depressed arch. Unfortunately, the original panel has been lost, its text now unknown.[28] Upon entering, the user finds

Healing by Design

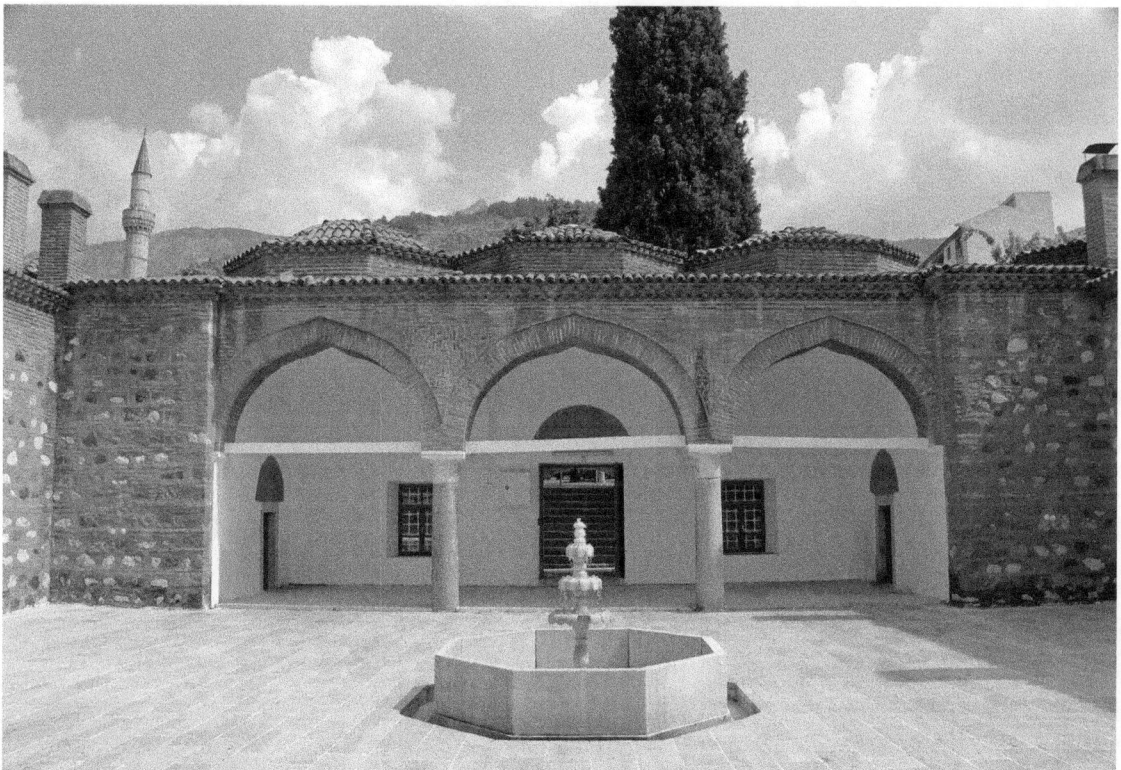

Figure 16.4 Portico of the Hafsa Sultan Darüşşifası. Kılıç, *Şifahaneler*, 247

himself in the portico surrounding the first courtyard, which measures 27 × 11.5 meters. The porticoes consist on their short side of five domed units supported by columns with fine muqarnas capitals carrying flat pointed arches and nine on its long side, but these do not preface patient cells. Yet, the corner units have been turned into self-contained rooms by means of dividing walls, and in the southwestern corner a staircase leads down to the lower level. When turning right or left, the user will find entrances to two dome-capped building units—a large double-domed room connected to the bakery to the left, or a suite of rooms that likely served the hospital administration, or as an infirmary/pharmacy that catered to patients with minor ailments that did not necessitate a stay[29]—as well as entrances to the outdoor service areas. Yet, in spite of this diversification of plan, Mimar Sinan maintained the customary appearance of a symmetrical and portico-encircled courtyard with a central water feature—a square pool with four lions that no longer exists.[30]

Through a passage directly across the entrance, the user can enter the second courtyard, which measures 25 × 15 m (Figure 16.6). The porticoes here are deeper and capped with larger domes, supported by the same columns and muqarnas capitals as in the first courtyard, counting seven units on the long side and five on the short side. On three sides, the porticoes are encircled by square (patient) rooms, almost all of which have a fireplace and window openings towards the portico as well as toward the outside, which due to the hillside and the hospital's substructure are placed high up on the northern exterior wall. The rooms located in three corners are accessed by diagonally placed doorways, while the fourth room in the southwestern corner communicates only with the first courtyard. In the second courtyard's center, a water feature must have existed where a polygonal pool had been placed during subsequent modifications and renovations. In the middle of the shorter sides, Mimar Sinan inserted passages to the outer service courtyard and to a lower-level entrance

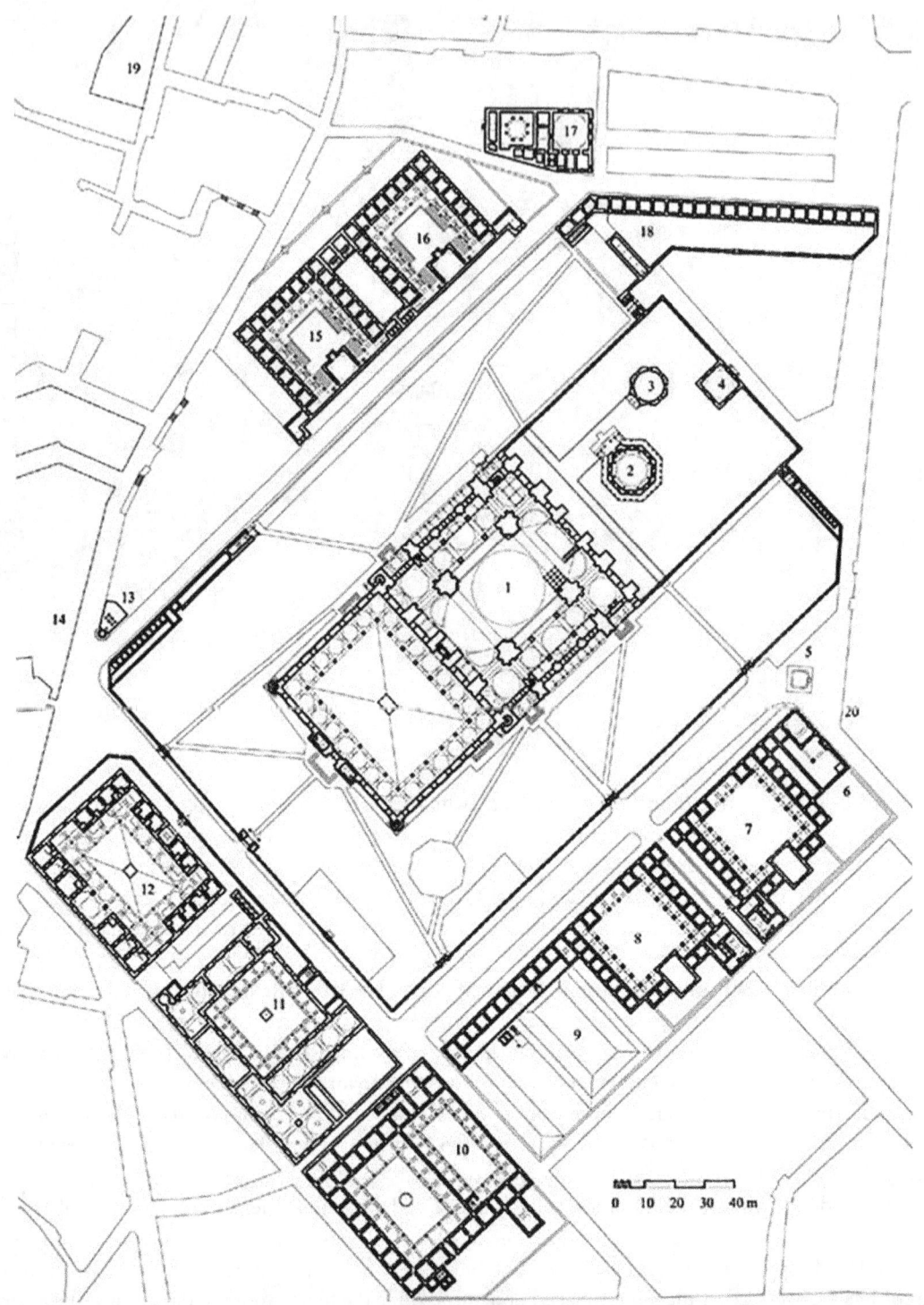

Figure 16.5 Overall plan of the Süleymaniye Mosque Complex, Istanbul. No. 10 indicates the *darüşşifa*. Necipoğlu, *The Age of Sinan*, 205

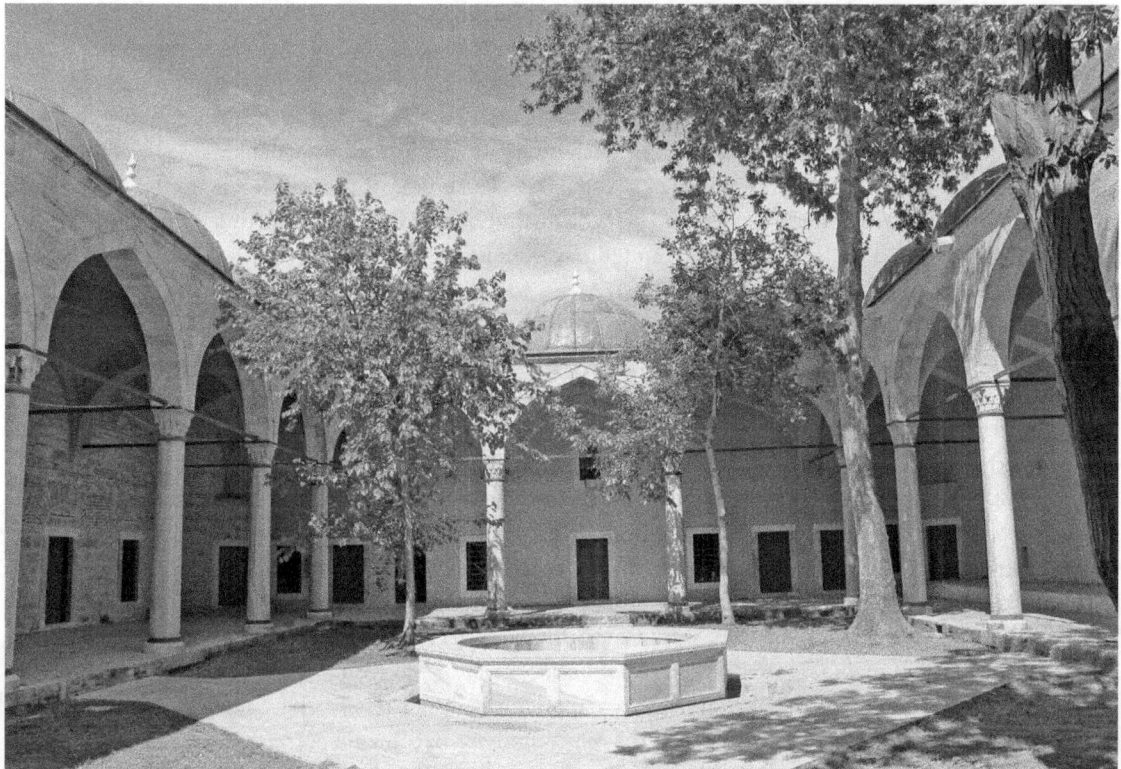

Figure 16.6 Second courtyard of the Süleymaniye Darüşşifası. Kılıç, *Şifahaneler*, 273

in the eastern exterior wall by means of a staircase. The lower level, which ensured that the main level was at the same elevation as the other mosque complex dependencies in spite of the sloping terrain, included a row of shops underneath the northern row of patient cells, as well as a long, barrel-vaulted room, lit and ventilated through small slit windows from above. Overall, the unified appearance of the courtyards seems to have been the paramount architectural feature on which Mimar Sinan hinged all other design decisions.

The Hospitals' Users

As mentioned above, good design practice pays attention to the variety of the users' sensory experiences of the architectural space. Logically, then, a crucial question follows such an assertion: who were the users of Hafsa Sultan's and Süleyman the Magnificent's and the many other hospitals? And, given that sensory perception is very much conditioned by culture, how were their experiences shaped by their values, their preceding knowledge and prior experiences? While the patient may come to mind first in discussing the *darüşşifa*'s users, it was in fact the hospital staff who would have perused the space in a much more long-term and sustained manner and that therefore should be counted as the first group. The doctors, surgeons, ophthalmologists, pharmacists, administrators, store clerks, nurses, assistants, doormen, laundrymen, hamam staff, and janitors would have spent a considerable portion of their lives, if not their entire working lives, inside the *darüşşifa*'s walls.

From the perspective of building usage duration, patients only make up the second group. They were usually Muslim male adults suffering from physical or mental illness.[31] Shefer-Mossensohn has convincingly argued that "family was the prime agent in distributing health and medical care[;] hospitalization, then, signaled the absence or the dysfunction of a family ... People of means were patients in a hospital if they had no family ... or they may have been strangers in a faraway place."[32] Evidence for the claim that travelers, merchants, and strangers made up the majority of patients can also be found in the hospital's frequent proximity to other mosque complex dependencies that served non-locals. A particular case in point is that of the Atik Valide Mosque Complex, which is situated at the terminus of the Silk Route on the Asian shore of the Bosphorus. The Atik Valide Darüşşifası in fact constitutes part of the building unit housing the *imaret*, *tabhane* (refectory), and *han* (caravanserai), and it may even have communicated with the latter institutions through a connecting door that offered immediate access to ill travelers. These would have arrived with their pack animals through the large gate where the *han*'s master welcomed them, stabled their horses or camels in the spaces adjoining the gate area, and then limped through the main courtyard toward the *darüşşifa*'s side door, rather than exiting and walking around the building to the main door.

The third group of persons who derived benefit from hospitals consisted of the patrons. Through the good deed of erecting and endowing a monument that dispersed healthcare, they earned high status, legitimacy, and blessing. Yet, this group of users shall be excluded here, since the elite patrons neither would have worked in the hospitals they funded nor received care from them, for the highest-ranking patrons at court had access to a number of hospitals on the grounds of their palaces,[33] or they would have received a visit from the chief doctor (*hekimbaşı*) in their private quarters.[34]

The first and second group of users would have shared a very similar cultural background. As young Muslim boys, the staff members went to the *sibyan mektebi* to learn to read at least the most crucial Qur'an verses; they could acquire knowledge and skills as apprentices to masters working in different professions, as autodidacts, or within the family; they had the opportunity to become medrese students if they exhibited the intellectual abilities and inclination; in the case of the doctors, they had studied in a medical school (*tıp medresesi*); they could join the Ottoman military through different channels; they could become members of a Sufi order; regardless of their original ethnic and linguistic background, they must have known a modicum of Ottoman Turkish; they interacted with Ottoman officials; washed in a hamam on Thursday night and visited the mosque on Friday; bought necessities from a bazaar; sought food from *imaret*s when in need; and, if they traveled, used Ottoman roads, bridges, and caravanserais.[35] Over a lifetime, they would have been exposed to a great number of monuments very similar to Ottoman hospitals—that is, buildings made up of portico-fronted rooms surrounding a central courtyard—and the associations they made with them—learning, food, rest—accompanied them everywhere.

Sensory Experiences of Hospital Users

Although extracted from a tenth-century source and hence dating much earlier—but still linked to Ottoman medicine due to its shared Galenic heritage—a passage from a treatise on fevers caused by tuberculosis, authored by Ishaq ibn Sulayman al-Isra'ili (d. 932?), emphasizes the significance that Islamic physicians attached to the sensory experiences of patients:

> The patient's position inside the room should be in front of the opening to the ventilating window on bedding of linen or Tabaristan cloth. Rooms should be strewn with aromatic plants ... Running fountains should be installed in front of the patient so that he may listen to the gentle fall of water; for the splash of water, if light and gentle, will induce sleep. Continual use should be made of sandalwood and rose-water.[36]

The following paragraphs will take al-Isra'ili's recommendations—the touch of linen, the fragrance of aromatics and the breeze, the sound of falling water—as inspiration and break down Ottoman hospital users' experiences in terms of the five senses.

In the *darüşşifa*s, the users' sense of vision oriented around the standardized Ottoman architectural aesthetic: an entryway decorated with muqarnas and/or an inscription, solid stone and/or brick walls, roof-tile- or lead-covered domes, and columns with muqarnas or Turkish triangle capitals. While Ottoman hospitals often lacked windows toward the outside, and therefore rarely incorporated the inspiring views for which the Topkapı Palace and Mimar Sinan's buildings are famous,[37] their interior design did not lack visual interest. A fountain or pool and a courtyard garden would have enlivened the architectural space, and, although we do not know which plants grew in the hospital gardens, it is likely that in addition to greenery and shrubs they would have included fragrant, flowering plants. At this point, another reference to Roger Ulrich's groundbreaking study, "View through a Window May Influence Recovery from Surgery," is elucidative.[38] Ulrich examined how the physiological effects of a view onto natural scenery on patients recovering from gallbladder surgery compared to those of a view against a brick wall and thereby laid the groundwork for evidence-based hospital design. It seems a foregone conclusion that those patients who could enjoy a window view of plants required less pain medication and recovered more quickly.

The sense of vision also encapsulates the elements of natural light and shade within the *darüşşifa*. Even though daylight is an important ingredient in good design to promote well-being, in a Mediterranean setting, the harsh glare and oppressive heat of a summer midday sun may be uncomfortable, especially for those inpatients who required the services of the ophthalmologist. The porticoes, therefore, provided a shady refuge from too much light without forcing the inpatients and doctors to retreat completely indoors (Figure 16.7). A further issue in the context of vision is the element of visual privacy. This concerned not only the privacy of the patients, whose maladies may have caused painful embarrassment, thus further curtailing their already diminished well-being, from other patients and staff, but also privacy from the surrounding urban space, to be discussed in greater details below.

In terms of the acoustic environment, Ottoman hospitals could offer its staff and patients a controlled soundscape behind the barrier of its walls. Indeed, current medical research also now pays attention to how unwanted, unpredictable, and uncontrollable sounds cause detrimental effects for both patients and staff. In physiological terms, these include elevated blood pressure and heart and respiratory rate, as well as skin conductance. Among the negative psychological effects are irritation, anxiety, tension, sadness, depression, stress, and fatigue.[39] Disruptive city noise that may have led to such effects could be shut out to a certain extent, although of course the call to prayer still served as a marker of time and communal belonging and as a reminder of God's omnipresence (and hoped-for mercy and benevolence in times of sickness). To enhance the restful acoustic environment, the fountain in the central courtyard would have burbled away. Indeed, in commenting on the Hospital of Qalawun in Cairo that he visited in 1672, Evliya Çelebi remarked on a practice that one also expects to have occurred in its Ottoman counterparts: "Some of those who are ill relax next to the flowing ornamental fountains when they are close to recovering their health."[40] Given the Ottomans' great love of birds, as evidenced in the birdhouses incorporated in the walls of many Ottoman monuments and the existence of aviaries in the Topkapı Palace,[41] Ottoman patients certainly would have enjoyed the presence of songbirds visiting the courtyard garden and bathing in the water feature. Indeed, Evliya Çelebi in his 1652 description of the Hospital of Bayezid II in Edirne remarked that in spring the mentally ill patients there listen to the touching voices of birds within the garden and are compelled to join in their singing.[42]

In addition to natural sounds such as birdsong, the patients of a few select *darüşşifa*s could also enjoy man-made pleasant sounds in the form of music. Music therapy was a regular and fixed element of

Health and Architecture

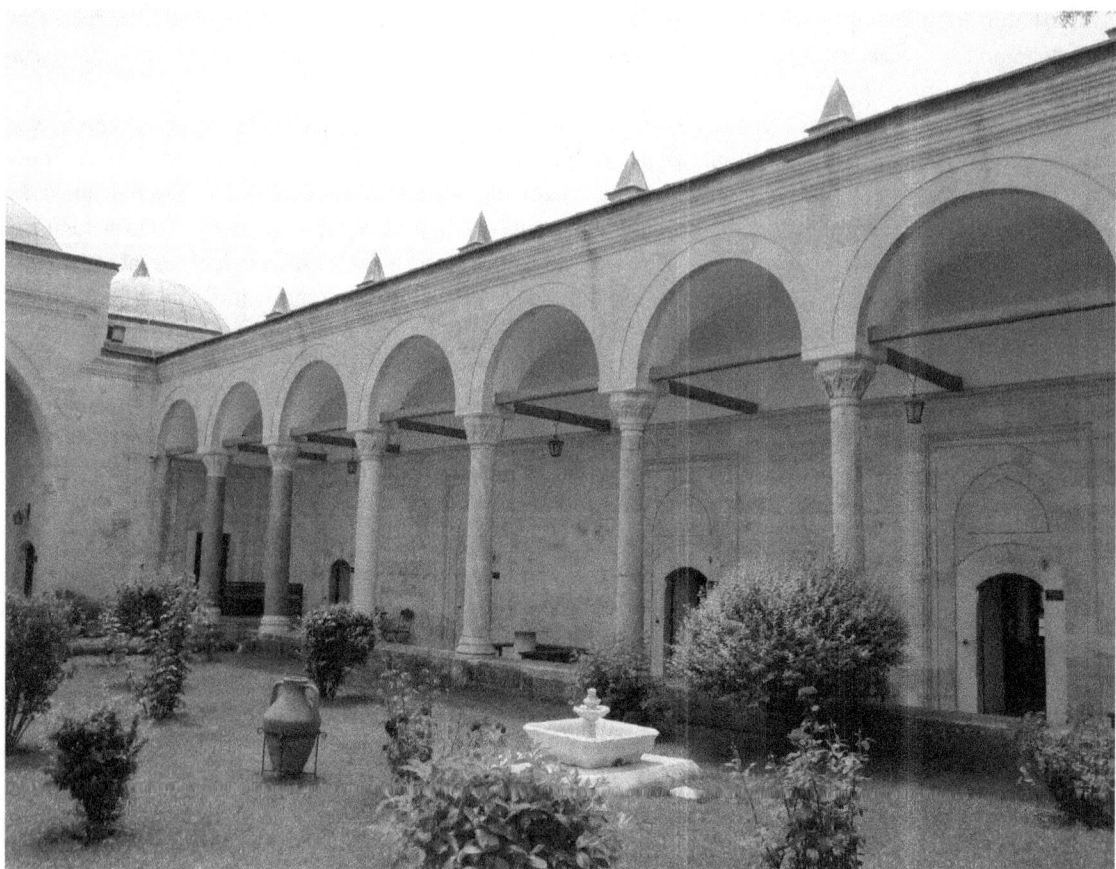

Figure 16.7 Portico of the Hospital of Bayezid II. Photo: Nina Ergin

treatment in the Hospital of Bayezid II in Edirne, for instance, which employed ten professional musicians. Evliya Çelebi describes the group as follows:

> The deceased and blessed Bayezid Veli appointed ten vocalists and instrumentalists in order to cure the patients and nourish their souls. Three of them are vocalists. One of them is a flute [*ney*] player, one is a violinist [*keman*], one is a panpipe [*musikar*] player, one is a dulcimer [*santur*] player, one is a harp [*çeng*] player, and another is the lute [*'ud*] player. They come three times a week and perform for the lunatics and patients. By the grace of God, the patients relax and are pleased by the sound of music. In fact, in the knowledge of music, the tonal modes of *nevâ*, *rast*, *dügâh*, *segâh*, *çargâh*, and *suzinâk* are especially for them. But if [the musician] decides on *rast* while [playing] in the modes of *zengûle* or *bûselik*, it breathes life into people. There is nourishment for the soul in every instrument and in every mode.[43]

The principles underlying Ottoman music therapy of the type described by Evliya derived from ancient Greek knowledge, mediated through Arab-Muslim scholarship, as well as pre-Ottoman Turkish and Byzantine practices.[44] Within the context of Galenic medicine, appropriately chosen music not only could improve the patient's mental well-being, but also through its harmonic and rhythmic qualities was held to have the power to (re)balance and regulate the humors in the human body. Hence, it was important to select the right tonal mode (*makam*) appropriate to the specific time of day and the specific disease to be effective. Following in the footsteps of earlier scholars such as Farabi (d. 950), the Ottoman poet-doctor Şuuri Hasan (d. 1693/4) in his *Ta'dîlü'l-Emzice* classified the various *makam*s based on their effectiveness for different diseases—Uşşak, for instance, was to help with pain from gout and to make the patient sleepy.[45]

Because music was a rather rare form of therapy, its performance did not shape the hospitals' architectural form, with one possible exception: the Hospital of Bayezid II. According to Arslan Terzioğlu, the dome-capped apsidal niche opposite the entrance from the second courtyard to the hexagonal main block served as a type of stage, and the domed space enhanced the acoustic qualities of the music played there (Figure 16.8).[46] It measures 4.3 × 4.8 meters, and its floor level is elevated at a height of 0.45 meters. Long stone benches against the lateral walls offer a place to sit comfortably. The three windows at the back look toward the exterior, but two more lead into the patient rooms located left and right of the niche. While it is tempting indeed to assign a stage function to this niche with a platform, there is no concrete evidence to either prove or disprove this claim. Unfortunately, the endowment deed is of no help in this matter, either, as the preserved versions do not mention the hospital's interior space.[47]

Much like the soundscape, so too would odors be under relatively greater control than in the world outside the hospital. The large number of cleaning staff in many of these institutions, from laundrymen to janitors, and the *vakfiye* documents' emphasis on the patients, their clothes, and their bedding being kept clean, demonstrate the significance that Ottomans attached not only to physical hygiene but also to the removal of olfactory nuisances created, for instance, by all manners of bodily secretions.[48] In fact, for Ottomans, the business of laundering textiles was not complete without fumigating the freshly washed items with pleasant-smelling incense (*buhûr*).[49] Hospital gardens, then, also created a pleasant olfactory diversion, depending on the scent of the plants grown there. In reference to the Hospital of Bayezid II, Evlia Çelebi remarked that the fragrant flowers in the garden brought pleasure to the mentally ill.[50] Thus, we may say that the hospital garden perfumed the body, mind, and soul of the patients, as much as of the staff who constantly had to deal with illness and suffering and therefore were in need of relief as much as the patients were.

The sense of touch was stimulated primarily by human touch via the physicians, hamam attendants, and servants or caretakers all putting their hands on the patients in the course of their interactions. Even patients may have touched each other regularly, whether inadvertently due to crowding, or intentionally to comfort and console each other. Hospital architecture provided a container and context for such "healing touch," but it also stimulated the haptic sense through the building's materials, as users touched stone and brick walls, whether left uncovered or plastered, the cool and smooth marble columns, wooden doors with metal door rings, and wooden window shutters or window grilles fashioned from iron; the plants they could touch and maybe even pick in the courtyard garden; and the water feature into which they could let their hands dangle. The sensation of temperature also deserves consideration here, both warm and cold. The existence of a courtyard, porticoes, and indoor rooms offered three different options as to where to locate inpatients, depending on whether they could sit or lie on bedding. In hot weather and under a blazing sun, the well-ventilated porticoes around the central water feature with its cooling effect as well as the cells offered a cooler environment. In cool but sunny weather, patients could be moved into the sun, so that they were warmed by its rays. During cold weather, the cells with their individual fireplaces must have constituted the preferred location for patients and staff alike. If the hospital had its own hamam—as did the Süleymaniye and Atik Valide Darüşşifası—then the sense of touch (and temperature sensation) was also stimulated there. Galenic medicine, as it was taught to and practiced by the doctors there, assigns great importance to balneotherapy as a therapeutic measure to restore humoral balance, and the hamams incorporated were used for that purpose: if a patient was determined to suffer from an excess of dry and cold humor, then a visit to a bathhouse staffed with a knowledgeable attendant was the cure prescribed.[51] Moreover, a small-scale research study by Zeki Karagülle conducted on the physiological effects of a hamam treatment has shown that the thermal and haptic

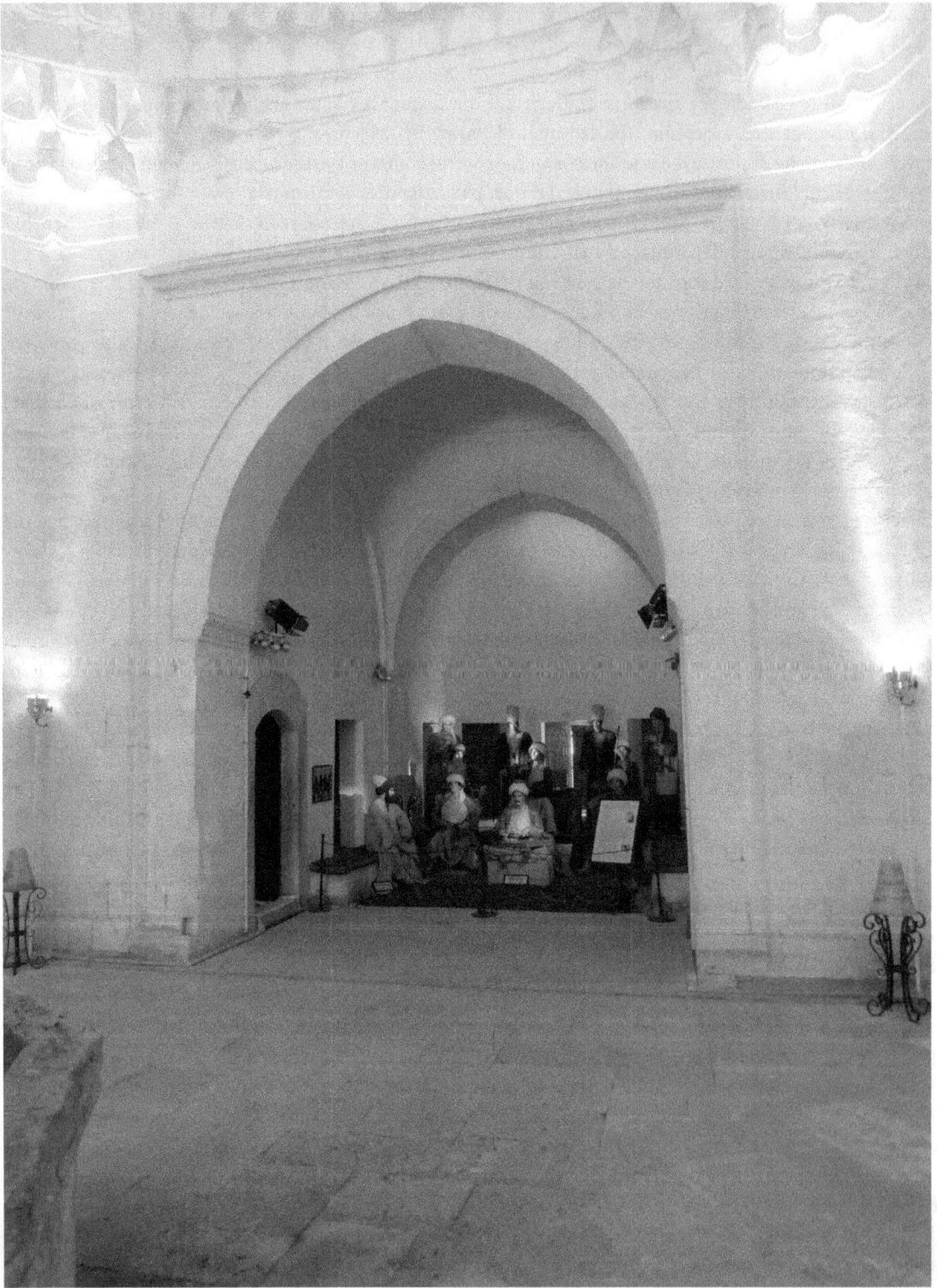

Figure 16.8 "Stage" in the Hospital of Bayezid II. Photo: Nina Ergin

stimulation of the body surface as a result of the sweating, scrubbing, and washing produces a decrease in pain sensation, in addition to mental relaxation and well-being.[52] It has also been argued that compassionate and gentle touching by the *darüşşifas*' healthcare staff, as it was stipulated in so many *vakfiyes*,[53] produced a healing, or at least somewhat relieving, effect.[54]

The sense of taste may not appear to be particularly relevant in connection to an architectural monument, but in fact the patients would have formed a strong association between the building and the types of medicines and food items they consumed there—very much like Evliya Çelebi formed strong associations between the mosque complexes he visited on his travels and the food served in their *imarets*.[55] A pharmacist prepared the medicine based on the doctor's orders in a room that served as dispensary and medicine storage, and patients receiving especially vile concoctions to ingest (or painful applications of salves) may have shuddered merely upon seeing the door to that room. Hospitals that were a dependency of a mosque complex with a soup kitchen would have received staff and inpatient meals from there,[56] but in a number of cases the *darüşşifa* itself employed a cook whose task it was to prepare dietetic meals after the doctor's directions in the hospital's own kitchen.[57] Beyond merely removing hunger and assisting the therapeutic process, hospital food was intended to produce the sensation of pleasurable satiation, if one takes the following statement from the *vakfiye* of the Atik Valide Complex at face value: "and they [the cooks] pay particular attention that the food is cooked well, in such a way that it brings appetite to the patients."[58]

Healing by Design: Four Qualities of Successful Hospital Space

Harnessing the curative powers of positive sensory experiences, such as those described in the preceding paragraphs, and preventing, or at least controlling, negative ones that decrease the patients' overall well-being, constitutes the primary underlying principle of "healing by design." In an article with the same title published in *The New England Journal of Medicine*, C. Robert Horsburgh discusses four qualities of space that have rendered a number of U.S. hospitals built in the 1980s and 1990s a success in terms of user satisfaction. The first of these qualities consists of *orientation*, including "access, the ability to find and gain entrance to a building, and internal orientation, the ability to locate a destination within a building."[59] Ottoman hospitals' location in cities, usually as part of or in close proximity to a mosque complex, ensured that the users easily found and gained access to the building. The construction material—stone and brick—immediately distinguished them from the majority of the urban fabric that was comprised of wooden residences and shops. Unlike most medieval Islamic hospitals, including Seljuk Anatolian ones, which boasted high gates with elaborate ornamentation such as muqarnas, Ottoman *darüşşifa* entrances were more modest, but still easy enough to identify, for instance by way of their epigraphic panels. Having passed the entrance, the interior of a typical *darüşşifa* can be captured and understood at a single glance: patient quarters line up around the perimeter, and healthcare providers could be found in a room differentiated by its size and roof cover, usually a much larger dome. Probably a doorman or staff member gave arriving patients directions, but, even if that was not the case, a single tour around the courtyard oriented visitors as to the location of the different facilities—unlike in large modern hospitals, which are notoriously labyrinthine and difficult to navigate, especially in times of physical and emotional distress.

The second user-friendly quality consists of *connection*—that is, "the quality of the interaction between people and their environment."[60] At first sight, Ottoman hospitals seem to have removed the sick from the healthy population by means of high walls and the employment of doormen to enforce a separation from the surrounding urban space and to prevent patients and others from willfully wandering in and out. Yet, there is more nuance to the aspect of connection, as it can further be subdivided into connection with nature and connection with other humans. Good design allows for a gradual transition from community at one end of the continuum, to privacy and isolation at the other end. Typical Ottoman hospitals offer such a transition: a communal area in the courtyard and under the porticoes, where patients could socialize if they desired to do so, but also more private areas in the form of small patient rooms, where they could withdraw. These considerations may also explain Mimar Sinan's choice to divide the Süleymaniye Darüşşifası's space into two courtyards, separating the administration wing of this busy teaching hospital in the first courtyard from the actual patients' area in the second and transitioning from public to semi-public to a more controlled and intimate space. Moreover, the lower-level, barrel-vaulted room for the mentally ill separated the potentially disturbing and even dangerous from those who needed quiet and comfort to recover. (As far as the customary proximity between the patients' beds needed for a basic level of comfort is concerned, we have unfortunately no evidence.)[61] Transition and potential separation equally apply to connection with nature: the garden in the central courtyard offered interaction with plants and exposure to fresh air and natural light, but the rooms also allowed patients to sever that connection with nature. Windows in patient rooms were generally small and high up on the wall—the building component housing the mental Hospital of Bayezid II in Edirne being a notable exception, maybe because it was deemed important for the mental patients to have visual access to the world outside—and therefore the fenestration permitted only little natural light and views. Isolation from nature would have been necessitated, for instance, for patients with eye diseases that made bright light painful.

The architectural quality of *scale* reflects itself in the building's overall size, the size of its different components, and especially its size in comparison to the human figure. Depending on a building's size, its users may feel small, insignificant, and overwhelmed—as is likely to happen with enormous modern hospitals with several hundred beds and endless corridors—or claustrophobic and cramped—as happens in buildings with low-ceilinged small rooms and without windows, for example. Ideally, however, a hospital user should feel comfortable and connected to their surroundings. Even the largest Ottoman hospitals, such as the Süleymaniye or the Atik Valide Darüşşifası, are of a size that could not have accommodated more than approximately sixty inpatients, based on the number of rooms with assumed double- and occasional triple-occupancy. As already noted, Ottoman *darüşşifa* entrances were not large and imposing, unlike some entrances to mosque courtyards. Hospital courtyards measured no more than 25 × 15 meters at most, creating a space that one could quite easily capture visually and traverse physically. Mimar Sinan, for example, could have planned the Süleymaniye Darüşşifası with one very large courtyard instead of two and thereby created a much simpler and faster-to-build design; however, by dividing the area, he prevented a loss of orientation and human scale, which otherwise would have inevitably occurred. Although the Süleymaniye and the Atik Valide hospitals were spread over two stories, this still did not make them into towering monuments that dwarfed their users. Patient rooms were small and measured usually 5 × 5 meters, thus offering a small-scale but not cramped space for cocooning.

Regardless of its function, every building conveys some kind of *symbolic meaning*. In present-day hospitals, rational science and the technological skill contained therein are emphasized by means of construction materials—concrete, glass, steel—and streamlined facades. Such an environment usually conveys the sense that one is not an individual person, but a medical case. Ideally, such dehumanization should not occur. To quote Horsburgh, "since patients and their families need to concentrate their energies on healing, architects [should] design hospitals to provide an atmosphere of security, cleanliness and physical comfort. In this way, patients are encouraged not to worry about safety, sanitation, or physical discomfort."[62] In the *darüşşifa*s, due to the limited number of entrances and windows, the presence of a doorman, the existence of storage space that could also accommodate a patient's belongings, and the frequent employment of a steward/scribe watching over the storage, patients could feel safe and secure. This was especially important since the mere fact of being cared for in a hospital usually implied being far away from one's family, or completely without a family, as mentioned above. Physical comfort was ensured with the variety of spaces to which patients had recourse, based on the individually most suitable environment in terms of temperature, light, and level of interaction with others: courtyard garden, portico, or indoor space. Cleanliness was easily maintained due

Healing by Design

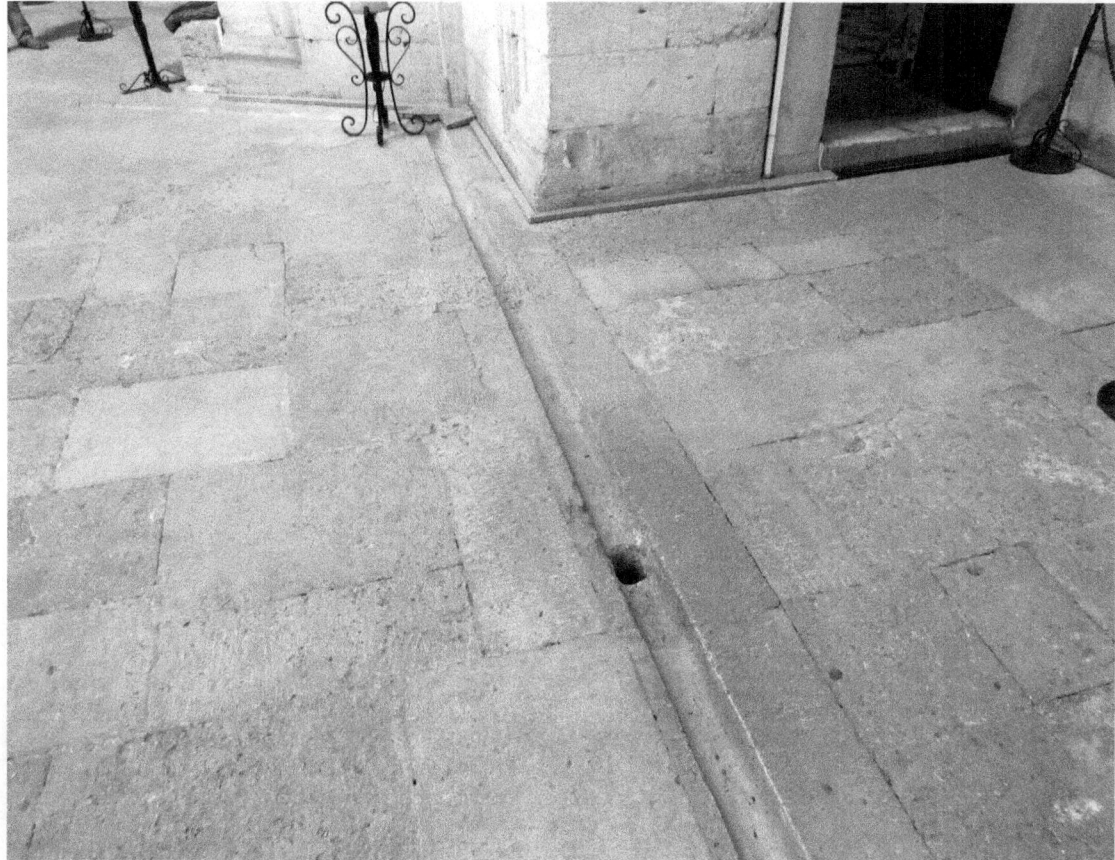

Figure 16.9 Water runnel in the Hospital of Bayezid II. Photo: Nina Ergin

to a number of factors: the usage of easy-to-clean building material, such as marble in the hamam interior; a layout that avoids awkward and difficult-to-clean corners; adequate water supply and drainage, as can be seen in the runnels of the Hospital of Bayezid II (Figure 16.9); and the existence of cleaning staff. As to the last most hospitals had a sizable cadre of cleaning personnel on hand. For instance, the Süleymaniye Darüşşifası employed four caretakers (*kayyum*), two janitors (*odacı*), and two laundrymen (*esvapcı*) with a daily salary of 3 *akçe* each.[63] Here, I would like to argue that the most significant symbolic meaning of Ottoman hospitals, however, was the sense of familiar surroundings that they evoked, a point to which I will return below.

Conclusion

In summary, orientation, connection, scale, and symbolic meaning all worked together to create a strong sense of comforting familiarity for the typical *darüşşifa* patient. This typical patient and hospital user was likely to be a traveler far away from home, but, due to his previous experiences and exposure to Ottoman culture, familiar with the appearance and layout of the dependencies of Ottoman mosque complexes, such as caravanserais, *imaret*s (Figure 16.10), and imperially sponsored *tekke*s: a modest entrance, maybe with an epigraphic panel, leading into a courtyard with a water feature, surrounded by porticoes that fronted rows of cells and with a larger room or *eyvan* serving as a focal point for shared activities, be they teaching, conducting rituals, or treating patients. Ottoman hospital architecture was rarely innovative—maybe with the

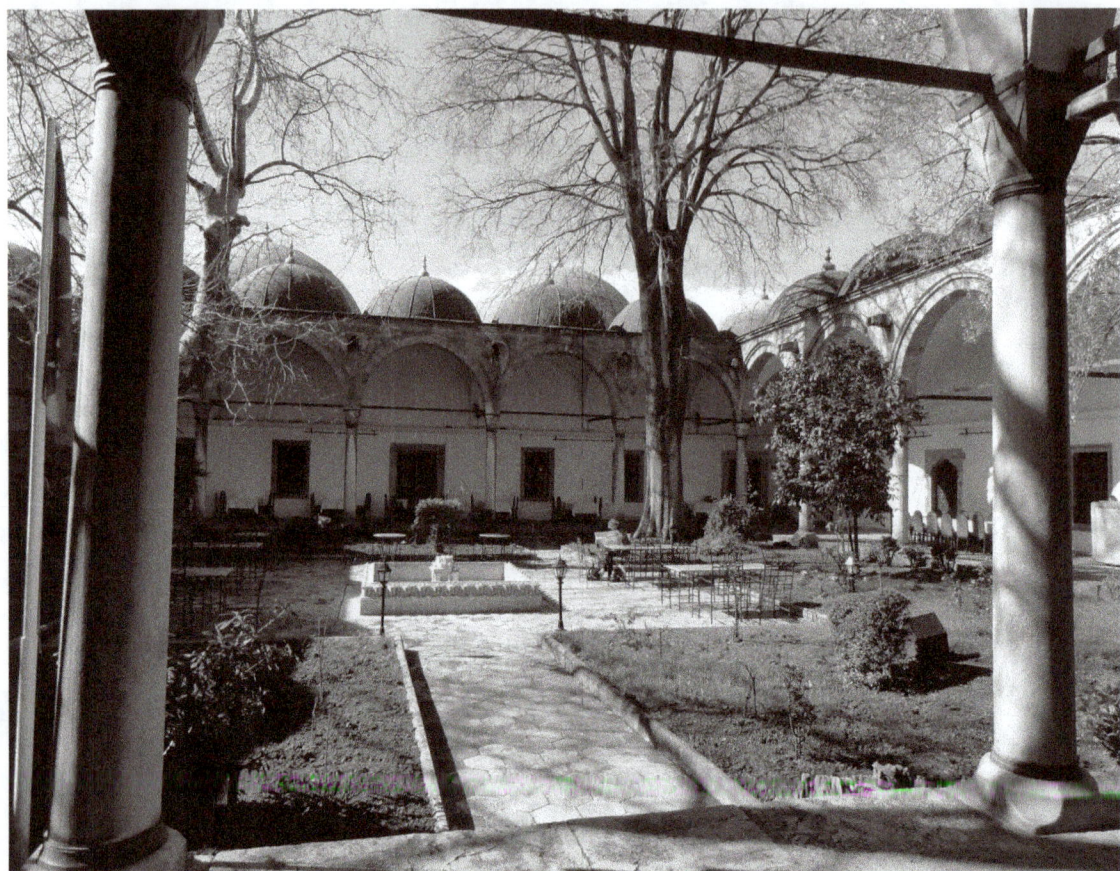

Figure 16.10 Courtyard of the Süleymaniye's *imaret*. Photo: Nina Ergin

exception of the Hospital of Bayezid II—but that was not the point to the question of whether the users, staff, and patients alike considered their built environment a successful one: easy to recognize as a building housing a charitable institution enhancing the well-being of its beneficiaries, easy to access, easy to navigate, providing spaces that allowed for privacy as much as different levels of social interaction, built at a scale that neither dwarfed nor cramped its users, and safe, clean, and comfortable.

Such a balanced and comforting environment was also in keeping with the principles of Galenic medicine.[64] First of all, the four cosmic elements—earth, air, fire, and water—found their reflection in the four humors in the human body, and whether in the cosmos or in the individual body, only the right mixture resulted in an ideal balance. Through the earth, air, and water feature in the courtyard garden, and the fire in the fireplaces, Ottoman patients could come into direct contact with the primal elements, and in such a way that, for example, an imbalance caused by an excess of hot and dry humors could be counteracted through exposure to water. More than just offering small fountains and pools, hospitals, from medieval to Ottoman, were usually erected in the proximity of bathhouses; while Baker points out the lack of evidence for the existence of integrated hamams in medieval institutions,[65] in the early modern period a few select *darüşşifa*s on Ottoman territory did offer such hamams to their patients.

Furthermore, there were the six non-naturals that help to maintain the balance of the four humors: light and air, food and drink, work and rest, sleep and waking, excretions and secretions, and dispositions and states of the soul. Ottoman hospitals—or any imperial monument built on the same scheme—certainly provided the first pair of non-naturals, light and air: the large courtyard allowed for air flow and circulation even in the hospital's closed areas, and light in the quantity deemed appropriate to a patient's condition could be found in the open courtyard, underneath the porticoes, entering through the oculus in the central dome in case of a covered "courtyard,"[66] or filtering through the rooms' windows. The needed amount of rest, as well as the balance between sleep and waking, was facilitated by the hospital's controlled soundscape: gently falling water induced sleep, while birdsong entertained and, in some cases, music provided therapeutic relief. This overlaps with the last pair, on which Pormann and Savage-Smith have remarked: "one of the six non-naturals is the mental state of the patients, and, as such, it affects their health directly. Sadness and anxiety are to be avoided, and music, as well as pleasant company, and a quiet environment can contribute to the convalescence."[67]

To return to Frank Lloyd Wright's famous dictum on hospital architecture—"hospital patients should never be imbued with the idea that they are sick"—*darüşşifa* patients indeed received treatment in an architectural space that, by dint of its similarity to mosque courtyards, medreses, hans, *imaret*s, and the like, evoked sensory experiences and memories of charitable institutional spaces that were *not* related to disease. At the same time, specific building elements such as the generally forbidding exterior walls that prevented the seriously ill from fully interacting with healthy society did ratify the patients' condition as different from the rest of the world— more fragile, and in need of separation and protection. Maybe the term "healing by design" would exaggerate the contribution that Ottoman hospital architecture made to curing the patients; however, it is not too far-fetched to speak of "balancing and comforting them, and making them forget their condition by design."

Acknowledgments: An earlier version of this chapter was presented at the conference "The Ottomans and Health: A Comparative Perspective," organized by the Skilliter Centre for Ottoman Studies at Newnham College in 2013, and then subsequently published as "Healing by Design? An Experiential Approach to Early Modern Ottoman Hospital Architecture," *Turkish Historical Review* 6 (2015): 1–37. I wish to thank the editors of the journal for their permission to re-publish the article. I also thank the conveners of the conference, Director of the Skilliter Centre Kate Fleet, and Ebru Boyar, academic advisor to the Centre, for inviting me to participate and for creating such a congenial and productive atmosphere. The article has greatly benefited from the comments of the other participants and anonymous peer reviewers. Any mistakes that remain are my own.

Notes

1. R. M. Cunningham, Jnr., "Frank Lloyd Wright on Hospital Design: A Modern Hospital Interview with the World-Famous Architect," *Modern Hospital* 71 (1948): 51.
2. See G. B. Risse, *Mending Bodies, Saving Souls: A History of Hospitals* (New York: Oxford University Press, 1999). The best-preserved example of an *asclepieion* is located on the island of Kos. For an overview of Ancient Greek Medicine, see Vivian Nutton, *Ancient Medicine* (London: Routledge, 2004).
3. Roger Ulrich, "View through a Window May Influence Recovery from Surgery," *Science* 224 (1984): 420–1. For an overview of research and practice several years on, see idem, "Effects of Interior Design and Wellness: Theory and Recent Scientific Research," *Journal of Health Care Interior Design* 3 (1991): 97–109; and Roger Ulrich et al., "The Role of the Physical Environment in the Hospital of the 21st Century," The Robert Wood Johnson Foundation and the Center for Health Design, accessed July 20, 2014. http://www.healthdesign.org/chd/research/role-physical-environment-hospital-21st-century.
4. See, for example, C. Robert Horsburgh, Jnr., "Healing by Design," *The New England Journal of Medicine* 333 (1995): 735–40. An excellent overview of such new directions in hospital design, based on an eight-year-long research project, is Cor Waagenar, ed., *The Architecture of Hospitals* (Amsterdam: NAi Publishers, 2006). For the point that restorative environments experience a cycle of disappearance and rediscovery, see S. B. Warner Jr., "The Periodic Rediscoveries

of Restorative Gardens: 1100–Present," in *The Healing Dimensions of People-Plant Relations: Proceedings of a Research Symposium*, ed. M. Francis, P. Lindsey, and J. S. Rice (Davis: University of California, Davis, Center for Design Research, 1995), 5–12.

5. Gönül Cantay, *Anadolu Selçuklu ve Osmanlı Darüşşifaları* [Anatolian Seljuk and Ottoman Hospitals] (Ankara: Atatürk Kültür Merkezi Yayınları, 1992). For two popular publications that give a good survey over Ottoman hospitals, see Abdullah Kılıç, *Anadolu Selçuklu ve Osmanlı Şefkat Abideleri: Şifahaneler* (Istanbul: MedicalPark, 2012); and idem, *Karşılıksız Hizmetin Muhteşem Abideleri: İstanbul Şifahaneleri* (Istanbul: İstanbul Büyükşehir belediyesi Kültür A. Ş. Yayınları, 2009). The scope of this chapter does not include palace hospitals, which have been discussed, among others, in Arslan Terzioğlu, *Die Hofspitäler und andere Gesundheitseinrichtungen der osmanischen Palastbauten unter Berücksichtigung der Ursprungsfrage sowie ihre Beziehungen zu den abendländischen Hofspitälern* (Munich: Trofenik, 1979). The latter scholar's prolific work on various aspects of Ottoman and Republican Turkish medical history has been collected in his *Beiträge zur Geschichte der türkisch-islamischen Medizin, Wissenschaft und Technik*, 2 vols. (Istanbul: Isis, 1996).

6. Miri Shefer-Mossensohn, *Ottoman Medicine: Healing and Medical Institutions, 1500–1700* (Albany: SUNY Press, 2009), 162.

7. For an introduction to Galenic Humoralism, see Peter Pormann and Emilie Savage-Smith, *Medieval Islamic Medicine* (Edinburgh: Edinburgh University Press, 2007), 44–5.

8. *Darüşşifa* literally means "house of recovery/healing." Ottomans also interchangeably used *şifahane* ("house of recovery/healing"), *darüssıha* ("house of health"), and the Persian-derived *bimarhane* and *bimaristan* (both meaning "house for the ill"). See Yasser Tabbaa, "The Functional Aspects of Medieval Islamic Hospitals," in *Poverty and Charity in Middle Eastern Contexts*, ed. Michael Bonner, Mine Ener, and Amy Singer (Albany: SUNY Press, 2003), 96. *Timarhane* (Persian for "house of care") refers to a hospital for the mentally ill. Gary Leiser and Michael Dols, "Evliya Chelebi's Description of Medicine in 17th C. Egypt," *Sudhoffs Archiv* 71 (1987): 207. Here, I prefer to employ the first, now more commonly used term, throughout.

9. Shefer-Mossensohn, *Ottoman Medicine*, 146.

10. Wagenaar, *Architecture of Hospitals*, 255.

11. Early modern Ottoman hospitals inherited much from pre-Ottoman institutions in Anatolia and elsewhere in the Islamic world, and questions as to the extent to which the principles of "healing by design" were applied in earlier (Islamic and Byzantine) hospitals, the ways in which Ottomans adopted them, or how Ottoman hospitals contributed to their application elsewhere in the Islamic world, exceed the boundaries of this chapter, but constitute fruitful questions for further inquiry. Although not explicitly framed by the concept of "healing by design," Baker has already approached medieval Islamic hospitals (and therefore the first question above) from a similar angle: Patricia Baker, "Medieval Islamic Hospitals: Structural Design and Social Perceptions," in *Medicine and Space: Bodies, Surroundings and Borders in Antiquity and the Middle Ages*, ed. Patricia Baker, Han Nijdam, and Karine van't Land (Leiden: Brill, 2012), 245–72.

12. Excellent examples of interpretative approaches to Islamic hospitals in different temporal and geographical contexts include Tabbaa, "Functional Aspects of Medieval Islamic Hospitals"; and Baker, "Medieval Islamic Hospitals."

13. For an overview of the latter, see the review essay by Chris Gratien, "Ottoman Environmental History: A New Area of Middle East Studies," *Arab Studies Journal* 20 (2012): 246–54. Although "The Cultural History of Emotions in Premodernity II: Emotions East and West" was the topic of a 2011 conference in Istanbul (for the program, see www.chep2011.bilkent.edu.tr), very few publications have taken up the issue within Ottoman Studies since then. For one example, see Walter Andrews, "Ottoman Love: Preface to a Theory of Emotional Ecology," in *A History of Emotions, 1200–1800*, ed. Jonas Liliequist (London: Pickering & Chatto, 2012).

14. VGM, D. 1766, p. 137, as translated in Nina Macaraig, *The Çemberlitaş Hamamı in Istanbul: The Biographical Memoir of a Turkish Bath* (Edinburgh: Edinburgh University Press, 2018), 249.

15. The Atik Valide Darüşşifası had in fact also one employee staffing its small bath. According to the *vakfiye*, "one *külhancı* [furnace attendant] shall be appointed in order to heat the hamam prepared for the patients and to massage the patients in the hamam and to look after other tasks related to the hamam." VGM, D. 1766, p. 158, as translated in Macaraig, *Çemberlitaş Hamamı*, 273.

16. Shefer-Mossensohn, *Ottoman Medicine*, 171.

17. Cf. Baker, "Medieval Islamic Hospitals," 269.

18. In the Bimaristan al-Nuri in Damascus, erected in 1154, one of the four *eyvan*s was likely used as place of study, a claim supported by the existence of storage niches that must have contained books. See Baker, "Medieval Islamic Hospitals," 258–9.

19. Due to limitations of space, only little attention can be paid to Ottoman hospital gardens, which constitute a major topic in themselves. For a discussion of these gardens and their therapeutic effects, see Shefer-Mossensohn, *Ottoman Medicine*, 159–66. On the contemporary context, see C. Cooper Marcus and M. Barnes, *Gardens in Healthcare Facilities: Uses, Therapeutic Benefits, and Design Recommendations* (Martinez: Center for Health Design, 1995).
20. See Nina Ergin, "'And in the Soup Kitchen Food Shall Be Cooked Twice Every Day': Gustatory Aspects of Ottoman Mosque Complexes," in *Rethinking Place in South Asian and Islamic Art, 1500–Present*, ed. Rebecca Brown and Deborah Hutton (New York: Routledge, 2016), 17–37. For the argument for a "hierarchy" of food quality (which can be considered in parallel to a hierarchy of architectural form), see Amy Singer, "The 'Michelin Guide' to Public Kitchens in the Ottoman Empire," in *Starting with Food: Culinary Approaches to Ottoman History*, ed. Amy Singer (Princeton: Markus Wiener, 2011), 69–92.
21. Gülru Necipoğlu, *The Age of Sinan: Architectural Culture in the Ottoman Empire* (Princeton: Princeton University Press, 2005), 292.
22. Cantay, *Darüşşifalar*.
23. For a more extensive discussion of this monument, see Cantay, *Darüşşifalar*, 88–91, pls. 147–57; and Nihad Yörükoğlu, *Manisa Bimarhanesi* (Istanbul: İsmail Akgün Matbaası, 1948). For a virtual tour of the monument, see http://www.mekan360.com/360fx_darussifamanisa-manisa-merkez.html (accessed July 20, 2014). As of November 2013, the building has opened its doors as a medical history museum connected to Celal Bayar Üniversitesi. On the number of patients and staff, as well as the latters' tasks, see Yörükoğlu, *Manisa Bimarhanesi*, 17–18.
24. The inscription reads as follows: *Bu dârı mâder-i Sultân Süleyman/binâ etti ki çây-ı menfaattır/bu hayrın bânisi fahrü'l-kuzât ol/emânet dârı ehl-i mekremettir/su'âl olunsa itmâm binâsı/de târîhi makâm-ı 'afiyettir*. The chronogram in the last line adds up to AH 946/1539 AD. Yörükoğlu, *Manisa Bimarhanesi*, 15.
25. For a comprehensive biography and discussion of his oeuvre, see Necipoğlu, *The Age of Sinan*.
26. Because the hospital, like most others, has served different functions over time, the monument's structure has been modified a great deal. Although renovations were completed as of summer 2014, the building has not yet been opened to the public. For a more extensive discussion of this monument, see Cantay, *Darüşşifalar*, 91–6, pls. 179–205.
27. Medical schools represent a separate topic and are therefore not considered here. For a study with a comprehensive bibliography, see Nil Sarı, "Educating the Ottoman Physician," in *History of Medicine Studies*, ed. Nil Sarı and Hüsrev Hatemi (Istanbul: [n.p.], 1988), 40–64, accessed July 21, 2014, http://www.fstc.org.uk/node/55.
28. The current panel reads *matba'a-yı 'askeriyye 1305* and, together with the *tuğra* of Sultan Abdülhamid, dates back to 1887/8.
29. Cf. Baker, "Medieval Islamic Hospitals," 266.
30. Cantay, *Darüşşifalar*, 97.
31. For this reason, I will refer to the hospital users as "he." On a more in-depth discussion of gender aspects in Ottoman healthcare, see Miri Shefer-Mossensohn, "Charity and Hospitality: Hospitals in the Ottoman Empire in the Early Modern Period," in *Poverty and Charity in Middle Eastern Contexts*, ed. Michael Bonner, Mine Ener, and Amy Singer (Albany: SUNY Press, 2003), 131–3; idem, *Ottoman Medicine*, 128–32.
32. Shefer-Mossensohn, *Ottoman Medicine*, 121.
33. See the above-mentioned Terzioğlu, *Hofspitäler und andere Gesundheitseinrichtungen der osmanischen Palastbauten*, as well as Nil Sarı, Gül Akdeniz, and Ramazan Tuğ, "Topkapı ve Galata Sarayı Enderun Hastanesi," in *IV. Türk Tıp Tarihi Kongresi, Istanbul, 18–20 Eylül 1988: Kongreye Sunulan Bildiriler* (Ankara: TTK, 2002), 187–201; and Vildan Özkan Göksoy, "Topkapı Sarayında 'Cariyeler Hastanesi,'" in *I. Türk Tıp Tarihi Kongresi, Istanbul, 17–19 Şubat 1988: Kongreye Sunulan Bildiriler* (Ankara: TTK, 1992), 193–8.
34. For a comprehensive study of Ottoman chief doctors, see Ali Haydar Bayat, *Osmanlı Devleti'nde Hekimbaşılık Kurumu ve Hekimbaşılar* (Ankara: Atatürk Kültür Merkezi, 1999).
35. Cf. Nina Ergin, "The Albanian Tellâk Connection: Labor Migration to the Hamams of Eighteenth-Century Istanbul, Based on the 1752 İstanbul Hamâmları Defteri," *Turcica* 43 (2011 [2012]): 248–9.
36. J. D. Latham and H. D. Isaacs, *Isaac Judaeus: On Fevers (The Third Discourse: On Consumption)* (Cambridge: Pembroke, 1981), sections 29–30. Amended translation from Pormann and Savage-Smith, *Medieval Islamic Medicine*, 57.
37. On the Topkapı Palace's viewscape, see Gülru Necipoğlu, "Framing the Gaze in Ottoman, Safavid and Mughal Palaces," *Ars Orientalis* 23 (1993): 303–42. For Mimar Sinan's viewscapes, see idem, *The Age of Sinan: Architectural Culture in the Ottoman Empire* (Princeton: Princeton University Press, 2005), 304–5, 323–4. On the theatrical aesthetic of Ottoman art and architecture, see Jale Nejdet Erzen, "Aesthetics and Aisthesis in Ottoman Art and Architecture," *Journal of Islamic Studies* 2 (1991): 1–24.

38. Ulrich, "View through a Window."
39. V. Blomkvist, C. A. Eriksen, T. Theorell, R. Ulrich, and G. Rasmanis, "Acoustics and Psychosocial Environment in Intensive Coronary Care," *Occupational Environmental Medicine* 62 (2005): e1–e8.
40. Gary Leiser and Michael Dols, "Evliya Chelebi's Description of Medicine in Seventeenth-Century Egypt, Part II: Text," *Sudhoffs Archiv* 72 (1988): 53.
41. On the birdhouses, see Cengiz Bektaş, *Kuş Evleri/Bird-Houses* (Istanbul: Arkeoloji ve Sanat Yayınları, 2000); and Rahşan Özen, "Bird Shelters in Turkey: Birdhouses and Dovecotes," *Kafkas Üniversitesi Veteriner Fakültesi Dergisi* 18 (2012): 1079–82. On the aviaries in the palace, see Gülru Necipoğlu, *Architecture, Ceremonial and Power: The Topkapı Palace in the Fifteenth and Sixteenth Centuries* (Cambridge, MA: MIT, 1991), 123.
42. Evliya Çelebi, *Evliya Çelebi Seyahatnamesi, 3. Cilt, 2. Kitap*, ed. Seyit Ali Kahraman and Yücel Dağlı (Istanbul: Yapı Kredi Yayınları, 2010), 609.
43. Evliya Çelebi, *Evliya Çelebi Seyahatnamesi, 3. Cilt, 2. Kitap*, 609–10. For a more extensive discussion of this passage, see Shefer-Mossensohn, *Ottoman Medicine*, 72–3.
44. For a comparative discussion of music therapy in the Byzantine, medieval Islamic, and medieval Western European hospitals, see Peregrine Horden, "Religion as Medicine: Music in Medieval Hospitals," in *Religion and Medicine in the Middle Ages*, ed. P. Biller and J. Ziegler (Woodbridge: York Medieval Press, 2001), 135–53. For more comprehensive studies, see idem, ed., *Music as Medicine: The History of Music Therapy since Antiquity* (Aldershot: Ashgate, 2000), and for the context of this chapter especially the article by Amnon Shiloah on "Jewish and Muslim Traditions of Music Therapy," 69–83; as well as Penelope Gouk, ed., *Musical Healing in Cultural Contexts* (Aldershot: Ashgate, 2000).
45. Ahmet Hakkı Turabi, "Hekim Şuûrî Hasan Efendi ve Ta'dîlü'l-Emzice adlı Eserinde Müzikle Tedavi Bölümü," *Marmara Üniversitesi İlahiyat Fakültesi Dergisi* 40 (2011): 153–66 (on Uşşak, see 163).
46. Arslan Terzioğlu, *Osmanlılarda Hastaneler, Eczacılık, Tababet ve Bunların Dünya Çapındaki Etkiler* (Istanbul: Kültür Bakanlığı, 1999).
47. For the *vakfiyes* related to Bayezid II's charitable institutions in Edirne, see VGM, D. 2113, p. 106 (no. 26), and D. 2148, pp. 59–82.
48. See, for example, the following passage from the title deed of the Atik Valide Complex: "And the founder set the condition that two male *çamaşırcı* [laundrymen] shall be appointed to this hospital. These will wash the laundry of the patients, such as bedding, covers, dirt, spills and stains, and they will clean dirt in the close proximity of the patients; and the salary of each of them shall be three dirhem." VGM, D. 1766, p. 158, as translated in Macaraig, *Çemberlitaş Hamamı*, 273.
49. C. G. Fisher and A. Fisher, "Topkapı Sarayı in the Mid-Seventeenth Century: Bobovi's Description," *Archivum Ottomanicum* 10 (1985): 47.
50. Evliya Çelebi, *Evliya Çelebi Seyahatnamesi, 3. Cilt, 2. Kitap*, 609.
51. According to Ibn Sina, the benefits of bathing are manifold for balancing the humors. A patient who needs to gain weight should visit the hamam after having eaten; this will produce a moderate increase of weight (Avicenna, *The General Principles of Avicenna's Canon of Medicine*, trans. Mazhar Shah [Karachi: Naveed Clinic, 1966], 196). Because the humid atmosphere in the hamam opens the pores, the skin can be cleansed most thoroughly. Furthermore, the humidity aids in the maturation and dispersal of waste matters in the body and gives physiological assistance in the excretion of these poisonous matters (308). Different types of massage also shaped the specific beneficial aspects of the bath: while hard massage makes the body firm and consequently removes fatigue, soft massage relaxes the body and induces sleep. The application of moderate massage helps to develop muscle tone, and prolonged massage is recommended to reduce the bather's weight. Rough massage with a *kese* or loofah sponge briskly draws the blood towards the skin and assists the body in the elimination of waste products (305). However, not all patients were advised to use balneotherapy indiscriminately, as massage in the hot environment could also disperse matters towards the flexures and weaker organs and thus produce inflammation; therefore, a person suffering from fever, injury, or inflammation was advised against a long hamam visit including a massage (197). Hence the need for a knowledgeable attendant who knew about potentially adverse effects of bathing as well as his massages.
52. Zeki Karagülle, "Health Effects of Hamams," paper presented at the symposium "Fürdö, Sauna, Hamam," Research Center for Anatolian Civilizations, Istanbul, April 25–6, 2009.
53. According to the title deed of the Atik Valide Complex, the doctors "will never use hard words when seeing the patients; they will treat every patient with kindness and politeness, as if they were their nearest family and relatives; they will encounter their patients with gentleness and with respect towards their condition, by taking the patients under the shadow of their compassion …" VGM, D. 1766, p. 156, as translated in Macaraig, *Çemberlitaş Hamamı*, 271.

54. Shefer-Mossensohn, *Ottoman Medicine*, 189.
55. See Ergin, "Gustatory Aspects of Ottoman Mosque Complexes."
56. On *imaret*s in general, see Nina Ergin, Christoph Neumann, and Amy Singer, eds., *Feeding People, Feeding Power: Imarets in the Ottoman Empire* (Istanbul: Eren, 2007); on the food served, see the chapter "Food for Feasts: Cooking Recipes in Sixteenth- and Seventeenth-Century Anatolian Hostelries (Imarets)" by Suraiya Faroqhi, as well as Singer, "Michelin Guide to Public Kitchens."
57. "And [Nurbanu Sultan, patron of the Atik Valide Mosque Complex] set the condition that two male *aşçı* [cooks] shall be appointed. They shall cook dishes which are good for the patients, in the way that a skillful and smart doctor trusts and relies on; … and the salary of each shall be three *dirhem*." VGM, D. 1766, p. 158, as translated in Macaraig, *Çemberlitaş Hamamı*, 273.
58. Ibid.
59. Horsburgh, "Healing by Design," 735.
60. Ibid., 736.
61. Cf. Baker, "Medieval Islamic Hospitals," 268.
62. Horsburgh, "Healing by Design," 738.
63. Kazım İsmail Gürkan, "Süleymaniye Darüşşifası," *Kanuni Armağanı* (Ankara: TTK, 1979), 263.
64. A comparative study of how Galenic principles were expressed in architectural form in Islamic versus medieval and early modern European hospitals has not yet been undertaken, but constitutes a *desideratum*.
65. Baker, "Medieval Islamic Hospitals," 267.
66. This was the case in the hospital in Divriği as well as of Bayezid II. See Baker, "Medieval Islamic Hospitals," 260.
67. Pormann and Savage-Smith, *Medieval Islamic Medicine*, 48.

CHAPTER 17
ARCHITECTURAL PRESCRIPTIONS
JOHNS HOPKINS MEDICINE AND THE SHIFT FROM THE PRE-MODERN TO THE MODERN HOSPITAL
Stuart W. Leslie

The Hôtel-Dieu (651), the enormous Parisian hospital that stood for a millennium on the banks of the Seine, might be considered the last of the ancients, and Johns Hopkins Hospital (1889) in Baltimore the first of the moderns. Adjoining Notre-Dame Cathedral and predating it by six hundred years, Hôtel-Dieu embodied the pre-modern ideals of the hospital, offering "charity, care, and convalescence" to the sick poor, but little medical treatment.[1] Even as a public institution after the sixteenth century, the Hôtel-Dieu retained its medieval character, with its seemingly endless open wards, conspicuous chapels, and nurses drawn from religious orders—a place where piety had priority over healing. Johns Hopkins Hospital, by contrast, was built from scratch on the principles of modern laboratory medicine, an avowedly secular, private institution organized and run by its medical faculty. Its campus, designed by a distinguished physician in line with the latest medical theories, sought to bring together the best recent German, French, and British ideas about medical teaching, research, and practice.

Erwin Ackerknect, in his study *Medicine at the Paris Hospital, 1794–1848*, suggests that the Hôtel-Dieu's "hospital medicine" marked a sharp break between the "library and bedside" medicine that preceded it and the "laboratory medicine" that would follow. Only in a large municipal hospital like the Hôtel-Dieu, he argues, could the defining features of hospital medicine—physical examinations, autopsies, and statistics—develop under the guiding hand of physicians. And only there would medicine and surgery, essentially separated at birth in the ancient world, come together in the modern.[2]

After a devastating fire at the Hôtel-Dieu in 1772, the French king appointed a distinguished committee of the Paris Academy of Sciences to propose designs for a new municipal hospital. In one way or another, all of the plans, including one drafted by surgeon Jacques Tenon and royal architect Julien David Le Roy, incorporated some version of a pavilion design, with patients housed in detached, self-contained wards with a relatively small number of beds. The pavilions would promote healing and combat contagion by isolating patients from one another and by providing them with as much fresh air, heat, and light as possible.[3] Tenon had spent his career at the Hôtel-Dieu and knew its horrors first-hand. Dedicated to serving anyone and everyone in need, the Hôtel-Dieu packed in the suffering four, five, or six to a bed and did little to segregate patients by disease or prognosis, lumping together the insane with lying-in women, the contagious with the chronic, adults with children, those awaiting surgery with those trying to recover from it, making it "the most unhealthy and most uncomfortable of all hospitals," with mortality rates exceeding 20 percent—shockingly high even for its time.[4]

Tenon could see the future, and wrote about it in his muckraking classic, *Memoirs of the Hospitals of Paris* (1788). Had Tenon's farsighted ideas prevailed—envisioning the hospital as "an instrument to facilitate cure," one administered by a medical staff, organized around clinical practice and patient care, and devoted to research and teaching—a new version of the Hôtel-Dieu, rather than Johns Hopkins, might have provided the model for the modern hospital. Instead, Tenon's Enlightenment-inspired conception of hospitals remained a literary masterpiece only, a casualty of the French Revolution, along with all the plans for new hospitals proposed by the Academy members.[5] The Johns Hopkins Hospital would be the opportunity to build what Tenon could only dream of, a hospital designed for "laboratory medicine."

Linking the Medical School and the Teaching Hospital

American public hospitals, though never built on the scale of their European counterparts, such as the London Hospital (1752), were founded on similar designs and missions. They had their roots in the Pennsylvania Hospital (1751), founded by Benjamin Franklin and physician Thomas Bond.[6] These hospitals, though often admirable civic landmarks, were administered by lay trustees as charitable institutions for the worthy poor, with little input from physicians. For admission they usually required a written testimonial from some "respectable" person, and often turned away those suffering from contagious or incurable diseases, those with ailments considered signs of moral failing such as alcoholism or venereal disease, and African-Americans and recent immigrants. Devoted as much to spiritual as to physical healing, these hospitals had strict "rules of order" aimed at social control and character-building, with an explicit sectarian message, including mandatory chapel attendance.[7] Benjamin West's monumental painting, "Christ Healing the Sick in the Temple" (1811) commissioned as a fundraiser by the trustees of the Philadelphia Hospital, perfectly expressed the hospital's mission of saving bodies and souls. West's painting turned out to be so popular that admission fees collected in the "picture house" he designed for it actually paid for the hospital's new building. To this day the painting has pride of place in the hospital, now as part of the University of Pennsylvania Health System.[8] Charles Bulfinch's Massachusetts General Hospital (1818) fit the same pattern, though its role as the first teaching hospital for Harvard University's medical school made it distinctive. Architecturally, it anticipated Bulfinch's later redesign of the U.S. Capitol Building (1846), his most famous commission.

Johns Hopkins Medicine, including its hospitals, clinics, and outpatient facilities, its schools of medicine, nursing, and public health, its research buildings and its science and technology park, now sprawls across more than eighty buildings on 100 acres in east Baltimore. Virtually a city unto itself, the campus rises above and has often been at odds with the impoverished neighborhood surrounding it. For more than a century, Johns Hopkins has defined and redefined modern medicine, establishing itself as one of the best-known and highest-ranked medical centers in the world. Today it is not only the city's but also the state's largest private employer, with 30,000 faculty, researchers, and staff on the main medical campus alone, and another 20,000 in satellite hospitals and institutes in the greater Baltimore region. The original hospital's signature dome has long since been overshadowed by a confusing jumble of buildings of every size, description, and style, whether the oddly coupled, if visually striking, Sheikh Zayed Tower and Bloomberg Children's Center (2012) by Perkins+Will, with a glass curtain wall inspired by Impressionist paintings and a curated art collection, or the otherwise anonymous brick labyrinths named for long-dead physicians and their grateful patients.

Though not exactly "architecture without architects"—even if most of the architects are more obscure than the names on the buildings—Johns Hopkins Medicine is closer in character to a small city with poorly enforced zoning than to any sort of planned community (Figure 17.1). As any first-time patient or first-year medical student can attest, simply finding your way to the right building and department can be a daunting challenge. Hopkins succeeds despite a seemingly deliberately arcane architecture. To a practiced eye, however, the campus is a palimpsest of modern medicine, where every era has literally built upon, and been influenced by, what has come before. Read closely, and the architecture of Hopkins Medicine reveals a richly layered archive of how the modern hospital has taken the form it has, not just at Johns Hopkins but at

Health and Architecture

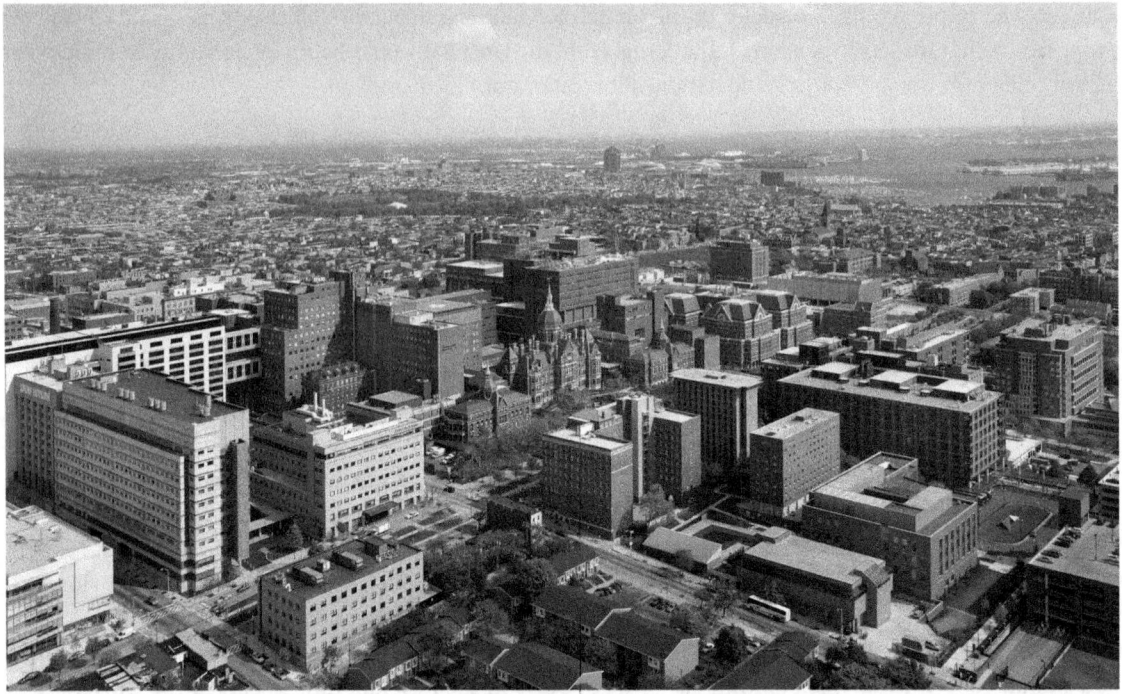

Figure 17.1 Johns Hopkins Medicine, a twenty-first-century city within a city. Note the original dome near the middle of the complex, with the School of Nursing to its right. Photo: Keith Weller, Courtesy of Johns Hopkins Medicine

urban campuses across the country, the University of Pittsburgh Medical Center, the Cleveland Clinic, and the University of California, San Francisco Medical Center.[9]

When, in 1873, Baltimore merchant and philanthropist Johns Hopkins instructed the trustees who would administer his estate to establish a university and a hospital that would bear his distinctive name, he could not have known that they would end up creating the first modern hospital, and a national, even international, model for those to follow.[10] A graduate of the school of hard knocks, Hopkins himself knew virtually nothing about universities, and very little about hospitals. Neither did his trustees, local businessmen, bankers, lawyers, and judges, none of whom had much, if any, previous experience with higher education or modern medicine. Yet they would prove themselves remarkably shrewd in seeking out the best professional advice of the day and putting it into practice. By design, Hopkins had assembled two overlapping boards of trustees, one for his university and one for his hospital, and split the unprecedented endowment of $7 million between them. Rather than envisioning the university and hospital as independent institutions, Hopkins saw them as mutually reinforcing, connected not merely by proximity but even more importantly by a new medical school that would be an integral part of both. That fundamental idea—a medical school embedded within a research university and controlling its own teaching hospital—though embryonic in Hopkins's will—would ultimately distinguish Johns Hopkins as the first fully modern hospital. From its opening in 1889 to the present, it has exemplified, for better and worse, how scientific medicine could be organized and administered, and also what it could look like. Architecturally and medically, Johns Hopkins Medicine's greatest contribution would not be any single innovation but rather the flexibility to adapt, improve, improvise, and combine best practice from many sources and then, through its faculty and graduates, spread those ideas to other hospitals and medical schools.

In preparing his will, Hopkins had given considerable thought to his hospital's purpose, location, and civic obligations. He had already purchased the site from the city, a large parcel of land that had previously housed a public hospital and later an insane asylum. He also specified the hospital's desired size (400 beds) and the population it would serve, "the indigent sick of this city and its environs, without regard to sex, age or color," a radical proposition in a segregated city of a former slave state but very much in line with Hopkins's Quaker heritage. Paying patients should also be admitted, he wrote, as their fees could help to offset the cost of providing care to charity patients. In addition, he directed the trustees to construct on the hospital grounds a home for orphaned African-American children and a school for the female nurses who would be placed in charge of patient care in the hospital wards. Hopkins offered no architecture guidance beyond landscaping the grounds so "as to afford solace to the sick and be an ornament to the section of the city in which the grounds are located."[11]

The trustees, taking seriously their benefactor's imperative to construct a hospital equal to any in North America or Europe, consulted five physicians with extensive experience in hospital planning, including the superintendent of Massachusetts General and the designer of the new Roosevelt Hospital in New York. While not an architectural competition in a strict sense, the trustees did ask the five physicians for detailed "practical suggestions for hospital design and administration, patient distribution, medical care, hospital hygiene, and the relationship of the schools of medicine and nursing to the hospital."[12]

Deciding to share what they had learned from the planning competition with the medical profession at large, the trustees published all five proposals. The one submitted by John Shaw Billings clearly impressed them the most. Billings, the Assistant Surgeon General during the Civil War, had directed two major hospitals and led a study of military hospitals. Billings's experience with military hospitals and his highly regarded studies of "hospitalism" (diseases contracted and spread within the hospital itself), made him an obvious choice to advise the trustees. They asked him, in consultation with local architect John Niernsee, to take charge of the design and construction of the Johns Hopkins Hospital, borrowing as he saw fit from the other plans. To prepare for the project, the trustees sent Billings on a fact-finding trip to Europe to study the latest hospital designs and to confer with medical authorities there.

Billings, already a strong proponent of Florence Nightingale's pavilion designs for military hospitals, returned even more committed to them having studied the latest example first-hand at St. Thomas' Hospital in London, the design of which was inspired by Nightingale's experience as a nurse during the Crimean War. Billings, though fully aware of the latest European ideas about germ theory, nonetheless held that, however germs might pass from one person to the next, the pavilion plan offered the best defense (Figure 17.2).

For Billings, a modern hospital should be what he called "a sort of laboratory of heating and ventilation," and he would build that idea into the Johns Hopkins Hospital.[13] His original plan called for a large administrative building flanked by paying wards for male and female patients, with a series of parallel common ward pavilions arrayed behind them, with sun rooms on the southern exposure. Billings also included a building for the nursing school, a surgical amphitheater, a dispensary for ambulatory patients, and a laundry and bathhouse. As proposed, the design would have been properly symmetrical, with the pavilions facing one another across a central quadrangle. Financial difficulties truncated the original campus design, so that only the north pavilions would be completed. Among the notable architectural features in Billings's final plan were an octagonal ward for surgical patients, designed for disinfection, and an isolation ward with private rooms, each with its own chimney and ventilation and heating control.

Completed in 1889, the Queen Anne style administration building (now named for Billings), in red brick and sandstone trim with a towering octagonal dome and cupola, dominated the city's eastern skyline and gave

Health and Architecture

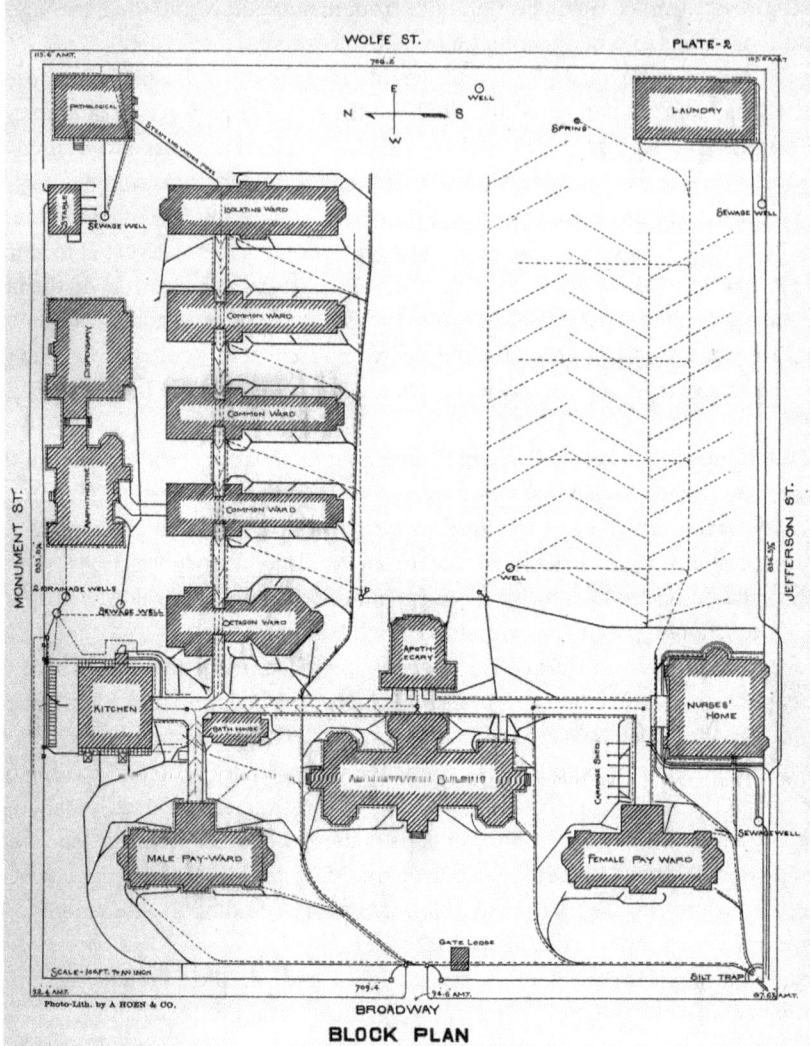

Figure 17.2 John Shaw Billings's final plan for the Johns Hopkins medical campus. The pathology laboratory, the first building to be completed, is at the upper left, with the octagon ward pavilion closest to the administrative building and the isolating ward furthest away. Courtesy Institute of the History of Medicine Historical Collection, Johns Hopkins Medical Institutions

the hospital a public face befitting its founder's stature in the community. No one disputed Billings's claim that "these are the best built buildings of their kind in the world," though the state-of-the-art ventilation and heating system, so complex it took the nursing staff six weeks to master, added significantly to the hospital's cost and had been rendered largely obsolete by the aseptic practices introduced by the faculty Billings himself had helped recruit (Figure 17.3).

As Billings understood all too well, even the best medical care could not by itself overcome longstanding prejudices against the hospital. At a time when all but the poorest patients still insisted on being treated at home, paying patients would expect a familiar domestic environment. The university's president, Daniel Coit Gilman, who simultaneously served as the hospital's first director, recognized this, and so instructed the

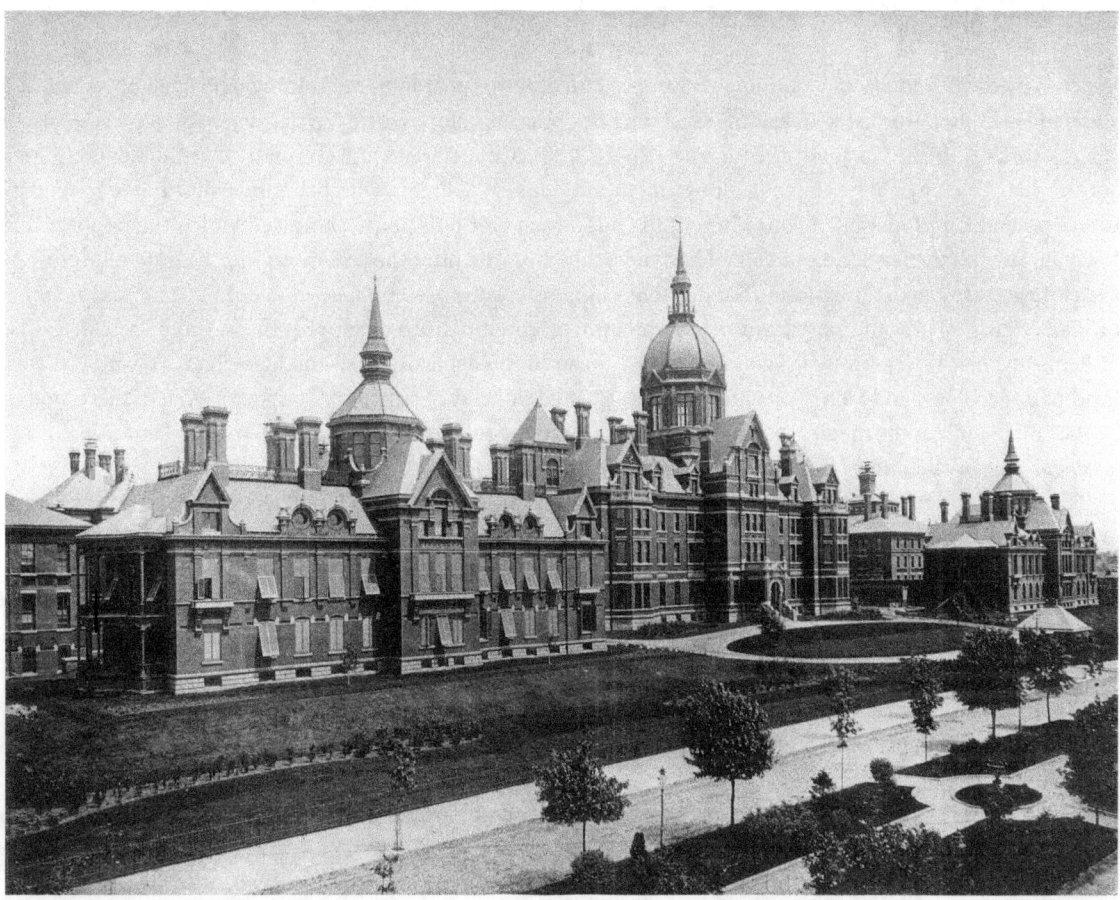

Figure 17.3 The Johns Hopkins Hospital at its opening in 1889. The administration building, with the signature dome and cupola, is at the center, with the paying wards for male and female patients, topped with turrets, to either side. Front view of buildings from northeast. Photo by Frederick Gutekunst, 1889, #295061, Courtesy of The Alan Mason Chesney Medical Archives of The Johns Hopkins Medical Institutions

hospital's administrators to study modern hotel management and operations and to outfit its private wards with all the comforts of a good hotel.[14]

Billings had initially accepted an appointment to the future medical school faculty, while the trustees hoped to persuade him to take helm of the hospital. When continuing fiscal challenges put the opening of the medical school on indefinite hold, Billings resigned his faculty appointment and returned to direct the Surgeon General's Library. He continued to advise the trustees on the appointment of the founding faculty, however, which perhaps left an even more enduring mark on modern medicine than did his hospital design. As Billings wrote: "The hospital should not only teach the best methods of caring for the sick now known, but aim to increase knowledge and thus benefit the whole world by its diffusion."[15] In short, Johns Hopkins should be a center for biomedical research and teaching as well as patient care. To that end, Billings helped recruit a small but top-notch faculty trained in the best European laboratories and medical schools, starting with William H. Welch, the intellectual cornerstone for the hospital and its medical school.

Health and Architecture

Organizing Specialized Institute and Clinics

Welch, a medical graduate of Columbia University, had done his postdoctoral training in Pierre Louis's famous clinic in Paris, then studied with leading German physiologists before setting up his own pathology laboratory at New York's Bellevue Hospital. The medical experts in the United States and Germany that Gilman consulted agreed that Welch would be an ideal appointment for Hopkins. Gilman, with his unmatched ability to size up future potential and his stated commitment to "build men, not buildings," promised Welch the opportunity to create an entirely new kind of hospital and medical school, an offer the ambitious Welch could not refuse.[16] Welch proved to be just the master builder that Hopkins required, someone who could recruit and retain a brilliant young faculty and raise funds from philanthropic foundations to support them. From the University of Pennsylvania, Welch brought William Osler as head of the department of medicine and Howard Kelly as head of gynecology, and from Bellevue, William Halsted as head of surgery. Along with Welch, these would be the "Big Four" for the medical school and hospital, and the subject of John Singer Sargent's famous painting *The Four Doctors* that now hangs in the school's medical library, which is named after Welch.

For modern medicine, to "build men" also meant new buildings for research, teaching, and patient care. Welch's Pathology Building, designed by Baltimore architect George Archer, would be the first structure completed on the medical campus, three years before the opening of the hospital and seven years before the opening of the medical school. Under Welch and his assistant William T. Councilman, that laboratory became the training ground for a generation of accomplished pathologists and future leaders at Hopkins and at other leading hospitals and medical schools. Set at the very corner of the property, the freestanding pathology building would be a vital link between the medical school and the hospital and the first of many "institutes" that would mark the indebtedness of Hopkins to the German model of laboratory-based biomedicine.[17]

Only a generous donation from a group of local women philanthropists, led by railroad heiress Mary Elizabeth Garrett, allowed the medical school to open when it did in 1893. The gift, an early example of "coercive philanthropy," stipulated unprecedentedly high academic standards for medical school applicants, and equal admission for women.[18] In recognition of the gift, the medical school commissioned the Women's Fund Building, again from Archer, to house its anatomy department under Franklin P. Mall, one of Welch's early pathology fellows. Mall considered textbooks such as *Gray's Anatomy* feeble crutches compared with having students do dissections for themselves. He refused to give conventional lectures or any other structured instruction. Instead, he assigned the students a cadaver, then told them the human body was their textbook and that their job was figuring out how to read it for themselves. Archer designed the Women's Fund Building to reinforce Mall's unique instructional methods, with small dissection rooms and laboratories to encourage self-guided learning. Archer added a second no-frills brick building for physiology (Figure 17.4).

As Katherine Carroll has shown, architecturally, Johns Hopkins became the American prototype of the German model of clustered biomedical institutes, independent though interconnected through the medical school and the hospital. Hopkins would continue to add institutes as the generosity of grateful patients and benefactors allowed—the Brady Urological Institute (1915), the Wilmer Eye Institute (1925), and the Children's Rehabilitation Institute (1937), now the Kennedy-Krieger Institute. Given limited space on an increasingly crowded urban campus, Hopkins consolidated its institutes into the hospital complex, aligning research, teaching, and clinical medicine as best it could.

W. T. Councilman, Welch's protégé, brought the "institute design" with him when he joined the Harvard medical school faculty. Its new medical campus, completed in 1906 by Shepley, Rutan, and Coolidge, "created the formally organized, comprehensive plant that had eluded the medical educators at Johns Hopkins," mostly

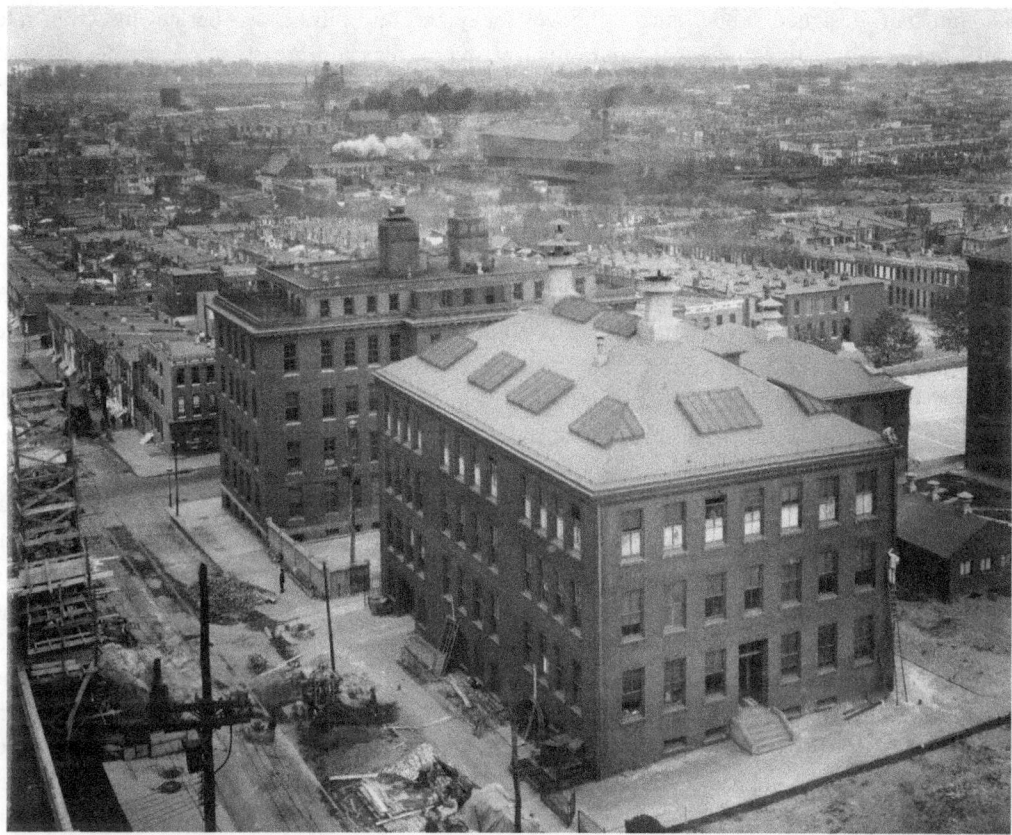

Figure 17.4 Johns Hopkins University School of Medicine, Women's Fund Memorial Building under renovation, 1915. The Hunterian Laboratory (anatomy) and the Women's Fund Building (physiology), exemplified the institute model of German medicine, with each department in its own building. #117177, Courtesy of The Alan Mason Chesney Medical Archives of The Johns Hopkins Medical Institutions

because Hopkins lacked sufficient financial resources.[19] As Councilman pointed out in an article, "Ideas and Methods of New Medical School," it was by design that Harvard medical students worked their way through the curriculum—anatomy, histology, physiology—in the same order as they worked their way through the complex of buildings.

Surgery, recently transformed by advances in anesthesia and antisepsis, brought paying patients and prestige to modern hospitals, and so merited its own building at Hopkins. William Halsted, like other aspiring American physicians of his generation, undertook a self-directed course of postgraduate education in Europe, mostly in Vienna. He subsequently took a position in surgery at Bellevue Hospital, where he rebuilt the surgical pavilion at his own expense to the specifications for the antiseptic surgical techniques set out by Joseph Lister. Undeniably gifted, Halsted had become addicted to cocaine while using it as an ophthalmological anesthetic. Welch recognized his genius and offered Halsted a fresh start at Hopkins. Halsted never entirely kicked his drug habit, with a lifelong dependence on cocaine and morphine that did astonishingly little to dull his surgical brilliance.[20]

For a generation, Halsted's operating room would be perhaps the most important surgical space in the world. There, he perfected aseptic surgery, including elaborate protocols for sterilizing instruments, patients, and staff; designed rubber surgical gloves for nurses and physicians that cut infection rates to less than 1 percent; developed new techniques for treating hernias and breast cancer; pioneered vascular surgery; and taught the best of the next generation of surgeons, at least those willing to put up with his infamously cranky personality for the chance to learn from a master. Halsted's residents included Harvey Cushing and Walter Dandy, who together invented neurosurgery, and Hugh Hampton Young, who literally wrote the book on *The Practice of Urology* and whose perineal prostatectomy revolutionized surgery for prostate cancer.[21]

Halsted's surgical innovations could only succeed within their own carefully controlled space.[22] In 1904 a new surgical building at Hopkins was constructed for Halsted, who inaugurated it with an "All Star" operation featuring his former residents and associates. The adjoining Hunterian Laboratory was for experimental surgery on animals. Halsted firmly believed that the laboratory mattered as much for surgery as for any other medical specialty. Each procedure began in the Hunterian and he followed each case, success or failure, all the way to the pathology laboratory, including the fatal complications from gallstone surgery he performed on his good friend Mall (Figure 17.5).

Hopkins also had to accommodate a new style of clinical medicine. William Osler, a once-in-a-generation diagnostician, considered the bedside rather than the laboratory or the dissecting table the most important space of medical instruction.[23] "The student begins with the patient, continues with the patient, and ends his studies with the patient, using books and tools as means to an end," Osler explained. To that end he initiated grand rounds, where he had his medical students examine the patients for themselves, and added clerkships for fourth-year medical students, giving them charge of their own ward beds where they diagnosed and treated patients under Osler's supervision. Osler also introduced the idea of residents—so-called because they had rooms in the hospital itself—for the best recently graduated medical students, who then served as senior assistants to department heads. On Saturdays, Osler held a general clinic in the hospital amphitheater, the precursor to today's Mortality and Morbidity conferences. The faculty and students discussed the week's most challenging cases, missed diagnoses, and fatalities, with elaborate blackboard charts of patient outcomes, often with one of those patients in the room as Exhibit A. Under Osler and his successors, the ward became a space for diagnosis and treatment rather than for rest and recuperation as it had been in Billings's original designs.

Hopkins incorporated what elsewhere had been freestanding specialty clinics into its main medical campus. Pediatrician-in-Chief Clemens von Pirquet planned and supervised the construction of the Harriett Lane Home (1912) for invalid children, the first of its kind attached to a medical school and teaching hospital. The Phipps Psychiatric Clinic (1912) under founding director Adolf Meyer redefined psychiatry as a clinical- and laboratory-based specialty. Like Harriett Lane, the Phipps would be the first clinic of its type on a medical campus. Contemporary asylums such as Calvert Vaux's Sheppard and Enoch Pratt Hospital (1891) north of Baltimore still relied on the Kirkbride Plan, with its distinctive echelons designed to provide maximum sunshine, fresh air, and privacy for patients who would be housed there indefinitely.[24] Meyer, by contrast, intended the Phipps for clinical observation, diagnosis, and treatment. Given a million dollars from philanthropist Henry Phipps to build and staff the new clinic, Meyer and his architect Grosvenor Atterbury jointly planned "clinical, teaching, research and treatment facilities" that would "set a standard for all to follow."[25] Atterbury spent two months studying the latest European psychiatric clinics in person before drafting the final plans. His five-story structure, echoing the Queen Anne style of the administration building in front of it, had the same kind of laboratories, clinical lecture halls, and wards as the rest of the hospital. And it shared the same expectations, namely, that mental illness, like any other disease, could be treated with modern medical science.

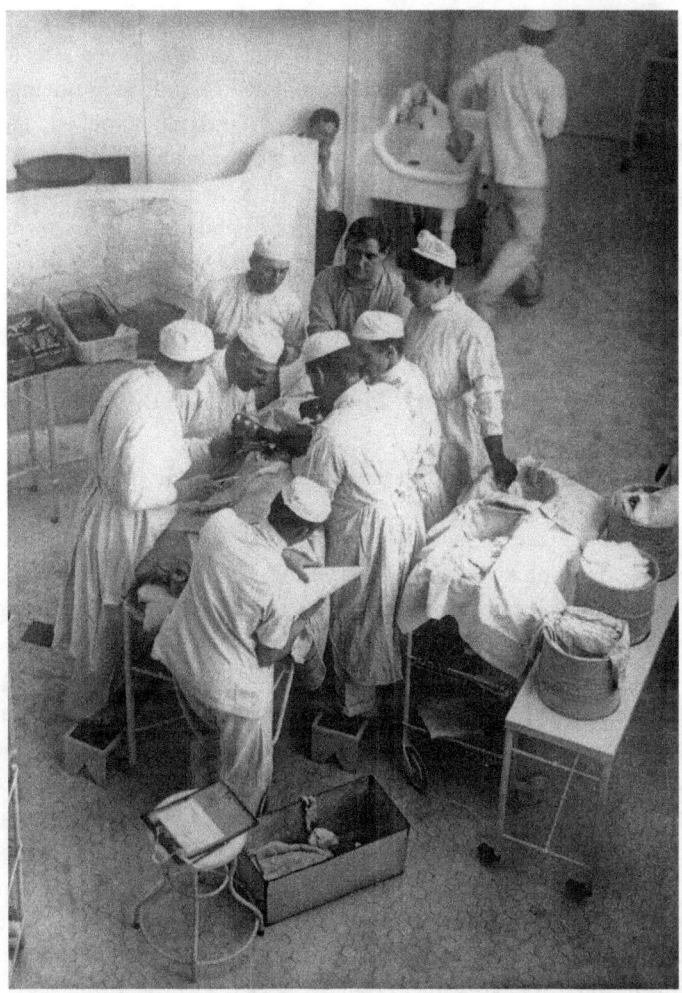

Figure 17.5 Chief of surgery William Halsted and his "All Star" team performing an operation in their new surgical theater, 1904. Designed for aseptic surgery, Halsted's operating room had strict protocols for sterilizing instruments, garments, and all surfaces. Note the rubber gloves on the nurse and physicians. Courtesy of The Alan Mason Chesney Medical Archives of The Johns Hopkins Medical Institutions

A Machine for Healing

Much as the Flexner Report (1910) established the Johns Hopkins medical school as a model for all others to emulate—a "small but ideal medical school, embodying in a novel way, adapted to American conditions, the best features of medical education in England, France, and Germany"—so, too, would Johns Hopkins Hospital set the standard for a new generation of university medical centers constructed in the 1920s, most notably at Vanderbilt, Rochester, and Duke.[26] At Vanderbilt, Hopkins medical graduate and dean of medicine G. Canby Robinson, with funding from the Rockefeller Foundation aimed at bringing modern medicine to the South, designed an entirely new medical campus that architecturally integrated the medical school and hospital more successfully than Hopkins's patchwork campus could ever have done. Opened in 1925,

Robinson's "unified medical school-hospital" carefully coordinated the preclinical and clinical departments, the laboratories and wards, all within a single structure.[27] During the planning phase, Robinson spent several years at Johns Hopkins consulting with its administrators and medical staff and studying its layout. He adopted the Hopkins curriculum, with minor tweaks, and staffed his new medical school and hospital with more than a dozen former Hopkins faculty.[28] The University of Rochester also consulted with, and borrowed freely from, the Hopkins model in designing its new medical school curriculum and its teaching hospital, though Strong Memorial Hospital (1926) adapted its architectural plan from Vanderbilt. Rochester hired so many current and former Hopkins faculty that they proudly considered themselves "a small edition of the Johns Hopkins Medical School." Duke chose Wilburt Davidson, assistant dean at Hopkins, as the dean of its new medical school. Davidson sought the advice of the superintendent of the Johns Hopkins Hospital in planning the Duke University Hospital (1930), again with the Vanderbilt architectural design clearly in mind. Considered "the most complete Hopkins colony," Duke hired Hopkins-trained faculty for thirty of its forty-six original positions.[29]

The modern hospital, "a medical, technological health factory," differs so radically from its predecessor, "a charitable, environmentally therapeutic, reformative waystation," in form and function, and in social and economic significance, that it may require entirely new interpretive strategies to make sense of it.[30] How best can historians understand the hospital functionally as well as aesthetically, as a series of choices about how to incorporate the latest medical theories into practical design? One approach, following Annemarie Adams, would be looking at the hospital as a performative space that structures the interactions of physicians, nurses, patients, and staff.[31]

Jeanne Kisacky explicitly considers the modern hospital as a kind of factory for healing, first as a *machine à guérir*, a space that would heal patients by controlling such environmental factors as ventilation, temperature, and exposure to sunlight, later as a "sorting machine" that could place patients and staff into appropriate categories and spaces for diagnosis, therapy, research, and training, and finally "as an attractive factory" where control of information would be as essential as access to the latest medical technology. Certainly, there are striking parallels between hospitals and factories as distinctly modern architectures that reflected and reinforced innovations in scientific management, plant layout, labor organization, standardization, and cost efficiency within a highly contested space where the "one best way" was never certain or final. The most intriguing example of the hospital as factory might well be the Henry Ford Hospital (1920) by architect Albert Kahn, better known for his automotive factories, designed as a deliberate experiment in "Fordist" medicine and staffed largely with physicians recruited from Johns Hopkins. Like performative space, the factory analogy underscores workers—nurses, technicians, and orderlies as well as physicians—and how changing architectural prescriptions affected where and how (and how well) they did their jobs.

The challenge will be scaling up methodologies intended for individual buildings to modern medical centers, cities within cities. Instead of thinking about modern hospitals as matters of individual architects and particular buildings, architectural historians will have to situate them within a wider (sub)urban context where so-called "eds and meds"—research universities and major teaching hospitals—often dominate the economic as well as the physical landscape of modern cities. Places such as Houston's Texas Medical Center, or Johns Hopkins Medicine, are no longer architecture in the conventional sense but rather exercises in urban planning where administrators, developers, philanthropists, and politicians— not physicians and healthcare experts—call the shots. Studying them will require attention not only to architecture, medicine, and public health but also to the political economy of twenty-first-century cities, where race, class, and access to healthcare are the key variables and where hospital design can heighten socioeconomic disparity and community tension.[32]

Notes

1. Roy Porter, *Blood and Guts: A Short History of Medicine* (New York: Norton, 2002), 135–52 provides an astute overview of the hospital from ancient to modern times.
2. Erwin Ackerknecht, *Medicine at the Paris Hospital, 1794–1848* (Baltimore: Johns Hopkins University Press, 1967), 15.
3. John D. Thompson and Grace Goldin, *The Hospital: A Social and Architectural History* (New Haven: Yale University Press, 1975), 118–42 covers the history of the Hôtel-Dieu and the architectural competition in some detail.
4. Ackerknecht, *Medicine at the Paris Hospital*, 16–17.
5. Louis S. Greenbaum, "'Measure of Civilization': The Hospital Thought of Jacques Tenon on the Eve of the French Revolution," *Bulletin of the History of Medicine* 49, no. 1 (Spring 1975): 43–56.
6. Kristin Graham, *A History of Pennsylvania Hospital* (London: History Press, 2008).
7. Charles Rosenberg, *The Care of Strangers: The Rise of America's Hospital System* (New York: Basic Books, 1987) is the definitive social history of the nineteenth-century American hospital.
8. "Christ Healing the Sick in the Temple," The Penn Art Collection, accessed November 1, 2018. http://artcollection.upenn.edu/collection/art/897/christ-healing-the-sick-in-the-temple/.
9. Andrew Simpson, "Health and Renaissance: Academic Medicine and the Remaking of Modern Pittsburgh," *Journal of Urban History* 41 (2015): 19–27 opens up an important comparative conversation, as does his dissertation, Andrew Simpson, *The Medical Metropolis: Health Care and Economic Transformation in Pittsburgh and Houston* (Philadelphia: University of Pennsylvania Press, 2019).
10. Guenter Risse, *Mending Bodies, Saving Soul: A History of Hospitals* (New York: Oxford University Press, 1999) includes an excellent chapter on the hospital's origins and early years. Thompson and Goldin, *The Hospital*, 175–93 also highlights its architectural contributions.
11. Alan M. Chesney, *The Johns Hopkins Hospital and The Johns Hopkins University School of Medicine: The Early Years, 1867–1893* (Baltimore: Johns Hopkins Press, 1943), 13–16 quotes Hopkins's letter to the trustees in full.
12. Gert Brieger, "The Original Plans for the Johns Hopkins Hospital and Their Historical Significance," *Bulletin of the History of Medicine* 39, no. 6 (November–December 1965): 518–28.
13. Alistair Fair, "'A Laboratory of Heating and Ventilation': The Johns Hopkins Hospital as Experimental Architecture, 1870–90," *The Journal of Architecture* 19, no. 3 (2014): 357–81.
14. Risse, *Mending Bodies, Saving Souls*, 408.
15. Ibid., 404.
16. Donald Fleming, *William H. Welch and the Rise of Modern Medicine* (Boston: Little, Brown, 1954) remains the best short biography with an emphasis on Welch's institution-building.
17. Katherine L. Carroll, "Creating the Modern Physician: The Architecture of American Medical Schools in the Era of Medical Education Reform," *Journal of the Society of Architectural Historians* 75, no. 1 (March 2016): 48–73 makes a compelling case for how architecture reflected and reinforced the modern medical curriculum at Johns Hopkins, Harvard, Syracuse, Vanderbilt, and Columbia.
18. Kathleen Waters Sander, *Mary Elizabeth Garrett: Society and Philanthropy in the Gilded Age* (Baltimore: Johns Hopkins University Press, 2008).
19. Carroll, "Creating the Modern Physician," 54–8 covers the evolution of the Harvard plan in detail.
20. Howard Markel, *An Anatomy of Addiction: Sigmund Freud, William Halsted, and the Miracle Drug, Cocaine* (New York: Pantheon, 2011).
21. Michael Bliss, *Harvey Cushing: A Life in Surgery* (New York: Oxford University Press, 2005); Hugh Hampton Young, *Hugh Young: A Surgeon's Autobiography* (New York: Harcourt Brace, 1940).
22. Thomas Schlich, "Surgery, Science, and Modernity: Operating Rooms and Laboratories as Spaces of Control," *History of Science* 45, no. 3 (2007): 231–56.
23. Michael Bliss, *William Osler: A Life in Medicine* (Toronto: University of Toronto Press, 1999) is the best modern biography, though Harvey Cushing, who worked closely with Osler during his time at Hopkins, won the Pulitzer Prize for his two-volume biography, *The Life of Sir William Osler* (Oxford: Clarendon Press, 1925).
24. Carla Yanni, *The Architecture of Madness* (Minneapolis: University of Minnesota Press, 2007).
25. Susan D. Lamb, *Pathologist of the Mind: Adolf Meyer and the Origins of American Psychiatry* (Baltimore: Johns Hopkins University Press, 2014), 107.
26. Kenneth Ludmerer, "Understanding the Flexner Report," *Academic Medicine* 85 (February 2010): 193–6, and Ludmerer, *Learning to Heal: The Development of American Medical Education* (New York: Basic Books, 1985).

27. Carroll, "Creating the Modern Physician," 62–6.
28. A. McGehee Harvey et al., *A Model of Its Kind: A Centennial History of Medicine at Johns Hopkins*, vol. 1 (Baltimore: Johns Hopkins University Press, 1989), 220–5 covers the Hopkins/Vanderbilt, Rochester, and Duke connections.
29. Ibid., 222.
30. Jeanne Kisacky, *Rise of the Modern Hospital: An Architectural History of Health and Healing, 1870–1940* (Pittsburgh: University of Pittsburgh Press, 2017), 297 is the best recent survey, at least for the American context. See also Stephen Verderber and David Fine, *Healthcare Architecture in an Era of Radical Transformation* (New Haven: Yale University Press, 2000), a more conventional architectural history.
31. Annemarie Adams, *Medicine by Design: The Architect and the Modern Hospital, 1893–1943* (Minneapolis: University of Minnesota Press, 2008) reconstructs modern medical practice from the built environment itself, though not expressly with "performative space" in mind. Though mostly discussed by literary scholars, performativity has attracted some attention from architectural theorists. For an architect's perspective, see Michael Hensel, *Performance-Oriented Architecture: Rethinking Architectural Design and the Built Environment* (Hoboken, NJ: Wiley, 2013).
32. Kisacky, *Rise of the Modern Hospital*, and Simpson, "Making the Medical Metropolis" are important steps in the right direction.

BIBLIOGRAPHY

Chapter 1. Places of Care and Healing: Context, Design, and Development in History

Allen, Nigel. "Hospice to Hospital in the Near East: An Instance of Continuity and Change in Late Antiquity." *Bulletin of the History of Medicine* 64, no. 3 (1990): 446–62.

Amster, Ellen J. *Medicine and the Saints: Science, Islam, and the Colonial Encounter in Morocco, 1877–1956*. Austin: University of Texas Press, 2013.

Anonymous. "Household Medicine in Ancient Rome." *The British Medical Journal* 1, no. 2140 (1902): 39–40.

Appleby, Andrew B. "The Disappearance of Plague: A Continuing Puzzle." *Economic History Review* 33 (1980): 161–73.

Barr, J. "Vascular Medicine and Surgery in Ancient Egypt." *Journal of Vascular Surgery* 60, no. 1 (July 2014): 260–3.

Bastos, Cristiana. "Medical Hybridisms and Social Boundaries: Aspects of Portuguese Colonialism in Africa and India in the Nineteenth Century." *Journal of Southern African Studies* 33, no. 4, Histories of Healing (December 2007): 767–82.

Behr, Charles Allison. *Aelius Aristides and The Sacred Tales*. Amsterdam: Adolf M. Hakkert, 1968.

Bhattacharya, Jayanta. "The Hospital Transcends into Hospital Medicine: A Brief Journey through Ancient, Medieval and Colonial India." *Indian Journal of History of Science* 52, no. 1 (2017): 28–53.

Binet, J. "Drogue et mystique: le Bwiti de Fangs (Cameroon)." *Diogéne* 86 (1974): 34–57.

Bowers, Barbara S. *The Medieval Hospital and Medical Practice*. London: Routledge, 2017.

Brewer, Harry. "Historical Perspectives on Health: Early Arabic Medicine." *Journal of Social Health* 124 (2004): 184–7.

Buklijaš, Tatjana. "Medicine and Society in the Medieval Hospital." *Croatian Medical Journal* 49, no. 2 (2008): 151–4.

Burford, Alison. *The Greek Temple Builders at Epidauros*. Liverpool: Liverpool University Press, 1969.

Carod, F. J. and C. Vazquez-Cabrera. "Pensamiento mágico y epilepsia en la medicina tradicional indígena." *Revista de Neurologia* 26, no. 154 (1998): 1064–8.

Columella, Lucius J. M. *On Agriculture (De Re Rustica)*. Translated by H. Boyd Ash. Cambridge, MA: Harvard University Press, 1960, vol. 3.

Cook, Constance A. "The Pre-Han Period." In *Chinese Medicine and Healing: An Illustrated History*, edited by T. J. Hinrichs and Linda L. Barnes, 5–29. Cambridge, MA: The Belknap Press of Harvard University Press, 2013.

Crislip, A. T. *From Monastery to Hospital: Christian Monasticism & the Transformation of Health Care in Late Antiquity*. Ann Arbor: University of Michigan Press, 2005.

Da Mota, Clarice Novaes and Rodrigo de Azeredo. *Os filhos de jurema na floresta dos espíritos: ritual e cura entre dois grupos indígenas do nordeste Brasileiro*. Maceió, Brazil: EDUFAL, 2007.

"Dominik Wujastyk." *Academia*. https://ualberta.academia.edu/DominikWujastyk/talks. [Unpublished paper.] Accessed May 16, 2019.

Dupras, T. L., L. J. Williams, M. De Meyer, C. Peeters, D. Depraetere, B. Vanthuyne, and H. Willems. "Evidence of Amputation as Medical Treatment in Ancient Egypt." *International Journal of Osteoarchaeology* 20, no. 4 (July/August 2010): 405–23.

Ebeid, N. I. *Egyptian Medicine in the Days of the Pharaohs*. Cairo: General Egyptian Book Organization, 1999.

Edelstein, Emma, J. Ludwig Edelstein, and Gary B. Ferngren. *Asclepius: Collection and Interpretation of the Testimonies*. Baltimore: Johns Hopkins University Press, 1998.

Edler, Flávio and MRF da Fonseca. "Saber erudito e saber popular na medicina colonial." *Cadernos da ABEM* 2 (2006): 8–9.

Emden, A. B. *A Biographical Register of the University of Oxford, A.D. 1501 to 1540*. Oxford: Clarendon Press, 1974.

Estes, J. Worth. *Medical Skills of Ancient Egypt*. Canton, MA: Science History Publications, 1993.

Bibliography

Falconer, Julia. "The Use of Forest Resources in Traditional Medicine." In *The Major Significance of "Minor" Forest Products: The Local Use and Value of Forests in the West African Humid Forest Zone*, edited by Carla R. S. Koppell. Rome: Food and Agriculture Organization of the United Nations, 1990. http://www.fao.org/3/t9450e/t9450e04.htm#1.3%20The%20use%20of%20forest%20resources%20in%20traditional%20medicine. Accessed December 15, 2019.

Franco, Renato Júnio. "O modelo luso de assistência e a dinâmica das Santas Casas de Misericórdia na América portuguesa." *Revista Estudos Históricos* 27, no. 53 (2014): 5–25.

Garcia, Élfego Rolando López. "Historia de la Farmacia en Guatemala." Master's thesis, Universidad Complutense de Madrid Facultad de Farmacia, Madrid, 2012.

Garlands, Robert. *Introducing New Gods: The Politics of Athenian Religion*. Ithaca: Cornell University Press, 1992.

Getz, Faye. *Medicine in the English Middle Age*. Princeton: Princeton University Press, 1998.

Hajar, Rachel. "The Air of History (Part II) Medicine in the Middle Ages." *Heart Views* 13, no. 4 (2012): 158–62.

Henderson, John. *The Renaissance Hospital: Healing the Body and Healing the Soul*. New Haven and London: Yale University Press, 2006.

Higham, Charles. *The Civilization of Angkor*. London: Weidenfeld & Nicolson, 2001.

Hinrichs, T. J. "The Song and Jin Periods." In *Chinese Medicine and Healing: An Illustrated History*, edited by T. J. Hinrichs and Linda L. Barnes, 97–127. Cambridge, MA: The Belknap Press of Harvard University Press, 2013.

Horden, Peregrine. *Hospitals and Healing from Antiquity to the Later Middle Ages*. London: Routledge, 2008.

Iglésias, Francisco. "Encontro de Duas Culturas: América e Europa." *Estudos Avançados* 6, no. 14 (1992): 23–37.

Iwasa, Kiyoshi. "Hospitals of Japan: History and Present Situation." *Medical Care* 4, no. 4 (October–December 1966): 214–46.

Jacques, Jouanna. "Egyptian Medicine and Greek Medicine." In *Greek Medicine from Hippocrates to Galen: Selected Papers*, translated by Neil Allies, edited by Philan der Eijk, 3–20. Boston: Leiden, 2012.

Jan Meulenbeld, Gerrit. *A History of Indian Medical Literature IA*. Groningen: Egbert Forsten, 1999.

Jennings, Michael. "Healing of Bodies, Salvation of Souls: Missionary Medicine in Colonial Tanganyika, 1870s–1939." *Journal of Religion in Africa* 38, fasc. 1 (2008): 27–56.

Junqueira, Carmen. "Pajés E Feiticeiros." *Estudos Avançados* 18, no. 52 (2004): 289–302.

"Kamaiurá." *Kamaiurá—Povos Indígenas No Brasil*. https://pib.socioambiental.org/pt/Povo·Kamaiurá. Accessed April 9, 2019.

Ka-wai, Fa. "The Period of Division and the Tang Period." In *Chinese Medicine and Healing: An Illustrated History*, edited by T. J. Hinrichs and Linda L. Barnes, 65–96. Cambridge, MA: The Belknap Press of Harvard University Press, 2013.

Khaulah, Liya and Ahmad Ramli. "Contributions of Islamic Civilization to the Mathematics Development." *Proceedings of the Second Conference on Arabic Studies and Islamic Civilization, Kuala Lumpur, Malaysia* (2017), 199–208.

Kleisiaris, C. F., C. Sfakianakis, and I. V. Papathanasiou. "Health Care Practices in Ancient Greece: The Hippocratic Ideal." *Journal of Medical Ethics and History of Medicine* 7, no. 6 (March 2014).

Kleine, C. "Buddhist Monks as Healers in Early and Medieval Japan." *Japanese Religions* 37, no. 1/2 (2012): 13–38.

Koithan, Mary and Cynthia Farrell. "Indigenous Native American Healing Traditions." *The Journal for Nurse Practitioners* 6, no. 6 (2010): 477–8.

Lawrence, Clifford Hugh. *Medieval Monasticism: Forms of Religious Life in Western Europe in the Middle Ages*. 2nd ed. London: Longman, 1989.

Lindberg, David C. *The Beginnings of Western Science: The European Scientific Tradition in Philosophical, Religious, and Institutional Context, Prehistory to A.D. 1450*. 2nd ed. Chicago: University of Chicago Press, 2007.

Lo, Vivienne. "The Han Period." In *Chinese Medicine and Healing: An Illustrated History*, edited by T. J. Hinrichs and Linda L. Barnes, 31–63. Cambridge, MA: The Belknap Press of Harvard University Press, 2013.

Lunde, Per and Christine Stone. "Early Islamic Hospitals: In the Hospital Bazaar." *Health and Social Service Journal* 91, no. 4777 (December 1981): 1548–51.

MacNalty, Arthur Salusbury. "The Renaissance and its Influence on English Medicine, Surgery and Public Health." In *The Thomas Vicary Lecture for 1945*, 8–30. London: Christopher Johnson, 1946.

Mark, J. J. "Egyptian Medical Treatments." *Ancient History Encyclopedia* (February 20, 2017). https://www.ancient.eu/article/51/egyptian-medical-treatments/. Accessed September 2, 2019.

Mauk, Kristen L. and Mary Hobus, *Nursing as Ministry*. Burlington, MA: Jones & Bartlett Learning, 2019.

McHugh, T. "Establishing Medical Men at the Paris Hôtel-Dieu, 1500–1715." *Social History of Medicine* 19, no. 2 (2006): 209–24.

McIntosh, Marjorie K. *Autonomy and Community: The Royal Manor of Havering, 1200 –1500*. Cambridge: Cambridge University Press, 1986.

Med-Help. "Renaissance Medicine." http://www.med-help.net/med-renaissance-medicine.html. Accessed January 20, 2019.

Medical News Today. "What Was Medieval and Renaissance Medicine?" https://www.medicalnewstoday.com/articles/323533.php. Accessed January 20, 2019.

Miller, Andrew C. "Jundi-Shapur, Bimaristans, and the Rise of Academic Medical Centres." *Journal of the Royal Society of Medicine* 99, no. 12 (December 2006): 615–17.

Miller, Timothy S. *The Birth of the Hospital in the Byzantine Empire*. Baltimore: Johns Hopkins University Press, 1997.

Miranda, Carlos Alberto Cunha. *A Arte De Curar Nos Tempos Da Colônia: Limites E Espaços Da Cura*. Recife: Editora Universitária UFPE, 2011.

"Moctezuma." *Aztec History*. http://www.aztec-history.com/moctezuma.html. Accessed April 9, 2019.

Mokgobi, M. G. "Understanding Traditional African Healing." *African Journal of Physical Health Education and Recreation Dance* 20, suppl. 2 (September 2014): 25–34.

Montague, Joel. "Hospitals in the Muslim Near East: A Historical Overview." In *Mimar* 14 (1984): 20–7.

Mossensohn, Miri Shefer. "Hospitals and Medical Institutions." *The Oxford Encyclopedia of Philosophy, Science, and Technology in Islam*, 2018. https://www.oxfordreference.com/view/10.1093/acref:oiso/9780199812578.001.0001/acref-9780199812578-e-79?rskey=HxK7Co&result=78. Accessed April 10, 2018.

Musisi, Seggane and Nakanyika Musisi. "The Legacies of Colonialism in African Medicine." Lecture. The Impact of Decolonization and the End of Cold War on Health Development in Africa, Kenya, Nairobi. February 6, 2007. https://www.who.int/global_health_histories/seminars/nairobi02.pdf?ua=1. Accessed September 9, 2019.

Nagamia, Husain. "Islamic Medicine History and Current Practice." *International Institute of Islamic Medicine* 2 (March 2003): 19–30.

Nardi, Antonio E., Adriana Cardoso Silva, Jaime E. Hallak, and José A. Crippa. "A Humanistic Gift from the Brazilian Emperor D. Pedro II (1825–1891) to the Brazilian Nation: The First Lunatic Asylum in Latin America." *Arquivos De Neuro-Psiquiatria* 71, no. 2 (2013): 125–6.

Niangoran-Bouah, George. "Le Silence dans les traditions de culture Africaine." *Revue Ivoirienne d'Anthropologie et de Sociologie* 3 (1983): 6–11.

Nkwi, Walter Gam. "The Sacred Forest and the Mythical Python: Ecology, Conservation, and Sustainability in Kom, Cameroon, c. 1700–2000." *Journal of Global Initiatives: Policy, Pedagogy, Perspective* 11, no. 2 (April 2017): 31–47.

Nyanto, Salvatory Stephen. "Indigenous Beliefs and Healing in Historical Perspective: Experiences from Buha and Unyamwezi, Western Tanzania." *International Journal of Humanities and Social Science* 5, no. 10 (October 2015): 189–201.

Oda, Galdini Raimundo, Maria Ana and Paulo Dalgalarrondo. "História Das Primeiras Instituições Para Alienados No Brasil." *História, Ciências, Saúde—Manguinhos, Rio De Janeiro* 12, no. 3 (September–November 2005): 983–1010.

On Line Editora, ed. *Guia Segredos Do Império 03—O Povo Asteca*. March 22, 2017.

Orme, Nicholas and Margaret Elise Graham Webster. *The English Hospital 1070–1570*. New Haven: Yale University Press, 1995.

Oumeish, Youssef. "The Philosophical, Cultural, and Historical Aspects of Complementary, Alternative, Unconventional, and Integrative Medicine in the Old World." *Archives of Dermatology* 134, no. 11 (December 1998): 1373–86.

Pormann, Peter E. and Emilie Savage-Smith. *Medieval Islamic Medicine*. Edinburgh: Edinburgh University Press, 2007.

Porter, Dorothy. *Health, Civilization and the State: A History of Public Health from Ancient to Modern Times*. London: Routledge, 1999.

Pringle, Yolana. "Crossing the Divide: Medical Missionaries and Government Service in Uganda, 1897–1940." *Beyond the State: The Colonial Medical Service in British Africa*, edited by Anna Greenwood, 19–38. Manchester: Manchester University Press, 2016.

Ragab, Ahmed. *The Medieval Islamic Hospital: Medicine, Religion, and Charity*. Cambridge: Cambridge University Press, 2015.

Rawcliffe, Carole. "Hospital Nurses and their Work." In *Daily Life in the Middle Ages*, edited by Richard Britnell, 43–65. Stroud: Sutton Publishing, 1998.

Rey, Philippe-Marius. "O Hospício de Pedro II e os Alienados no Brasil (1875)." *Revista Latinoamericana de Psicopatologia Fundamental* 15, no. 2 (2012): 382–403.

Bibliography

Risse, Guenter B. *Mending Bodies, Saving Souls: A History of Hospitals*. New York: Oxford University Press, 1999.

Risse, Guenter B. *Mending Bodies, Saving Souls*. Oxford: Oxford University Press, 2011.

Ritter, Edith K. "Medical Expert (*asipu*) and Physician (*asu*). Notes on Two Complementary Professions in Babylonian Medicine." *Assyriological Studies* 16 (1965): 299–321.

Rodini, Mohammad. "Medical Care in Islamic Medical Care in Islamic Tradition during the Middle Ages." *International Journal of Medicine and Molecular Medicine* 7 (June 2012): 2–14.

Rubin, Miri. *Charity and Community in Medieval Cambridge*. Cambridge: Cambridge University Press, 1987.

Sant'Anna, J. Firmino. "O problema da assistência médico-sanitária ao indígena em Africa." *Revista Médica de Angola* 2, no. 4 (1924): 73–200.

Sakai, Shizu. "History of Medical Care at Inpatient Facilities in Japan." *The Journal of the Japan Medical Association* 54, no. 6 (2011): 351–6.

Santos. F. Ferreira dos. "Assistência médica aos Indígenas e processos práticos da sua hospitalização." *Revista Médica de Angola* 2, no. 4 (1924), Special issue dedicated to the First West Africa Tropical Medicine Conference: 51–71.

Savage-Smith, Emilie. *A Brochure to Accompany an Exhibition in Celebration of the 900th Anniversary of the Oldest Arabic Medical Manuscript in the Collections of the National Library of Medicine*. Oxford: University of Oxford, 1994.

Sayili, Aydin. "The Emergence of the Prototype of the Modern Hospital in Medieval Islam." Foundation for Science Technology and Civilisation, December 2006.

Scherer, Johan H. "The Ha of Tanganyika." *Anthropos* 54, no. 5/6 (1959): 841–904.

Sigaud, José Francisco Xavier. "Reflexões sobre o trânsito livre dos doidos pelas ruas da cidade do Rio de Janeiro." *Revista Latinoamericana de Psicopatologia Fundamental* 8, no. 3 (2005): 559–62.

Sihn, Kyu-hwan. "Reorganizing Hospital Space: The 1894 Plague Epidemic in Hong Kong and the Germ Theory." *Korean Journal of Medical History* 26, no. 1 (2017): 59–94.

Slack, Paul. "The Disappearance of Plague: An Alternative View." *Economic History Review* 34 (1981): 469–76.

Speziale, Fabrizio, ed. *Hospitals in Iran and India, 1500–1950s*. Brill: Leiden, 2012.

Stone, Per Lunde Christine. "Early Islamic Hospitals: In the Hospital Bazaar." *Health and Social Service Journal* 91 (1981): 1548–51.

Stow, John. *A Survey of London. Reprinted from the Text of 1603*, edited by C. L. Kingsford. Oxford, 1908, British History Online. http://www.british-history.ac.uk/no-series/survey-of-london-stow/1603. Accessed December 31, 2020.

Strocchia, Sharon T. "Caring for the 'Incurable' in Renaissance Pox Hospitals." In *Hospital Life: Theory and Practice from the Medieval to the Modern*, edited by Laurinda Abreu and Sally Sheard, 67–92. Bern: Peter Lang, 2013.

Talbot, Charles H. "Medicine." In *Science in the Middle Ages*, edited by David C. Lindberg, 391–428. Chicago: University of Chicago Press, 1978.

Verma, R. L. "The Growth of Greco-Arabian Medicine in Medieval India." *India Journal of History of Science* 5, no. 2 (1970): 347–63.

Voigts, Linda E. "Anglo-Saxon Plant Remedies and the Anglo-Saxons." *Isis: A Journal of the History of Science Society* 70, no. 2 (1979): 250–68.

Wagenaar, Cor. *Architecture of Hospitals*. Rotterdam: Netherlands Architecture Institute, 2006.

Weisz, George. "The Emergence of Medical Specialization in the Nineteenth Century." *Bulletin of the History of Medicine* 77, no. 3 (2003): 536–75.

Williams, Carlos Rivera. "Historia de la medicina y cirugía en América: La Civilización Maya." *Revista Medica Hondureña* 75, no. 3 (July/August 2007): 152–8.

Wujastyk, Sominik. *The Roots of Ayruveda: Selections from Sanskrit Medical Writings*. New Delhi: Penguin, 2003.

Xuanzang. *Si-Yu-Ki: Buddhist Records of the Western World*, trans. Samuel Beal, vol. 1, London: Trubner & Co., 1884.

Yazdani, Ghulam. *Bidar: Its History and Monuments*. Oxford: Oxford University Press, 1944.

I. Religiosity: Healthcare in Religious Context

Chapter 2. The Hospital Design in History: The Dichotomy of Religious and Secular Contexts

Angelis, Pietro de. *The Hospital of Santo Spirito in Saxia*. Rome: Biblioteca Lancisiana, 1960.

Barry, J. and C. Jones, eds. *Medicine and Charity*. London: Routledge, 1991. Bianchi, Francesco. "Italian Renaissance Hospitals: An Overview of the Recent Historiography." *Mitteilungen des Instituts für Oestereiche Geschichtsforschung* 115 (January 2007): 394–403.

Bonastra, Quim and Gerard Jori. "El uso de Google Earth para el estudio de la arquitectura hospitalaria, (i) de los asclepiones a los hospitales medievales." *Ar@cne, Revista Electronica de Recursos en Internet Sobre Geografia y Ciencias Sociales Universidad de Barcelona* 122 (July 1, 2009). http://www.ub.es/geocrit/aracne/aracne-122.

Bourdieu, Pierre. "Social Space and Symbolic Power." *Social Theory* 7 (1989): 14–25.

Burford, Alison. *The Greek Temple Builders at Epidauros: A Social and Economic Study of Building in the Asklepian Sanctuary*. Liverpool: Liverpool University Press, 1969.

Bynum, William F. and Roy Porter, eds. *Companion Encyclopedia of the History of Medicine*. 2 vols. London: Routledge, 1993.

Compton, Michael T. "The Union of Religion and Health in Ancient Asklepieia." *Journal of Religion and Health* 37, no. 4 (1998): 212–301.

Conan, Michel, ed. *Middle East Gardens: Traditions, Unity and Diversity*. Washington, DC: Dumbarton Oaks, 2007.

Cooper Marcus, Clare and Marni Barnes. *Healing Gardens: Therapeutic Benefits and Design Recommendations*. New York: Wiley, 1999.

Craemer, Ulrich. *Das Hospital als Bautyp des Mittelalters*. Koeln: Kohlhammer, 1963.

D'Andrea, David M. *Civic Christianity in Renaissance Italy: The Hospital of Treviso, 1400–1530*. Rochester, NY: University of Rochester Press, 2007.

Eliade, Mircea. *Shamanism: Archaic Techniques of Ecstasy*. Translated by W. R. Trask. Princeton: Princeton University Press, 1964.

Ferngren, Gary B. *Medicine and Health Care in Early Christianity*. Baltimore: Johns Hopkins University Press, 2009.

Graham, Charlotte. *The Hospital of Santo Spirito in Sassia*. Rome: Foreign Study Program, 1975.

Granshaw, Lindsay and Roy Porter, eds. *The Hospital in History*. London: Routledge, 1989.

Greer, R. "Hospitality in the First Five Centuries of the Church." *Medieval Studies* 10 (1974): 29–48.

Henderson, John. *The Renaissance Hospital: Healing the Body and Healing the Soul*. New Haven: Yale University Press, 2006.

Horden, Peregrine. "How Medicalized were Byzantine Hospitals?" *Medicina e Storia* 10 (2008): 45–74.

Horn, Walter, Ernest Born, Wolfgang Braunfels, Charles W. Jones, and A. Hunter Dupree. *The Plan of St. Gall: A Study of the Architecture, Economy, and Life in a Paradigmatic Carolingian Monastery*. 3 vols. Berkeley: University of California Press, 1979.

Jetter, Dieter. "Das Mailänder Ospedale Maggiore und der kreuzförmige Krankenhausgrundriss." *Sudhoffs Archiv* 44 (1960): 64–75.

Kostof, Spiro. *A History of Architecture: Settings and Rituals*. New York: Oxford University Press, 1995.

Kuilman, Marten. *Quadralectic Architecture: A Panoramic Review* (August 2013). quadralectics.wordpress.com.

Lachmund, J. and G. Stollberg, eds. *The Social Construction of Illness*. Stuttgart: F. Steiner Verlag, 1992.

Leistikow, Dankwart. *Ten Centuries of European Hospital Architecture, A Contribution to the History of Hospital Architects*. Ingelheim: Böhringer, 1967.

Marberry, Sara O., ed. *Innovations in Healthcare Design*. New York: John Wiley & Sons, 1995.

Miller, Timothy S. *The Birth of the Hospital in the Byzantine Empire*. Baltimore: Johns Hopkins University Press, 1997.

Miller, T. S. "From Poorhouse to Hospital." *Christian History* 101 (2011). christianhistoryinstitute.org/magazine/article/frompoorhousetohospitalchristianhistoryinstitute.org/magazine/article/frompoorhousetohospital

Park, K. and J. Henderson. "The First Hospital among Christians: The Ospedale di Santa Maria Nuova in Early Sixteenth-Century Florence." *Medical History* 35 (1991): 164–88.

Pawlick, Peter R. "Responsibilities and Goals of Hospital History. A Personal Retrospect from the Viewpoint of a Hospital Architect and Historian." *Historia Hospitalium* 29 (2014): 425–33.

Pevsner, Nikolaus. *A History of Building Types*. London: Thames & Hudson, 1976.

Prior, L. "The Architecture of the Hospital: A Study of Spatial Organization and Medical Knowledge." *British Journal of Sociology* 39 (1988): 86–113.

Proshansky, H. M., W. H. Ittelson, and L. G. Rivlin, eds. *Environmental Psychology: People and their Physical Settings*. 2nd ed. New York: Holt, Rinehart & Winston, 1970.

Quadflieg, R. "Die oberitalienische Hospitalreform des 15. Jahrhunderts und ihre Bauten." *Sudhoffs Archiv* 67 (1983): 25–38.

Risse, Guenter B. "Asclepius at Epidaurus: The Divine Power of Healing Dreams." May 13, 2008. https://ucsf.academia.edu/GuenterRisse/papers. Accessed December 31, 2020.

Risse, Guenter B. "Imhotep and Medicine: A Reevaluation." *The Western Journal of Medicine* 144 (1986): 622–4.

Risse, Guenter B. *Mending Bodies, Saving Souls: A History of Hospitals*. New York: Oxford University Press, 1999.

Bibliography

Risse, Guenter B. "Patients: Historical Perspectives." November 2015. https://ucsf.academia.edu/GuenterRisse/papers. Accessed December 31, 2020.
Risse, Guenter B. "Shamanism: The Dawn of a Healing Profession." *Wisconsin Medical Journal* 71 (1972): 18–23.
Ritter, E. K. "Magical Expert (*ashipu*) and Physician (*asu*). Notes on Two Complementary Professions in Babylonian Medicine." *Assyriological Studies* 16 (1965): 299–321.
Rowland, Ingrid. *Vitruvius: Ten Books of Architecture*. Cambridge: Cambridge University Press, 2001.
Siraisi, Nancy G. *Medieval and Early Renaissance Medicine: An Introduction to Knowledge and Practice*. Chicago: University of Chicago Press, 1990.
Thompson, John D. and Grace Goldin. *The Hospital: A Social and Architectural History*. New Haven: Yale University Press, 1975.
Tyson, Martha M. *The Healing Landscape: Therapeutic Outdoor Environments*. New York: McGraw-Hill, 1998.
Unschuld, Paul U. *Medicine in China: A History of Ideas*. Berkeley: University of California Press, 1985.
Vogler, W. "Historical Sketch of the Abbey of St. Gall." In *The Culture of the Abbey of St. Gall. An Overview*, edited by J. C. King and P. W. Tax, 9–23. Stuttgart: Belser Verlag 1991.
Wagenaar, Cor, ed. *The Architecture of Hospitals*. Rotterdam: NAi Booksellers, 2006.
White, Michael L. *The Social Organization of Christian Architecture*. Valley Forge: Trinity Press, 1996.
Winkelman, Michael. *Shamanism: A Biopsychological Paradigm of Consciousness and Healing*. Santa Barbara, CA: Praeger, 2010.
Zeisel, John. *Sociology and Architectural Design*. New York: Russell Sage Foundation, 1975.

Chapter 3. A Plan for the King and the Sick: Portuguese Hospital Architecture during the Age of Exploration

Abreu, Laurinda. "O que nos ensinam os regimentos hospitalares? Um estudo comparativo entre os Hospitais das Misericórdias de Lisboa e do Porto (séculos XVI e XVII)." In *A Solidariedade nos Séculos: A Confraternidade e as Obras*, edited by Santa Casa da Misericórdia do Porto, 267–85. Porto: Santa Casa da Misericórdia do Porto e Alêtheia Editores, 2009.
Abreu, Laurinda. *Political and Social Dynamics of Poverty, Poor Relief and Health Care in Early-Modern Portugal*. New York: Routledge, 2016.
Albala, Ken. *Eating Right in the Renaissance*. Berkeley: University of California Press, 2002.
Alberti, Leon Battista. *On the Art of Building in Ten Books*. Translated by Joseph Rykwert, Neil Leach, and Robert Tavernor. Cambridge, MA: MIT Press, 1998.
Antunes, Cátia. "Early Modern Ports, 1500–1750." *European History Online (EGO)* (2010): n.p.
Araújo, Renata de. *Lisboa: A Cidade e o Espetáculo na Época dos Descobrimentos*. Lisbon: Livros Horizontes, 1993.
Baini, Laura. "Ipotesi sull'origine della tipologia cruciforme per gli ospedali del XV secolo." In *Processi accumulativi, forme e funzioni: Saggi sull'architettura lombarda del Quattrocento*, edited by Luisa Giordano, 59–102. Florence: La Nuova Italia Editrice, 1996.
Baldasso, Renzo. "Function and Epidemiology in Filarete's Ospedale Maggiore." In *The Medieval Hospital and Medical Practice*, edited by Barbara S. Bowers, 107–20. Burlington, VT: Ashgate, 2007.
Bianchi, Francesco and Marek Słoń. "Le riforme ospedaliere del Quattrocento in Italia e nell'Europa centrale." *Ricerche di storia sociale e religiosa* 35 (2006): 7–45.
Bock, Nicolas. "Patronage, Standards, and *Transfert Culturel*: Naples between Art History and Social Science Theory." *Art History* 31 (2008): 594–7, 601–2.
Braga, Paulo Drumond. "A crise dos estabelecimentos de assistência aos pobres nos finais da idade média," *Revista Portuguesa de História* 26 (1991): 175–90.
Brandão de Buarcos, João. *Grandeza e Abastança de Lisboa em 1552*. Edited by José da Felicidade Alves. Lisbon: Livros Horizontes, 1990.
Campbell, Stephen J. "Artistic Geograghies." In *The Cambridge Companion to the Italian Renaissance*, edited by Michael Wyatt, 17–39. Cambridge: Cambridge University Press, 2014.
Carmona, Mario. *O Hospital Real de Todos-os-Santos da Cidade de Lisboa*. Lisbon: n.p., 1954.
Carpo, Mario. *Architecture in the Age of Printing: Orality, Writing, Typograph, and Printed Images in the History of Architectural Theory*. Translated by Sarah Benson. Cambridge, MA: MIT Press, 2001.

Carvalho, Augusto da Silva. *Crónica do Hospital de Todos-os-Santos*. Lisbon: n.p., 1949.
Cavallo, Sandra. *Charity and Power in Early Modern Italy: Benefactors and their Motives in Turin, 1541–1789*. Cambridge: Cambridge University Press, 1995.
Cavallo, Sandra and Tessa Storey. *Healthy Living in Late Renaissance Italy*. Oxford: Oxford University Press, 2013.
Cesariano, Cesare. *Di Lucio Vitruvio Pollione de Architectura libri dece*. 10 vols. Como: G. da Ponte, 1521.
Clarke, Georgia. "Vitruvian Paradigms." *Papers of the British School at Rome* 70 (2002): 319–46.
Correia, Fernando da Silva. *Subsídios para a história da saúde pública portuguesa do Século XV a 1822*. Oporto: n.p., 1958.
Daupiás, Nuno. *Cartas de Privilégio, Padrões, Doações e Mercês Régias ao Hospital Real de Todos-os- Santos (1492–1775): Subsídios para a sua história*. Lisbon: Imprensa Portuguesa, 1959.
De la Mare, Albinia. "Notes of the Portuguese Patrons of the Florentine Book Trade in the Fifteenth Century." In *Cultural Links between Portugal and Italy in the Renaissance*, edited by Kate Lowe, 167–81. Oxford: Oxford University Press, 2000.
De Marinis, Tammaro. *La biblioteca napoletana dei re d'Aragona*. 2 vols. Verona: Stamperia Valdonega, 1969.
Dias, Bernardo Santos. "A História na medida do Presente. O Ospedale della Misericordia di Parma." MA thesis, Universidade do Porto, 2015–16.
Ficino, Marsilio. *Consiglio contra la pestilenzia*. Florence: San Jacopo a Ripoli, 1481.
Filarete. *Treatise on Architecture; being the treatise by Antonio di Piero Averlino, known as Filarete*. 2 vols. Translated by John R. Spencer. New Haven: Yale University Press, 1965.
Finoli, Anna Maria. "Nota al testo." In Filarete, *Tratatto di architettura*. Vol. 2, edited by Anna Maria Finoli and Liliana Grassi, cvii–cxxix. Milan: Edizioni Il Polifilo, 1972.
Foster, Philip. "Per il disegno dell'Ospedale di Milano." *Arte Lombarda* 18 (1973): 1–22.
Franchini, Lucio. "Introduzione." In *Spedali Lombardi del Quattrocento: Fondazione, trasformazioni, restauri*, edited by Lucio Franchini, 11–72. Como: Edizioni New Press, 1995.
Frommel, Christoph L. "Introduction: The Drawings of Antonio da Sangallo the Younger: History, Evolution, Method, Function." In *The Architectural Drawings of Antonio da Sangallo and His Circle*. Vol. 1, edited by Christoph L. Frommel and Nicholas Adams, 1–60. Cambridge, MA: MIT Press, 1994–2000.
Frommel, Christoph L. and Nicholas Adams, eds. *The Architectural Drawings of Antonio da Sangallo and His Circle*. 2 vols. Cambridge, MA: MIT Press, 1994–2000.
Giordano, Luisa. "On Filarete's *Libro Architettonico*." In *Paper Palaces: The Rise of the Renaissance Architectural Treatise*, edited by Vaughan Hart and Peter Hicks, 51–65. New Haven: Yale University Press, 1998.
Giovannoni, Gustavo. *Antonio da Sangallo il Giovane*. 2 vols. Rome: Tipografia Regionale, 1959.
Gorini, Raffaella. "Gli ospedali Lombardi del XV secolo. Documenti per la loro storia." In *Processi accumulativi, forme e funzioni: Saggi sull'architettura lombarda del Quattrocento*, edited by Luisa Giordano, 11–58. Florence: La Nuova Italia Editrice, 1996.
Grassi, Liliana. *Lo 'Spedale di Poveri' del Filarete: Storia e restauro*. Milan: Università degli Studi di Milano, 1972.
Gschwend, Annemarie Jordan and Kate Lowe, eds. *A Cidade Global: Lisboa no Renascimento/The Global City: Lisbon in the Renaissance*. Lisbon: Museu Nacional de Arte Antiga, 2017.
Gschwend, Annemarie Jordan and Kate Lowe. "Princess of the Seas, Queen of Empire: Configuring the City and Port of Renaissance Lisbon." In *The Global City: On the Streets of Renaissance Lisbon*, edited by Annemarie Jordan Gschwend and Kate Lowe, 12–35. London: Paul Holberton Publishing, 2015.
Gschwend, Annemarie Jordan and Kate Lowe. "Sítios globais da Lisboa renascentista." In *A Cidade Global: Lisboa no Renascimento/The Global City: Lisbon in the Renaissance*, edited by Annemarie Jordan Gschwend and Kate Lowe, 32–59. Lisbon: Museu Nacional de Arte Antiga, 2017.
Gschwend, Annemarie Jordan and Kate Lowe, eds. *The Global City: On the Streets of Renaissance Lisbon*. London: Paul Holberton Publishing, 2015.
Henderson, John. *The Renaissance Hospital: Healing the Body and Healing the Soul*. New Haven: Yale University Press, 2006.
Henderson, John, Peregrine Horden, and Alessandro Pastore. "Introduction. The World of the Hospital: Comparisons and Continuities." In *The Impact of Hospitals, 300–1200*, edited by John Henderson, Peregrine Horden, and Alessandro Pastore, 15–56. Oxford: Peter Lang, 2007.
Herrmann, Eva Maria et al. In *Enclose | Build: Walls, Facade, Roof*, edited by Alexander Reichel and Kerstin Schultz. Basel: Birkhäuser, 2015.
Höfler, Janez. "New Light on Andrea Sansovino's Journey to Portugal." *The Burlington Magazine* 134 (1992): 234–8.
Jütte, Robert. *Poverty and Deviance in Early Modern Europe*. Cambridge: Cambridge University Press, 2006.

Bibliography

Kalina, Pavel. "European Diplomacy, Family Strategies, and the Origins of Renaissance Architecture in Central and Eastern Europe." *Artibus et Historiae* 30 (2009): 173–90.

Leite, Ana Cristina. "Hospital Real de Todos-os-Santos. Uma Obra Moderna." In *Omnia Sanctorum. Histórias da História do Hospital Real de Todos-os-Santos e seus sucessores*, edited by Jorge Penedo, 18–39. Lisbon: By the Book, 2012.

Leite, Ana Cristina. "O Hospital Real de Todos-os-Santos." In *Hospital Real de Todos-os-Santos: Séculos XV a XVIII*, edited by Paulo Pereira, 5–19. Lisbon: Museu Rafael Bordalo Pinheiro, 1993.

Lowe, Kate, ed. *Cultural Links between Portugal and Italy in the Renaissance*. Oxford: Oxford University Press, 2000.

Lowe, Kate, ed. "Foreign Descriptions of the Global City: Renaissance Lisbon from the Outside." In *The Global City: On the Streets of Renaissance Lisbon*, edited by Annemarie Jordan Gschwend and Kate Lowe, 37–55. London: Paul Holberton Publishing, 2015.

Marías, Fernando. "Arquitectura y Sistema hospitalario en Toledo en el siglo XVI." In *Tolède et l'expansion urbaine en Espagne, 1450–1650: actes du colloque organisé par la Junta de Comunidades de Castilla-La Mancha et la Casa de Velázquez, Tolède-Madrid, 21–23 mars 1988*, 49–68. Madrid: Recontres de la Casa de Velázquez, 1991.

Moita, Irisalva. "As escavações de 1960 que puseram a descoberto parte das ruínas do Hospital Real de Todos-os-Santos." In *Hospital Real de Todos-os-Santos: Séculos XV a XVIII*, edited by Paulo Pereira, 20–2. Lisbon: Museu Rafael Bordalo Pinheiro, 1993.

Moita, Irisalva. "A imagem e a vida da cidade." In *Lisboa quinhentista: A imagem e a vida da cidade*, edited by Irisalva Moita, 9–22. Lisbon: Câmara Municipal de Lisboa, 1983.

Moita, Irisalva. "Hospital Real de Todos-os-Santos (relatório das escavações a que mandou proceder a CML de 22 de agosto a 24 de setembro 1960)." *Revista Municipal* 101–11 (1964–6).

Moita, Irisalva. "O Hospital Real de Todos-os-Santos: Enfermarias—Aposentadorias—Serviços." In *Hospital Real de Todos-os-Santos: Séculos XV a XVIII*, edited by Paulo Pereira, 40–8. Lisbon: Museu Rafael Bordalo Pinheiro, 1993.

Moreira, Rafael. "O Hospital Real de Todos-os-Santos e o Italianismo de D. João II." In *Hospital Real de Todos-os-Santos: Séculos XV a XVIII*, edited by Paulo Pereira, 23–30. Lisbon: Museu Rafael Bordalo Pinheiro, 1993.

Pereira, Paulo, ed. *Hospital Real de Todos-os-Santos: Séculos XV a XVIII*. Lisbon: Museu Rafael Bordalo Pinheiro, 1993.

Pevsner, Nikolaus. *A History of Building Types*. Princeton: Princeton University Press, 1976.

Rijo, Delminda Maria Miguéns. "Palácio dos Estaus de Hospedaria Real a Palácio da Inquisição e Tribunal do Santo Ofício." *Cadernos do Arquivo Municipal* 5 (2016): 19–49.

Robey, Jessica. "From the City Witnessed to the Community Dreamed: The *Civitates Orbis Terrarum* and the Circle of Abraham Ortelius and Joris Hoefnagel." Ph.D. diss., University of California, Santa Barbara, 2006.

Safley, Thomas Max. "Introduction." In *Reformation of Charity: The Secular and Religious in Early Modern Poor Relief*, edited by Thomas Max Safley, 1–14. Boston: Brill, 2003.

Salgado, Abílio José and Anastásia Mestrinho Salgado, eds. *Regimento do Hospital de Todos-os-Santos (Edição Fac-Similada)*. Lisbon: Comissão Organizadora do V Centenário da Fundação do Hospital de Todos-os-Santos, 1992.

Salgado, Anastásia Mestrinho. *O Hospital de Todos-os-Santos: Assistência à pobreza em Portugal no século XVI; A irradiação da assistência médica para o Brasil, Índia e Japão*. Lisbon: By the Book, 2015.

Soyer, François. *The Persecution of the Jews and Muslims of Portugal: King Manuel I and the End of Religious Tolerance (1496–7)*. Boston: Brill, 2007.

Spencer, John. "Introduction." In *Treatise on Architecture; being the treatise by Antonio di Piero Averlino, known as Filarete*. Vol. 1, *The Translation*. Translated by John R. Spencer, xvii–xxxvii. New Haven: Yale University Press, 1965.

Spencer, John. Review of *Antonio Averlino detto il Filarete. Tratatto di Architettura*, by Anna Maria Finoli and Liliana Grassi. *Art Bulletin* 57 (1975): 131–3.

Terpstra, Nicholas. *Cultures of Charity: Women, Politics, and the Reform of Poor Relief in Renaissance Italy*. Cambridge, MA: Harvard University Press, 2013.

Vasari, Giorgio. *Le vite de' più eccellenti pittori, scultori ed architettori*. 9 vols. Edited by Gaetano Milanesi. Florence: G. C. Sansoni, 1878–85.

Vitruvius. *Ten Books on Architecture*. Translated by Ingrid D. Rowland. New York: Cambridge University Press, 1999.

Vulpi, Valentina. "Finding Filarete: The Two Versions of the Libro architettonico." In *Raising the Eyebrow: John Onians and World Art Studies: An Album Amicorum in his Honour*, edited by Lauren Golden, 329–39. Oxford: Archaeopress, 2001.

Wallerstein, Immanuel. *The Modern World System: Capitalist Agriculture and the Origins of the European World Economy in the Sixteenth Century*. New York: Academic Press, 1974.

Welch, Evelyn. *Art and Authority in Renaissance Milan*. New Haven: Yale University Press, 1995.

Wilkinson, Catherine. *The Hospital of Cardinal Tavera in Toledo*. New York: Garland Publishing, 1977.

Chapter 4. Healing of the Poor: The Hospital of Our Lady of Potterie in Bruges and the Miracle Book (c. 1520–1)

Brown, Andrew. *Civic Ceremony and Religion in Medieval Bruges c. 1300–1520.* Cambridge: Cambridge University Press, 2011.

Brown, Andrew and Jan Dumolyn, eds. *Medieval Bruges, c. 850–1550.* Cambridge: Cambridge University Press, 2018.

Delepierre, Octabe. *Guide indispensable dans la ville de Bruges ou description des monuments curieux et objets d'art que renferme cette ville.* Bruges: Bogaert, 1847.

Depoorter, Matthias. *The Hospital Museum, Bruges.* Ludion: Antwerp, 2016.

Duclos, A. "M. Verschelde's werk aan de Potterie." *Rond den Heerd* 17, no. 7 (1882): 49–53.

Fantazzi, Charles, ed. *A Companion to Juan Luis Vives.* Boston and Leiden: Brill, 2008.

González, Enrique. "Fame and Oblivion." In *A Companion to Juan Luis Vives*, edited by Charles Fantazzi, 359–414. Leiden: Brill, 2008.

Grell, Ole and Andrew Cunningham. *Health Care and Poor Relief in Protestant Europe 1500–1700.* London: Routledge, 1997.

Harmening, Dieter. "Mirakelbildzyklen—Formen und Tendenzen von Kultpropaganda." *Bayerisches Jahrbuch für Volkskunde* (1976/7): 53–6.

Jütte, Robert. "Poor Relief and Social Discipline in Sixteenth-Century Europe." *European Studies Reviews* 11 (1981): 25–52.

Kawahara, Atsushi. "Imaging Medieval Charity: Social Ritual and Poor Relief in Late Medieval Ghent." *Journal of Social Sciences and Humanities* 257 (1995): 1–32.

Lane, Barbara. *Hans Memling: Master Painter in Fifteenth-Century Bruges.* Turnhout: Brepols, 2009.

Ljungqvist, Frederik. "Female Shame, Male Honor: The Chastity of Code in Juan Luis Vives' De institutione feminae Christianae." *Journal of Family History* 37, no. 2 (2012): 139–54.

Maertens, Alfons. *Onze Lieve Vrouw der Potterie.* Brussels: S. Pietersabdij, 1937.

Maréchal, Griet. *De sociale en politieke gebondenheid van het Brugse hospitaalwezen in de middeleeuwen.* Kortelijk-Heule: UGA, 1978.

Maréchal, Griet. "Geschiedenis van het hospitaal van Onze Lieve Vrouw van de Potterie te Brugge in de middeleeuwen." MA thesis, Ghent University, 1964.

Nijkamp, Marlies. "Mijrakelen van onse lieue vrauwe te potterije: Studie naar de functie van een zestiende-eeuws Brugs manuscript." MA thesis, Rijksuniversiteit Groningen, 2014.

Pannier, Charlotte. "De mirakeltekeningen van Onze-Lieve-Vrouw van de Potterie te Brugge. Hun situering ten opzichte van XVIe en XVIIe eeuwse Westvlaamse mirakelvoorstellingen van Onze-Lieve-Vrouw. Schilderijen en wandtapijten." MA thesis, Ghent University, 1978.

Rosweydus, Heribertus. "Kerckeliicke historie van Nederlandt." In *Generale kerckelycke historie van de gheboorte onses H. Iesu Christi tot het Iaer MDCXXIV*, edited by Caesar Baronius, Part 2. Antwerp: Jan Cnobbaert, 1623.

Spicker, Paul, ed. and trans. *The Origins of Modern Welfare: Juan Luis Vives, De Subventine Pauperum, and City of Ypres, Forma Subventionis Pauperum.* Oxford: Peter Lang, 2010.

Taisne, Philippus. "Onse Lieve Vrauwe van Potterye toevlucht der sondaeren, en van alle behoeftighe menschen, het oudste mirakeleus beeldt van ons Nederlant, door veel jonsten vermaert, ende te Brugghe besonderlyk vereert." Bruges, 1666. Reprinted in *Van Blindekens naar de Potterie: een eeuwenoude Brugse belofte*, edited by Jean Meulemeester et al., 156–97. Bruges: Jong Kristen Onthaal voor toerisme, 1980.

Tournoy, Gilbert. "Towards the Roots of Social Welfare: Joan Lluís Vives's De subventione pauperum." *City* 8, no. 2 (2004): 266–73.

Travill, A. "Juan Luis Vives: A Humanistic Medical Educator." *Canadian Bulletin of Medical History* 4, no. 1 (1987): 53–76.

Travill, A. "Juan Luis Vives: The De Subventione Pauperum." *Canadian Bulletin of Medical History* 4, no. 2 (1987): 165–81.

Van de Putte, Felix. *Histoire de Notre-Dame de la Poterie.* Bruges: Imprimerie de Vandecasteele-Werbrouck, 1843.

Vives, Juan Luis. *Concerning the Relief of the Poor or Concerning Human Need, a Letter Addressed to the Senate of Bruges by Juan-Luis Vivès January 6, 1526.* Translated by Margaret Sherwood. New York: The New York School of Philanthropy, 1917.

Vives, Juan Luis. *De subventione pauperum sive de humanis necessitatibus, libri II. Introduction, Critical Edition, Translation and Notes.* Edited and translated by Constant Matheeussen and Charles Fantazzi. Leiden: Brill, 2002.

Bibliography

Chapter 5. 'The Love of Friends Made This in the Cause of Humanity': Therapeutic Environment in Quaker Asylum Design at the York Retreat

Abrams, M. H. *Natural Supernaturalism: Tradition and Revolution in Romantic Literature*. New York and London: W. W. Norton & Co. 1973.

Ackerman, James S. *The Villa: Form and Ideology of Country Houses*. London: Thames & Hudson, 1990.

Adams, Annmarie. *Medicine by Design: The Architect and the Modern Hospital 1893–1943*. Minneapolis and London: University of Minnesota Press, 2008.

Addison, Joseph. *The Spectator*, 195, October 13, 1711. https://www.gutenberg.org/files/12030/12030-h/SV1/Spectator1.html#section195. Accessed January 6, 2021.

Aikin, John. *A View of the Life, Travels, and Philanthropic Labors of the late John Howard, Esquire L.L.D. F.R.S.* Philadelphia: John Ormrod, 1794.

Aikin, John. *Thoughts on Hospitals*. London: Joseph Johnson, 1771.

Akehurst, Ann-Marie. "Architecture and Philanthropy: Building Hospitals in Eighteenth-Century York." Ph.D. diss., University of York, 2009.

Akehurst, Ann-Marie. "'The Body Natural as well as the Body Politic stands indebted': The Hospital—Foundation, Funding and Form." In *Architectural Theory and Practice, Companion to Architecture in the Age of the Enlightenment*, vol. 2, edited by Caroline van Eck and Sigrid de Jong. Chichester: John Wiley & Sons, 2017.

Akehurst, Ann-Marie. "'Inward Light': Taking Architecture Seriously with the Early Religious Society of Friends." In *Places of Worship in Britain and Ireland, 1689–1840*, edited by Paul Barnwell and Mark Smith. Donington: Shaun Tyas forthcoming.

Akehurst, Ann-Marie. "The York Retreat, 'a Vernacular of Equality.'" In *Built from Below: British Architecture and the Vernacular*, edited by Peter Guillery, 73–98. London and New York: Routledge, 2010.

Alexander, William. *Observations on the Construction and Fitting up of Meeting Houses*. York: William Alexander, 1820.

Andrews, Gavin T. "(Re)Thinking the Dynamics between Healthcare and Place: Therapeutic Geographies in Treatment and Care Practices." *Area* 36, no. 3 (September 2004): 307–18.

Anonymous. *Account of the Rise and Progress of the Asylum Proposed to be erected in Philadelphia*. Philadelphia: Kimber and Conrad, 1814.

Arnold, Dana. *The Spaces of the Hospital: Spatiality and Urban Change in London 1680–1820*. London and New York: Routledge, 2013.

Bachelard, Gaston. *The Poetics of Space*. Translated by Maria Jolas. Boston: Beacon Press, 1964.

Baer, Leonard D. and Wilbert M. Gesler. "Reconsidering the Concept of Therapeutic Landscapes in J. D. Salinger's 'The Catcher in the Rye.'" *Area* 36, no. 4 (December 2004): 404–13.

Barclay, Robert. *An Apology for the True Christian Divinity, Being an Explanation and Vindication of the Principles and Doctrines of the People Called Quakers*. 5th ed. London: T Sowle, 1703.

Barry, Jonathan and Colin Jones, eds. *Medicine and Charity before the Welfare State*. London and New York: Routledge, 1991.

Bellers, John. *An Essay toward the Improvement of Physick*. London: J. Sowle, 1714.

Bentham, Jeremy. *Panopticon: or, the Inspection-House*. Dublin: Thomas Byrne, 1791.

Bewley, Thomas. *Madness to Mental Illness. A History of the Royal College of Psychiatrists*. Online archive 1, William Tuke (1732–1822). https://www.rcpsych.ac.uk/docs/default-source/about-us/library-archives/archives/william-tuke-1732-1822.pdf?sfvrsn=e21108e9_4. Accessed January 6, 2021.

Brett, David. *The Plain Style*. Cambridge: The Lutterworth Press, 2004.

Brooks Kelley, Donald. "'A Tender Regard to the Whole Creation': Anthony Benezet and the Emergence of an Eighteenth-Century Quaker Ecology." *The Pennsylvania Magazine of History and Biography* 106, no. 1 (1982): 69–88.

Butler, David M. *Quaker Meeting Houses of the Lake Counties*. London: Friends Historical Society, 1978.

Cantor, Geoffrey. "Aesthetics in Science, as Practiced by Quakers in the Eighteenth and Nineteenth Centuries." *Quaker Studies* 4 (1999): 1–20.

Cantor, Geoffrey. "The Bible, the Creation and Inward Light: Tensions within Quaker Science." http://www.fundacionorotava.org/media/web/files/page147__10_ing_Cantor_QuakerScience.pdf. Accessed January 6, 2021.

Castell, Robert. *Villas of the Ancients Illustrated*. London, 1728.

Christie, W. "The Modern Athenians: The Edinburgh Review in the Knowledge Economy of the Early Nineteenth Century." *Studies in Scottish Literature* 39, no. 1 (2013): 115–38.

Colvin, Howard. *A Biographical Dictionary of British Architects 1600–1840*. New Haven and London: Yale University Press, 2008.

Cornaro, Alvise. *Discorsi della Vita Sobria*. Translated Robert Urie. Glasgow, 1770.

Dandelion, Ben Pink. *An Introduction to Quakerism*. Cambridge: Cambridge University Press, 2007.

d'Antonio, Patricia. *Founding Friends: Families, Staff, and Patients at the Friends Asylum in Early Nineteenth-Century Philadelphia*. Pennsylvania: Lehigh University Press, 2006.

Digby, Anne. "Changes in the Asylum: The Case of York, 1777–1815." *Economic History Review* 36, no. 2 (May 1983): 218–39.

Digby, Anne. "Tuke, William (1732–1822), Philanthropist and Founder of the York Retreat." *Oxford Dictionary of National Biography*. September 23, 2004. https://www-oxforddnb-com.sheffield.idm.oclc.org/view/10.1093/ref:odnb/9780198614128.001.0001/odnb-9780198614128-e-27810. Accessed January 6, 2021.

Donawerth, Jane. "Women's Reading Practices in Seventeenth-Century England: Margaret Fell's 'Women's Speaking Justified.'" *The Sixteenth Century Journal* 37, no. 4 (Winter, 2006): 985–1005.

Ellwood, Thomas. ed. *A Journal or Historical Account of the life, travels, sufferings, Christian experiences and labour of love in the work of the ministry, of that ancient, eminent and faithful servant of Jesus Christ, George Fox*. London: Thomas Northcott, 1694.

Fens-de Zeeuw, Lyda. *Lindley Murray (1745–1826), Quaker and Grammarian*. Utrecht: LOT, 2011.

Filarete. *Codex Magliabechianus*, Tractate on Architecture. 1456.

Fox, George. *To the Parliament of the Common-wealth of England*. London: Simmons, 1659.

Garvan, Anthony N. B. "Proprietary Philadelphia as Artifact." In *The Historian and The City*, edited by Oscar Handlin and John Burchard, 177–210. Cambridge, MA: MIT Press, 1966.

Gerlach-Spriggs, Nancy, Richard Enoch Kaufman, and Sam Bass Warner, Jnr. *Restorative Gardens: The Healing Landscape*. New Haven, CT: Yale University Press, 1998.

Gesler, Wilbert M. *Healing Places*. Lanham, Boulder, New York and Oxford: Rowman and Littlefield, 2003.

Glover, Mary R. *The Retreat, York: An Early Experiment in the Treatment of Mental Illness*. York: William Sessions, 1984.

Goldie, Mark. 2005 "Cambridge Platonists (act. 1630s–1680s)." *Oxford Dictionary of National Biography*. September 22, 2005. https://www-oxforddnb-com.sheffield.idm.oclc.org/view/10.1093/ref:odnb/9780198614128.001.0001/odnb-9780198614128-e-94274 Accessed January 6, 2021.

Guibbory, Achsah. *The Map of Time: Seventeenth-Century English Literature and Ideas of Pattern in History*. Urbana: University of Illinois Press, 1986.

Henderson, John. *The Renaissance Hospital: Healing the Body and Healing the Soul*. New Haven and London: Yale University Press, 2008.

Hickman, Clare. "The Picturesque at Brislington House, Bristol: The Role of Landscape in Relation to the Treatment of Mental Illness in the Early Nineteenth-Century Asylum." *Garden History* 33, no. 1 (Summer 2005): 47–60.

Hill, Christopher. *The World Turned Upside Down: Radical Ideas During the English Revolution*. London: Penguin, 1972.

Hoppit, Julian. "King, Gregory (1648–1712), Herald and Political Economist." *Oxford Dictionary of National Biography*. September 23, 2004. https://www-oxforddnb-com.sheffield.idm.oclc.org/view/10.1093/ref:odnb/9780198614128.001.0001/odnb-9780198614128-e-15563. Accessed January 6, 2021.

Howard, John. *An account of the principal lazarettos in Europe; with various papers relative to the plague: Together with Further Observations on Some Foreign Prisons and Hospitals*. London: Johnson, Dilly and Cadell, 1791.

Hunt, Harold Capper. *A Retired Habitation: A History of the Retreat at York*. London: H. K. Lewis and Co., 1932.

Ingle, H. Larry. 2004 "Fox, George (1624–1691), a Founder of the Religious Society of Friends (Quakers)." *Oxford Dictionary of National Biography*. September 23, 2004. https://www-oxforddnb-com.sheffield.idm.oclc.org/view/10.1093/ref:odnb/9780198614128.001.0001/odnb-9780198614128-e-10031 Accessed January 6, 2021.

Imbert, Jean, ed. *Histoire des Hôpitaux en France*. Toulouse: Privat, *c*. 1982.

Jones, Kathleen. *Lunacy, Law, and Conscience 1744–1845: The Social History of the Care of the Insane*. London: Routledge and Kegan Paul, 1955.

Kearns, Robin A. and W. M. Gesler. *Culture/Place/Health*. London: Routledge, 2001.

Leistikow, Dankwart. *Ten Centuries of European Hospital Architecture: A Contribution to the History of Hospital Architecture*. Ingelheim-am-Rhein: C. H. Boehringer Sohn, 1967.

Lidbetter, Hubert. *The Friends Meetinghouse*. 2nd ed. York: William Sessions, 1979.

London Friends' Institute. *Biographical Catalogue*. London: [n.p.], 1888.

Marcus, Clare Cooper and Marni Barnes, eds. *Healing Gardens: Therapeutic Benefits and Design Recommendations*. Chichester: John Wiley & Sons, 1999.

Bibliography

McWhir, Anne. "Scott, John (1730–1783), Poet and Writer." *Oxford Dictionary of National Biography*. September 23, 2004. https://www-oxforddnb-com.sheffield.idm.oclc.org/view/10.1093/ref:odnb/9780198614128.001.0001/odnb-9780198614128-e-24891. Accessed January 6, 2021.

Mendieta, Eduardo and Jonathan Vanantwerpen, eds. *The Power of Religion in the Public Sphere*. New York: Columbia University Press, 2011.

Morris, Robert. *Rural Architecture: Consisting of Regular Designs of Plans and Elevations for Buildings in the Country*. London: printed for the author, 1750.

Nelson, Robert. *Address to Persons of Quality and Estate*. London: G. James, 1715.

Pallasmaa, Juhanni, *The Embodied Image: Imagination and Imagery in Architecture*. Chichester: John Wiley & Sons, 2011.

Penn, William. *Some Fruits of Solitude, in Reflections and Maxims Relating to the Conduct of Human Life*. London, 1702.

Pevsner, Nikolaus. *A History of Building Types*. Princeton: Princeton University Press, 1976.

Pike, Joseph. *Some Account of the Life of Joseph Pike*. London: Darton and Harvey, 1838.

Porter, Roy. *Madmen: A Social History of Madhouses, Mad-Doctors and Lunatics*. Stroud: Tempus, 2004.

Raistrick, Arthur. *Quakers in Science and Industry*. York: Sessions Book Trust, 1993.

Rendel Harris, J. "The Attitudes of the Society of Friends towards Modern Thought." In *Report of the Proceedings of the Conference of Members of the Society of Friends, Held, by Direction of the Yearly Meeting, in Manchester from Eleventh to the Fifteenth of Eleventh Month, 1895*. London: Headley Brothers, 1896.

Richardson, Harriet, ed. *English Hospitals and their Design 1660–1948*. Swindon: Royal Commission on the Historical Monuments of England, 1998.

Risse, Guenter B. *Hospital Life in Enlightenment Scotland*. Cambridge: Cambridge University Press, 1986.

Risse, Guenter B. *Mending Bodies, Saving Souls: A History of Hospitals*. Oxford and New York: Oxford University Press, 1999.

Rutherford, Sarah. "Landscapes for the Mind: English Asylum Designers, 1845–1914. *Garden History* 33, no. 1 (Summer 2005): 61–86.

Savage, Robert J. G. "Natural History of the Goldney Garden Grotto, Clifton, Bristol." *Garden History* 17, no. 1 (Spring 1989): 1–40.

Scott, John. *The Poetical Works of John Scott Esq.* London: J. Buckland, 1782.

Scull, Andrew. *The Most Solitary of Afflictions: Madness and Society in Britain 1700–1900*. New Haven and London: Yale University Press, 1993.

Sessions, William Kaye. *The Tukes of York in the Seventeenth, Eighteenth and Nineteenth Centuries*. London: Friends Home Service Committee, 1971.

Smith, Nigel. 2004. "Whitehead, George (1637–1724), Quaker Leader and Writer." *Oxford Dictionary of National Biography*. September 23, 2004. https://www-oxforddnb-com.sheffield.idm.oclc.org/view/10.1093/ref:odnb/9780198614128.001.0001/odnb-9780198614128-e-29287. Accessed January 6, 2021.

Steere, Douglas Van, ed. *Quaker Spirituality: Selected Writings*. London: SPCK, 1984.

Stevenson, Christine. "Carsten Anker Dines with the Younger George Dance, and Visits St Luke's Hospital for the Insane." *Architectural History*, 44, *Essays in Architectural History, Presented to John Newman* (2001): 153–61.

Stevenson, Christine. *Medicine and Magnificence: Hospital and Asylum Architecture 1660–1820*. New Haven and London: Yale University Press, 2000.

Stevenson, Christine. "Robert Hooke's Bethlem." *Journal of the Society of Architectural Historians* 55 (1996): 254–75.

Stevenson, Christine. *The City and the King: Architecture and Politics in Restoration London*. New Haven and London: Yale University Press, 2013.

Thompson, John D. and Grace Goldin. *The Hospital: A Social and Architectural History*. New Haven and London: Yale University Press, 1975.

Tolles, Frederick B. *Meeting House and Counting House: The Quaker Merchants of Colonial Philadelphia 1682–1763*. New York and London: Norton and Co., 1948.

Tolles, Frederick B. "'of the Best Sort but Plain': The Quaker Esthetic." *American Quarterly* 11, no. 4 (Winter 1959): 484–502.

Tuke, Samuel. *A Description of the Retreat: An Institution Near York, for Insane Persons of the Society of Friends*. York: William Alexander, 1813.

Turner, Harold W. *From Temple to Meeting House: Phenomenology and Theology of Places of Worship*. The Hague: Mouton, 1979.

Vergil. *Georgics*, II, 459–69. http://sabidius.com/index.php/prolegomenon/item/1326-virgil-georgics-book-ii. Accessed October 23, 2018.

Wade Martins, Susanna. *The English Model Farm: Building the Agricultural Ideal, 1700–1914*. Macclesfield: Windgather Press, 2002.
Waln, Robert, Jnr., *An Account of the Asylum for the Insane Established by the Society of Friends Near Frankford, in the Vicinity of Philadelphia*. Philadelphia: Benjamin and Thomas Kite, 1825.
Walvin, James. *The Quakers: Morals and Money*. London: John Murray, 1997.
Weiner, D. B. "'Le Geste de Pinel': The History of a Psychiatric Myth." In *Discovering the History of Psychiatry*, Mark Micale, 232–47. Oxford: Oxford University Press.
Weiner, D. B. "Philippe Pinel's 'Memoir on Madness' of December 11, 1794: A Fundamental Text of Modern Psychiatry." *American Journal of Psychiatry* 149, no. 6 (June 1992): 725–32.
Wordsworth, William. Preface to Poems, 1815. Paragraph 29 at https://en.wikisource.org/wiki/Poems_(Wordsworth,_1815)/Volume_1#vii. Accessed January 6, 2021.
Wragg, Brian and Giles Worsley. *The Life and Works of John Carr*. York: Oblong Press, 2000.
Wright, Sheila. *Friends in York: The Dynamics of Quaker Revival 1780–1860*. Keele: Keele University Press, 1995.
Yanni, Carla. *The Architecture of Madness: Insane Asylums in the United States*. Minneapolis and London: University of Minnesota Press, 2007.

II. Polity: Public Health and Politics

Chapter 6. *Dar al-Shifa'* or *Bimaristan*? Islamic Hospitals of Damascus, Sivas, and Cairo in the Twelfth and Thirteenth Centuries

Arnold, Felix. *Islamic Palace Architecture in the Western Mediterranean: A History*. Oxford: Oxford University Press, 2017.
Bakir, Betül and Ibrahim Başağaoğlu. "How Medical Functions Shaped Architecture in Anatolian Seljuk Darüşşifas (Hospitals) and Especially in the Divriği Turan Malik Darüşşifa." *Journal of the International Society for the History of Islamic Medicine* 5, no. 10 (2006): 64–82.
Behrens-Abouseif, Doris. *Cairo of the Mamluks: A History of the Architecture and its Culture*. London: I.B.Tauris, 2007.
Behrens-Abouseif, Doris. *Islamic Architecture in Cairo: An Introduction*. Leiden: Brill, 1989.
Bosworth, Clifford Edmund. *The New Islamic Dynasties: A Chronological and Genealogical Manual*. Edinburgh: Edinburgh University Press, 1996.
Çetintaş, Sedat. *Sivas Darüşşifası*. Istanbul: Ibrahim Horoz Basımevi, 1953.
Cevdet, M. "Sivas Darüşşifası vakfiyesi ve tercümesi." *Vakıflar Dergisi* 1 (1938): 35–38.
Chipman, Leigh. "Islamic Pharmacy in the Mamlūk and Mongol Realms: Theory and Practice." *Asian Medicine* 3 (2007): 265–78.
Coste, Pascal. *Architecture arabe au Monuments de Kaire*. Paris: Firmin Didot Frère, 1839.
Crowe, Yoland. "Divriği: Ulu Cami and Hospital." Ph.D. diss., University of London, 1973.
Dişli, Gülşen and Zühal Özcan. "An Evaluation of Heating Technology in Anatolian Seljuk Period Hospitals (Darüşşifa)." *METU Journal of the Faculty of Architecture* 33, no. 2 (2016): 183–200.
Dols, Michael W. "Insanity and its Treatment in Islamic Society." *Medical History* 31 (1987): 1–14.
Dols, Michael W. "The Origins of the Islamic Hospital: Myth and Reality." *Bulletin of the History of Medicine* 61 (1987): 367–90.
Elgood, Cyril. *A Medical History of Persia and the Eastern Caliphate*. Cambridge: Cambridge University Press, 1951.
Gabriel, Albert. *Monuments turcs d'Anatolie*. Paris: E. de Boccard, 1934.
Herzfeld, Ernst. "Damascus: Studies in Architecture: 1." *Ars Islamica* 9 (1942): 1–53.
Hirschler, Konrad. *The Written Word in the Medieval Arabic Lands: A Social and Cultural History of Reading Practices*. Edinburgh: Edinburgh University Press, 2012.
Karimullah, Kamran I. "Avicenna and Galen, Philosophy and Medicine: Contextualising Discussions of Medical Experience in Medieval Islamic Physicians and Philosophers." *Oriens* 45 (2017): 105–49.
Khadr, M. "Deux actes de WAQF d'un Qaraḫānide d'Asie centrale." *Journal Asiatique* 255 (1967): 305–34.
Kuban, Doğan. *Ottoman Architecture*. Woodbridge: Antique Collectors' Club, 2010.
Lev, G. and Yaacov Lev. "Politics, Education, and Medicine in Eleventh Century Samarkand. A Waqf Study." *Wiener Zeitschrift für die Kunde des Morgenlandes* 93 (2003): 119–45.

Bibliography

McClary, Richard Piran. *Rum Seljuq Architecture, 1170–1220: The Patronage of Sultans*. Edinburgh: Edinburgh University Press, 2017.
Munajid, Salaheddine. *Bimaristan de Nur-ed-Din*. Damascus: n.p., 1946.
Northrup, Linda S. "Qalāwūn's Patronage of the Medical Sciences in Thirteenth-Century Egypt." *Mamluk Studies Review* 5 (2001): 119–40.
Önkal, Hakkı. *Anadolu Selçuklu Türbeleri*. Ankara: Atatürk Kültür Merkezi, 1996.
Özcan, Zühal and Gülşen Dişli. "Refrigeration Technology in Anatolian Seljuk and Ottoman Period Hospitals." *Gazi University Journal of Science* 27, no. 3 (2014): 1015–21.
Pitchon, Véronique. "Food and Medicine in Medieval Islamic Hospitals: Preparation and Care in Accordance with Dietetic Principles." *Food & History* 14, no. 1 (2016): 13–33.
Pormann, Peter E. and Emily Savage-Smith. *Medieval Islamic Medicine*. Edinburgh: Edinburgh University Press, 2007.
Rabbat, Nasser. *Mamluk History through Architecture: Monuments, Culture and Politics in Medieval Egypt and Syria*. London: I.B.Tauris, 2010.
Ragab, Ahmed. *The Medieval Islamic Hospital: Medicine, Religion and Charity*. Cambridge: Cambridge University Press, 2015.
Shoshan, Boaz. "The State and Madness in Medieval Islam." *International Journal of Middle Eastern Studies* 35 (2003): 329–40.
Sözen, Metin. *Anadolu Medreseleri: Selçuklular ve Beylikler Devri*. Vol. 1. Istanbul: Istanbul Teknik Üniversitesi Mimarlık Fakültesi, 1970.
Tabbaa, Yasser. "The Architectural Patronage of Nur al-Din (1146–1174)." Ph.D. diss., New York University, 1982.
Trépanier, Nicolas. *Foodways and Daily Life in Medieval Anatolia*. Austin: University of Texas Press, 2014.
Ulmann, Manfred. *Islamic Medicine*. Edinburgh: Edinburgh University Press, 1978.

Chapter 7. The Body of the City: Medicine and Urban Renewal in Sixtus IV's Rome

Ackerman, James S. "The Planning of Renaissance Rome, 1450–1580." In P. A. Ramsey, *Rome in the Renaissance: The City and the Myth*, 3–17. Binghamton, NY: Center for Medieval & Early Renaissance Studies, 1982.
Alberti, Leon Battista. *On the Art of Building in Ten Books*. Translated by Joseph Rykwert, Neil Leach, and Robert Tavernor. Cambridge, MA: MIT Press, 1988.
Albertini, Francesco. *Opusculum de mirabilibus novae et veteris urbis Romae* [1510] (Basel: [n.p.], 1519), fol. 75v. https://books.google.com/books?id=bsJbAAAAQAAJ. Accessed May 30, 2018.
Alteri, Giancarlo. "Il Giubileo di Sisto IV attraverso alcune testimonianze numismatiche dirette e indirette." In *Sisto IV: Le Arti a Roma nel Primo Rinascimento*, edited by Fabio Benzi, 151–4. Rome: Edizioni dell'Associazione Culturale Shakespeare and Company, 2000.
Alveri, Gasparo. *Roma in ogni stato*. 2 vols. Rome: Fabio Falco, 1664. https://books.google.com/books?id=s0kokCu_dugC. Accessed July 5, 2018.
Archambault, Paul. "The Analogy of the 'Body' in Renaissance Political Literature." *Bibliothèque d'Humanisme et Renaissance* 29, no. 1 (1967): 21–53.
Averlino, Antonio (Filarete). *Treatise on Architecture*. Translated by John R. Spencer. 2 vols. New Haven and London: Yale University Press, 1965.
Barkan, Leonard. *Nature's Work of Art: The Human Body as Image of the World*. New Haven and London: Yale University Press, 1975.
Benzi, Fabio. *Sisto IV Renovator Urbis: Architettura a Roma 1471–1484*. Rome: Officina, 1990.
Benzi, Fabio, ed. *Sisto IV: Le Arti a Roma nel Primo Rinascimento*. Rome: Edizioni dell'Associazione Culturale Shakespeare and Company, 2000.
Berlier, Stéphane. "Niccolò da Reggio traducteur du *De usu partium* de Galien. Place de la traduction latine dans l'histoire du texte." *Medicina nei secoli* 25, no. 3 (2013): 957–78.
Bertino, Antonio. "Arte e storia nelle medaglie di Sisto IV e di Giulio II." In *Sisto IV e Giulio II mecenati e promotori di cultura*, edited by Silvia Bottaro, Anna Dagnino, and Giovanna Rotondi Terminiello, 127–35. Savona: Coop Tipograf, 1985.

Bibliography

Bianca, Concetta. "Francesco della Rovere: Un Francescano tra teologia e potere." In *Un pontificato ed una città: Sisto IV (1471–1484)*, edited by Massimo Miglio, Francesca Niutta, Diego Quaglioni, and Concetta Ranieri, 19–46. Vatican City: Associazione Roma nel Rinascimento, 1986.

Blondin, Jill E. "Constructing History: The Visual Legacy of Pope Sixtus IV." Ph.D. diss., University of Illinois, Urbana-Champaign, 2002.

Blondin, Jill E. "Power Made Visible: Pope Sixtus IV as 'Urbis Restaurator' in Quattrocento Rome." *The Catholic Historical Review* 91, no. 1 (January 2005): 1–25.

Boyle, Leonard E. O.P. "Sixtus IV and the Vatican Library." In *Rome: Tradition, Innovation and Renewal. A Canadian International Art History Conference, 8–13 June 1987*, edited by C. Brown, J. Osborne and C. Kirwin, 65–73. Victoria, BC: University of Victoria, 1991.

Buddensieg, Tillman. "Die Statuenstifting Sixtus' IV. im Jahre 1471." *Römisches Jahrbuch für Kunstgeschichte* 20 (1983): 34–73.

Burroughs, Charles. *From Signs to Design: Environmental Process and Reform in Early Renaissance Rome*. Cambridge, MA: MIT Press, 1990.

Bynum, Caroline Walker. *Wonderful Blood: Theology and Practice in Late Medieval Northern Germany and Beyond*. Philadelphia: University of Pennsylvania Press, 2007.

Cantatore, Flavia. "La Biblioteca Vaticana nel palazzo di Niccolò V." In *Storia della Biblioteca Vaticana I: Le origini della Biblioteca Vaticana tra umanesimo e rinascimento (1447–1534)*, edited by Antonio Manfredi, 383–412. Vatican City: Biblioteca Apostolica Vaticana, 2010.

Cantatore, Flavia. "Sisto IV committente di architettura a Roma tra magnificenza e conflitto." In *Congiure e conflitti. L'affermazione della signoria pontificia su Roma nel Rinascimento: politica, economia e cultura*, edited by Myriam Chiabò, Maurizio Gargano, Anna Modigliani, and Patricia Osmond, 313–26. Rome: Roma nel Rinascimento, 2014.

Cassiani, Maria Alessandra. "L'Ospedale di Santo Spirito in Sassia: cultura francescana e devozione nel ciclo pittorico della corsia sistina." In *Sisto IV: Le Arti a Roma nel Primo Rinascimento*, edited by Fabio Benzi, 167–73. Rome: Edizioni dell'Associazione Culturale Shakespeare and Company, 2000.

Ceen, Allan. "The Quartiere de' Banchi and Urban Planning in Rome in the First Half of the Cinquecento." Ph.D. diss., University of Pennsylvania, 1977.

Chaney, Edward P. de G. "Giudizi inglesi su ospedali italiani, 1545–1789." In *Timore e carità: i poveri nell'Italia moderna*, edited by Giorgio Politi, Mario Rosa, and Franco della Peruta, 77–101. Cremona: Biblioteca Statale, 1982.

Colonna, Flavia. "Distribuzione urbana e tipologie degli edifici assistenziali." In *Roma: Le trasformazioni urbane nel Quattrocento*. Vol. 2, *Funzioni urbane e tipologie edilizie*, edited by Giorgio Simoncini, 159–71. Rome: Leo S. Olschki, 2014.

Colonna, Flavia. *L'ospedale di Santo Spirito in Sassia: Lo sviluppo dell'assistenza e le trasformazioni architettonico-funzionali*. Rome: Edizioni Quasar, 2009.

Colonna, Flavia. "Paolo II Barbo e un suo possibile intervento nel quattrocentesco ospedale di S. Spirito." *Il Veltro: Rivista della civiltà italiana* 45, no. 5–6 (2001): 331–9.

Cosmacini, Giorgio. *Storia della medicina e della sanità in Italia dalla peste europea alla Guerra Mondiale, 1348–1918*. Rome and Bari: Laterza, 1987.

Cunningham, Andrew. *The Anatomical Renaissance: The Resurrection of the Anatomical Projects of the Ancients*. Aldershot, Hants.: Scolar, 1997.

De Angelis, Pietro. *L'architetto e gli affreschi di Santo Spirito in Saxia*. Rome: Nuova Tecnica Grafica, 1961.

De Angelis, Pietro. *L'Ospedale di Santo Spirito in Saxia*. 2 vols. Rome: Tipografia Dario Detti, 1962.

De' Liuzzi, Mondino. *Anatomia*. Translated by Sebastiano Manilio. [Venice, 1492.] In *Medicina medievale: Testi dell'Alto Medioevo*, edited by Luigi Firpo, 165–204. Turin: L'Unione Tipografico-Editrice Torinese, 1972.

Dei Conti, Sigismondo. *Le storie de' suoi tempi dal 1475 al 1510*. 2 vols. Rome: [Ministero di Agricoltura, Commercio e Industria]; Florence: G. Barbèra, 1883–5. https://books.google.com/books?id=R1YhHQAACAAJ. Accessed July 2, 2018.

Della Rovere, Francesco. *Tractatus de sanguine Christi*. Rome: Giovanni Filippo Lignamine, 1472.

Di Fonzo, Lorenzo. "Sisto IV. Carriera scolastica e integrazioni biografiche (1414–84)." *Miscellanea Francescana* 86, no. 2–4 (1986): 1–491.

D'Onofrio, Cesare. *Acque e fontane di Roma*. Rome: Staderini, 1977.

Bibliography

Durling, Richard J. "A Chronological Census of Renaissance Editions and Translations of Galen." *Journal of the Warburg and Courtauld Institutes* 24, no. 3–4 (1961): 230–305.

Esposito, Anna. "Assistenza e organizzazione sanitaria nell'Ospedale di Santo Spirito." *Il Veltro: Rivista della civiltà italiana* 45, no. 5–6 (September–December 2001): 201–14.

Esposito, Anna. "Gli ospedali romani tra iniziative laicali e politica pontificia (secc. XIII–XV)." In *Ospedali e città. L'Italia del Centro-Nord, XIII–XVI secolo*, edited by Allen J. Grieco and Lucia Sandri, 233–51. Florence: Casa Editrice Le Lettere, 1997.

Ettlinger, Leopold. *The Sistine Chapel before Michelangelo: Religious Imagery and Papal Primacy*. Oxford: Clarendon Press, 1965.

Fagiolo, Marcello and Maria Luisa Madonna. *Roma 1300–1875. La città degli anni santi: Atlante*. Milan: A. Mondadori, 1985.

Fortuna, Stefania. "The Latin Editions of Galen's *Opera omnia* (1490–1625) and Their Prefaces." *Early Science and Medicine* 17, no. 4 (2012): 391–412.

French, R. K. "*De iuvamentis membrorum* and the Reception of Galenic Physiological Anatomy." *Isis* 70, no. 1 (March 1979): 96–109.

Galen. *On the Natural Faculties*. Translated by Arthur John Brock. Cambridge, MA: Harvard University Press, 1963.

Galen. *On the Usefulness of the Parts of the Body*. Translation and introduction by Margaret Tallmadge May. 2 vols. Ithaca, NY: Cornell University Press, 1968.

Galenus, Claudius (Galen). *De usu partium*. Paris: Simonis Colinaei, 1528. https://hdl.handle.net/2027/uc1.31378008366729. Accessed June 1, 2018.

Gargano, Maurizio. "Ponte Sisto a Roma, nuove acquisizioni (1473–1475)." *Quaderni dell'Istituto di storia dell'architettura* 21 (1994): 29–38.

Grafton, Anthony, ed. *Rome Reborn: The Vatican Library and Renaissance Culture*. Exhibition catalog. Washington, DC: Library of Congress, 1993.

Grafton, Anthony. "The Vatican and Its Library." In *Rome Reborn: The Vatican Library and Renaissance Culture*, edited by Anthony Grafton, 3–45. Washington, DC: Library of Congress, 1993.

Grant, Edward, ed. *A Source Book in Medieval Science*. Cambridge, MA: Harvard University Press, 1974.

Guerrini, Paola. "L'epigrafia sistina come momento della 'restauratio urbis.'" In *Un pontificato ed una città: Sisto IV (1471–1484)*, edited by Massimo Miglio, Francesca Niutta, Diego Quaglioni, and Concetta Ranieri, 453–79. Vatican City: Associazione Roma nel Rinascimento, 1986.

Henderson, John. *The Renaissance Hospital: Healing the Body and Healing the Soul*. New Haven and London: Yale University Press, 2006.

Horrigan, J. Brian. "Imperial and Urban Ideology in a Renaissance Inscription." *Comitatus* 9 (1978): 73–86.

Howe, Eunice D. "A Temple Facade Reconsidered: Botticelli's *Temptation of Christ*,." In P. A. Ramsey, *Rome in the Renaissance: The City and the Myth*, 209–21. Binghamton, NY: Center for Medieval & Early Renaissance Studies, 1982.

Howe, Eunice D. "Appropriating Space: Women's Place in Confraternal Life at Santo Spirito in Sassia, Rome." In *Confraternities and the Visual Arts in Renaissance Italy: Ritual, Spectacle, Image*, edited by Barbara Wisch and Diane Cole Ahl, 235–58. Cambridge: Cambridge University Press, 2000.

Howe, Eunice D. *Art and Culture at the Sistine Court: Platina's "Life of Sixtus IV" and the Frescoes of the Hospital of Santo Spirito*. Vatican City: Biblioteca Apostolica Vaticana, 2005.

Howe, Eunice D. "L'ospedale di Santo Spirito come città ideale." *Il Veltro: Rivista della civiltà italiana* 45, no. 5–6 (2001): 341–52.

Howe, Eunice D. *The Hospital of Santo Spirito and Pope Sixtus IV*. New York: Garland, 1978.

Isidore of Seville. *The Etymologies of Isidore of Seville*. Translated by Stephen A. Barney, W. J. Lewis, J. A. Beach, and Oliver Berghoff. Cambridge and New York: Cambridge University Press, 2006.

Jackson, Donald F. "Greek Medicine in the Fifteenth Century." *Early Science and Medicine* 17, no. 4 (2012): 378–90.

Kajanto, Iiro. *Papal Epigraphy in Renaissance Rome*. Helsinki: Suomalainen Tiedeakatemia, 1982.

Karmon, David. "Restoring the Ancient Water Supply System in Renaissance Rome: The Popes, the Civic Administration, and the Acqua Vergine." *The Waters of Rome* 3 (August 2005): 1–13.

Kent, Dale. *Cosimo de' Medici and the Florentine Renaissance: The Patron's Oeuvre*. New Haven and London: Yale University Press, 2000.

Keyvanian, Carla. *Hospitals and Urbanism in Rome, 1200–1500*. Leiden and Boston: Brill, 2015.

Lee, Egmont. *Sixtus IV and Men of Letters*. Rome: Edizioni di Storia e Letteratura, 1978.

Lowic, Lawrence. "The Meaning and Significance of the Human Analogy in Francesco di Giorgio's Trattato." *Journal of the Society of Architectural Historians* 42, no. 4 (December 1983): 360–70.

Magnuson, Torgil. *Studies in Roman Quattrocento Architecture*. Stockholm: Almquist & Wiksell, 1958.

Maier, Anneliese. "Alcuni autografi di Sisto IV." In *Ausgehendes Mittelalter: Gesammelte Aufsätze zur Geistesgeschichte des. 14. Jahrhunderts*, 2 vols., 2: 135–40. Rome: Edizioni di Storia e Letteratura, 1967.

Manfredi, Antonio. "La nascita della Vaticana in età umanistica da Niccolò V a Sisto IV." In *Storia della Biblioteca Vaticana I: Le origini della Biblioteca Vaticana tra umanesimo e rinascimento (1447–1534)*, edited by Antonio Manfredi, 147–236. Vatican City: Biblioteca Apostolica Vaticana, 2010.

Manfredi, Antonio, ed. *Storia della Biblioteca Vaticana I: Le origini della Biblioteca Vaticana tra umanesimo e rinascimento (1447–1534)*. Vatican City: Biblioteca Apostolica Vaticana, 2010.

Martin, Gregory. *Roma Sancta*. Edited by George Bruner Parks. Rome: Edizioni di storia e letteratura, 1969.

Martini, Francesco di Giorgio. *Trattati di architettura ingegneria e arte militare*. Edited by Corrado Maltese. Milan: Il Polifilo, 1967.

Meyer, Starleen Kay. "The Papal Series in the Sistine Chapel: The Embodiment, Vesting and Framing of Papal Power." Ph.D. diss., University of Southern California, 1998.

Miarelli Mariani, Gaetano, Tiziana Cianfa, Riccardo dalla Negra, Paola Grifoni, Stefano Marani, and Maria Piera Sette. *Ponte Sisto (1475–1975; 1877–1977): Ricerche e proposte*. Rome: Multigrafica Editrice, 1977.

Miglio, Massimo, Francesca Niutta, Diego Quaglioni, and Concetta Ranieri, eds. *Un pontificato ed una città: Sisto IV (1471–1484)*. Vatican City: Associazione Roma nel Rinascimento, 1986.

Modigliani, Anna. "L'approvigionamento annonario e i luoghi del commercio alimentare." In *Roma: Le trasformazioni urbane nel Quattrocento*. Vol. 2, *Funzioni urbane e tipologie edilizie*, edited by Giorgio Simoncini, 29–63. Rome: Leo S. Olschki, 2014.

Moli Frigola, Montserrat. "Iakobo." In *Scrittura, biblioteche e stampa nel Quattrocento: Aspetti e problemi*, edited by C. Bianca, P. Farenga, G. Lombardi, A.G. Luciani, and M. Miglio, 183–203. Vatican City: Scuola Vaticana di Paleografia, Diplomatica e Archivistica, 1980.

Müntz, Eugène. *Les Arts à la cour des papes pendant le XVe et le XVIe siècle. Troisième partie: Sixte IV–Léon X*. Paris: E. Thorin, 1882.

Müntz, Eugène and Paul Fabre. *La Bibliothèque du Vatican au XVe siècle d'après des documents inédits*. Paris: Ernest Thorin, 1887.

Nicholas of Cusa. *The Catholic Concordance*. Translated by Paul E. Sigmund. Cambridge and New York: Cambridge University Press, 1995.

Nussbaum, Martha Craven. *Aristotle's* De Motu Animalium: *Text with Translation, Commentary and Interpretive Essays*. Princeton: Princeton University Press, 1978.

Pacifici, Vincenzo. *Un carme biografico di Sisto IV del 1477*. Tivoli: Società Tibertina di Storia e Arte, [1923]. https://hdl.handle.net/2027/njp.32101073446377. Accessed May 30, 2018.

Paravicini-Bagliani, Agostino. *The Pope's Body*. Translated by David S. Peterson. Chicago and London: University of Chicago Press, 2000.

Pastor, Ludwig. *The History of the Popes from the Close of the Middle Ages*. Vol. 4. St. Louis, MO: B. Herder, 1923.

Pellecchia, Linda. "The Contested City: Urban Form in Early Sixteenth-Century Rome." In *Cambridge Companion to Raphael*, edited by Marcia Hall, 59–94. Cambridge: Cambridge University Press, 2005.

Pepper, Simon. "Body, Diagram, and Geometry in the Renaissance Fortress." In *Body and Building: Essays on the Changing Relation of Body and Architecture*, edited by George Dodds and Robert Tavernor, 115–25. Cambridge, MA and London: MIT Press, 2002.

Pesenti, Tiziana. "The *Libri Galieni* in Italian Universities in the Fourteenth Century." *Italia medioevale e umanistica* 42 (2001): 119–47.

Piacentini, Paola Scarcia. "Ricerche sugli antichi inventari della Biblioteca Vaticana: I codici di lavoro di Sisto IV." In *Un pontificato ed una città: Sisto IV (1471–1484)*, edited by Massimo Miglio, Francesca Niutta, Diego Quaglioni, and Concetta Ranieri, 115–78. Vatican City: Associazione Roma nel Rinascimento, 1986.

Pinto, John. *The Trevi Fountain*. New Haven and London: Yale University Press, 1986.

Pollali, Angeliki. "Human Analogy in *Trattati I*: The *Ragione* of Modern Architecture." In *Reconstructing Francesco di Giorgio Architect*, edited by Berthold Hub and Angeliki Pollali, 59–84. Frankfurt am Main: Peter Lang, 2011.

Presciutti, Diana Bullen. "Dead Infants, Cruel Mothers, and Heroic Popes: The Visual Rhetoric of Foundling Care at the Hospital of Santo Spirito, Rome." *Renaissance Quarterly* 64, no. 3 (2011): 752–99.

Bibliography

Ramsey, P. A. *Rome in the Renaissance: The City and the Myth*. Binghamton, NY: Center for Medieval & Early Renaissance Studies, 1982.

Scaccia Scarafoni, Camillo. "L'antico statuto dei 'Magistri Stratarum' e altri documenti relativi a quella magistratura." *Archivio della Società Romana di Storia Patria* 50 (1927): 239–308. https://hdl.handle.net/2027/uc1.31175029518324. Accessed May 15, 2018.

Schraven, Minou. "Founding Rome Anew: Pope Sixtus IV and the Foundation of Ponte Sisto, 1473." In *Foundation, Dedication and Consecration in Early Modern Europe*, edited by Minou Schraven and Maarten Delbeke, 129–50. Leiden: Brill, 2012.

Sennett, Richard. *Flesh and Stone: The Body and the City in Western Civilization*. New York and London: W. W. Norton, 1994.

Simoncini, Giorgio. *Roma: Le trasformazioni urbane nel Quattrocento*. Vol. 1, *Topografia e urbanistica da Bonifacio IX ad Alessandro VI*. Rome: Leo S. Olschki, 2014.

Simoncini, Giorgio, ed. *Roma: Le trasformazioni urbane nel Quattrocento*. Vol. 2, *Funzioni urbane e tipologie edilizie*. Rome: Leo S. Olschki, 2014.

Siraisi, Nancy G. "Life Sciences and Medicine in the Renaissance World." In *Rome Reborn: The Vatican Library and Renaissance Culture*, edited by Anthony Grafton, 169–97. Washington, DC: Library of Congress, 1993.

Siraisi, Nancy G. *Medieval & Early Renaissance Medicine: An Introduction to Knowledge and Practice*. Chicago and London: University of Chicago, 1990.

Spezzaferro, Luigi. "Ponte Sisto." In *Via Giulia: una utopia urbanistica del '500*, edited by Luigi Salerno, Luigi Spezzaferro, and Manfredo Tafuri, 521–6. Rome: A. Staderini, 1975.

Tomei, Piero. "Le strade di Roma e l'opera di Sisto IV." *L'Urbe* 2 (1937): 12–20.

Toscano, Gennaro. "La miniatura 'all'antica' tra Roma e Napoli all'epoca di Sisto IV." In *Sisto IV: Le Arti a Roma nel Primo Rinascimento*, edited by Fabio Benzi, 249–87. Rome: Edizioni dell'Associazione Culturale Shakespeare and Company, 2000.

Verdi, Orietta. "Da ufficiali capitolini a commissari apostolici: I maestri delle strade e delle edifici di Roma tra XIII e XVI secoli." In *Il Campidoglio e Sisto V*, edited by Luigi Spezzaferro and Maria Elisa Tittoni, 54–63. Rome: Edizioni Carte Segrete, 1991.

Watanabe, Morimichi. *The Political Ideas of Nicholas of Cusa with Special Reference to his De concordantia catholica*. Geneva: Librairie Droz, 1963.

Weiss, Roberto. *The Medals of Pope Sixtus IV (1471–1484)*. Rome: Edizioni di Storia e Letteratura, 1961.

Westfall, Carroll William. *In this Most Perfect Paradise: Alberti, Nicholas V, and the Invention of Conscious Urban Planning in Rome, 1447–55*. University Park, PA: Pennsylvania State University Press, 1974.

Chapter 8. Spaces of Healing in the Early Modern Portuguese Empire: Changing Public Health and Hospital Buildings on Mozambique Island

Abreu, Laurinda. *Pina Manique. Um reformador no Portugal das Luzes*. Lisbon: Gradiva, 2013.

Abreu, Laurinda. "Training Health Professionals at the Hospital de Todos os Santos (Lisbon) 1500–1800." In *Hospital Life: Theory and Practice from the Medieval to the Modern*, edited by Laurinda Abreu and Sally Sheard, 119–37. Bern: Peter Lang, 2013.

Adams, Annmarie. *Medicine by Design: The Architect and the Modern Hospital, 1893–1943*. Minneapolis: University of Minnesota Press, 2008.

Andrade, Banha de. "Fundação do Hospital Militar de S. João de Deus, em Moçambique." *Stvdia* 1 (1958): 77–89.

Andrade, Banha de. "O hospital de Moçambique durante a administração dos Almoxarifes." *Portugal em África* 13, no. 78 (1956): 357–70.

Andrade, Banha de. "O Hospital de Moçambique durante a administração dos religiosos de S. João de Deus." *Portugal em África* 13, no. 77 (1956): 261–89.

Andrade, Banha de. "Os Hospitaleiros de S. João de Deus na Índia." *Portugal em África* 14, no. 80 (1957): 107–19.

Arnold, Dana. *The Spaces of the Hospital: Spatiality and Urban Change in London 1680–1820*. New York: Routledge, 2013.

Arnold, David. "Introduction. Tropical Medicine before Manson." In *Warm Climates and Western Medicine: The Emergence of Tropical Medicine, 1500–1900*, edited by David Arnold, 1–19. Amsterdam and Atlanta: Rodopi, 1996.

Bibliography

Arnold, David. *Science, Technology and Medicine in Colonial India*. Cambridge: Cambridge University Press, 2004.

Arnold, David. "The Place of 'the tropics' in Western since 1750." *Tropical Medicine and International Health* 2, no. 4 (1997): 303-13.

Arquivo Português Oriental 5, no. 2 (1865).

Arrizabalaga, Jon. "Medical Theory and Surgical Practice: Coping with the French Disease in Early Renaissance Portugal and Spain." In *Hospital Life: Theory and Practice from the Medieval to the Modern*, edited by Laurinda Abreu and Sally Sheard, 93-117. Bern: Peter Lang, 2013.

Arrizabalaga, Jon, John Henderson, and Roger French. *The Great Pox: The French Disease in Renaissance Europe*. New Haven and London: Yale University Press, 1997.

Axelson, Eric. *Portuguese in South-East Africa 1600-1700*. Johannesburg: Witwatersrand University Press, 1969.

Baldasso, Renzo. "Function and Epidemiology in Filarete's Ospedale Maggiore." In *Medieval Hospital and Medical Practice*, edited by Barbara S. Bowers, 107-22. Aldershot: Ashgate, 2007.

Bastos, Cristiana. "Hospitais e sociedade colonial. Esplendor, ruína, memória e mudança em Goa." *Ler História* 58 (2010): 61-80.

Bastos, Cristiana. "Together and Apart: Catholic Hospitals in Plural Goa." In *Hospitals in Iran and India, 1500-1950*, edited by Fabrizio Speziale, 133-57. Leiden: Brill, 2012.

Borges, Augusto Moutinho. *Reais Hospitais Militares em Portugal (1640-1834)*. Coimbra: Imprensa da Universidade de Coimbra, 2009.

Botelho, Sebastião Xavier. *Memória estatística sobre os domínios portugueses na África Oriental*. Lisbon: Tipografia José Baptista Morando, 1835.

Boxer, C. R. "Moçambique Island and the 'carreira da Índia.'" *Stvdia* 8 (1961): 95-132.

Capela, José. *O tráfico de escravos nos portos de Moçambique, 1733-1904*. Porto: Afrontamento, 2002.

Chakrabarti, Pratik. "'Neither of meate nor drink, but what the Doctor alloweth': Medicine amidst War and Commerce in Eighteenth-Century Madras." *Bulletin of the History of Medicine* 80, no. 1 (2006): 1-38.

Cheminade, Christian. "Architecture and Medicine in the Late 18th Century: Ventilation in Hospitals, from the Encyclopédie to the Debate on the Hôtel-Dieu in Paris." *Recherches sur Diderot et sur l'Encyclopédie* 14 (1993): 85-109.

Correia, Gaspar. *Lendas da Índia*. Coimbra: Imprensa da Universidade de Coimbra, 1921.

Estes, J. Worth. "Food as Medicine." In *The Cambridge World History of Food*, edited by Kenneth F. Kiple and Kriemhild Conèe Ornelas, vol. 2, 1534-53. Cambridge: University of Cambridge Press, 2000.

Dias, Pedro. "Algumas Misericórdias no Estado da Índia. Apontamentos para a História da Construção dos seus Edifícios." In *A Misericórdia de Vila Real e as Misericórdias no Mundo de Expressão Portuguesa*, edited by Natália Marinho Ferreira-Alves, 555-62. Porto: CEPESE, 2011.

Flandrin, Jean-Louis and Massimo Montanari, eds. *Histoire de l'Alimentation*. Paris: Fayard, 1996.

Fonseca, Pedro Quirino da. "Algumas Descobertas de Interesse Histórico-arqueológico na Ilha de Moçambique." *Monumenta* 8 (1972): 55-71.

Fonseca, Pedro Quirino da. "Breves Notas Sobre a Evolução da Habitação e Construção em Moçambique." *Monumenta* 4 (1968): 45-48.

Foucault, Michel. *The Birth of the Clinic*. London: Routledge, 2003.

Foucault, Michel. "The Politics of Health in the Eighteenth Century." In Michel Foucault, *Power/Knowledge*, edited by Colin Gordon, 166-82. New York: Pantheon Books, 1980.

Garlake, Peter S. *The Early Islamic Architecture of the East African Coast*. London: Oxford University Press, 1966.

Gracias, Fátima da Silva. *Health and Hygiene in Colonial Goa, 1510-1961*. New Delhi: Concept Publishing, 1994.

Harrison, Mark. *Climates and Constitutions: Health, Race, Environment and British Imperialism in India, 1600-1850*. New Delhi: Oxford University Press, 1999.

Henderson, John. *The Renaissance Hospital: Healing the Body and Healing the Soul*. New Haven: Yale University Press, 2006.

Henderson, John, Peregrine Horden, and Alessandro Pastore, eds. *The Impact of Hospitals, 300-2000*. Oxford: Peter Lang, 2007.

Herédia, Manuel Godinho de. *O lyvro de plantaforma das fortalezas da India*. Lisbon: Ministério da Defesa, 1999.

Ilha de Moçambique. Relatório—Report 1982-85. Maputo: Secretaria de Estado da Cultura—Moçambique & Arkitektskolen i Aarhus—Danmark, n.d.

Bibliography

Jordanova, Ludmilla. "Earth Science and Environmental Medicine: The Synthesis of the Late Enlightenment." In *Images of the Earth: Essay in the History of the Environmental Sciences*, edited by Ludmilla Jordanova and Roy Porter, 119–46. Chalfont St. Giles: British Society for the History of Science, 1979.

Kessel, Anthony. *Air, the Environment and Public Health*. Cambridge: Cambridge University Press, 2010.

Kisacky, Jeanne. *Rise of the Modern Hospital. An Architectural History of Health and Healing, 1870–1940*. Pittsburgh: University of Pittsburgh Press, 2017.

Lemos, Maximiano de. *História da Medicina em Portugal*. Lisbon: Dom Quixote & Ordem dos Médicos, 1991.

Lindemann, Mary. *Medicine and Society in Early Modern Europe*. Cambridge: Cambridge University Press, 2010.

Lobato, Alexandre. "Ilha de Moçambique: Notícia Histórica." *Arquivo* 4 (1988): 79–83.

Lobato, Alexandre. *Ilha de Moçambique. Panorama Histórico*. Lisbon: AGU, 1967.

Matos, Artur Teodoro de. "A Glimpse of the Hospitallers of Diu in the late 18th Century." In *Goa and Portugal: History and Development*, edited by Charles J. Borges, Oscar Guilherme Pereira, and Hannes Stubbe, 231–7. New Delhi: Concept Publishing, 2000.

Meier, Prita. *Swahili Port Cities: The Architecture of Elsewhere*. Bloomington, IN: Indiana University Press, 2016.

Newitt, Malyn. *A History of Mozambique*. London: Hurst & Company, 1995.

Newitt, Malyn. "Mozambique Island: The Rise and Decline of a Colonial Port City." In *Portuguese Colonial Cities in the Early Modern World*, edited by Liam Matthew Brockey, 105–27. Aldershot: Ashgate, 2008.

Pacheco, António Fernando. "De Todos-Os-Santos a São José: Textos e Contextos do 'esprital grande de Lixboa'." MA diss., New University of Lisbon, 2008.

Pataca, Ermelinda. "Entre a engenharia militar e a arquitetura médica: representações de Alexandre Rodrigues Ferreira sobre a cidade de Belém no final do século XVIII." *História, Ciências, Saúde. Manguinhos* 25, no. 1 (2018): 89–113.

Pearson, Michael N. *Port Cities and Intruders: The Swahili Coast, India, and Portugal in the Early Modern Era*. Baltimore: Johns Hopkins University Press, 1998.

Pereira, Paulo, ed. *O Hospital Real de Todos os Santos: 500 Anos. Catálogo*. Lisbon: Câmara Municipal de Lisboa, 1993.

Petersen, Andrew. *Dictionary of Islamic Architecture*. London and New York: Routledge, 2002.

Pinho, Joana Maria Balsa Carvalho de. "As Casas da Misericórdia: confrarias da Misericórdia e a arquitectura quinhentista portuguesa." Ph.D. diss., University of Lisbon, 2012.

Porter, Roy. "The Eighteenth Century." In *The Western Medical Tradition: 800 BC–1800 AD*, edited by Laurence I. Conrad, Michael Neve, Viviane Nutton, Roy Porter, and Andrew Wear, 371–475. Cambridge: Cambridge University Press, 1995.

Prior, James. *Voyage along the Eastern Coast of Africa, to Mosambique, Johanna and Quilloa; St. Helena; to Rio de Janeiro, Bahia, and Pernambuco in Brazil in the Nysus Frigate*. London: Printed for Sir Richard Phillips and Co., 1819.

Ramos, Luís A. de Oliveira. "Do Hospital Real de Todos os Santos. A história hospitalar portuguesa." *Revista da Faculdade de Letras* 10 (1993): 333–50.

Rego, A. da Silva, ed. *Documentação para a história do padroado português do Oriente. India*. Lisbon: AGU, 1953.

Richardson, Harriet, ed. *English Hospitals, 1660–1948: A Survey of Their Architecture and Design*. Swindon: Royal Commission on the Historical Monuments of England, 1998.

Risse, Guenter B. *Mending Bodies, Saving Souls. A History of Hospitals*. New York: Oxford University Press, 1999.

Rodrigues, Eugénia. "As Misericórdias de Moçambique e a administração local, c. 1606–1763." In *O reino, as ilhas e o mar oceano. Estudos em homenagem a Artur Teodoro de Matos*, edited by Avelino de Freitas de Menezes and João Paulo Oliveira e Costa, vol. 2, 709–29. Lisbon: CHAM, 2007.

Rodrigues, Eugénia. "Crossing the Indian Ocean: African Slaves and Medical Knowledge in Goa." In *Learning from Empire: Medicine, Knowledge and Transfers under Portuguese Rule*, edited by Poonam Bala, 74–96. Newcastle upon Tyne: Cambridge Scholars Publishers, 2018.

Rodrigues, Eugénia. "Eating and Drinking at the Royal Hospital of Mozambique Island: Medicine and Diet Change Between the End of the 18th and the Early 19th Century." *Afriques. Débats, méthodes et terrains d'histoire* 5 (2014). http://afriques.revues.org/1553. Accessed January 30, 2015.

Rodrigues, Eugénia. "Moçambique e o Índico: a circulação de saberes e práticas de cura." *Métis: História & Cultura* 19 (2011): 15–42.

Rodrigues, Eugénia. *Portugueses e Africanos nos Rios de Sena. Os Prazos da Coroa em Moçambique nos Séculos XVII e XVIII*. Lisbon: Imprensa Nacional-Casa da Moeda, 2013.

Rodrigues, Eugénia, and Miguel Brito. "Colonização e polícia médica em Moçambique no final do período moderno." In *Saber Tropical em Moçambique. História, Memória e Ciência*, edited by Ana Cristina Roque and Eugénia Rodrigues. Lisbon: IICT (CDRom edition), 2013.

Rodrigues, Lisbeth de Oliveira. "Os hospitais portugueses no Renascimento (1480–1580): o caso de Nossa Senhora do Pópulo das Caldas da Rainha." Ph.D. diss., University of Minho, 2013.

Rosen, George. *From Medical Police to Social Medicine: Essays on the History of Health Care*. New York: Science History Publications, 1974.

Sá, Isabel dos Guimarães. *Quando o rico se faz pobre: Misericórdias, caridade e poder no império português 1500–1800*. Lisbon: CNCDP, 1997.

Salt, Henry. *A Voyage to Abyssinia, and Travels Into the Interior of that Country, Executed Under the Orders of the British Government, in the Years 1809 and 1810*. Philadelphia: M. Carey; Boston: Wells & Lilly, 1816.

Santos, João dos. *Etiópia Oriental e Vária História de Cousas Notáveis do Oriente*. Lisbon: CNPCDP, 1999.

Sheriff, Abdul, and Javed Jafferji. *Zanzibar Stone Town: An Architectural Exploration*. Zanzibar: Gallery, 1998.

Silva, André Costa Aciole da. "'Queremos e mandamos ... que o dito hospital ... cure os enfermos ...': poder e medicina no hospital de Nossa Senhora do Pópulo (séc. XVI–XVII)." Ph.D. diss., Federal University of Goiás, 2015.

Sousa, Germano de. *História da Medicina Portuguesa durante a Expansão*. Lisbon: Temas e Debates, 2013.

Steyn, Gerald. "The Lamu House—An East African Architectural Enigma." *South African Journal of Art History* 17 (2003): 157–80.

Stevenson, Christine. *Medicine and Magnificence: British Hospital and Asylum Architecture, 1660–1815*. New Haven: Yale University Press, 2000.

Wald, Erica. *Vice in the Barracks: Medicine, the Military and the Making of Colonial India, 1780–1868*. Basingstoke: Palgrave Macmillan, 2014.

Chapter 9. From Exigency to Civic Pride: The Development of Early Australian Hospitals

"Adelaide—Hospitals." In *The Manning Index of South Australian History*, State Library of South Australia. http://www.slsa.sa.gov.au/manning/adelaide/hospital/hospital.htm. Accessed August 20, 2018.

Bigge, John Thomas. *Report on State of the Colony of New South Wales*. London, 1822.

Bolton, G. C. and Prue Joske. *History of the Royal Perth Hospital*. Nedlands, WA: University of Western Australia Press, 1982.

Caring for Convicts and the Community: A History of the Parramatta Hospital. Westmead, NSW: Cumberland Area Health Service, 1988.

Considine and Griffiths Architects. *Royal Perth Hospital Precinct Conservation Plan*. Cottesloe, WA: Considine and Griffiths, September 1995.

Cummins, C. J. "The Colonial Medical Service: I. The General Hospital, Sydney 1788–1848." *Modern Medicine of Australia* (January 7, 1974): 11–24.

Cummins, C. J. *A History of Medical Administration in New South Wales 1788–1973*. Sydney: Health Commission of New South Wales, 1979.

Goad, Philip and Julie Willis, eds. *The Encyclopedia of Australian Architecture*. Melbourne: Cambridge University Press, 2012.

Herman, Morton. *The Early Australian Architects and Their Work*. Sydney: Angus & Robertson, 1954.

Historical Records of Australia. Sydney: Library Committee of the Commonwealth Parliament, 1914.

Kerr, James Semple. *Design for Convicts: An Account of Design for Convict Establishments in the Australian Colonies during the Transportation Era*. Sydney: Library of Australian History, 1984.

King, Stuart and Julie Willis. "The Australian Colonies." In *Architecture and Urbanism in the British Empire*, edited by G. A. Bremner, 318–55. Oxford: Oxford University Press, 2016.

"Laying the Foundation." *Port Phillip Gazette and Settler's Journal*, March 21, 1846.

Linn, Rob. *Frail Flesh & Blood: The Health of South Australian since Earliest Times*. Woodville, SA: The Queen Elizabeth Hospital Research Foundation, 1993.

Memmott, Paul. *Gunyah, Goondie & Wurley: The Aboriginal Architecture of Australia*. St Lucia, Qld: University of Queensland Press, 2007.

Morison, Margaret Pitt. "Settlement and Development: The Historical Context." In *Western Towns and Buildings*, edited by Margaret Pitt Morison and John White, 1–9. Nedlands, WA: University of Western Australia Press, 1979.

Bibliography

Phillip, Arthur. *The Voyage of Governor Phillip to Botany Bay.* Sydney: Angus and Robertson, 1970.
Rimmer, W. G. *Portrait of a Hospital: The Royal Hobart.* Hobart: Royal Hobart Hospital, 1981.
Thompson, John D. and Grace Goldin. *The Hospital: A Social and Architectural History.* New Haven and London: Yale University Press, 1975.
Tibbits, George and Angela Roenfeldt. *Port Phillip Colonial.* Clifton Hill, Vic.: Port Phillip Colonial, 1989.
Tyrer, John H. *History of the Brisbane Hospital and its Affiliates.* Brisbane: Boolarong Publication, 1993.
Watson, J. Frederick. *The History of the Sydney Hospital from 1811 to 1911.* Sydney: Government Printer, 1911.
Webb, Carolyn. "Stone the Crows: Image of a Cocky Found in 13th Century Manuscript." *The Age,* June 25, 2018. https://www.theage.com.au/national/victoria/stone-the-crows-image-of-a-cocky-found-in-13thc-manuscript-20180625-p4znnt.html. Accessed February 1, 2019.

III. Typologies: Places of Health in History

Chapter 10. House of Misericórdia: Healthcare and Welfare Architecture in Sixteenth-Century Portugal.

Afonso, José Ferrão. *A Igreja Velha da Misericórdia de Barcelos e cinco Igrejas de Misericórdias de Entre-Douro e Minho: Arquitectura e paisagem urbana (c. 1534–1635).* Barcelos: Santa Casa da Misericórdia de Barcelos, 2012.
Afonso, José Ferrão. "Regressando a Alberti. As igrejas das Misericórdias de Entre Douro e Minho, de Vila do Conde a Penafiel: arquitectura e paisagem urbana." In II Jornadas de Estudos sobre as Misericórdias *As Misericórdias quinhentistas,* 123–51. Penafiel: Câmara Municipal de Penafiel, 2009.
Beirante, Maria Ângela. *Confrarias Medievais Portuguesas.* Lisbon: s.n., 1990.
Chorão, Maria José. *Os forais de D. Manuel: 1496–1520.* Lisbon: ANTT, 1990.
Cidade, Hernani. *A literatura portuguesa e a expansão ultramarina: as ideias, os sentimentos, as formas de arte (séculos XV e XVI).* Lisbon: Agência Geral das Colónias, 1943.
Coelho, Maria Helena da Cruz. "As confrarias medievais portuguesas: espaços de solidariedade na vida e na morte." In *Cofradías, gremios, solidariedades en la Europa medieval.* Estella, Pamplona: Governo de Navarra, 1992.
Correia, Fernando Silva. *Origens e formação das Misericórdias Portuguesas.* Lisbon: Livros Horizonte, 1999.
D. Manuel e a sua época: actas. Guimarães: Câmara Municipal de Guimarães, 2004.
Dias, João José Alves. *Ordenações manuelinas, 500 anos depois: os dois primeiros sistemas (1512–1519).* Lisbon: BNP, 2012.
Ferrão, José Eduardo Mendes. *A aventura das plantas e os Descobrimentos Portugueses.* Lisbon: Instituto de Investigação Científica e Tropical, Comissão Nacional para a Comemoração dos Descobrimentos Portugueses, 1999.
Ferreira-Alves, Natália (ed.). *A Misericórdia de Vila Real e as Misericórdias do mundo de expressão portuguesa.* Porto: CEPESE, 2011.
Fortuna, A. Matos. *Misericórdia de Palmela: vida e factos.* Lisbon: Edição da Santa Casa da Misericórdia de Palmela, 1990.
Gonçalves, António Nogueira. *Inventário artístico de Portugal: distrito de Aveiro, zona sul.* Lisbon: Academia Nacional de Belas Artes, 1959.
Gouveia, António Camões. "Portugal e a Europa: a sociedade e as relações diplomáticas de Tordesilhas aos Pirenéus." *Revista ICALP* 15 (1989): 89–95.
Gschwende, Annemarie Jordan and K. J. P. Lowe eds., *The Global City: On the Streets of Renaissance Lisbon.* London: Paul Holberton, 2015.
Hooykaas, Reijer. *O humanismo e os descobrimentos: na ciência e nas letras portuguesas do século XVI.* Lisbon: Gradiva, 1983
Leitão, Henrique. *Os Descobrimentos portugueses e a ciência europeia.* Lisbon: Alêtheia, 2009 [English version: *The Portuguese Discoveries and the Science in Europe*].
Leitão, Henrique (ed.). *360º Ciência descoberta.* Lisboa: Fundação Calouste Gulbenkian, Universidade de Lisboa, Museu de Marinha, 2013.
Martínez, Pedro Soares. *História diplomática de Portugal.* Coimbra: Almedina, 2010.
Moreira, Rafael. "As Misericórdias: um património artístico da humanidade." In *500 Anos das Misericórdias Portuguesas: solidariedade de geração em geração,* 135–64. Lisbon: Comissão para as Comemorações dos 500 anos das Misericórdia, 2000.

No tempo das Feitorias: a arte portuguesa na Época dos Descobrimentos. 2 vols. Lisbon: Museu Nacional de Arte Antiga, 1992.
Noé, Paula. "As igrejas de Misericórdia do distrito de Coimbra: ensaio de classificação tipológica." *Monumentos* 25 (September 2006): 198–207.
Noé, Paula. "O Inventário do Património Arquitectónico das Misericórdias: ensaio tipológico: as Igrejas da Misericórdia do Distrito de Viana do Castelo." In Jornadas de Estudo, *As Misericórdias como Fontes Culturais e de Informação*. Penafiel: Câmara Municipal de Penafiel, Arquivo Municipal de Penafiel, 2001.
Noé, Paula. *Património Arquitectónico: Igrejas de Misericórdia (version 1.0)*. Lisbon: Instituto de Reabilitação Urbana, Instituto de Gestão do Património Arquitectónico e Arqueológico, 2010. http://www.monumentos.gov.pt.
Os descobrimentos portugueses e a Europa do Renascimento: XVII Exposição europeia de arte, ciência e cultura. 6 vols. Lisbon: Presidência do Conselho de Ministros, 1983.
Paiva, José Pedro (coord.). *Portugaliae Monumenta Misericordiarum*. Lisbon: Centro de Estudos de História Religiosa da Universidade Católica Portuguesa, União das Misericórdias Portuguesas, 2002–4.
Paiva, José Pedro and Giuseppe Marcocci. *História Geral da Inquisição Portuguesa (1536–1821)*. Lisbon: Esfera dos Livros, 2013.
Pinho, Joana Balsa de. "A Casa da Misericórdia: as confrarias da Misericórdia e a arquitectura portuguesa quinhentista." Ph.D. diss., University of Lisbon, 2012.
Sá, Isabel dos Guimarães. *As Misericórdias portuguesas de D. Manuel I a Pombal*. Lisbon: Livros Horizonte, 2001.
Sá, Isabel Guimarães. *Quando o rico se faz pobre: Misericórdias, caridade e pobreza no império português 1500–1800*. Lisbon: Comissão Nacional para a Comemoração dos Descobrimentos Portugueses, 1997.
Saraiva, António José e Óscar Lopes, *História da literatura portuguesa*. 17th edn. Porto: Porto Editora, 2017.
Sousa, Ivo Carneiro. *A Rainha D. Leonor (1458–1525): Poder, Misericórdia, Religiosidade e Espiritualidade no Portugal do Renascimento*. Lisbon: Fundação Calouste Gulbenkian, Fundação para a Ciência e Tecnologia, 2002.
Sousa, Ivo Carneiro. *V Centenário das Misericórdias Portuguesas*. Lisbon: CTT—Correios de Portugal, 1998.
Sphera Mundi: arte e cultura no tempo dos descobrimentos. Lisbon: Caleidoscópio, 2015.
Soyer, François. *A Perseguição aos Judeus e Muçulmanos de Portugal—D. Manuel I e o Fim da Tolerância Religiosa (1496–1497)*. Lisbon: Edições 70, 2013.

Chapter 11. Making the Home a Healing Space: Self-Cultivating Practices in Late Imperial China

Anonymous. *Jiye liangfang* (A Collection of Good Recipes). Late Qing manuscript held at the Berlin State Library. Staatsbibliothek Berlin. Unschuld 8210.
He Bian, *Know Your Remedies: Pharmacy and Culture in Early Modern China*, Princeton: Princeton University Press, 2020.
Bray, Francesca. *Technology and Gender: Fabrics of Power in Late Imperial China*. Berkeley: University of California Press, 1997.
Bray, Francesca. *Technology, Gender and History in Imperial China: Great Transformation Reconsidered*. New York: Routledge, 2013.
Brokaw, Cynthia J. *Commerce in Culture: The Sibao Book Trade in the Qing and Republican Periods*. Cambridge, MA: Harvard University Press, 2007.
Chen Hsiu-fen. *Yangsheng yu xiushen: Wan Ming wenren de shenti shuxie yu shesheng jishu* (Nourishing Life and Cultivation: Writing the Literati's Body and Techniques for Preserving Health in the Late Ming). Taipei: Daoxiang chubanshe, 2009.
Clunas, Craig. *Superfluous Things: Material Culture and Social Status in Early Modern China*. Honolulu: University of Hawaii Press, 2004.
Cullen, Christopher. "Patients and Healers in Late Imperial China: Evidence from the *Jinpingmei*." *History of Science* 31 (1993): 99–150.
Furth, Charlotte. *A Flourishing Yin: Gender in China's Medical History: 960–1665*. Berkeley: University of California Press, 1999.
Gaoyangshi. *Yifang bianlan* (A Convenient Survey of Medical Recipes). Nineteenth-century manuscript held at the Berlin State Library. Staatsbibliothek Berlin. Unschuld 8453.

Bibliography

Gao Lian. *Zunsheng bajian* (Eight Essays on Cultivating Life). Yashang zhai, 1591.
Hanson, Marta. "Merchants of Medicine: Huizhou Mercantile Consciousness, Morality, and Medical Patronage in Seventeenth-Century China." In *East Asian Science: Tradition and Beyond*, edited by K. Hashimoto et al., 207–14. Osaka: Kansai University Press, 1995.
Hanson, Marta and Gianna Pomata. "Medicinal Formulas and Experiential Knowledge in the Seventeenth-Century Epistemic Exchange between China and Europe." *ISIS* 108, no. 1 (2017): 1–25.
Kleinman, Arthur. *Patients and Healers in the Context of Culture: An Exploration of the Borderland between Anthropology, Medicine and Psychiatry*. Berkeley: University of California Press, 1980.
Leong, Elaine. "Collecting Knowledge for the Family: Recipes, Gender and Practical Knowledge in the Early Modern English Household." *Centaurus* 55, no. 2 (2013): 81–103.
Leong, Elaine. "Making Medicines in the Early Modern Household." *Bulletin of the History of Medicine* 82 (2008): 145–68.
Leung, Angela. *Shishan yu jiaohua: Ming Qing de cishan zuzhi* (Philanthropy and Moral Transformation: Ming-Qing Philanthropic Organizations). Taipei: Lianjing chuban shiye gongsi, 1997.
Mann, Susan. *The Talented Women of the Zhang Family*. Berkeley: University of California Press, 2007.
Mao Xiang. *Chaomin shiwenji* (Collection of Poems and Essays by Chaomin). Printed 1661–1722. Zhongguo jiben guji ku, Beijing ai ru sheng shuzihua jishu yanjiu zhongxin, 2009. http://dh.ersjk.com. Accessed January 5, 2020.
Meyer-Fong, Tobie. *What Remains: Coming to Terms with Civil War in 19th Century China*. Stanford: Stanford University Press, 2013.
Pu Songling. *Yaosui shu* (Book of Drugs and Demons). Prefaced 1706, transcribed 1937. Manuscript held at Keio University.
Rowe, William T. *China's Last Empire: The Great Qing*. Cambridge, MA: The Belknap Press of Harvard University Press, 2009.
Rowe, William T. *Hankow: Conflict and Community in a Chinese City, 1796–1895*. Stanford: Stanford University Press, 1992.
Schonebaum, Andrew. *Novel Medicine: Healing, Literature and Popular Knowledge in Early Modern China*. Seattle: University of Washington Press, 2016.
Shi Chengjin. *Chuanjia bao* (Family Treasures Handed Down). First printed 1739. Repr. edited by Jin Qinghui and Yan Mingxun. Tianjin: Tianjin shehui kexueyuan chubanshe, 1992.
Unschuld, Paul and Zheng Jinsheng, eds. *Chinese Traditional Healing: The Berlin Collections of Manuscript Volumes from the 16th through the Early 20th Century*. Leiden: Brill, 2012.
Wu, Yi-Li. *Reproducing Women: Metaphor, Medicine, and Childbirth in Late Imperial China*. Berkeley: University of California Press, 2010.
Wu, Yi-Li. "The Bamboo Grove Monastery and Popular Gynecology in Qing China." *Late Imperial China* 21, no. 1 (2000): 41–76.
You Zi'an. *Shan yu ren tong: Ming Qing yilai de cishan yu jiaohua* (In Company with Goodness: Charity and Morality in China). Beijing: Zhonghua shuju, 2005.
Zhang, Ying. "Household Healing: Rituals, Recipes, and Virtues in Late Imperial China." Ph.D. diss., Johns Hopkins University, 2017.
Zhu Xi. *Xiaoxue jicheng* (A Collection of Elementary Learning). Edited by He Shixin. Kyoto: Fogetsu Shozaemon, 1658.

Chapter 12. For Care and Salvation: Leprosy Hostels in Pre-Modern Japan, c. 1200–1800

Buraku Mondai Kenkyūjo, eds. *Buraku no rekishi: Kinki hen*. Kyoto: Buraku Mondai Kenkyūjo Shuppanbu, 1982.
Buraku Mondai Kenkyūjo, eds. *Burakushi shiryō senshū*, Vol. 1: *Kodai chūsei hen*. Kyoto: Buraku Mondai Kenkyūjo Shuppanbu, 1988.
Fujino, Yutaka, ed. *Kanagawa no burakushi*. Tokyo: Fuji Shuppan, 2007.
Fujiwara, Yoshiaki. "Chūsei zenki no byōsha to kyūsai: Hinin ni kansuru isshiki ron." In *Rettō no bunkashi*, edited by Amino Yoshihiko et al., 79–114. Tokyo: Nihon Editāsukūru Shuppanbu, 1986.
Goble, Andrew Edmund. *Confluences of Medicine in Medieval Japan: Buddhist Healing, Chinese Knowledge, Islamic Formulas, and Wounds of War*. Honolulu: University of Hawaii Press, 2011.

Goodwin, Janet R. *Alms and Vagabonds: Buddhist Temples and Popular Patronage in Medieval Japan*. Honolulu: University of Hawaii Press, 1994.

Goodwin, Janet R. "Outcasts and Marginals in Medieval Japan." In *The Routledge Handbook of Premodern Japanese History*, edited by Karl F. Friday, 296–309. London and New York: Routledge, 2017.

Katsuyuki, Kōno. *Shōgaisha no chūsei*. Kyoto: Bunrikaku, 1987.

Kawata, Nobuo. "Jōdoji Jōdodō oyobi Kitayama Jūhachikenko kenchiku no jissoku hōkokusho." *Tōkyō geijutsu daigaku bijutsu gakubu kiyō* 11 (1976): 1–40.

Kierstead, Thomas. "Outcasts before the Law: Pollution and Purification in Medieval Japan." In *Currents in Medieval Japanese History: Essays in Honor of Jeffrey P. Mass*, edited by Gordon M. Berger et al., 267–97. Los Angeles: Figueroa Press, 2009.

Kobayashi, Shigefumi. "Kodai-chūsei no 'raisha' to shūkyō." In *Reikishi no naka no raisha*, edited by Fujino Yutaka. Miyuru Shuppan, 1996.

Kokuritsu Hansenbyō Shiryōkan, eds. *Ippen hijirie Gokurakuji ezu ni miru Hansenbyō kanja: Chūsei zenki no kanja he no manazashi to shōgun*. Higashimurayama: Kokuritsu Hansenbyō Shiryōkan, 2014.

Kōno, Katsuyuki. *Shōgaisha no chūsei*. Kyoto: Bunrikaku, 1987.

Leung, Angela Ki Che. *Leprosy in China: A History*. New York: Columbia University Press, 2009.

Naimusho, eds., *Shiseki chōsa hōkokusho*, no. 4: "Nara-ken ka ni okeru shitei shiseki." Tokyo: Naimushō, 1928.

Nara Daigaku Sōgō Kenkyūjo, eds. *Nara Daibutsumae ezuya Tsutsui-ke kokusei ezu shūsei*. Nara: Nara Daigaku Sōgō Kenkyūjo, 2002.

Nara-ken shiseki shōchi chōsakai hōkokusho, no. 7. Nara-ken, 1920.

Niunoya, Tetsuichi. *Kebiishi: Chūsei no kegare to kenryoku*. Tokyo: Heibonsha, 1986.

Ōyama, Kyōhei. *Nihon chūsei nōsonshi no kenkyū*. Tokyo: Iwanami Shoten.

Quinter, David. *From Outcastes to Emperors: The Shingon Ritsu Sect and the Mañjúsrī Cult in Medieval Japan*. Leiden and Boston: Brill, 2015.

Sawa, Riichiro. "Nihon saisho no raibyōin ni tsuite." *Kyoto iji eisei shinbun* 110 (1902): 3–5.

Shibuya Kuritsu Shoto Bijutsukan. *Chūsei shomin shinkō no kaiga: Sankei mandara, jigokue, otogizōshi*.Tokyo: Shibuya Kuritsu Shoto Bijutsukan, 1993.

Shinmura, Taku. "Kodai ni okeru seyaku hiden'in ni tsuite." *Nihonshi* 343 (1976): 54–67.

Shinmura, Taku. *Shi to yamai to kango no shakaishi*. Tokyo: Hōsei Daigaku Shuppankyoku, 1989.

Shōzen, Kajiwara. *Ton'isho*. Tokyo: Kagaku Shoin, 1986.

Suzuki, Takao. *Hone kara mita Nihonjin: Kobyōrigaku ga kataru rekishi*. Tokyo: Kōdansha Sensho, 1998.

The Lotus Sutra. Translated by Burton Watson. New York: Columbia University Press, 1993.

Williams, Duncan Ryūken. *The Other Side of Zen: A Social History of Sōtō Zen Buddhism in Tokugawa Japan*. Princeton: Princeton University Press, 2009.

Yokota, Noriko. "'Monoyoshi' kō: Kinsei Kyōto no raisha ni tsuite." *Nihonshi kenkyū* 352 (1991): 1–29.

Chapter 13. Purity and Progress: The First Maternity Hospitals in the United States

"A Brief History of Obstetrical Care at Pennsylvania Hospital." Penn Medicine website. http://www.uphs.upenn.edu/paharc/timeline/1801/tline10.html. Accessed December 18, 2017.

Adams, Annmarie. *Architecture in the Family Way: Doctors, Houses, and Women, 1870–1900*. Montreal: McGill-Queen's University Press, 1996.

The American Lady's Medical Pocket-Book, and Nursery-Adviser. Philadelphia: James Kay, 1833. https://archive.org/details/47020250R.nlm.nih.gov. Accessed November 19, 2019.

Annual Reports of the Board of Managers of the New York Asylum for Lying-In Women, 1824–55. Samuel J. Wood Library of the New York-Presbyterian/Weill Cornell Medical Center. Archive.org (note: titles vary by year). https://archive.org/stream/newyorkasylumfor1824newy#page/n5/mode/2up/search/building. Accessed December 19, 2017.

Barker-Benfield, G. J. *The Horrors of the Half-Known Life: Male Attitudes toward Women and Sexuality in Nineteenth-Century America*. New York: Harper & Row, 1976.

Beach, W. *An Improved System of Midwifery, Adapted to the Reformed Practice of Medicine*. New York: n.p., 1847.

Bibliography

Beck, John B. "An Historical Sketch of the State of Medicine in the American Colonies, from their First Settlement to the Period of the Revolution," *Assembly* 174 (1850): 41–93.

Blundell, James. *The Principles and Practice of Obstetricy*. Edited by Thomas Castle. London: E. Cox, 1834.

Board of Managers, *Address of the Board of Managers of the Preston Retreat*. Philadelphia: Merrihew and Gunn, 1836.

Bryan, James. *Report on the State of the Lying-In Hospitals in Europe*. Philadelphia: King and Baird, 1845.

Bryan, James. *The Progress of Medicine During the First Half of the Nineteenth Century* (Lecture, Philadelphia College of Medicine, March 17, 1851). Philadelphia: Grattan & M'Lean, 1851.

Bull, Thomas. *Hints to Mothers for the Management of Health during the Period of Pregnancy and in the Lying-In Room*. New York: Wiley & Putnam, 1842.

Burdett, Henry C. *Hospitals and Asylums of the World*, vol. 4 London: J. & A. Churchill, 1893. https://archive.org/stream/hospitalsasylums04unse#page/n7/mode/2up/search/lying-in. Accessed November 19, 2019.

Churchill, Fleetwood. *Observations on the Diseases Incident to Pregnancy and Childbed*. Dublin: Martin Keene and Son.

"College of Physicians Report." Printed in W. Robert Penman, *The Public Practice of Midwifery in Philadelphia*. Philadelphia: Transactions & Studies of the College of Physicians of Philadelphia, 1969.

Denig, George. *The Domestic Instructor in Midwifery: Containing Directions for the Proper Treatment of Sexual Diseases of Women; for the Management of Pregnancy, Labor & Child-Bed; Also, for the Treatment of New-Born Infants, Compile or the Advantage and Use of Such as Have Not Access to a Physician*. M'Conellsburg, Bedford County, PA: n.p., 1838.

Dewees, William Potts. *A Treatise on the Diseases of Females*. Philadelphia: Carey, Lea, & Blanchard, 1837.

Dubrow, Gail Lee and Jennifer B. Goodman, eds. *Restoring Women's History through Historic Preservation*. Baltimore: Johns Hopkins University Press, 2003.

Ferguson, Eugene S. "An Historical Sketch of Central Heating: 1800–1860." In *Building Early America*, edited by Charles E. Peterson. Apple Valley, MN: Astragal Press, 1999.

Ferguson, Robert. *Essays on the Most Important Diseases of Women (Part I: Puerperal Fever)*. London: John Murray, 1839.

Gooch, Robert. *An Account of Some of the Most Important Diseases Peculiar to Women*. 2nd ed. Philadelphia: Ed. Barrington and Geo. D. Hawell, 1848.

Goodell, William. *On the Means Employed at the Preston Retreat for the Prevention and Treatment of Puerperal Diseases*. Philadelphia: Collins, 1874.

Hodge, Hugh L. *Introductory to the Course on Obstetrics, and Diseases of Women and Children, in the University of Pennsylvania*. Philadelphia: T. B. Town, 1836.

Ingersoll, Joseph R. *An Address Delivered at the Opening of the Wills Hospital for Indigent Blind, March 3, 1834*. Philadelphia: James Kay, Jun. & Co. 1834.

Irving, Frederick C. "Highlights in the History of the Boston Lying-In Hospital," *Canadian Medical Association Journal* 54 (February 1946): 174–8. https://www.ncbi.nlm.nih.gov/pmc/articles/PMC1582583/. Accessed November 19, 2019.

Kirkbride, Thomas S. *Notice of Some Experiments in Heating and Ventilating Hospitals by Steam and Hot Water*. Philadelphia: T. K. and P. G. Collins, 1850.

Kisacky, Jeanne. *Rise of the Modern Hospital: An Architectural History of Health and Healing, 1870–1940*. Pittsburgh: University of Pittsburgh Press, 2017.

Kobrin, Frances E. "The American Midwife Controversy: A Crisis of Professionalism." *Bulletin of the History of Medicine* 40 (1966): 350–63.

Lawrence, Charles. *History of the Philadelphia Almshouse and Hospitals*. Philadelphia: n.p., 1905.

Leavitt, Judith Walzer. *Brought to Bed: Childbearing in America, 1750–1950*. New York: Oxford University Press, 1986.

Leiby, James. *A History of Social Welfare and Social Work in the United States*. New York: Columbia University Press, 1978.

Manuel, Diana E., ed. *Walking the Paris Hospitals: Diary of an Edinburgh Medical Student, 1834–1835*. London: Wellcome Trust Centre for the History of Medicine at UCL, 2004.

Griscom, John H. *The Uses and Abuses of Air: Showing its Influence in Sustaining Life, and Producing Disease: With Remarks on the Ventilation of Houses, and the Best Methods of Securing a Pure and Wholesome Atmosphere Inside of Dwellings, Churches, Court-Rooms, Workshops, and Buildings of All Kinds*. New York: J. S. Redfield, 1850.

Maunsell, Henry. *The Dublin Practice of Midwifery*. London: Longmans, Green, and Co., 1871.

Mauriceau, A. M. *The Married Woman's Private Medical Companion*. New York: Joseph Trow, 1847.

MayGrier, J. P. *Midwifery Illustrated*. New York: Harper, 1834.

McCalman, Janet. *Sex and Suffering: Women's Health and a Women's Hospital*. Baltimore: Johns Hopkins University Press, 1999.

McGregor, Deborah Kuhn. *From Midwives to Medicine: The Birth of American Gynecology*. New Brunswick: Rutgers University Press, 1988.

Meigs, Charles D. *Females and their Diseases: A Series of Letters to His Class*. Philadelphia: Lea and Blanchard, 1848.

Meigs, Charles D. *The Philadelphia Practice of Midwifery*. Philadelphia: James Kay, Jun. & Brother, 1842.

Moore, George. *An Enquiry into the Pathology, Causes, and Treatment of Puerperal Fever*. London: Samuel Highley, 1836.

Nightingale, Florence. *Introductory Notes on Lying-In Institutions*. London: Longmans, Green, and Co., 1871. https://archive.org/details/introductorynot00nighgoog. Accessed November 19, 2019.

Price, Eli K. *The Address Delivered at the Laying of the Corner-Stone of the Preston Retreat, July 17, 1837*. Philadelphia: John Richards, 1837.

Quiroga, Virginia A. Metaxas. *Poor Mothers and Babies: A Social History of Childbirth and Child Care Hospitals in Nineteenth-Century New York City*. New York: Garland, 1989.

Ryan, Thomas. *The History of Queen Charlotte's Lying-In Hospital*. London: Hutchings and Crowley, 1885. https://archive.org/details/historyofqueench00ryan. Accessed November 19, 2019.

Spaulding, Jonah. *The Female's Guide to Health: Containing an Address to the Married Lady, with a Complete Treatise on Female Complaints, and Midwifery, to which is Added a Few Remarks on the Management of Infants*. Skowhegan, ME: Sentinel Office, 1837.

Taylor, Jeremy. *The Architect and the Pavilion Hospital: Dialogue and Design Creativity in England, 1850–1914*. London: Leicester University Press, 1997.

Thomas, T. Gaillard. "A Century of American Medicine, 1776–1876: Obstetrics and Gynaecology." *American Medical Science* 72 (July 1876): 133–70. https://catalog.hathitrust.org/Record/002073179. Accessed November 19, 2019.

Thompson, John D. and Grace Goldin. *The Hospital: A Social and Architectural History*. New Haven: Yale University Press, 1975.

Tredgold, Thomas. *Principles of Warming and Ventilating Public Buildings, Dwelling-Houses, Manufactories, Hospitals, Hot-Houses, and Conservatories*. London: Josiah Taylor, 1824.

Vogel, Morris J. *The Invention of the Modern Hospital: Boston, 1870–1930*. Chicago: University of Chicago Press, 1980.

Warrington, J. *The Nurse's Guide. Containing a Series of Instructions to Females Who Wish to Engage in the Important Business of Nursing Mother and Child in The Lying-In Chamber*. Philadelphia: Thomas, Cowperthwait and Co., 1839.

Wertz, Richard W. and Dorothy C. Wertz. *Lying-In: A History of Childbirth in America*. New York: The Free Press, 1977.

Williams, William H. *America's First Hospital: The Pennsylvania Hospital, 1751–1841*. Wayne, PA: Haverford House, 1976.

IV. Architecture: Designing Spaces of Healing

Chapter 14. Health as Harmony: The *Pellegrinaio* Cycle of Santa Maria della Scala in Siena

Alberti, Leon Battista. *On Painting: A New Translation and Critical Edition*. Translated Rocco Sinisgalli. Cambridge, NY: Cambridge University Press, 2011.

Alberti, Leon Alberti. *On the Art of Building in Ten Books*. Translated by Joseph Rykwert, Neil Leach, and Robert Tavernor. Cambridge, MA: MIT Press, 1988.

Averlino, Antonio di Piero. *Antonio Averlino detto il Filarete: trattato di architettura*. Translated by Anna Maria Finoli and Liliana Grassi. 2 vols. Milan: Il Polifilo, 1972.

Averlino, Antonio di Piero. *Filarete's Treatise on Architecture: Being the Treatise by Antonio di Piero Averlino, Known as Filarete*. Translated by John R. Spencer. 2 vols. New Haven: Yale University Press, 1965.

Banchi, Luciano. *Statuti volgari de lo spedale di Santa Maria Vergine di Siena scriti l'Anno MCCV: e ora per la prima volta pubblieati*. Siena: I. Gati Editore, 1864.

Bloch, Amy. *Lorenzo Ghiberti's Gates of Paradise: Humanism, History, and Artistic Philosophy in the Italian Renaissance*. New York: Cambridge University Press, 2016.

Bibliography

Carlotti, Mariella and Bernhard Scholz. *Ante gradus: quando la certezza diventa creativa: gli affreschi del Pellegrinaio di Santa Maria della Scala a Siena*. Florence: Società editrice fiorentina, 2011.

Costa, Elda and Laura Ponticelli. "L'iconografia del Pellegrinaio nello Spedale di Santa Maria della Scala di Siena." *Iconographia* 3 (2004): 110–47.

Dunlop, Anne. *Painted Palaces: The Rise of Secular Art in Early Renaissance Italy*. Pennsylvania: Pennsylvania State University Press, 2009.

Fahy, Everett. "Italian Painting before 1500," *Apollo* 107 (1978): 377–88.

Gage, Frances. *Painting as Medicine in Early Modern Rome: Giulio Mancini and the Efficacy of Art*. University Park, PA: The Pennsylvania State University Press, 2016.

Galen. *On the Structure of the Art of Medicine; The Art of Medicine; On the Practice of Medicine to Glaucon*. Translated by Ian Johnston. The Loeb Classical Library, 523. Cambridge MA: Harvard University Press, 2016.

Gowland, Angus. "Medicine, Psychology and the Melancholic Subject in the Renaissance." In *Emotions and Health*, edited by Elena Carrera, 185–219. Leiden: Brill, 2013.

Henderson, John. *The Renaissance Hospital: Healing the Body and Healing the Soul*. New Haven: Yale University Press, 2006.

Hills, Helen. "Architecture and Affect: Leon Battista Alberti and Edification." In *Representing Emotions: New Connections in the Histories of Art, Music and Medicine*, edited by Penelope Gouk and Helen Hills, 89–108. Burlington, VT: Ashgate, 2005.

Horden, Peregrine. "A Non-Natural Environment: Medicine Without Doctors and the Medieval European Hospital." In *Hospitals and Healing from Antiquity to the Later Middle Ages*, edited by Peregrine Horden, 133–45. Burlington, VT: Ashgate, 2008.

Hourihane, Colum. *King David in the Index of Christian Art*. Princeton: Princeton University Press, 2002.

Howe, Eunice D. *Art and Culture at the Sistine Court: Platina's "Life of Sixtus IV" and the Frescoes of the Hospital of Santo Spirito*. Vatican City: Biblioteca Apostolica Vaticana, 2005.

Hub, Berthold. 'Vedete come e bella la cittade quando e ordinata': Politics and the Art of City Planning in Republican Siena." In *Art as Politics in Late Medieval and Renaissance Siena*, edited by Timothy B. Smith and Judith B. Steinhoff. Farnham: Ashgate, 2012.

Krinsky, Carol Herselle. "Representations of the Temple of Jerusalem before 1500," *Journal of the Warburg and Courtauld Institutes* 33 (1970): 1–19.

Norman, Diana. "'Santi cittadini': Vecchietta and the Civic Pantheon in Mid-Fifteenth-Century Siena." In *Art as Politics in Late Medieval and Renaissance Siena*, edited by Timothy B. Smith and Judith B. Steinhoff. Farnham: Ashgate, 2012.

Paolucci, Giulio and Giuliano Pinto. "Gli 'infermi' della Misericordia di Prato (1409–1491)." In *Società del bisogno: povertà e assistenza nella Toscana medievale*, edited by Giuliano Pinto, 101–29. Florence: Salimbeni, 1989.

Park, Katherine. *Doctors and Medicine in Early Renaissance Florence*. Princeton: Princeton University Press, 1985.

Piccinni, Gabriella and Lucia Travaini. *Il Libro del pellegrino: Siena, 1382–1446: affari, uomini, monete nell'Ospedale di Santa Maria della Scala*. Naples: Liguori, 2003.

Piccinni, Gabriella and Laura Vigni. "Modelli di assistenza ospedaliera tra Medioevo ed Età Moderna: quotidianità, amministrazione, conflitti nell' ospedale di Santa Maria della Scala di Siena." In *La Società del bisogno: povertà e assistenza nella Toscana medieval*, edited by Giuliano Pinto, 131–74. Florence: Salimbeni, 1989.

Piccinni, Gabriella and Carla Zarrilli. *Arte e assistenza a Siena: le copertine dipinte dell'Ospedale di Santa Maria della Scala*. Ospedaletto, Pisa: Pacini editore per Santa Maria della Scala, 2003.

Scharf, Friedhelm. *Der Freskenzyklus des Pellegrinaios in S. Maria della Scala zu Siena: Historienmalerei und Wirklichkeit in einem Hospital der Frührenaissance*. Hildsheim: G. Olms, 2001.

Sordini, Beatrice. *Dento l'antico ospedale: Santa Maria della Scala, uomini, cose e spazi di vita nella Siena medievale*. Siena: Protagon, 2010.

Starn, Randolph. *Ambrogio Lorenzetti: The Palazzo Pubblico, Siena*. New York: George Braziller, 1994.

Strehlke, Carl Brandon. "Domenico di Bartolo." Ph.D. diss., Columbia University, 1986.

Terrien, Samuel L. *The Iconography of Job through the Centuries: Artists as Biblical Interpreters*. University Park, PA: Pennsylvania State University Press, 1996.

Whitley, Antonia. "Concepts of Ill Health and Pestilence in Fifteenth-Century Siena." Ph.D. diss., University of London, 2004.

Chapter 15. Uterus House: Incubating Obstetrics in Early Modern Bologna

Alexander, John. "The Educational Buildings of Pius IV: Variations upon a Building Type in Urban Monuments." *Landscape and Urban Planning* 73 (2005): 89–109.

Baidada, Enrica. "Notizie sull'origine e lo sviluppo della Specola bolognese e della sua strumentazione negli archivi cittadini." In *Gli strumenti nella storia e nella filosofia della scienza*, edited by G. Tarozzi, 129–38. Bologna: Litosei, 1983.

Bollette, Giuseppe Gaetano and Giuseppe Maria Angelleli. *Notizie dell'origine, e progressi dell'Instituto delle scienze di Bologna e sue accademie … nuovamente compilate.* Bologna: Istituto delle Scienze, 1780.

Bortolotti, Marco. "Insegnamento, ricerca e professione nel museo ostetrico di Giovanni Antonio Galli." In *I materiali dell'Istituto delle Scienze, Catalogo della Mostra*. Bologna: Accademia delle Scienze, 1979.

Bortolotti, Marco and Viviana Lanzarini. *Ars obstetricia bononiensis: Catalogo ed inventario del Museo Ostetrico Giovan Antonio Galli*. Bologna: CLUEB, 1988.

Caffaratto, T. M. *Storia dell'Ospedale S. Anna di Torino (Opera di Maternità)*, supplement to *Annali dell'Ospedale Maria Vittoria di Torino* 63, no. 7–8 (1970).

Cavazza, Marta. *Settecento inquieto: Alle origini dell'Istituto delle Scienze di Bologna*. Bologna: Il Mulino, 1990.

Ceccarelli, Francesco and Pier Luigi Cervellati. *Da un palazzo a una città: La vera storia della moderna Università di Bologna*. Bologna: Il Mulino, 1987.

Corradi, Alfonso. *Dell'ostetricia in Italia dalla metà dello scorso secolo fino al presente*. Bologna: Gamberini e Parmeggiani, 1874.

Coyecque, Ernest. *L'Hôtel-Dieu de Paris au Moyen-Age. Histoire et documents*. Vol. 1. Paris: Champion, 1889.

Dacome, Lucia. *Malleable Anatomies: Models, Makers, and Material Culture in Eighteenth-Century Italy*. Oxford: Oxford University Press, 2017.Dacome, Lucia. "Women, Wax and Anatomy in the 'Century of Things.'" *Renaissance Studies* 21, no. 4 (2007): 522–50.

Fabbri, Giambattista. "Antico museo ostetrico di Giovanni Antonio Galli, restauro fatto alle sue preparazioni in plastica e nuova conferma della suprema importanza dell'ostetrica sperimentale; con appendice." *Memorie della Accademia delle scienze dell'Istituto di Bologna* 2, ser. 3 (1872): 129–66.

Fabbri, Giambattista. "Rendiconti accademici, Sessione ordinaria, 16 Gennaio 1873." *Bullettino delle scienze mediche* 15, ser. 5 (1873): 383–5.

Ferrari, Giovanna. "Public Anatomy Lessons and the Carnival: The Anatomy Theatre of Bologna." *Past & Present* 117 (1987): 50–106.

Filippini, Nadia Maria. "Assistenza al parto nel primo Ottocento: Appunti sull'intervento istituzionale." In *Le culture del parto*, edited by Ann Oakley, 63–70. Milan: Feltrinelli, 1985.

Filippini, Nadia Maria. "The Church, the State and Childbirth: The Midwife in Italy during the Eighteenth Century." In *The Art of Midwifery: Early Modern Midwives in Europe*, edited by Hilary Marland, 152–75. London: Routledge, 1994.

Filippini, Nadia Maria. "Gli ospizi per partorienti e i reparti di maternità tra il Sette e l'Ottocento." In *Gli ospedali in area padana fra Settecento e Novecento*, edited by Maria Luisa Betri and Edoardo Bressan, 395–411. Milan: Feltrinelli, 1992.

Findlen, Paula. "Science as a Career in Enlightenment Italy: The Strategies of Laura Bassi." *Isis* 84, no. 3 (1993): 441–69.

Foucault, Michel, et al. *Les Machines à guérir: Aux origines de l'hôpital moderne*. Brussels and Liège: Mardaga, 1979.

Franchetti, Daniela. *La scuola ostetrica pavese tra Otto e Novecento*. Milan: Cisalpino, 2012.Fratello, Bernardo, et al. "Una collezione settecentesca del Museo di Anatomia dell'Università di Modena e Reggio Emilia. I modelli ostetrici realizzati in terracotta da Giovan Battista Manfredini." *Museologia scientifica memorie* 2 (2008): 215–20.

Frize, Monique. *Laura Bassi and Science in 18th-Century Europe: The Extraordinary Life and Role of Italy's Pioneering Female Professor*. Berlin: Springer, 2013.

Griffini, Romolo. "Sul progetto di regolamento organico dell'ospizio provinciale degli esposti e delle partorienti di Milano." *Annali universali di medicina* 206, no. 618 (December 1868): 465–563.

Habermas, Jürgen. *The Structural Transformation of the Public Sphere: An Inquiry into a Category of Bourgeois Society*. Translated by T. Burger. Cambridge, MA: MIT Press, 1991.

Henderson, John. *The Renaissance Hospital: Healing the Body and Healing the Soul*. New Haven: Yale University Press, 2006.

Lalande, Jérôme. *Voyage d'un François en Italie, Fait dans les années 1765 & 1766*. Vol. 2. Venice, 1769.

Bibliography

Lanzarini, Viviana. "La scuola ostetrica di Giovan Antonio Galli e la sua collezione didattica." In *Nascere a Siena: Il parto e l'assistenza alla nascità dal medioevo all'età moderna*, edited by Francesca Vannozzi, 25–34. Siena: Protagon, 2005.
Lefebvre, Henri. *The Production of Space*. Translated by Donald Nicholson-Smith. Oxford: Basil Blackwell, 1991.
Lines, David A. "Reorganizing the Curriculum: Teaching and Learning in the University of Bologna." *History of Universities* 26, no. 2 (2012): 1–59.
Logan, Gabriella Berti. "Women and the Practice and Teaching of Medicine in Bologna in the Eighteenth and Early Nineteenth Centuries." *Bulletin of the History of Medicine* 77, no. 3 (2003): 506–35.
Medici, Michele. "Elogio di Gian-Antonio Galli." *Memorie della Reale Accademia delle Scienze dell'Istituto di Bologna* 8 (1857): 423–50.
Medici, Michele. *Memorie storiche intorno le accademie scientifiche e letterarie della città di Bologna*. Bologna: Sassi nelle Spaderie, 1852.
Messbarger, Rebecca. *The Lady Anatomist: The Life and Work of Anna Morandi Manzolini*. Chicago: University of Chicago Press, 2010.
Monari, Daniela. "Palazzo Bocchi: il quadro storico e l'intervento del Vignola." *Il Carrobbio* 6 (1980): 263–72.
Newman, Karen. *Fetal Positions: Individualism, Science, Visuality*. Stanford: Stanford University Press, 1996.
Pancino, Claudia. *Il bambino e l'acqua sporca: Storia dell'assistenza al parto dalle mammane alle ostetriche (secoli XVI–XIX)*. Milan: Franco Angeli, 1984.
Roli, Renato. "Il Palazzo Poggi, il Palazzo Malvezzi, la Biblioteca." In *I luoghi del conoscere: I laboratori storico e i musei dell'università di Bologna*, Vol. 2, edited by Franca Arduini et al., 18–31. Bologna: Banca del Monte, 1988.
Roversi, Giancarlo. *Palazzi e case nobili del '500 a Bologna: La storia, le famiglie, le opera d'arte*. Casalecchi di Reno: Grafis, 1986.
Sexton, Kim. "Academic Bodies and Anatomical Architecture in Early Modern Bologna." In *Architecture and the Body, Science and Culture*, edited by Kim Sexton, 139–56. London: Routledge, 2017.
Schmidt, Johann Karl Schmidt. "Zu Vignolas Palazzo Bocchi in Bologna." *Mitteilungen des Kunsthistorischen Institutes in Florenz* 13, no. 1–2 (1967): 83–94.
Tafuri, Manfredo. *Venice and the Renaissance*. Translated by J. Levine. London: MIT Press, 1989.
Thompson, John D. and Grace Goldin. *The Hospital: A Social and Architectural History*. New Haven: Yale University Press, 1975.
Tonelli, Gualtiero. "Sul teatro anatomico dell'Archiginnasio. Chi furono i padrini?" *Strenna storica bolognese* 28 (1978): 381–400.
Vannozzi, Francesca. "Una palestra per la didattica ostetrica: Il ricovero di maternità." In *Figure femminili (e non) intorno alla nascita: La storia in Siena dell'assistenza alla partoriente e al nascituro, XVIII–XX secolo*, edited by Francesca Vannozzi, 225–43. Siena: Protagon, 2005.
Wilson, Adrian. *The Making of Man-Midwifery: Childbirth in England, 1660–1770*. Cambridge, MA: Harvard University Press, 1995.
Wilson, Bronwen and Paul Yachnin, eds. *Making Publics in Early Modern Europe: People, Things, Forms of Knowledge*. New York: Routledge, 2010.
Zanotti, Francesco Maria. *De Bononiensi Scientiarum et Artium Instituto atque Academia commentarii*. Vol. 3. Bologna, 1755.

Chapter 16. Healing by Design: An Experiential Approach to Early Modern Ottoman Hospital Architecture

Andrews, Walter. "Ottoman Love: Preface to a Theory of Emotional Ecology." In *A History of Emotions, 1200–1800*, edited by Jonas Liliequist, 21–47. London: Pickering & Chatto, 2012.
Avicenna, *The General Principles of Avicenna's Canon of Medicine*. Translated by Mazhar Shah. Karachi: Naveed Clinic, 1966.
Baker, Patricia. "Medieval Islamic Hospitals: Structural Design and Social Perceptions." In *Medicine and Space: Bodies, Surroundings and Borders in Antiquity and the Middle Ages*, edited by Patricia Baker, Han Nijdam, and Karine van't Land, 245–72. Leiden: Brill, 2012.
Bayat, Ali Haydar. *Osmanlı Devleti'nde Hekimbaşılık Kurumu ve Hekimbaşılar*. Ankara: Atatürk Kültür Merkezi, 1999.

Bektaş, Cengiz. *Kuş Evleri/Bird-Houses*. Istanbul: Arkeoloji ve Sanat Yayınları, 2000.
Blomkvist, V., C. A. Eriksen, T. Theorell, R. Ulrich, and G. Rasmanis. "Acoustics and Psychosocial Environment in Intensive Coronary Care." *Occupational Environmental Medicine* 62 (2005): e1–e8.
Cantay, Gönül. *Anadolu Selçuklu ve Osmanlı Darüşşifaları*. Ankara: Atatürk Kültür Merkezi Yayınları, 1992.
Çelebi, Evliya. *Evliya Çelebi Seyahatnamesi, 3. Cilt, 2. Kitap*. Edited by Seyit Ali Kahraman and Yücel Dağlı. Istanbul: Yapı Kredi Yayınları, 2010.
Cooper Marcus, C. and M. Barnes. *Gardens in Healthcare Facilities: Uses, Therapeutic Benefits, and Design Recommendations*. Martinez: Center for Health Design, 1995.
Cunningham, R. M., Jnr. "Frank Lloyd Wright on Hospital Design: A Modern Hospital Interview with the World-Famous Architect." *Modern Hospital* 71 (1948): 51–4.
Ergin, Nina. "'And in the Soup Kitchen Food Shall Be Cooked Twice Every Day': Gustatory Aspects of Ottoman Mosque Complexes." In *Rethinking Place in South Asian and Islamic Art, 1500–Present*, edited by Rebecca Brown and Deborah Hutton, 17–37. New York: Routledge, 2016.
Ergin, Nina. "The Albanian Tellâk Connection: Labor Migration to the Hamams of Eighteenth-Century Istanbul, Based on the 1752 İstanbul Hamâmları Defteri." *Turcica* 43 (2011 [2012]): 229–54.
Ergin, Nina, Christoph Neumann, and Amy Singer, eds. *Feeding People, Feeding Power: Imarets in the Ottoman Empire*. Istanbul: Eren, 2007.
Erzen, Jale Nejdet. "Aesthetics and Aisthesis in Ottoman Art and Architecture." *Journal of Islamic Studies* 2 (1991): 1–24.
Fisher, C. G. and A. Fisher. "Topkapı Sarayı in the Mid-Seventeenth Century: Bobovi's Description." *Archivum Ottomanicum* 10 (1985): 5–81.
Gouk, Penelope, ed. *Musical Healing in Cultural Contexts*. Aldershot: Ashgate, 2000.
Gratien, Chris. "Ottoman Environmental History: A New Area of Middle East Studies." *Arab Studies Journal* 20 (2012): 246–54.
Gürkan, Kazım İsmail. "Süleymaniye Darüşşifası." In *Kanuni Armağanı*, 259–67. Ankara: TTK, 1979.
Horden, Peregrine. "Religion as Medicine: Music in Medieval Hospitals." In *Religion and Medicine in the Middle Ages*, edited by P. Biller and J. Ziegler, 135–53. Woodbridge: York Medieval Press, 2001.
Horden, Peregrine, ed. *Music as Medicine: The History of Music Therapy since Antiquity*. Aldershot: Ashgate, 2000.
Horsburgh, C. Robert, Jnr. "Healing by Design." *The New England Journal of Medicine* 333 (1995): 735–40.
Karagülle, Zeki. "Health Effects of Hamams." Paper presented at the symposium *Fürdö, Sauna, Hamam*, Research Center for Anatolian Civilizations, Istanbul, April 25–6, 2009.
Kılıç, Abdullah. *Anadolu Selçuklu ve Osmanlı Şefkat Abideleri: Şifahaneler*. Istanbul: MedicalPark, 2012.
Kılıç, Abdullah. *Karşılıksız Hizmetin Muhteşem Abideleri: İstanbul Şifahaneleri*. Istanbul: İstanbul Büyükşehir belediyesi Kültür A. Ş. Yayınları, 2009.
Latham, J. D. and H. D. Isaacs. *Isaac Judaeus: On Fevers (The Third Discourse: On Consumption)*. Cambridge: Pembroke, 1981.
Leiser, Gary and Michael Dols. "Evliya Chelebi's Description of Medicine in 17th C. Egypt." *Sudhoffs Archiv* 71 (1987): 197–216.
Leiser, Gary and Michael Dols. "Evliya Chelebi's Description of Medicine in Seventeenth-Century Egypt, Part II: Text." *Sudhoffs Archiv* 72 (1988): 49–68.
Macaraig, Nina. *The Çemberlitaş Hamamı in Istanbul: The Biographical Memoir of a Turkish Bath*. Edinburgh: Edinburgh University Press, 2018.
Necipoğlu, Gülru. *Architecture, Ceremonial and Power: The Topkapı Palace in the Fifteenth and Sixteenth Centuries*. Cambridge, MA: MIT, 1991.
Necipoğlu, Gülru. "Framing the Gaze in Ottoman, Safavid and Mughal Palaces." *Ars Orientalis* 23 (1993): 303–42.
Necipoğlu, Gülru. *The Age of Sinan: Architectural Culture in the Ottoman Empire*. Princeton: Princeton University Press, 2005.
Nutton, Vivian. *Ancient Medicine*. London: Routledge, 2004.
Özen, Rahşan. "Bird Shelters in Turkey: Birdhouses and Dovecotes." *Kafkas Üniversitesi Veteriner Fakültesi Dergisi* 18 (2012): 1079–82.
Özkan Göksoy, Vildan. "Topkapı Sarayında 'Cariyeler Hastanesi.'" In *I. Türk Tıp Tarihi Kongresi, Istanbul, 17–19 Şubat 1988: Kongreye Sunulan Bildiriler*, 193–8. Ankara: TTK, 1992.

Bibliography

Pormann, Peter, and Emilie Savage-Smith. *Medieval Islamic Medicine*. Edinburgh: Edinburgh University Press, 2007.
Risse, G. B. *Mending Bodies, Saving Souls: A History of Hospitals*. Oxford: Oxford University Press, 1990.
Sarı, Nil. "Educating the Ottoman Physician." In *History of Medicine Studies*, edited by Nil Sarı and Hüsrev Hatemi, 40–64. Istanbul: [n.p.], 1988.
Sarı, Nil, Gül Akdeniz, and Ramazan Tuğ. "Topkapı ve Galata Sarayı Enderun Hastanesi." In *IV. Türk Tıp Tarihi Kongresi, Istanbul, 18–20 Eylül 1988: Kongreye Sunulan Bildiriler*, 187–201. Ankara: TTK, 2002.
Shefer-Mossensohn, Miri. "Charity and Hospitality: Hospitals in the Ottoman Empire in the Early Modern Period." In *Poverty and Charity in Middle Eastern Contexts*, edited by Michael Bonner, Mine Ener, and Amy Singer, 121–43. Albany: SUNY Press, 2003.
Shefer-Mossensohn, Miri. *Ottoman Medicine: Healing and Medical Institutions, 1500–1700*. Albany: SUNY Press, 2009.
Shiloah, Amnon. "Jewish and Muslim Traditions of Music Therapy." In *Music as Medicine: The History of Music Therapy since Antiquity*, edited by Peregrine Horden, 69–83. Aldershot: Ashgate, 2000.
Singer, Amy. "The 'Michelin Guide' to Public Kitchens in the Ottoman Empire." In *Starting with Food: Culinary Approaches to Ottoman History*, edited by Amy Singer, 69–92. Princeton: Markus Wiener, 2011.
Tabbaa, Yasser. "The Functional Aspects of Medieval Islamic Hospitals." In *Poverty and Charity in Middle Eastern Contexts*, edited by Michael Bonner, Mine Ener, and Amy Singer, 95–119. Albany: SUNY Press, 2003.
Terzioğlu, Arslan. *Beiträge zur Geschichte der türkisch-islamischen Medizin, Wissenschaft und Technik*. 2 vols. Istanbul: Isis, 1996.
Terzioğlu, Arslan. *Die Hofspitäler und andere Gesundheitseinrichtungen der osmanischen Palastbauten unter Berücksichtigung der Ursprungsfrage sowie ihre Beziehungen zu den abendländischen Hofspitälern*. Munich: Trofenik, 1979.
Terzioğlu, Arslan. *Osmanlılarda Hastaneler, Eczacılık, Tababet ve Bunların Dünya Çapındaki Etkiler*. Istanbul: Kültür Bakanlığı, 1999.
Turabi, Ahmet Hakkı. "Hekim Şuûrî Hasan Efendi ve *Ta'dîlü'l-Emzice* adlı Eserinde Müzikle Tedavi Bölümü." *Marmara Üniversitesi İlahiyat Fakültesi Dergisi* 40 (2011): 153–66.
Ulrich, Roger. "Effects of Interior Design and Wellness: Theory and Recent Scientific Research." *Journal of Health Care Interior Design* 3 (1991): 97–109.
Ulrich, Roger. "View through a Window May Influence Recovery from Surgery." *Science* 224 (1984): 420–1.
Ulrich, Roger et al. "The Role of the Physical Environment in the Hospital of the 21st Century." The Robert Wood Johnson Foundation and the Center for Health Design. http://www.healthdesign.org/chd/research/role-physical-environment-hospital-21st-century. Accessed July 20, 2014.
Waagenar, Cor, ed. *The Architecture of Hospitals*. Amsterdam: NAi Publishers, 2006.
Warner Jr, S. B. "The Periodic Rediscoveries of Restorative Gardens: 1100–Present." In *The Healing Dimensions of People-Plant Relations: Proceedings of a Research Symposium*, edited by M. Francis, P. Lindsey, and J. S. Rice, 5–12. Davis: University of California, Davis, Center for Design Research, 1995.
Yörükoğlu, Nihad. *Manisa Bimarhanesi*. Istanbul: İsmail Akgün Matbaası, 1948.

Chapter 17. Architectural Prescriptions: Johns Hopkins Medicine and the Shift from the Pre-Modern to the Modern Hospital

Ackerknecht, Erwin. *Medicine at the Paris Hospital, 1794–1848*. Baltimore: Johns Hopkins University Press, 1967.
Adams, Annemarie. *Medicine by Design: The Architect and the Modern Hospital, 1893–1943*. Minneapolis: University of Minnesota Press, 2008.
Bliss, Michael. *Harvey Cushing: A Life in Surgery*. New York: Oxford University Press, 2005.
Bliss, Michael. *William Osler: A Life in Medicine*. Toronto: University of Toronto Press, 1999.
Brieger, Gert. "The Original Plans for the Johns Hopkins Hospital and Their Historical Significance." *Bulletin of the History of Medicine* 39, no. 6 (November–December 1965): 518–28.
Carroll, Katherine L. "Creating the Modern Physician: The Architecture of American Medical Schools in the Era of Medical Education Reform." *Journal of the Society of Architectural Historians* 75, no. 1 (March 2016): 48–73.
Chesney, Alan M. *The Johns Hopkins Hospital and The Johns Hopkins University School of Medicine: The Early Years, 1867–1893*. Baltimore: Johns Hopkins Press, 1943.
Fair, Alistair. "'A Laboratory of Heating and Ventilation': The Johns Hopkins Hospital as Experimental Architecture, 1870–90." *The Journal of Architecture* 19, no. 3 (2014): 357–81.

Fleming, Donald. *William H. Welch and the Rise of Modern Medicine*. Boston: Little, Brown, 1954.

Graham, Kristin. *A History of Pennsylvania Hospital*. London: History Press, 2008.

Greenbaum, Louis S. "'Measure of Civilization': The Hospital Thought of Jacques Tenon on the Eve of the French Revolution" *Bulletin of the History of Medicine* 49, no. 1 (Spring 1975): 43–56.

Harvey, A. McGehee et al., *A Model of Its Kind: A Centennial History of Medicine at Johns Hopkins*. Vol. 1. Baltimore: Johns Hopkins University Press, 1989.

Hensel, Michael. *Performance-Oriented Architecture: Rethinking Architectural Design and the Built Environment*. Hoboken, NJ: Wiley, 2013.

Kisacky, Jeanne. *Rise of the Modern Hospital: An Architectural History of Health and Healing, 1870–1940*. Pittsburgh: University of Pittsburgh Press, 2017.

Lamb, Susan D. *Pathologist of the Mind: Adolf Meyer and the Origins of American Psychiatry*. Baltimore: Johns Hopkins University Press, 2014.

Ludmerer, Kenneth. *Learning to Heal: The Development of American Medical Education*. New York: Basic Books, 1985.

Ludmerer, Kenneth. "Understanding the Flexner Report." *Academic Medicine* 85 (February 2010): 193–6.

Markel, Howard. *An Anatomy of Addiction: Sigmund Freud, William Halsted, and the Miracle Drug, Cocaine*. New York: Pantheon, 2011.

Osler, William. *The Life of Sir William Osler*. Oxford: Clarendon Press, 1925.

Porter, Roy. *Blood and Guts: A Short History of Medicine*. New York: Norton, 2002.

Risse, Guenter. *Mending Bodies, Saving Soul: A History of Hospitals*. New York: Oxford University Press, 1999.

Rosenberg, Charles. *The Care of Strangers: The Rise of America's Hospital System*. New York: Basic Books, 1987.

Sander, Kathleen Waters. *Mary Elizabeth Garrett: Society and Philanthropy in the Gilded Age*. Baltimore: Johns Hopkins University Press, 2008.

Schlich, Thomas. "Surgery, Science, and Modernity: Operating Rooms and Laboratories as Spaces of Control." *History of Science* 45, no. 3 (2007): 231–56.

Simpson, Andrew. "Health and Renaissance: Academic Medicine and the Remaking of Modern Pittsburgh." *Journal of Urban History* 41 (2015): 19–27.

Simpson, Andrew. *The Medical Metropolis: Health Care and Economic Transformation in Pittsburgh and Houston* (Philadelphia: University of Pennsylvania Press, 2019).

Thompson John D. and Grace Goldin. *The Hospital: A Social and Architectural History*. New Haven: Yale University Press, 1975.

Verderber, Stephen and David Fine. *Healthcare Architecture in an Era of Radical Transformation*. New Haven: Yale University Press, 2000.

Yanni, Carla. *The Architecture of Madness*. Minneapolis: University of Minnesota Press, 2007.

Young, Hugh Hampton. *Hugh Young: A Surgeon's Autobiography*. New York: Harcourt Brace, 1940.

INDEX

Note: Page numbers in *italics* refer to figures.

abaton 3
Abrams, M.H. 86
Abreu, Laurinda 41
Abu Jafar Al-Mansour (Caliph) 7
Abu-l-Fadl Muhammad al-Harithi 102
Academy of the Unquiet (Bologna) 268
Accademia Ermatena (Bologna) 268
Ackerknect, Erwin 302
Acqua Vergine (Rome) 123
Adams, Annemarie 312
Adelaide hospitals (Australia) 173–4
Adriaens, Pieter 66, *68*
'Adud al-Dawla (Sultan) 99
Aelius Aristides 2
Africa
    colonial medicine in 13–14
    places of healing in 8
    Portuguese involvement in 43
air quality/airflow. *See* ventilation
'Alam al-Din Sanjar al-Shuja'i 107
Alberti, Leon Battista 38, 252, 253
    Della tranquilllità dell'animo 253
    On Painting (*Della pittura*) 254
    Pellegrinaio cycle 241
Albertini, Francesco 116
Alcochete House of Misericórdia (Portugal) *192*
Aleppo 101, 102, 108
Alexander, William 80
Alexandria (Egypt) 221
All Saints Royal Hospital (Lisbon) 138
Allgemeines Krankenhaus (Vienna) 223
Almeida, Luis de 9
almshouses
    in America 222–3, 225–7, 229, 233
    in England 12, 77, 87
    in India 10
    in Japan 9
    in the Middle Ages 4
Alvares, José 149
Amasya 104

Americas
    almshouses in 222–3, 225–7, 229, 233
    Aztec civilization 11, 15
    Inca civilization 11
    Mayan civilization 11
    pre-colonial civilizations 11
Anatolia 4, 279
    hospitals in 100, 104, 112
    See also Ottoman Empire
anatomy 12
Anatomy Theater (Bologna) 267–8, 270
ancient civilizations 2–4
Ancient Egypt 2
    healers in 26–7
Ancient Greece 2–3, 279
    abaton 3
    healers in 27
    musical knowledge 290
    temples of healing (Asclepieia) 2–3
Ankyoji temple (Japan) 213
Anthony (saint) 75
aqueducts 3, 121, 123–4
Archer, George 308
Archer, John Lee 169
Archiginnasio (Bologna) 267, 268
architectural materials
    adobe 146
    ashlar masonry 284
    brass 102
    brick 83, 104, 127, 165, 168, 282, 292
    copper 65
    limestone 57
    macuti palm leaves 146, *146*, 153
    marble 30, 103, 108, 127, 231, 292, 294
    mecrusse wood (Lebombo ironwood) 143
    mortar 143
    mosaics 30
    palm thatch 146
    plaster 83, 143
    stone 77, 83, 140, 143, 168, 188, 282, 292

Index

stucco 83, 104
terracotta pipes 39
tile 29–30, 216–17, 282
timber 83, 165
tombstones 42
wood 16, 38, 143, 146, 165, 292
architectural styles
  Buddhist 218
  courtyard plan 28, 39, 76, 281
  cruciform 29–30, 35, 38, 41, 44–5, 48, 49, 76, 108, 126, 138
  Doric 231
  double-cross design 30, 47, 48, 76
  early Christian 28–32
  hip-and-gable roof 213, 216
  Ionic 227
  Islamic 100–12
  Italianate 227
  loggia facade 76
  Manueline (16th century Portuguese) 44
  in the Middle Ages 37
  monastery architecture 262
  Palladian 227
  patterned after classical villas 86
  pavilion design 305
  polygonal 282
  Quadralectic 25
  Queen Anne 305, 310
  Regency 169, *170*
  T-shaped 30
  Tudor Gothic 174–5, *174*
  U-plan 76, 146, 227
  wrap-around veranda 214
  See also hospital architecture
architecture
  building and repurposing structures for specific uses 182–3
  and the human body 121
  on Mozambique island 143–5, *144*, *145*, 155
  religious 186, 188
  salutary function of 252
  as vehicle for God's work 81
  See also hospital architecture
Arez hospital (Portugal) 187
Argentina 11
Aristotle 120
Arnold, Dana 87, 138, 149
Asclepieia/Asclepieion 2–3
Asclepius/Asclepios 2, 27, 279
Ashrafiya Library (Damascus) 101
Asia, places of healing in 8–9. *See also* China; Japan
asylums
  Bethlem Hospital 76–9

  in Constantinople 85
  design of 77, 81–5, 90
  Kirkbride plan 310
  regulation of 77
  Sheppard and Enoch Pratt Hospital 310
  St. Luke's *78*, 81
  in Tasmania 169
  See also Retreat Asylum (York)
Atik Valide Darüşşifası (Istanbul) 281, 282, 288, 294
  ground plan *280*
Atik Valide Mosque Complex (Istanbul) 281, 293
Atkinson, Peter the Elder 81, 83, 88
Atterbury, Grosvenor 310
Augustine of Hippo (saint) 58
Austin, James 172–3
Australia
  Colonial Hospital (Perth) 172–3, *172*
  colonial settlement in 163
  hospital in Tasmania 169
  hospitals in 162–75
  hospitals in Adelaide 173–4
  hospitals in free settlements (Western and South Australia) 171–3
  Liverpool Hospital 168–9, *168*
  Melbourne hospitals 173–5, *174*
  Melbourne Lying-in Hospital 227
  Moreton Bay Hospital 170–1
  New Norfolk convict hospital 169
  New South Wales governor's residence *174*
  as penal colony 163, 170–1
  "Rum Hospital" 165–9, *166*
  Swan River Colony 171
  Sydney General Hospital 163–6, *164*
Averlino, Antonio di Pietro 241
Averlino, Antonio (il Filarete) *36*, 38
Avicenna (ibn Sina) 7, 251
Avignon papacy 116
Aztec Empire 11, 15

Babelegisi 8
Baghdad, hospitals in 7, 99
Bapedi tribe 8
Bartolo, Domenico di 243–4, *244*, 247, *249*, 251
  The Distribution of Alms 247
  Job 247
  Solomon 247
  Tobit 247
Bartolomei, Giacomo 265–6, 272
Basil of Caesarea (saint) 4, 29
Basileiados 29
Bass, H. 87
Bassi, Laura 265, 268
Bastos, Cristiana 14

Index

Bath (England) 75
bathhouses 3, 108, 214, *215*, 282, 292, 296, 305. *See also* hammams
bathing
   in America 305
   in ancient Greece 3
   in ancient Rome 3
   of babies 66
   benefits of 300 n. 51
   in Cambodia 10
   in Constantinople 5
   as cure 9
   in India 10
   in Indonesia 14
   in Islamic hospitals 108, 112, 282, 289, 292, 296, 298n15
   in Italy 31, 122
   in Japan 213, 214, *215*, 217
Bayn al-Qasrayn (Cairo) 107
Beccari, Jacopo Bartolomeo 265, 272
Beja (Portugal), hospital of Our Lady of Piedade 187
Belgium, hospitals in 5–6. *See also* Our Lady of Potterie (hospital of)
Bellers, John 77
Bellevue Hospital (New York) 308, 309
Benedict of Nursia 29, 119
Benjamin of Tuleda 99
Bentham, Jeremy 85
Benzi, Ugo 254
Bethlem Hospital (London) 76–9, 81
Bevans, John 81, 83
Beyazit Ii complex (Edirne) 107
Bhattacharya, Jayanta 10
Billings, John Shaw 305–7, *306*
bimaristans 7, 100
biomedical institutes, German model 308, *309*
biomedical research 307
biomedicine 88, 308
Blatternbaus (pox houses) 13
Bloomberg Children's Center (John's Hopkins) 303, *304*
Blore, Edward *174*
Bocchi, Achille 268
Bologna (Italy) 268
   Anatomy Theater 267–8, 270
   Archiginnasio 267, 268
   Institute of the Sciences 263, *264*, 265, 268, 274
   map *267*
   Palazzo Marsili 268, *269*
   Palazzo Poggi *264*, 268, 270, 274
   Torre della Specola 268
   See also Casa Nascentori
Bond, Thomas 303
Book of Drugs and Demons (*Yao sui shu*) 204

Bootaert, Andries 64, 66
Borgo Santo Spirito (Rome) 122
borning/birthing rooms 221–2. *See also* maternity hospitals
botanical gardens 6, 11, 142, 202. *See also* hospital gardens
botanical medicine 6, 11, 142, 202
Botelho, Sebastião Xavier 153
Boyle, Robert 77
Brady Urological Institute (Johns Hopkins) 308
Braga (Portugal), hospital of St. Mark's 187
Brandolini, Aurelio 118
Braun, Georg *40*, 45, *46*
Brazil 11, 15–16
British Colonial Medical Service 14
British Lying-In Institution 233
Brothers Hospitallers of Saint John of God 141–2, 145, 147, 149, 153, 155
Bruges (Belgium) 57, 58. *See also* Our Lady of Potterie (hospital of)
Brunelleschi, Filippo 76, 127
Buddhism 9, 10, 210, 211–12
   charity 212
   institutions of care 213–15, 219
   Manjusri Bodhisattva 212, 214
   Ritsu Precept sect 212
   Shingon sect 212
   Tendai sect 214
Buha tribe 8
Bulfinch, Charles 303
Bunyan, John 86
burials, in Japan 211–2
Buzzichelli, Gilvanni di Francesco 243
Byzantine Empire 4–5, 28–9, 279

Cairo (Egypt) 99, 100, 101, 107–11. *See also* al-Mansur Hospital (Cairo)
Caldas da Rainha (Portugal) 138
Calza, Luigi 266
Cambodia 10
Campo de' Fiori (Rome) 122
Cantay, Gönül 279
Caraka-Samhita (CS) 10
Carr, John 79, 83
Carre, Victor 64
Carroll, Katherine 308
Casa da Misericórdia (Portugal) 183. *See also* Misericórdias (Portugal)
Casa das Boubas (Portugal) 54 n 71
Casa Nascentori (Bologna) 260, *261*, 262, 263, 268, 270, 272
   architecture of 266–8, 270
   location of 266–7

Index

map *267*
passage from street to courtyard *273*
Cassels, Richard 227
Cassini, Giovanni 260
Castell, Robert 86
Catholic Reformation 182
Çelebi, Evliya 108, 289–90, 292
cemeteries 30
Cesariano, Cesare 48
Channing, Walter 225
charity
    Buddhist 212
    Christian 5, 63, 77–8, 125, 244
    and hospitals 77–8
    Islamic 7, 99, 112
    in the Renaissance 13
Charlemagne 4
Charlotte (Queen of Cyprus) 128
Chen Xunzhai 201–2, 204
childbirth 165, 221
    borning/birthing rooms 221–2
    in the home 221–2, 224, 234
    See also maternity hospitals
Children's Rehabilitation Institute (Johns Hopkins) 308
China
    cultivating life in 198–9
    healers in 26
    homes as spaces of healing 197–207
    medical pluralism in 197
    places of healing in 9
    See also Hong Kong
Chinese medical theory 210
cholera 13
"Christ Healing the Sick in the Temple" (West) 303
Christianity
    Armenian 99
    and care for the poor 5, 69–70, 75
    charity 5, 63, 77–8, 125, 244
    Christians as body of Christ 121
    in Europe 76
    Jesuits in the Americas 15
    missionaries in Africa 14
    missionaries in Japan 9–10
    Neoplatonised 86
    nursing religious orders 32
    Papal Schism 116
    philanthropic efforts 28
    Protestant Reformation 76
    relics of Christ 119
    role of prayer in healing 141
    and social welfare 63
    See also Religious Society of Friends (Quakers)
Church and Convent of St. John (Mozambique) 145–6
Church of Good Health (Mozambique) 145
churches/chapels
    attached to cathedrals and monasteries 150–1, *150*
    connected to hospitals 5, 31, 45, 47–8, 57–8, 140, 186–8, *189*, 190, *192*, 302
Çifte Madrasa (Kayseri) 104
City of London Lying-in Hospital for Married Women 227, *228*
Civitates orbis terrarium (Braun and Hogenberg) 45, *46*
classicism 84
Cleveland Clinic 304
Colino, Adamo *246*, *248*
Collie, Alexander 171
Colonial Hospital (Perth, Australia) 172–3, *172*
colonial medicine 13–14
Columella 3
Confrarias da Misericórdia. *See* Misericórdias (Portugal)
Constantinople (Turkey) 4–5, 85
Cornaro, Alvise 83
Corsia Sistina (Hospital of Santo Spirito, Rome) 127–8, *129*
Coste, Pascal 108
cottage hospitals 162
Cotter, Thomas 173
Councilman, William T. 308–9
County Asylum Act (1808) 80
courtyards 3, 4, 13
    in ancient hospitals 27–30
    in Australian hospitals 169
    at Casa Nascentori 266, 267, 272
    in cruciform hospital plans 38–9
    in Islamic hospitals 99, 101, 103–4, 106–8, 111
    in maternity hospitals 227
    in Mozambique 140, 146, 152, 156
    in Ottoman hospitals 281–5, 287–9, 291–7
    in Portuguese hospitals 44–5, 47
    in Rome 126, 127, 128
    in Santa Maria della Scala 253, 255
Crichton, James 171
crusades 6
cruzeiros 190, 193
cupolas 76, 222, 226, 305, *307*
Cushing, Harvey 310

Dacome, Lucia 265
Damascus (Syria) 101–4, 107. *See also* al-Nuri Hospital (Damascus)
Dance, George (the Younger) 81, 85
Dandy, Walter 310
Danişmendids 104
Dao Xuan 9
dar al-shifa' (house of healing/cure) 100
dar al-sihha (house of health) 100

Index

darüşşifası. See Ottoman hospitals
Davidson, Wilburt 312
De concordantia catholica (Nicholas of Cusa) 124
De facultatibus naturalibus (Galen) 120
de la Rive, Charles-Gaspard 82, 84
De sanguine Christi (Sixtus IV) 119–20
De Subventione Pauperum (Juan Luis Vives) 57, 62–3, 70
De usu partium (Galen) 120
Debret, Jean Baptiste 15
Delepierre, Octave 59–60
dental surgery 247
depression 111
Description of the Retreat: An Institution Near York (Tuke) 75, 79–81, 82, 88, 90
diarrhea 111
Digby, Anne 89
Dioscorides 6
disease. *See* epidemics; illness
dissection 268, 270, 308, 310
Divriği 104
Dom João II (Prince/King of Portugal) 41, 42–3, 44, 182
Dom Manuel (King of Portugal) 42–3, 44, 181–2
domes
    over the altar 128
    in American hospitals 230
    in Australia 169
    on European hospitals 29, 31, 39, 226
    in France 226
    in Italy 30, 31, 39, 247
    Johns Hopkins Hospital 303, *304, 307*
    muqarnas 102, 103
    octagonal 30, 247, 305
    Ottoman 279, 281, 282, 283, 285, 289, 291, 293
    on towers 169
Dong Qichang 201–2
dos Santos, Ferreira 14
Dotti, Francesco *269*
Dublin Lying-In Hospital 227, *229*, 230
Duke University Hospital (Durham, North Carolina) 311–12

Effects of Good Government (Lorenzetti) *250*
Egas, Enrique 35
Egypt. *See* Ancient Egypt; Cairo (Egypt)
Eison (Eizon) 212, 214
elixirs and medicines
    home preparation of *198,* 199–207
    recipes for *203, 205,* 208 n 34, 208 n 36
    utensils used to make 206
Ellwood, Thomas 86
Encarnação, Vicente da (Friar) 148–9
England
    cottage hospitals in 162
    early hospitals in 5, 12

Enlightenment 11, 90, 148, 302
environmentalism 148
Epidauros (Greece) 75
epidemics 15, 26, 29, 74, 76, 226. *See also* illness; plague
Essentials for Rebirth in Paradise (Ōjoyoshu) (Genshin) 214
Estremoz hospital (Portugal) *187*
Eugenius IV (pope) 243
Europe
    in the early modern era 11–12
    medieval 4–6
    See also England; France; Germany; Italy; Portugal; Spain
Évora (Portugal) 87
exorcism 9

Fabbri, Giambattista 266
Fang people 8
Fang Xiangxian 201
Farabi 291
Fatih Darüşşifası (Istanbul), ground plan *280*
Febbrari, Francesco 266, 270, 276 n. 30
fevers 44, 111, 119, 224, 252, 288
Ficino, Marsilio 39, 254
Filarete (Averlino, Antonio) 30, *36,* 38, 39, 41, 47, 76, 121, 241, 245, 247, 250–3, 255
    Treatise on Architecture 40–1, *40,* 45, 48–9
Flemmyng, Robert 119
Flexner Report 311
Florence (Italy) 12, 38, 49, 127
    Ospedale degli Innocenti 26, 127
    Santa Maria Nuova 30, 43, 138, 252
Fordist medicine 312
Foster, Philip 48
Foucault, Michel 74
fountains 1, 7, 28, 99, 101, 108, 111, 112
    in Ottoman hospitals 281, 283, 288, 289, 296
    Trevi 123
Four Doctors, The (Sargent) 308
Foveaux, Joseph 167
Fox, George 87
Francesco di Giorgio Martini 121
Franklin, Benjamin 303

Gage, Frances 254
Galen 120, 123, 124, 141, 251–2, 279, 288, 290
Galletti, Giuseppe 266
Galli, Angelo Camillo 266, 272
Galli, Giovanni Antonio 260, 268, 270, 272, 274
    influence of 265–6
    obstetrical models 262, *263,* 265, 270, 274–5
    See also Casa Nascentori
Galvani, Luigi 270
Gao Lian 198

gardens. *See* hospital gardens; landscaping
Garrett, Mary Elizabeth 308
Genealogical Tree of the Kings and Queens of Portugal 46
Genealogy of the Royal Houses of Spain and Portugal 45, *46*
Genshin 214
Gerarts, Marcus 58
germ theory 225, 305
Germany, hospitals in the early modern era 12–13
Gesler, Wilbert M. 75, 81, 83, 85, 86, 87, 88
Getz, Faye 6
Gevher Nesibe 104
Gevher Nesibe Hospital (Kayseri) 104, 107
Gilman, Daniel Coit 306–7, 308
Giovanni, Gualteri di *246*, 248
Gloucester Infirmary 86
God's Hostels. *See* Hostels of God
Gokurakuji (Japan) 214, 217, 218
　facilities of care at *215*
Goodwin, Janet 212
Greece. *See* Ancient Greece
Greenway, Francis 168
Guarani tribe 11
Guatemala, colonial medicine in 15
Guesdon, Alfred *36*
Guillaume d'Estouteville 122, 125

Hafsa Sultan Darüşşifası (Manisa) 282–4
　entrance *284*
　ground plan *280*
　portico *285*
Hafsa Sultan Mosque Complex (Manisa) 282
　plan of *283*
Halsted, William 308, 309–10, *311*
Hamilton, Alexander 225
hammams 100, 107, 111. *See also* bathhouses
Hammurabi of Babylon 2
Hannyaji temple (Japan) 214
Harmening, Dieter 60
harmony and medicine 251–2
Harriett Lane Home (Johns Hopkins) 310
Harun Al-Rashid (Caliph) 7
Harvard University medical school Boston) 303, 308–9
Harvey, William 12
Haseki Sultan Darüşşifası (Istanbul) 282
　ground plan *280*
He Cide 201
He Lianggong 201
healers
　holy men as 5–6
　in the medieval world 6
　traditional (African) 8
healing 1
　by design 279, 293–5
　and religion 26–7
　as social activity 87
healing places. *See* asylums; home medical practices; hospitals
Hebron (Palestine), hospitals in 107
Henderson, John 12
Henry Ford Hospital 312
herbal medicine. *See* botanical medicine
Herodotus 2
hiden'in (mercy houses) 9, 213, 214
Hill, Lamel 82
Hinduism 10
Hippocrates 39, 141, 148, 251–2
Hippocratic Oath 2
Hobart Hospital (Tasmania) 169, *170*
Hogenberg, Frans *40*, 45, *46*
Holanda, António de 45, *46*
Holy Ghost God House (Heilige Geest Godshuius, Bruges) 58
Holy Spirit hospital (Évora, Portugal) 187
Holy Spirit hospitals (Portugal) 186–7
home medical practices
　childbirth 221–2, 224, 234
　in China 197–207
　cultivating life 207 n. 7
　cultivating virtue 200–2, 207
　medicine chambers 199–200
　preparation of medicines *198*, 199–207, *203*, *205*
　setting up domestic spaces 199–200
Hong Kong, colonial medicine in 15
Hong Kong Government Civil Hospital 15
Hooke, Robert, 77, 81
Hôpital Saint-Jacques (Besançon) 76
Hopkins, Johns 304–5
Horsburgh, C. Robert 293
Hospice de la Salpêtrière (Paris) 80, 226
hospital architecture 44, 86
　based on monastery architecture 262
　courtyard plan 28, 39, 76
　cruciform 29–30, 35, 38, 41, 44–5, 48, 49, 76, 108, 126, 138
　double-cross design 30, 47, 48, 76
　early Christian 28–32
　Hospital Real de Todos-os-Santos 42–4
　Islamic 100–12
　Johns Hopkins Medicine 303–4
　leprosy hostels 209, 215–8, *216*
　loggia facade 76
　mercy houses 213
　in the Middle Ages 37
　Our Lady of Potterie (hospital of) 57–9
　patterned after classical villas 86
　pavilion design 305

Index

polygonal 282
as restorative 279
selection of site 38–9
therapeutic 280
T-shaped 30
U-plan 76, 227
See also architectural styles
hospital gardens
at asylums 74, 77, 79–87
botanical 11
courtyard (central) 3, 28, 30, 294, 296
herbal 16
leprosy hostels 211
of medicinal plants 6, 11, 142, 202
monastic 6
Ottoman hospitals 279, 282–3, 289, 292, 294, 296
in Portugal 43
therapeutic 86–7, 152, 199, 279
hospital history
Africa (medieval) 8
Africa (colonial) 13–14
Americas (early) 11
Americas (colonial) 15–16
ancient Greece 2–3, 27–8
ancient times 2–4, 26–7
Asia (colonial) 14–15
Asia (medieval) 8–11
early Christian 28–31
early modern era 11–13, 75–6
Europe (medieval) 4–6
Islamic (medieval) 6–8
Mesopotamia 2, 26
pre-modern 31–2
Renaissance 11–13, 29–32
Roman Empire 3–4, 27–8
Hospital of Bayezid II (Edirne) 282, 289, 294–5
ground plan *280*
music in 291–2
portico *290*
"stage" area *291*
water runnels 294, *295*
Hospital of Qalawun (Cairo) 289
Hospital of Santo Spirito (Rome) 116, 117–18, 122, 125–30, 245, 252
east end and north facade *118*
elevations of east and north facades *127*
frescoes 116, 117–18, 119, 128, 130
functions and users 125–6
interior design 128
plan of *126*
residential courtyards 126–7
Hospital of St. Nicholas de Bruille (Tournai) 5–6
Hospital of the Pantocrator (Constantinople) 4–5

Hospital Real de Todos-os-Santos (Lisbon) 35, *37*, 41–2, 45, 47
construction of 42–4
reconstruction *43*
representations of 45, *46–7*, 47–8
hospitalism 305
hospitalitas 28
hospitals
in America 222–3
in Anatolia 279
associated with mosques 281
in Australia 162–75
in Central and South America 15–16
charitable mission of 63
churches/chapels in 5, 12, 16
cottage (England) 162
early design 29–30
as factory for healing 312–13
function and facilities 100–1
governmental involvement with 38, 41–3
interior design 31–2
in Iran 7
Islamic 6–8, 99–112, 293 (*see also* Ottoman hospitals)
medicalization of 38
military 167, 305
and Misericórdias 186–8
modern design 302
ospedale grande (general hospital) 38
Persian terms for 100
private ownership of 76
proximity to cathedrals 4, 76, 241–2
psychiatric 77
as reflections of culture 1
religious function of 29–30
religious management of 141
religious ownership of 76
and the rise of scientific medicine in Europe 75–6
in Rome 116–31
Seljuk Anatolian 293
Sultanic patronage of 104
voluntary 77
and the worship of God 5
See also maternity hospitals
Hostels of God 29, 31, 32
hot springs 5, 9, 17 n. 9
Hôtel-Dieu (Lyons) 226
Hôtel-Dieu (Paris) 76, 223, 225, 226, 265, 302
Hôtel-Dieu de Beaune (France) 75
Hôtels-Dieu (France) 4, 76
Houses of Life (Egypt) 2
Howard, John 81, 84
Howe, Eunice 117
humanism 62, 181

humanitarianism 87
humoral theory 39, 100, 102, 113 n. 22, 119, 121, 141, 252, 254, 279, 290, 292, 296, 300 n. 51
Hunter, William 224
Hunterian Laboratory (Johns Hopkins) *309*, 310
hygiene 7, 108, 247, 294
   social 221

Ibn Abi Usaybi'ah 101, 103, 111
Ibn al-Nafis 101
Ibn Jubayr 99, 101
Ibn Sina (Avicenna) 7, 251
Ibn Tulun 99
Ibrahim ibn Nasr 100
Il Lucchese 270
illness
   in ancient times 26
   cholera 13
   diarrhea 111
   fevers 44, 111, 119, 224, 252, 288
   emotional aspects of 26–7
   malarial fever 119
   pleurisy 119
   and poverty 37, 75, 108
   puerperal fever 225, 226, 233
   as punishment 26
   smallpox 13, 64
   supernatural contexts 25–6
   syphilis (pox) 12–13, 54 n. 71, 152
   in tropical regions 148
   tuberculosis 288
   typhus 13, 15
   See also epidemics; leprosy; plague
imarets 281, 282, 284, 288, 293, *296*, 297
Imhotep 27
Incas 11
incense 202, 214, 292
India
   almshouses in 10
   Estado da India 139, 141, 148
   healers in 26, 141
   influence on Mozambique 139–41, 143, 145, 148, 155
   places of healing in 10–1, 138
   See also Mozambique
indigenous medical traditions 16, 20 n. 102
indigenous people
   in the Americas 11, 16
   in Australia 172
infirmarium 29
Inner Light Protestants 86
Innocent III (pope) 125, 130
Insignia degli Anziani Consoli 268
Institute of the Sciences (Bologna) 263, *264*, 265, 268, 274

Inward Light 86, 94 n 71
Iraq, hospitals in 100
Islam
   charity 7, 99, 112
   influence in Portugal 143
   See also hospitals, Islamic; Ottoman hospitals
Islamic world
   in the early modern era 12
   healthcare in 6–8
Italy
   hospitals in the early modern era 12–13
   hospitals in the Renaissance 12
   social reform in 37–8
   See also Bologna; Milan; Rome
'Izz al-Din Kay Kawus I 100, 104, 107
'Izz al-Din Kay Kawus I Hospital (Sivas) 104–7
   courtyard 106
   entrance portal *106*
   iwans *105*
   plan of 104, *105*

Jackson, Samuel 174, *174*
Japan
   approach to sickness and death 210
   concern about pollution in 210–11
   leprosy hostels in 209–19
   leprosy in 209–10
   places of healing in 9–10
Jayavarman VII 10
Jennings, Michael 14
João II (Prince/King of Portugal) 41, 42–3, 44, 182
John Commenos II (Emperor) 5
Johns Hopkins Hospital (Baltimore, Maryland) 302–12
   1889 depiction *307*
   construction of 305–7
   link with medical school 303–307
   as "machine for healing" 311–312
   specialized institute and clinics 308–311
   See also Johns Hopkins Medicine
Johns Hopkins Medicine (Baltimore, Maryland) 303, *304*
   Billings's plan for *306*
   Brady Urological Institute 308
   Children's Rehabilitation Institute (Kennedy-Krieger Institute) 308
   Harriett Lane Home 310
   Hunterian Laboratory *309*, 310
   influence of 311–12
   organizing specialized institute and clinics 308–10
   Pathology Building 308
   Phipps Psychiatric Clinic 310
   urban planning in 312
   Wilmer Eye Institute 308

Index

Women's Fund Memorial Building 308, *309*
  See also Johns Hopkins Hospital (Baltimore)
Julius II (pope) 116
Jundi Shapur (Gundi Shapur, Iran) 7

Kahn, Albert 312
Kamayura (Kamaiura) tribe 11
Kariri-Xoco tribe 11
karma 209–10, 218
katagogion 27
Kayseri (Turkey) 100, 104, 107
Kelly, Howard 308
Kennedy-Krieger Institute (Johns Hopkins) 308
Keyvanian, Carla 123
khastakhana 100
Kiliç Arslan II (Sultan) 104
King, Gregory 77
Kirkbride plan 310
Kitayama Hall (Japan) 212–13
  architectural diagram *216*
  association with death and pollution 217–18
  establishment of 214–15
  plan of 217, 219
  residents of 217–18
  restoration of 209, *210*, 215
Kiyomizu Temple (Japan) 211–12, 216, 218
Kleinman, Arthur 197
Kleisiaris, C.F. 2
Kobayashi Shigefumi 214
Kofuku-ji 9
Kom tribe 8
Kōmyō (Empress) 212–13, 214
Kostof, Spiro 25

Lalande, Jérôme 265, 272
Lam, Alardus 58
landscaping 28, 74, 85–7, *86*, 305
  at the York Retreat 85–7
  See also hospital gardens
Last Judgment, The (Van der Weyden) 75
latrines 4, 5, 32, 39, 49, 100, 103, 281–2. *See also* sanitation; sewer systems
Laurens, Andries 66
lazarettos (pesthouses) 13, 29
Le Roy, Julien David 302
Leeds General Infirmary (England) 79
Lelli, Ercole 270, 274
Leo II (Armenia) 99
Leonardo Da Vinci 12
Leonor (Queen of Portugal) 15
Leontius (Bishop) 5
leprosaria/leprosariums 29, 209. *See also* leprosy hostels
leprosy 4, 64, 74
  as karmic retribution disease 209, 211
  in medieval Japan 209–12
  stigmatization of 211
  as Wind disease 210
leprosy hostels 29
  architectural form of 209, 215–18
  construction of 213
  in Japan 209–19
Levanti, Antonio 271
l'Hôpital Bicêtre (Paris) 80
Liber Chronicarum 116, *117*
lighting 28–9, 32, 252, 255, 296–7
Lindemann, Mary 141, 146
lion sculptures 104, 106, 285
Lippomano, Girolamo 37
Lisbon (Portugal) 35, 37, 41, 42, 45, *46*, 47
  depictions of *46–7*, 48
  as global metropolis 49
  panoramic view of *47*
  See also Hospital Real de Todos-os-Santos (Lisbon)
Lister, Joseph 309
Liverpool Hospital (Australia) 168–9, *168*
Lives of the Artists (Vasari) 48
London, England
  Bethlem Hospital 76–9
  City of London Lying-in Hospital for Married Women 227, *228*
  London Hospital 175
  St. Luke's Asylum *78*, 81
  St. Paul's Cathedral 81
  St. Thomas' Hospital 305
Lonsdale, William 17
Lorenzetti, Amgrogio 250
l'Orme, Philibert de 226
Lotus Sutra 211
Lourdes (France) 75
lying-in hospitals 226–9
  in Great Britain 227
  See also maternity hospitals
Lyon, France 76

Macquarie, Elizabeth 166
Macquarie, Lachlan 165–8, 175
madness 111. *See also* mental illness
Maertens, Alfons 61
Maestri di Pietra e di Legname 250–1
Maia e Vasconcelos, Vicente da 152
Mall, Franklin P. 308
Malvezzi, Sigismondo 274
Mamoru, Shimosaka 212
Manfredini, Giovan Battista 266
Manjusri Bodhisattva 212, 214
Manolini, Giovanni 265

al-Mansur Hospital (Cairo) 100, 107–11
   design and appearance 111
   entrance portal 108, *109*
   interior *110*
   plan of 108, *109*, 111
al-Mansur Qalawun 100, 101, 107
Manuel I (King of Portugal) 42–3, 44, 181–2
Manzolini. Giovanni *263*, 265, 270
Mao Xiang 201–2
al-Maqrizi 99, 111
Marseille, France 76
Marsili, Luigi Fernando 268
Marsilio, Agostino di *246*, *248*
Martin V (pope) 116
Martin, Gregory 126
Masai people 8
Masona (Bishop of Merida) 4
Massachusetts General Hospital 303, 305
maternity hospitals
   in Alexandria 221
   in the United States 221–34
   in Western Europe 221
   See also lying-in hospitals
Mayan civilization 11
medical education 112
medical policing 147–8
medical specialization
   Blatternbaus 13
   in Byzantine *xenons* 5
   experimental sciences 263
   Hospital of the Pantocrator 5
   in hospitals 16, 38, 149, 151, 152, 156, 247, 253
   in the Islamic world 7, 101
   Johns Hopkins 308
   mental illness 74, 75, 77, 84
   psychiatry 310
   in Renaissance Europe 12–13, 38, 125
   urology 310
   See also maternity hospitals; obstetricians; surgeons; surgery
Medici, Michele 270
Medicine at the Paris Hospital, 1794–1848) (Ackerknect) 302
Mehmed Aşık 282
Mehmed the Conqueror (Sultan) 279
Meigs, Charles 225
Melbourne hospitals (Australia) 173–5, *174*
Melbourne Lying-In Hospital (Australia) 227
Melo e Castro, Francisco de 148
Memoirs of the Hospitals of Paris (Tenon) 302
men
   as midwives 260, 262, 263
   treatment of 12, 44, 54 n 71

mental health facilities 294
   in Brazil 15–16
   in Dutch colonies 14
   See also asylums
mental illness 66, 74, 80, 108, 111, 310
mercy houses (*hiden'in*) 213, 214
Mesopotamian cultures 2, 26
Meulenbeld, Gerrit Jan 10
Meyer, Adolf 310
Middlesex Hospital (London) 175
midwifery schools 265. *See also* Casa Nascentori (Bologna)
midwives 224–5, 233, 235 n.16, 260, 274
   men as 260, 262, 263
   studying with Galli 263
   See also Casa Nascentori (Bologna)
Milan (Italy) 35, *36*, *40*
   depictions of *36*, *40*
   hospitals in 38
   pesthouse 13
   See also Ospedale Maggiore (Milan)
Mileham, James 165
military hospitals 167, 305
Miller, Timothy 5
Mills, Hannah *89*
Milton, John 86
Mimar Acem Ali *284*
Mimar Sinan 284, 285–6, 293, 294
Miracle Book of Our Lady of Potterie 56–7, 59–62, 63
   drawings from *60*, 61–2, *61*, 64, *65*, 66, *67*, 69
Misericórdia Church (Mozambique) 150–1, *150*
   Misericórdia hospital (Mozambique) 139, 140, 150–3, 155
   plan of 152–3
Misericórdias (Portugal) 138, 181
   Alcochete House of Misericórdia *192*
   artistic collections of 183
   building plans 183
   Casa da Misericórdia 183
   church (Tentúgal) 189
   concept of 183–4, 186
   design, space, and elements 188–90, 193
   entryway 190
   Estremoz hospital (Portugal) *187*
   facade 190, *191*
   healthcare, history, and art 182–3
   and hospitals 186–8
   iconic representations in 193
   interconnected spaces and functions 183–4
   interior space 190
   meeting room of the brothers 189–90, *189*, 193
   Misericórdia of Colares 186
   Montemor-o-Velho 185, *189*

Index

Proença-a-Nova House of Misericórdia *191*
Tentúgal House of Misericórdia *189*
use of space in 187
Vila do Conde *184*
as welfare institution 193
missionaries
　in Africa 14
　in Japan 9–10
　as providers of healthcare 141–2
Moffat, Robert 14
Monamoto Yoritomo 212
monasteries
　as architectural inspiration for hospitals 262, 275
　and artistic production 182
　built/restored by Sixtus IV 116, 119
　dissolution of (England) 12, 77
　infirmaries/hospitals in 1, 4, 9, 28, 58, 146
Mondini, Carlo 266, 270
Mondino de' Liuzzi 120, 124
Montemor-o-Velho House of Misericórdia (Portugal) *185*
　meeting room of the brothers *189*
Moore, George 226
Moral Management 88
moral therapy 80
Morandi, Anna *263*, 265, 270, 274
Moratti, Antonio 272
Moreton Bay Hospital (Queensland) 170–1
Mozambique
　carved entrance door 145
　church and convent of St. John 145–6
　Church of Good Health 145
　criticism of healthcare facilities 148–9
　first hospital 140–1, 155
　hospitals in 139–56
　map *142*, *147*, *154*
　Misericórdia Church 150–1, *150*
　multicultural character of 140, 156
　Order of Hospitallers 141–2
　pipe system on Misericórdia terrace *151*
　Portuguese factories in 139
　refurbishment of second hospital 151–3
　role in African trade 139
　role in support of navigation 139
　Santa Casa da Misericórdia 139, 140, 150–3, 155
　second hospital 143–53, 155–6
　Tower of São Gabriel 139–40
　view of street in the stone town *144*
Mughal Empire 11
Muhammad bin Tughluq 10
mujōdō (death halls; hospices) 213–14
muqarnas 102, 103, 104, 285, 289, 293
Murray, Lindley 81

music therapy 289–92
Mylne, Robert 227

Nara-zaka 214–15, 218
Nash, John 169
Natural Philosophy 86
Naudi (Dr.) 82
Neak Pean (Neak Poan) 10
Nelson, Robert 77
Nesibe, Gevher 100
neurosurgery 310
New Norfolk convict hospital (Tasmania) 169
New-York Asylum for Lying-in-Women 232–4, *232*
Niangoran-Bouah, Georges 8
Niccoló da Reggio 120
Nicholas of Cusa 121, 124
Nicholas V (pope) 116, 123, 124
Niernsee, John 305
Nightingale, Florence 81, 305
Nijkamp, Marlies 60
Ninshō 212, 213, 214, 218
Nobuo, Kawata 216
nosokomeion 29
Nur al-Din 100
Nur al-Din Mahmud 101
al-Nuri Hospital (Damascus) 101–4
　decorative elements 103–4, *103*
　Mamluk additions 103
　plan of 101, *102*, 104
　Qur'anic inscriptions 101

observatory tower 268, *269*
obstetricians 224–6
　training for 260, 262–3, 265–6, 272, 274–5
occupational therapy 14, 74
odors 292
O'Hearne, John 166
Ōjoyoshu (*Essentials for Rebirth in Paradise*) (Genshin) 214
ophthalmology 111
Order of Santiago 187
Order of Santo Spirito 122, 128
Orme, Nicholas 5
orphanages 9, 111, 222
Osler, William 308, 310
Ospedale degli Innocenti (Florence) 76, 127
Ospedale della Misericordia (Prato) 255–6 n 4, 256 n 8
Ospedale di San Matteo (Pavia) 38
Ospedale di Santa Maria Nuova (Florence) 266
Ospedale di Santo Spirito (Sassia) 30, 31
Ospedale Maggiore (Milan) 30, 35, 38–41, 47–9, 76, 126, 252, 255
　frescoes at 245

Ottoman Empire 11
Ottoman hospitals 279-97
   architectural form 281-7
   balancing six non-naturals 296-7
   connection in 293-4
   form and function of 281-2
   and the Galenic principles 296
   Hafsa Sultan Darüşşifası *280*, 282-4, *284*, *285*
   Haseki Sultan Darüşşifası *280*, 282
   Hospital of Qalawun 289
   innovations in 282
   orientation of 293
   patients 288, 295
   patrons 288
   qualities of successful hospital space 293-5
   scale 294, 296
   sensory experiences of hospital users 288-93
   staff members 287-8, 295
   Sultanahmed Darüşşifası *280*
   symbolic meaning 294-5
   users of 287-8
   See also Hospital of Bayezid II (Edirna); 'Izz al-Din Kay Kawus I Hospital (Sivas); Süleymaniye Darüşşifası
Our Lady of Piedade hospital (Beja, Portugal) 187
Our Lady of Potterie (hospital of, Bruges) 56
   architecture and history of 57-9
   Virgin Chapel 59
   welfare mission of 62-3
Our Lady of Potterie (statue) *56*, 57, 59-62, 69
   miracles of 56-7, 60-1, 64, *65*, 66, *67*, *68*, 69

Paço dos Estaus 44
Palazzo Bocchi (Bologna) 268
Palazzo dall'Archinnasio (Bologna) 274
Palazzo Marsili (Bologna) 268, *269*
Palazzo Poggi (Bologna) *264*, 268, 270, 274
Palazzo Pubblico (Siena) 250
Palladio, Andrea 83
Palmela (Portugal) 187-8
Panopticon (Bentham) 85
Papal Schism 116
Paracelsus 12
Paradise Lost and *Paradise Regained* (Milton) 86
Paré, Ambrose 12, 265
Paris Academy of Sciences 302
Parramatta Convict Hospital (Sydney) 167, *167*
pathology 308
patronage, cultural and institutional 118
Pedro II Hospice for the Alienated (Rio de Janeiro) 16
Pellegrinaio cycle (Santa Maria della Scala hospital, Siena) 241, 243, 252, 253-4
   architectural function of 254

   The Care and Marriage of Foundlings 243, 246-7, *249*
   The Care of the Sick 243, 253
   David 245, 247, *248*
   The Distribution of Alms 243
   The Expansion of the Hospital 243, 243-4, *244*, 245, *246*, 248, 250, *251*
   full view *242*
   The Investiture of the Rector by Beato Agostino Novello 243
   Job 245
   The Liberation of the Hospital and Indulgence of Pope Celestine III 243
   The Lunch for the Poor 241, 243
   site-specificity of 253-4
   Solomon 245, 246-7, *246*
   Tobit 245, 258 n 37
   The Vision of Sorore 243
Penn, William 83, 86
Pennsylvania Hospital 222-4, *223*, 225, 226, 303
Pereira do Lago, Baltazar 149
Pesellino (Francesco di Stefano) *250*
pesthouses (*lazaretto*) 13
Philadelphia Friends' Hospital 79, *79*
Phipps, Henry 310
Phipps Psychiatric Clinic (Johns Hopkins) 310
physical handicaps 66
physicians
   in Africa 14
   in China 9, 10
   Christ as physician 28
   in Constantinople 5
   diagnostic techniques 252
   Egyptian 2, 101
   in England 80
   in France 80
   Greek 7, 27, 39, 120
   Hindu 10
   and hospital design 302, 305
   in Italy 30, 84, 119-20
   and maternity care 224-7, 233-4, 265
   medical authority of 197
   in the medieval world 6
   in Mozambique 151-2, 155
   Muslim/Islamic 10, 117, 288
   Persian 7
   specializing in maternity care 224-6
   support for home production of medicine 204
   training for 223
   See also obstetricians; surgeons
Piazza Navona (Rome) 122
pilgrimage mandalas 212
Pilgrim's Progress 86
Pinel, Philippe 80, 89

Index

Pisano, Nicola 248
Pius II (pope) 252
places of healing
    homes as 197–207
    See also asylums; hospitals
plague 13, 15, 29, 42, 76. *See also* epidemics
Platonism 83, 93 n 39, 120, 253
Pliny 6, 86
Ponte Sant'Angelo (Rome) 116, 122, 123, 125
Ponte Sisto (Rome) 116, 122–3, *123*, 128, 130
pools 101, 103, 106, 296. *See also* bathing
Porta del Popolo (Rome) 122
Portel (Portugal)187
Portugal
    Arez hospital 187
    Caldas da Rainha 138
    Casa da Misericórdia 183
    and colonial medicine 14, 15
    hospital architecture in 35–50
    hospital of St. Marks (Braga) 187
    hospitals in 138
    period of Discoveries 181–2, 193
    Regulation for Chapels and Hospitals (Portugal) 182
    Rossio 43–4, 45, 49
    See also Misericórdias (Portugal); Mozambique
poverty
    caring for the poor 69–70
    and childbirth 221–2
    and healthcare 241, 243
    and the hospital 58, 63
    and illness 75, 108
    ministering to the poor 183
    in Portugal 182
    virtuous/vicious 222, 234
pox (syphilis) 12, 54 n. 71, 152
pox houses (*Blatternbaus*) 13
Preston, Jonas 229
Preston Retreat (Philadelphia) 229–31, *230*, *231*
Price, Eli 231
Pringle, Yolana 14
Prior, James 153
Proença-a-Nova House of Misericórdia (Portugal), exterior facade *191*
Protestant Reformation 76
psychiatric hospitals 77. *See also* asylums
psychiatry 310
public health
    and childbirth 221
    in Germany 13
    institutions and policies 1
    international 209
    in the Islamic world 6–7
    at Johns Hopkins 303, 312
    leprosy and 209, 218
    in Portugal 35, 42, 44, 49
    in the Renaissance 12–13
    in the Roman Empire 3
Pucci, Pietro di Giovanni *242*
puerperal fever 225, 226, 233

Quadralectic Architecture 25
Quakers. *See* Religious Society of Friends (Quakers)
Queen Charlotte's Lying-In Hospital (London) 227, 233
Quercia, Priamo della 243

radicalism 81
Rashid al-Din Tabib 100
rationalism 76, 85
Regulation for Chapels and Hospitals (Portugal) 182
Religious Society of Friends (Quakers) 74–5, 81, 83, 86, 87–8, 90–1, 93 n. 39
    engagement with nature 85–7
    See also York Asylum
Retreat Asylum (York). *See* York Asylum
Rey, Philippe-Marius 16
Richardson, Harriet 149
Rio de Janeiro, mental health facilities in 16
Risse, Guenter B. 13, 149
Rive, Charles-Gaspard de la 84
Robinson, G. Canby 311–12
Rochester medical center (New York) 311–12
Roman Empire 3–4, 86, 162
    military infirmaries 3–4
    places of healing in 27–8
    slave infirmaries 3
    valetudinarian 3, 27–8
Rome, Italy
    Borgo Santo Spirito 122
    health, medicine, and theology in 119–20
    hospitals in 116–31
    Piazza Navona 122
    Ponte Sant'Angelo 116, 122, 123, 125
    Ponte Sisto 116, 122–3, *123*, 128, 130
    Porta del Popolo 122
    restoration of 116, 118, 121–5, 128, 130–1
    Santa Maria dalla Pace 124
    Santa Maria del Popolo 122, 124, 128
    Sistine inscription from Via Florea 116, *117*
    St. Peter's Basilica 166, 122, 125
    Trevi Fountain 123
    Via Florea repairs 116
    view of (*Liber Chronicarum*) *117*
    See also Hospital of Santo Spirito (Rome)
Roosevelt Hospital (New York) 305
Rossio (Portugal) 43–4, 45, 49
Rosweydus, Heribertus 59, 61

Royal Hospital (Chelsea) 169
Royal Society (England) 77
Royal Society of Edinburgh 225
"Rum Hospital" (New South Wales) 165–9, *166*, 169
    design of 166–7
Rum Seljuq Empire 104

sacred groves 8
sacrifice 3, 27
Safavid Empire 11
Sala dei Nove 250
Salpêtrière (Paris) 226
Salt, Henry 143
salvation
    and Buddhism 218
    of the dying 213
    and leprosy 212–13
Sandri, Pietro 266
Sangallo, Antonio da (the Younger) 48
sanitation 3, 7, 42. *See also* latrines; sewer systems
Sansovino, Andrea 45
Santa Casa da Misericórdia (Mozambique) 139, 140, 150–3, 155
Santa Casa de Misericordia (Holy Mercy Houses) 15–16
Santa Maria dalla Pace (Rome) 124
Santa Maria de Nasova (Venice) 13
Santa Maria del Popolo (Rome) 122, 124, 128
Santa Maria della Morte (Bologna) 267
Santa Maria della Scala hospital (Siena) 43, 255
    Pellegrinaio cycle 241–55
Santa Maria della Vita hospital (Bologna) 267
Santa Maria Nuova (Florence) 30, 43, 138, 252
Santarém House of Misericórdia, church *192*
Santas Casas da Misericórdia (Holy Houses of Mercy). *See* Misericórdias (Portugal)
Sanusi (Sedupe) 8
São Cosme infirmary (Portugal) 44
São Vicente infirmary (Portugal) 44
Sargent, John Singer 308
Saulnier, Pierre 126, *127*
Savage, John 165
scale 294
Scarselli, Flaminio 274
Scattergood, Thomas 82
Sccrmcrs, Marjc 64
Schietere, Nicolaus 59
Scott, John 86–7
scurvy 140
Sebastian (saint) 75
secularism 90
Sennyūji temple (Japan) 213
sensory experiences
    acoustic 30, 289–92

    auditory 297
    of hospital users 288–93
    olfactory 292
    tactile 292
    taste 292–3
    visual 289
Seville (Spain) 41
sewer systems 13, 39, 121–2. *See also* latrines; sanitation
Seyaku-in 9
Shefer-Mossensohn, Miri 279, 287
Sheikh Zayed Tower (Johns Hopkins) 303, *304*
Sheppard and Enoch Pratt Hospital (Johns Hopkins) 310
Shi Chengjin 200–1, 202
Shigefumi, Kobayashi 214
Shihab al-Din al-Nuwayri 108
Shintennōjo temple (Japan) 213
Shitennoh-ji 9
Shizu Sakai 9
Siena, hospitals in 49. *See also* Santa Maria della Scala hospital (Siena)
Sigismondo de' Conti 122
Simoni, Luís Vicente de 153
Sisters of Charity 32
Sivas 104–7
Sixtus IV (pope) 30, 31, 116–19, 125, 245
    awareness of bodily systems 120–1
    De sanguine Christi 119–20, 124–5
    expanding the Hospital of Santo Spirito 125–6
    and the restoration of Rome 116, 118, 121–6, 128, 130–1
Sixtus V (pope) 116
Slantimorosi, Antonio 266
Sloane, John 169
smallpox 13, 64
smell, sense of 292
Smids, Kateline 64
Smith, John 83
social reform 9, 37, 79, 81, 90, 182, 221, 226
social welfare 28, 35, 42, 44, 49, 57, 62–3, 70, 162, 218
Some Fruits of Solitude (Penn) 86
sounds and noise 289–92, 297
Spain
    and colonial medicine 15
    hospitals in 4
Spellati statues 270, *271*
Spietaal van Onser Vrouw (Bruges) 58. *See also* Our Lady of Potterie (hospital of, Bruges)
spirit animals 11
spolia 102, 113 n. 10, 126
St. George's Hospital (London) 86
St. John's Hospital (Canterbury) 5
St. Luke's Asylum (London) *78*, 81
St. Mark's Hospital (Braga, Portugal) 187
St. Paul's Cathedral (London) 81

Index

St. Peter's Basilica (Rome) 116, 122, 125
St. Thomas' Hospital (London) 305
Stark, William 82
Stevenson, Christine 77
Stierman, Pieter Brant 66
Strickland, George 173
Strickland, W. 79
Strompers, Kateline 66
Strong Memorial Hospital (Rochester) 312
Su Shi 9
suffering 25, 26–27, 29, 32, 38, 165, *203*, 204, 292, 302, 303
    charity and 64
    in childbirth 225, 226, 231
    of the dead, 69
    from leprosy, 74, 209, 211, 212–15, 217–19
    pious, 247
    of the poor, 69
Süleyman II (Sultan) 279
Süleymaniye Darüşşifası (Istanbul) 281, 284–5, 293–4
    courtyard plan 281
    ground plan *280*
    imaret 296
    second courtyard *287*
Süleymaniye Mosque Complex (Istanbul), plan of *286*
Sultanahmed Darüşşifası (Istanbul), ground plan *280*
surgeons
    in Africa 8
    in ancient times 26
    in Australia 162–3, 165–6, 171, 173
    black 15
    in Brazil 15
    in England 77
    and hospital design 302
    in Italy 128
    in the medieval world 6, 32, 76
    in Mozambique 141–2, 149, 153
    Persian/Islamic 107, 112, 287
    specializing in obstetrics 260, 262–3, 265–7, 275
    training for 310
surgery 111, 260, 266, *311*
    and childbirth 262, 263
    dental 247
    at Johns Hopkins 309–10
    neuro- 310
    recovery from 279
Şuuri Hasan 291
Swan River Colony (Perth, Australia) 171
Sydney General Hospital (Australia) 163–6
    prefabricated second hospital 164–5, *164*
syphilis (pox) 12, 54 n. 71, 152

Tabriz, hospitals in 100
Taisne, Philippus 59, 61
Tanganyika (Tanzania) 14
Tasmania, hospitals in 168, 169
taste, sense of 292–3
Taylor, Charles 90
Ten Books on Architecture (Vitruvius) 38, 48
Tenon, Jacques 302
Tentúgal House of Misericórdia (Portugal), church *189*
Tetsuichi, Nyiunoya 211
Texas Medical Center (Houston) 312
The Construction of the Temple of Jerusalem (Pesellino) *250*
therapeutic environments 75, 79, 90
Thoros I (Armenia) 99
Tomb of the Physician at Saqqara 2
Torre della Specola (Bologna) 268
Toscano, João Domingos 152
touch, sense of 292
Tower of São Gabriel (Mozambique) 139–40
Trattato di architettura (Filarete). See *Treatise on Architecture* (Filarete)
Treatise on Architecture (Filarete) 36, 39, 40–1, *40*, 45, 48, 52 n. 35, 241, 245, 247
    Codex Magliabechiano 41, 45, 48
Tredgold, Thomas 230
Trevi Fountain (Rome) 123
Tron, Vicenzo 37
Tsumamuro 216–17
Tuke, Samuel 75, 79, 80, 81, 82, 83, 88, 89, 90
Tuke, William 86
Tungwah Hospital (Hong Kong) 15
Tupi-Guaranis 15
Tupinamba tribe 20 n. 102
turrets *307*
typhus 13, 15

Ulrich, Roger 279
University of California, San Francisco Medical Center 304
University of Pennsylvania 308
University of Pittsburgh Medical Center (Pennsylvania) 304
University of Rochester (New York) 311–12
urban sanitation 3. *See also* sanitation
urbanization 1, 31
    in England 77
    in Portugal 44
    in Western Europe 29
urology 310
uterus house. *See* Casa Nascentori (Bologna)

Index

Vagrancy Act (1744) 77
valetudinarium 3, 27–8
van der Rake, Loy 66
Van der Weyden, Rogier 75
van Eyck, Margareta 60
Vanderbilt medical center (Nashville, Tennessee) 311–12
Vasari, Giorgio 48
Vasconcelos e Almeida, José 151
Vaux, Calvert 310
Vecchietta 246–7
Venice (Italy) 13
ventilation
    in hospitals 19, 31, 70, 152, 162, 213, 217, 226–7, 230, 232, 292, 305–6, 312
    in maternity hospitals 225–6, 227
    windows for 29, 31, 38, 76, 82, 151, 252, 287, 288
    See also windows
verandas/verandahs 140, 143, 166–7, *167*, 168, 172, *172*, 173, 214, 227
Vergil 86
Verschelde, Karel 57
Vesalius, Andreas 12
Vienna (Austria) 223
View of Milan (Guesdon) *36*
Vila do Conde House of Misericórdia (Portugal) *184*
Vincent de Paul (saint) 32
visual elements 289
Vitruvius, Marcus 25, 32, 38–9, 48, 121
Vives, Juan Luis 57, 62–3, 66
von Pirquet, Clemens 310

al-Walid (Caliph) 101
Walter, Hubert (Archbishop) 6
Walter, Thomas U. 230–3
Warrington, Joseph 224
water sickness 64, *65*
water supply
    curative properties of 38, 39, 101
    in healthcare facilities 8, 10, 39–40, 108, 111–12, 116, 123–4, 252, 272, 274
    and hospital site selection 38–9, 252
    in Mozambique 139–40, 142, 143, 149, 151, *151*
    in Ottoman settings 279, 281–3, 285, 289, 292, 294, 295, *295*, 296
    for purification 3
    pipe system (Mozambique) *151*
    pools 101, 103, 106, 296
    sound of 288–9, 297
    stagnant 148, 149, 153
    See also bathing; fountains; hygiene
Watts, John 167

Webster, Margaret 5
Welch, William H. 307–8
Wentworth, D'Arcy 166
West, Benjamin 303
Westminster Infirmary (England) 77
wet-nurses 233
Wilkinson, Thomas 82
Wilmer Eye Institute (Johns Hopkins) 308
windows
    in Australian hospitals 162, 169, 172, 183
    decorated 31
    in Galli's house 262, 272
    glazed 272
    latticed 213
    leaded glass 29
    in the Milan pesthouse 13
    in Ottoman hospitals 281, 283, 285, 287, 289, 292, 294, 297
    of the *pellegrinaio* 243
    pointed-arch 57
    rose 127, 244
    round-headed 103, 173
    screens 103
    shutters/grilles 292
    slit 287
    stained glass 69
    triforate 127
    unglazed 77
    for ventilation 29, 31, 38, 76, 82, 151, 252, 287, 288
    See also ventilation
witchcraft 15
women
    healthcare for on Mozambique 153
    as philanthropists 308
    as scientists 265
    treatment of 12, 44, 54 n 71
    See also midwives
Women's Fund Memorial Building (Johns Hopkins) 308, *309*
Wren, Christopher 77, 169
Wright, Frank Lloyd 279, 297
Wyatt, Samuel 164

xenodochium 4
xenones 4–5, 28
Xuanzang 10

Yıldırım Darüşşifası (Istanbul), ground plan *280*
York County Hospital (England) 86
York Friends' Retreat. *See* York Retreat (England)
York Lunatic Asylum (England) 79, 88, 89

Index

York Retreat (England) 74, *78*, 78–9, 88, 90
    chamber story plan *85*
    design of 81
    ground story plan *82*
    natural environment 85–7
    plan and appearance 95–7
    Retreat Directors' Minute Book *89*
    social environment 87–8
    South front elevation *84*
    symbolic environment 88–90
Young, Hugh Hampton 310

Zafar Khan 10
Zanotti, Maria 260, 262, 270, 272
Zelada, Francesco Saverio de (Cardinal) 266

www.ingramcontent.com/pod-product-compliance
Lightning Source LLC
Chambersburg PA
CBHW080934300426
44115CB00017B/2808